Supportive Care in Respiratory Disease

Oxford University Press makes no representation, express or implied, that the drug dosages in this book are correct. Readers must therefore always check the product information and clinical procedures with the most up to date published product information and data sheets provided by the manufacturers and the most recent codes of conduct and safety regulations. The authors and the publishers do not accept responsibility or legal liability for any errors in the text or for the misuse or misapplication of material in this work.

Supportive Care in Respiratory Disease

Edited by

Sam H. Ahmedzai
Academic Unit of Supportive Care,
University of Sheffield,
Royal Hallamshire Hospital,
Sheffield, UK

Martin F. Muers
Department of Respiratory Medicine,
Leeds General Infirmary,
Leeds, UK

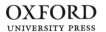
OXFORD
UNIVERSITY PRESS

OXFORD
UNIVERSITY PRESS

W F 145

Great Clarendon Street, Oxford OX2 6DP

Oxford University Press is a department of the University of Oxford.
It furthers the University's objective of excellence in research, scholarship,
and education by publishing worldwide in

Oxford New York

Auckland Cape Town Dar es Salaam Hong Kong Karachi Kuala Lumpur
Madrid Melbourne Mexico City Nairobi New Delhi Shanghai Taipei Toronto
With offices in

Argentina Austria Brazil Chile Czech Republic France Greece
Guatemala Hungary Italy Japan South Korea Poland Portugal Singapore
Switzerland Thailand Turkey Ukraine Vietnam

Oxford is a registered trade mark of Oxford University Press
in the UK and in certain other countries

Published in the United States
by Oxford University Press Inc., New York

© Oxford University Press, 2005

British Library Cataloguing in Publication Data

Data available

Library of Congress Cataloging in Publication Data

ISBN 0-19-263141-1

EAN code 9780192631411

10 9 8 7 6 5 4 3 2

Typeset by Integra Software Services Pvt. Ltd., Pondicherry, India
Printed in Great Britain
on acid-free paper by Biddles Ltd., King's Lynn, UK

Preface to the Supportive Care Series

Supportive care is the multidisciplinary holistic care of patients with chronic and life-limiting illnesses and their families – from the time around diagnosis, through treatments aimed at cure or prolonging life, and into the phase currently acknowledged as palliative care. It involves recognizing and caring for the side-effects of active therapies as well as patients' symptoms, co-morbidities, psychological, social and spiritual concerns. It also values the role of family carers and helps them in supporting the patient, as well as attending to their own special needs. Supportive care is a domain of health and social care that utilizes a network of professionals and voluntary carers in a 'virtual team'. It is increasingly recognized by healthcare providers and governments as a modern response to complex disease management, but so far it can lay claim to little dedicated literature.

This is therefore one volume in a unique new series of textbooks on supportive care, published by Oxford University Press which has already established itself as a leading publisher for palliative care. Unlike 'traditional' palliative care, which grew from terminal care of cancer patients, supportive care is not restricted to dying patients and neither to cancer. Thus this series covers the support of patients with a variety of long-term conditions, who are currently largely managed by specialist and general teams in hospitals and by primary care teams in community settings. It will therefore provide a practical guide to supportive care of the patient at all stages of the illness, providing up-to-date knowledge of the scientific basis of palliation and also practical guidance on delivering high quality multidisciplinary care across healthcare sectors. The volumes, edited by acknowledged leaders in the specific field of each volume, will bring together research, healthcare management, economics, and ethics through contributions from an international panel of experts of all disciplines. The underlying theme of all the books is the application of the latest evidence-based knowledge, in a humane way, for patients with advancing disease.

As Series Editors, we bring between us over four decades of research and clinical experience of acute medicine and palliative care. Our work has spanned St Christopher's Hospice and the Leicestershire Hospice in England – both of which have been inspirational leaders of traditional palliative care; the Academic Unit of Supportive Care at the University of Sheffield, England and the Harry Horvitz Center for Palliative Medicine in The Cleveland Clinic Foundation, USA. We have independently and jointly advocated the supportive care approach to cancer and other chronic disease management and are delighted to be collaborating on this series. We are both committed to delivering high quality of end-of-life care when it is necessary but we are constantly seeking to influence our colleagues in all relevant healthcare disciplines to adopt the principles of modern supportive care to benefit a wider range of patients at earlier stages of illness. We aim, through this series, to inform and inspire other doctors, nurses, allied health professionals, pharmacists, social and spiritual care providers, and students, to improve the quality of living for all patients and families in their care.

Sam Hjelmeland Ahmedzai
Professor of Palliative Medicine
Academic Unit of Supportive Care
The University of Sheffield
Royal Hallamshire Hospital
Sheffield, UK

Declan Walsh
Professor and Director
Harry Horvitz Center for Palliative Medicine
The Cleveland Clinic Foundation
Cleveland, Ohio, USA

Foreword

The starting point to support patients with any long-standing medical condition is to listen to them and understand those things which are compromising the quality of *their* lives. For one individual, it may be the burden of a particular symptom such as breathlessness; for another it may be the consequential limitation on some particular activity such as their inability to get upstairs or to get out and about. Different problems have different solutions.

This is a very timely book because it demonstrates the importance of the art as well as the science of medicine and brings the two together. In recent years there have been magnificent advances in the treatment of many lung conditions. Some of the world's most common diseases such as tuberculosis can be cured before there is irreparable damage to the lungs and immunization and antibiotics can prevent other forms of long-standing disabilities such as bronchiectasis following measles or whooping cough. Removal of damaging environmental agents including tobacco can reduce the burden of chronic obstructive pulmonary disease, many occupational lung diseases and lung cancer. Likewise anti-inflammatory medication can now transform other common and less common lung diseases if administered early enough. Advances in surgery can eliminate areas of localized disease, greatly improving symptoms and prolonging life. Indeed, flushed with the success of so many advances, made possible through modern scientific medicine in the pathogenesis and treatment of lung diseases, it is easy to overlook the burden of persisting symptoms and the compromise to normal life that a large number of patients are still compelled to endure.

The fact is that in spite of modern advances there remain a large number of patients with persisting conditions such as asthma which require continuing support, those with irreversible airways obstruction, destruction of alveolar units (eg emphysema) or lung scarring from a variety of causes, which result in loss of lung reserve and limit exercise through breathlessness and other pathophysiological mechanisms. Some patients have other bothersome symptoms such as chronic cough and sputum. In turn these often compromise sleep and lead to general debility. Such continuing symptoms often lead to social isolation, anxiety and depression and a general lack of self-esteem and confidence. All undermine the quality of life. Only too often, especially when doctors are under severe pressure of time, these patients are regarded as untreatable and simply left to their own devices without support until, often after years of unnecessary suffering and deteriorating health, the need for palliative care to ease their terminal distress is recognized. The importance of the distinction between supportive and palliative care cannot be overemphasized.

Of course many good doctors are well aware of the physical and psychological burden of chronic lung disease and over the years have tried their best to relieve their patients' symptoms. More recently there has been much more focused attention on the basic mechanisms underlying respiratory symptoms and this has led to the evaluation of a wide variety of techniques to improve respiratory performance as well as the development of scientific measurements to validate and quantify the improvements obtained in terms of quality of life, as well as the cost effectiveness of doing so. What has been lacking is a comprehensive and fully referenced book where all these advances in supportive medicine in respiratory disease are brought together.

This substantial book with contributions from many international specialists, reviews systematically the advances in this field across the whole range of lung diseases and sets new standards in both primary and secondary care to support patients with continuing respiratory disabilities. Indeed it goes much further because the principles of supportive medicine outlined here and the ways in which therapies may be evaluated are often equally applicable to those with non-respiratory disorders. In this way, this book makes a major contribution to the field of medical care of patients with chronic disease and emphasizes the responsibilities that doctors, other healthcare workers and society in general have for those who we are currently unable to cure, but for whom so much can still be done to lighten their burden.

Margaret Turner Warwick
November 2004

Preface

The care of patients with chronic respiratory disease has been central to medicine and health-care from the earliest times. Pulmonary infections are still one of the commonest forms of death and chronic chest diseases, and can cause major physical, psychological and social suffering for many months or years of life.

Palliative care has become well established in the wealthier countries and increasingly so in developing countries, to cater for the needs of both people who are dying – mainly from cancer – and those carers close to them. However, help is often needed long before this. In some cases a respiratory disease itself may not be the cause of death and so patients may be denied the benefits of conventional palliative care. It is for these reasons that we believe **supportive care**, with its broader remit and earlier interventions, is so important.

Supportive care is the multidisciplinary 'whole-person' care of patients and their families from the time of diagnosis, through treatments aimed at cure or prolonging life, into the advancing disease phase which is currently acknowledged as palliative care. It involves recognizing and caring for the side-effects of active therapies as well as patients' co-morbidities, and their psychological, social and spiritual concerns. It also values the role of family carers and helps them in supporting the patient, as well as attending to their special needs.

Unlike traditional palliative care, which grew from the terminal care of cancer patients, **supportive care** is neither restricted to dying patients nor to cancer. Thus this book covers the support of patients with a variety of long-term respiratory conditions, which are currently largely managed by respiratory and general medical teams in hospital and by primary care teams in community settings. The Editors and contributing authors therefore hope that this volume will provide a practical guide to the supportive care of respiratory patients at all stages of illness.

Symptoms such as breathlessness and cough are intrinsically common in patients with chronic and advancing disease. Pain is also a significant problem for patients, regardless of the diagnosis. Cancer, chronic cardiac and pulmonary disease, chronic infections, progressive neuromuscular disorders and degenerative disorders all give rise to varying degrees of respiratory distress which adversely affects the quality of life of both patients and families. In recent years, there have been significant advances in our understanding of how respiratory symptoms arise and in their palliation. This has led to practical ways of giving relief in hospitals, specialist palliative care units and at home. In this volume we have tried to emphasize comprehensively and critically the evidence base of this clinical progress and the scientific principles underlying it.

Throughout this book the authors have tried to emphasize the theoretical and empirical advances contributing to our knowledge base. Our design has been to examine the problems affecting respiratory patients from the point of view of first the mechanisms whereby symptoms are generated; next how they can be assessed and measured; and then how they can be palliated.

The first section starts with the editors charting the territory by discussing the concepts and theoretical basis of supportive care with a detailed discussion of its relation to palliation and palliative care; and of the basic anatomy and physiology of the respiratory system which is essential for understanding the topics of the later chapters. These are followed by further chapters on conceptual issues which apply throughout healthcare, namely quality of life and health economics. Complementary therapies, which are increasingly being incorporated into evidence-based healthcare are also discussed here.

The second section is on dyspnoea (breathlessness) with a total of 16 chapters on this important symptom. A 'state of the art' description of our current understanding of how dyspnoea is generated and modulated leads into discussions of how to assess and measure it in different scenarios. The management issues covered include the roles of rehabilitation and respiratory muscle training, occupational therapy, psychosocial therapies, complementary therapies and nutritional support as well as drug treatment and the role of oxygen. Special situations are discussed such as upper airways obstruction, diffuse obstructive and restrictive lung disease; neuromuscular disease including ALS/MND; and the 'hyperventilation' syndrome.

The third section is on cough and haemoptysis. There are chapters on the physiology and pathophysiology of cough and on the patient with chronic cough but 'normal' chest radiograph. These lead onto discussion of cough management in a variety of situations including cystic fibrosis and the approach to massive haemoptysis.

The fourth section is concerned with pain as it affects patients with respiratory disease. Once again it begins with a discussion of the mechanisms which produce pain in the thorax and this is followed by a chapter on the assessment of pain in both research and daily clinical practice. Two more chapters follow on the management of pain using drugs and neurolytic procedures respectively.

There then follow separate chapters on important specific diseases, which follow on respiratory distress in cancer patients and chronic infections. With respect to the latter we have focused on pulmonary aspects of HIV/AIDS and tuberculosis, as globally these now represent the most important infectious public health challenges for respiratory care.

Our authors represent a very wide range of specialist interests and come from many countries. They are well recognized authorities in their own subjects or have worked in leading centres researching and treating respiratory conditions. We hope that health professionals of all backgrounds, who work with respiratory patients, will find chapters of interest. One of the major developments of recent years has been the increasing role of specialist nurses, physiotherapists, technicians, occupational therapists, pharmacists and others in direct patient care and particularly we hope this book will appeal to them.

The Editors would like to emphasize their enormous gratitude to a large team of individuals who have helped to bring this volume and the new series to publication. We would like to start by thanking all the contributors and their assistants. We acknowledge the constant support and advice from our Commissioning Editors – initially Esther Hunt and Katherine Sugg who both worked with us on the preliminary design and latterly Catherine Barnes and her editorial assistants, who have overseen its completion.

Amanda Jones deserves our gratitude for collating and preparing the chapters edited by Martin in Leeds, and similarly Sue Button for working on chapters being edited by Sam in Sheffield. In addition, Sue has worked extensively with Oxford on bringing the whole volume together and producing the final manuscripts. We cannot overestimate the tremendous contribution that our secretaries have made in completing this work.

S.H.A.
M.F.M.
November, 2004

Contents

Contributors *xv*

Part I Supportive care in respiratory medicine

1 The nature of palliation and its contribution to supportive care *3*
   Sam H. Ahmedzai

2 Anatomy and physiology *39*
   Martin F. Muers

3 Quality of life – models and measures of quality of life *57*
   Michael E. Hyland and Samantha C. Sodergren

4 Complementary medicine for respiratory diseases *67*
   Jacqueline Filshie and Adrian White

5 Economics applied to respiratory supportive care *79*
   Niels Neymark

Part II Mechanisms and assessment of dyspnoea

6 Mechanisms of dyspnoea *93*
   Michael A. Gillette and Richard M. Schwartzstein

7 Assessment of dyspnoea in research *123*
   Helen R. Harty and Lewis Adams

8 Assessment of dyspnoea in clinical practice and audit *135*
   Eduardo Bruera and Catherine M. Neumann

Part III Management of dyspnoea

9 Drug therapies *147*
   Carol Davis

10 Oxygen and airflow *165*
   Sara Booth

11 Rehabilitation and exercise *189*
   Jane Lindsay and Roger Goldstein

12 Dyspnoea and respiratory muscle training *215*
   Hans Folgering and Yvonne Heijdra

13 Psychosocial therapies *229*
   Rod MacLeod

14 Nutrition and cachexia *239*
E.F.M. Wouters and A.M.W.J. Schols

15 Occupational therapy and environmental modifications *249*
Louise Sewell and Sally Singh

Part IV Dyspnoea in special situations

16 Upper airflow obstruction *265*
Martin R. Hetzel

17 Diffuse airflow obstruction and 'restrictive' lung disease *281*
Martin F. Muers

18 Neuromuscular and skeletal diseases *307*
John Shneerson

19 Dyspnoea in motor neurone disease (amyotrophic lateral sclerosis) *317*
David Oliver

20 Hyperventilation and disproportionate breathlessness *323*
William N. Gardner and Alex Lewis

Part V Cough and haemoptysis

21 Physiology and pathophysiology of cough *341*
John Myers

22 Chronic cough with a 'normal' chest radiograph *365*
J. Mark Madison and Richard S. Irwin

23 Massive haemoptysis: causes, assessment, and management *371*
Peter R. Mills and Jadwiga A. Wedzicha

24 The therapy of expectoration *381*
Alyn H. Morice

25 The management of cystic fibrosis *391*
John W. Wilson and Thomas Kotsimbos

Part VI Pain

26 Mechanisms of pain associated with respiratory disease *413*
Carla Ripamonti and Fabio Fulfaro

27 Pain in association with respiratory conditions: assessment
in research and clinical practice *427*
Nathan I. Cherny and Sam H. Ahmedzai

28 Treating severe pain in advanced lung disease *439*
Piotr Sobanski and Zbigniew Zylicz

29 Pain in association with respiratory disease
management: neurolytic procedures *453*
W.W.A. Zuurmond and J.J. de Lange

Part VII Specific diseases

30 Assessment and management of respiratory
symptoms of malignant disease *463*
Peter Hoskin and Sam H. Ahmedzai

31 Comprehensive supportive care in HIV pulmonary disease *487*
Elizabeth Bjorndal and Sam H. Ahmedzai

32 Chronic infections: pulmonary tuberculosis *515*
Suresh Kumar, Martin F. Muers, and Sam H. Ahmedzai

Contributors

Lewis Adams
School of Physiotherapy and Exercise Science,
Griffith University – Gold Coast Campus,
Queensland, Australia

Sam H. Ahmedzai
Academic Unit of Supportive Care,
University of Sheffield,
Royal Hallamshire Hospital,
Sheffield, UK

Elizabeth Bjorndal
The Margaret Centre,
Whipps Cross University Hospital,
Leytonstone, London, UK

Sara Booth
Palliative Care Service,
Oncology Centre,
Addenbrooke's NHS Trust,
Cambridge, UK

Eduardo Bruera
Department of Symptom Control and
Palliative Care,
University of Texas M.D. Anderson
Cancer Center,
Houston, Texas, USA

Nathan I. Cherny
Cancer Pain and Palliative Care Unit,
Department of Oncology,
Shaare Zedek Medical Center,
Jerusalem, Israel

Carol Davis
Countess Mountbatten House,
Moorgreen Hospital,
Southampton, UK

J.J. de Lange
Department of Anesthesiology,
Vrije Universiteit,
Amsterdam, The Netherlands

Jacqueline Filshie
Royal Marsden Hospital, Downs Road,
Sutton, Surrey, UK

Hans Folgering
Department of Pulmonology,
University of Nijmegen,
The Netherlands

Fabio Fulfaro
Medical Oncology Operative Unit,
University of Palmero,
Palmero, Italy

William N. Gardner
Department of Respiratory Medicine
and Allergy,
Guy's, King's and St Thomas's School
of Medicine,
London, UK

Michael A. Gillette
Division of Pulmonary and Critical Care
Medicine,
Department of Medicine,
Beth Israel Deaconess Medical Center
and Harvard Medical School,
Boston, USA

Roger Goldstein
West Park Hospital,
Toronto, Ontario, Canada

Helen R. Harty
Department of Physiology,
University College,
Dublin, Ireland

Yvonne Heijdra
Department of Pulmonology,
University of Nijmegen,
The Netherlands

Martin R. Hetzel
Bristol Royal Infirmary,
Bristol, and Department of Respiratory and
General Medicine,
University of Bristol, UK

Peter Hoskin
Mount Vernon Hospital,
Rickmansworth Road,
Northwood, Middlesex, UK

Michael E. Hyland
Department of Psychology,
University of Plymouth,
UK

Richard S. Irwin
Division of Pulmonary,
Allergy and Critical Care Medicine,
University of Massachusetts
Medical School,
Worcester, Mass, USA

Thomas Kotsimbos
Adult Cystic Fibrosis Service,
Department of Respiratory Medicine,
Alfred Hospital,
Prahran, Australia

Suresh Kumar
Institute of Palliative Medicine,
Medical College,
Calicut, Kerala, India

Alex Lewis
Department of Psychological Medicine
Guy's, King's and St Thomas's School
of Medicine,
London, UK

Jane Lindsay
Jane Lindsay and Associates,
Ottawa, Ontario, Canada

Rod MacLeod
Dunedin School of Medicine,
University of Otago,
PO Box 56, Dunedin, New Zealand

J. Mark Madison
Division of Pulmonary,
Allergy and Critical Care Medicine,
University of Massachusetts Medical School,
Worcester, Mass, USA

Peter R. Mills
Academic Department of Respiratory
Medicine,
St Bartholomew's and The Royal London
School of Medicine & Dentistry,
The London Chest Hospital,
London, UK

Alyn H. Morice
The University of Hull,
Academic Department of Medicine,
Castle Hill Hospital,
Cottingham,
East Yorkshire, UK

Martin F. Muers
Department of Respiratory Medicine,
Leeds General Infirmary,
Leeds, UK

John Myers
Barnet General Hospital,
Barnet, Herts, UK

Catherine M. Neumann
Department of Symptom Control
and Palliative Care,
University of Texas M.D. Anderson
Cancer Center,
Houston, Texas, USA

Niels Neymark
Scientific/medical writer,
Rixensart, Belgium

David Oliver
Wisdom Hospice,
St Williams Way,
Rochester, Kent and Kent Institute of
Medicine and Health Sciences,
University of Kent at Canterbury,
UK

Carla Ripamonti
Pain Therapy and Palliative Care Division,
National Cancer Institute,
Milan, Italy

A.M.W.J. Schols
Department of Respiratory Medicine,
University Hospital Maastricht,
Maastricht, The Netherlands

Richard M. Schwartzstein
Division of Pulmonary and Critical Care
Medicine,
Departments of Medicine,
Beth Israel Deaconess Medical Center and
Harvard Medical School,
Boston, Mass, USA

Louise Sewell
Pulmonary Rehabilitation Specialist,
University Hospitals of Leicester NHS Trust,
Glenfield Hospital,
Leicester, UK

John Shneerson
Respiratory Support and Sleep Centre,
Papworth Hospital,
Papworth Everard, Cambridgeshire,
UK

Sally Singh
Head of Cardiac and Pulmonary
Rehabilitation,
University Hospitals of Leicester NHS Trust,
Glenfield Hospital,
Leicester, UK

Piotr Sobański
Department of Cardiology,
Regional Hospital,
Bydgoszcz, Poland

Samantha C. Sodergren
Department of Psychology,
University of Plymouth,
UK

Jadwiga A. Wedzicha
Academic Department of Respiratory
Medicine,
St Bartholomew's and The Royal London
School of Medicine and Dentistry,
The London Chest Hospital,
London, UK

Adrian White
British Medical Acupuncture Society,
The Royal London Homoeopathic Hospital,
Greenwell Street, London
UK

John W. Wilson
Adult Cystic Fibrosis Service,
Department of Respiratory Medicine,
Alfred Hospital, Prahran, Australia

E.F.M. Wouters
Department of Respiratory Medicine,
University Hospital Maastricht, Maastricht,
The Netherlands

W.W.A. Zuurmond
Department of Anesthesiology,
Vrije Universiteit,
Amsterdam, The Netherlands

Zbigniew Zylicz
Comprehensive Cancer Centre,
Nijmegen, The Netherlands, and Chair of
Palliative Medicine,
The L. Rydygie University of Medical
Sciences
Bydgoszcz, Poland

The publishers would like to thank Kjersti Hjelmeland Brakstad for designing the covers for the Supportive Care series.

The editors would like to acknowledge the use of images taken from X-rays and CT scans loaned from Leeds General Infirmary, Royal Hallamshire Hospital and Rotherham General Hospital. We would also like to thank Dr Nubeel Qureshi for his assistance in preparing medical images.

Part I

Supportive care in respiratory medicine

Chapter 1

The nature of palliation and its contribution to supportive care

Sam H. Ahmedzai

Changing aims of medicine

Medicine has undergone significant changes throughout history, but perhaps none so dramatic as those in the 20th century. Particularly in the last 50 years, there has been a shift in focus from the restricted view of the physician at the bedside, in the clinic or at the operating table, to the broader vision of community and social networks. Public health medicine has become a major force in planning and delivering healthcare, whereas previously this was determined by the interests of individual practitioners, who worked largely in independent settings with little accountability or need to cooperate with other colleagues. The birth of the World Health Organization (WHO) and its subsequent influence on the public health policies of most countries can be seen as both a reflection and a driving force of this global change. The founding of the British National Health Service (NHS) in 1947 is another indicator of the shift in medical strategy away from the authority of the individual clinician towards organizations and teams operating in primary, secondary, and tertiary sectors.[1]

At the same time, paradoxically, other contemporary influences have made patients' views more powerful, which has led healthcare practitioners to think more carefully about the psychological and social implications of their actions. These influences include the rise of consumerism, at least in developed countries, and the growing disenchantment many people have felt with the unchallenged authority of medicine and nursing. In some countries, there has also been an increasing role for non-governmental organizations, or charities, which have become significant agencies for stimulating social reform, funding research, influencing policy and even competing with or at least supplementing state healthcare systems for providing direct medical care to the public. (The function of charities in the latter part of the 20th century is rather different from their role in the 19th century, when they were dominated by religious principles and were largely concerned with relieving the pitiful conditions of the very poorest people in society.) Examples of the modern organizations are the many national cancer leagues and international bodies, such as the International Union against Cancer (UICC), and the international hospice movement.

A central theme with all the diverse charitable organizations has been the recognition of the importance of individual patients and their families, and their needs at different stages of illness and the road to recovery. Parallel to the development of the charitable organizations has been the growing role for volunteers in health and especially social care. In many cases this aspect has been crucial to the charities' outreach work. Volunteers have been particularly important, for instance, in the implementation of hospice principles in Europe, Australia, India, south-east Asia and the Americas.

These shifts in healthcare thinking can be seen reflected in the changing aims of medicine. Table 1.1 shows how the originally simple purpose of medicine has moved from making a

Table 1.1 Changing aims of medicine

Older aims	Newer aims
	Prevention
Diagnosis	Early and accurate diagnosis
Cure	Cure
	Prolonging life
	Rehabilitation
Palliation	Palliation
Terminal care	End-of-life care
(Death seen as a failure and dying as usually terrible)	(Death seen as inevitable and dying as potentially tolerable)

diagnosis, followed by attempting a cure and if that were not possible, then trying to palliate the consequences, into broader and more humanistic objectives. The first of these modern objectives is the increasing investment into prevention and earlier detection of disease, reflecting the current view that earlier intervention with many diseases may result in a better chance of disease eradication. The case of cancer prevention has also been seen by MacDonald as an even longer-term investment in healthcare, with four stages: (1) prevention of disease; (2) prevention of advanced disease; (3) prevention of death; and (4) prevention of suffering.[2] Other key elements of the new aims of medicine include recognizing the value of prolonging life, even if the patient cannot be 'cured'; rehabilitation to enable people whose lives have been changed by disease (or treatment) to restore better function and reclaim personal and social roles; and the value placed on care at the end of life.

There is perhaps now greater honesty among physicians about the true chances of 'curability', with recognition that prolonging life is itself a worthy aim of medicine, even if the disease cannot be cured. In a similar vein, oncologists have realized that 'response rates' to anticancer therapies do not in themselves always translate into benefit for patients, and are therefore increasingly incorporating subjective endpoints such as symptom relief and quality of life as markers of their interventions.[3,4] MacDonald has stated this as a challenge to his fellow oncologists to see cancer management as more than curing cancer, or prolonging life, but also from the point of view of improving the **quality** of life of the patients.[5] We will return to this balance between quantity and quality of life later in this chapter. Of course, away from oncology and in the field of chronic disease management, notions of 'cure' are often meaningless. In the respiratory field, chronic obstructive pulmonary disease (COPD), pulmonary fibrosis, industrial lung diseases, neuromuscular disorders, and even some chronic infections such as bronchiectasis cannot be thought of as curable, and so a different attitude to their management has emerged.

Rehabilitation is becoming integral to the plan of disease management, in both acute and chronic conditions. Some rehabilitation is required because many treatment interventions, e.g. surgery, themselves compromise the independence of the patient. Other motivations for rehabilitation become partly justified by humane reasons of improving health, and partly by socio-economic arguments about restoring the patient to a former occupation, or allowing a family carer to resume work or being less reliant on outside help. Pulmonary rehabilitation in

COPD is a good example of these phenomena, and programmes are becoming widespread within respiratory disease services (see Chapter 11).

Although Table 1.1 shows that palliation is still a legitimate aim of medicine, it is interesting to briefly review here how the medical meaning of the word 'palliate' has itself changed over time. According to the *Compact Oxford English Dictionary*, one of the first recorded uses in the English language was:

> A wise physician will consider whether a disease be incurable; if he find it to be such, let him resort to palliation; and alleviate the symptom. Bacon, *Sylva*, 1626

One hundred years later, the following quote shows palliation in a less positive light:

> He is but half a physician: he hath palliated our sores and diseases, but he hath not removed them. Sharp, *Sermon*, 1714

Another century on, palliation has an even more derogatory connotation:

> These drugs at best are no more than palliative. Allbutt, Syst. Med. VIII. 887, 1889

The current dictionary definition of 'to palliate' is:

> To alleviate the symptoms of a disease without curing it; to relieve superficially or temporarily; to mitigate the sufferings of; to ease. *Oxford Concise Dictionary*

Leaving aside the fascinating etymological history of the word, the dictionary definition given above is not particularly helpful in the fuller clinical context that this volume will be considering. For this purpose, a more comprehensive definition is proposed:

> Medical palliation is the relief of a symptom or a problem associated with an illness, without necessarily curing the underlying disease process; and in the case of a life-threatening illness, without primarily attempting to prolong life.

The terms 'necessarily' and 'primarily' are important parts of this definition, but in clinical practice they may frequently be overruled. As will be seen throughout this volume, in many areas of medicine the best palliation may well be achieved through measures which are in fact designed to cure or to prolong life, by being directed against the underlying primary disease process. Examples are the impressive relief of physical symptoms of small-cell lung cancer through the use of life-prolonging cytotoxic chemotherapy; and the resolution of fever, cough, and haemoptysis with the use of combination antibiotics in pulmonary tuberculosis.

In many other cases, however, symptoms may be better controlled by interventions which act directly on them, by mitigating the pathological processes caused by the primary disease which give rise to symptoms remote from the primary disease site. An example of this is the management of nausea and vomiting which arises in some patients with squamous cell cancer of the lung. The mechanism of the emetic stimulus is hypercalcaemia, which is caused by the production of a parathormone-like substance from the tumour. Treating the hypercalcaemia systemically by means of intravenous bisphosphonates is dramatically helpful for reducing emesis (and other hypercalcaemia-related symptoms such as confusion), without any need to treat the primary cancer directly.[6]

A third mechanism of palliation is the relief of symptoms and other problems by interventions which are targeted not at the causative disease nor at its pathophysiological consequences, but directly tackle the subjective perception of the symptom or problem. The use of opioids such as morphine for pain control is an example of this mechanism. In the case of pain during angina, the distress is caused by ischaemia in the cardiac muscle. Morphine promptly relieves the pain, not by restoring blood supply (as would glyceryl trinitrate), nor by intervening in the pathology of coronary artery disease (as would cholesterol-reducing agents), but by its direct effect on the brain's perception of pain originating in visceral tissues. It does this by interacting with mu-opioid receptors in the brain and spinal cord, far from the site of the pathology. (Recently we have learnt that opioids do not always need to act centrally to give analgesia – there is increasing evidence that peripheral nerves in areas of tissue damage and inflammation acquire active opioid receptors which migrate down sensory axons; these may be targeted by morphine applied topically to the inflamed lesion.)[7,8]

Another way of relieving the nausea in a patient with hypercalcaemia could be the administration of a butyrophenone drug such as haloperidol. This works without having any impact on the underlying malignancy or the elevated serum calcium, but by modulating dopaminergic D2 receptors in the brainstem. There are examples of this third type of palliation in the field of psychological care: the relief of anxiety by the use of anxiolytic drugs, or by explanation and information. Thus it is not always strictly 'medical' palliation that may be helpful, but also the contributions from other healthcare disciplines such as nursing or psychology.

In order to improve the clarity in describing and attributing the palliative actions of healthcare interventions, a proposed new classification of palliative interventions is shown in Table 1.2. This table shows that to the three types of palliation described above, a fourth has been added, called type 1 or preventive palliation. This type of palliation is included for completeness, because it emphasizes that appropriate preventive measures can also relieve symptoms, even if they cannot stop the onset or progress of a disease. An example of this is the reduction in the number and duration of episodes of delirium in elderly hospital patients, by a programme which attended to good ambient light, noise reduction at night, and sleep deprivation (rather than the use of neuroleptic agents, which would represent type 3 palliation).[9] The purpose of introducing this taxonomy is to clarify the aims of palliation, so that we can better understand how to use different approaches to maximum advantage. The classification may also be useful in guiding us to use appropriate outcome measures to evaluate the potential benefit of different palliation techniques.

Table 1.2 A proposed classification of palliative interventions based on intention

Type of palliation	Intention	Example – cancer	Example – COPD
Type 1	Prevention/prophylaxis	Smoking prevention/cessation Cranial irradiation to prevent brain metastases	Smoking prevention or cessation Exercise programmes to prevent deconditioning
Type 2	Direct targeting of the primary disease process	Lobectomy Radiotherapy for bone metastases	α_1-Antitrypsin replacement Corticosteroid
Type 3	Manipulation of the pathophysiological consequences of the primary disease process	Bisphosphonate for symptoms of hypercalcaemia, e.g. nausea, confusion	Bronchodilator for airflow obstruction
Type 4	Alteration of the perception or secondary effects of the symptom	Drug treatments for symptoms of hypercalcaemia, e.g. emetic, neuroleptic	Therapies to reduce perception of dyspnoea, e.g. oxygen, opioid

Factors determining symptom perception and the success of palliation

So far I have considered how a palliative intervention may bring about its effect. There is another important aspect to this discussion, and that is the role of the individual's own psychic traits and state, and how that may affect the success or failure of an intervention. It is a commonplace observation in healthcare that no two patients respond with the same degree of pain to an injury, and even the same person may report different levels of pain with the same pathology at different times, depending on other conscious or subconscious processes. Increasing age is thought to be accompanied by reducing tendency to complain of some physical symptoms such as pain; and at the same time older people appear to require lower doses of analgesic drugs to achieve pain control. Recent studies have shown that not only do men and women report some symptoms to different extents,[10,11] but they also react differently to some classes of drugs.[12,13] The reasons for these findings are no doubt complex, and could include true differences in end-organ sensitivity, changes in metabolism of drugs, social conditioning and biases of observers.

Bruera has presented a helpful diagrammatic representation of how symptoms may be reported and modified in cancer patients (see Figure 8.1). Previously, Hyland proposed an elegant model of how 'quality of life' is conceptualized in an individual.[14] Ingham and Portenoy have also proposed an elaborate model to show the relationships between pain, symptoms, and quality of life.[15] I have combined elements of these theories together with my proposed four types of palliation, into a generic algorithm, which attempts to explain how and when palliation works – and when it may not work (Figure 1.1). The generic model could be used in several ways:

- As an educational tool for teaching healthcare professionals about the impact of disease on patients' lives and how other intrinsic and extrinsic factors modify that impact.
- As an information tool for explaining to patients themselves and their family carers, why and how specific palliative interventions are hoped to work, and to help them understand why some treatments may fail.
- To expose key aspects of the disease or patient's psychological condition which could be further researched to lead to more effective interventions for the future.

Care of dying patients

The final row in Table 1.1 represents a new objective for medicine, that of **end-of-life care**. It could be said that care of the dying has always been central to medicine, but it is fair to comment that it had to be included in medical care during the centuries before curative treatments were available. In the 16th century an anonymous author defined the role of a physician as

To cure sometimes, to relieve often, to comfort always.

The medical establishment subsequently adopted an increasingly distant position from patients with diseases which could not be cured, as was seen above in the evolution of the term 'palliation'. Only in the last two centuries has the care of a dying person been recognized by the body of physicians as a worthy end in itself. The origins of terminal or end-of-life care go back many hundreds of years, but it became an organizational reality only in the latter half of the 19th century in the first Christian hospice-like institutions of Ireland, France, and England.

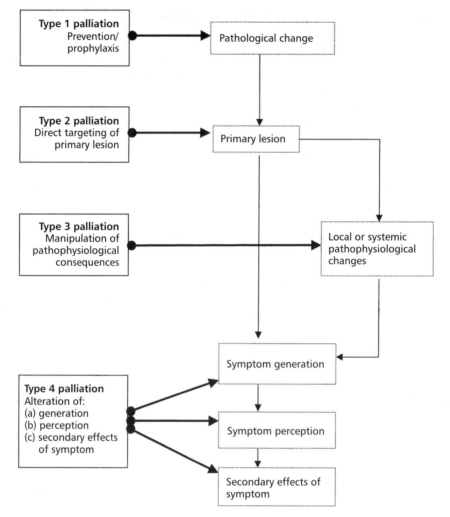

Fig. 1.1 Generic model of symptom perception and palliation.

A discussion of the hospice movement is beyond the scope of this volume, but its relevance and contribution to modern supportive care should never be underestimated.[16]

Why have end-of-life care and the recognition of comfort as a valid goal of healthcare become more widely recognized recently? Part of the explanation derives from the secular trends described earlier, and sociologists have commented on the public's concern with the increasing 'medicalization' of life and death, and the perceived 'sanitization' or 'sequestration' of the dying process.[17,18] Over the last 50 years, the tendency has been for most deaths in developed countries to occur in hospital, rather than at home. One reason for this is that the notion of 'home' and who resides there has itself changed because of demographic shifts. Seale has reported on this using data from two large studies in the UK, conducted in 1969 and in 1987.[19] These surveys involved interviews with the carers or others close to recently deceased people, whose names were taken randomly from death certificates.

In 1969 29% of deaths were of people aged under 65 years, but in 1987 this had fallen to 22%. In contrast, the proportion of deaths in people over the age of 75 rose over this period from 40% to 55%.

Even more telling are the statistics regarding who was living in the home of the deceased. In 1969, only 15% of those who died were living alone, and 85% were living with a spouse and/or others. By 1987, 32% of those who died were alone and only 68% were living with a spouse and/or other people. This picture of an ageing population which is increasingly isolated at the time of death is typical of industrialized societies. It is a major influence on the need for people to be hospitalized towards the end of their lives. For example, Hinton has analysed the medical and socio-demographic features which predicted hospice admission for terminal care, from a cohort of 415 patients who had been referred to a palliative home care team in London. Age of the patient was not an independent predictor, but living alone and having relatives who were 'unfit' themselves (i.e. not physically able to care) did predispose to terminal admissions.[20]

Non-industrialized societies may not have the same opportunities for admitting terminally ill patients to hospital or hospice, but in other ways they have embraced the concept of providing high-quality specialized end-of-life care. In India, for example, Rajagopal and Kumar have argued that the western hospice model cannot be widely implemented partly because of the sheer size of the terminally ill population (1 million cancer patients who mostly present with advanced incurable disease), but also because the hospice concept is not culturally suited to Indians.[21] In response, they describe the 'Calicut model', in which families are mobilized to assist the dying patient, aided by existing cancer services and boosted by non-governmental charitable organizations. In 1998 nine central and eastern European countries joined to make the 'Poznan declaration', which emphasized the desire to pursue palliative care but stressed the need for national policies, education and awareness programmes and improved drug availability.[22] Building more hospices was not a viable option here, as in many other parts of the world.

The unifying principle behind these international developments is the recognition that terminally ill patients (usually identified as having incurable cancer) have a need to receive good-quality care at the end of life. In the words of the preamble to the Poznan declaration,

> It is a human right to receive effective cancer pain relief and palliative care. It is unethical to tolerate unnecessary and unacceptable suffering.

Clearly this statement could equally apply to a patient with a potentially curable cancer, or to one with a progressive non-malignant chronic disease such as severe COPD or fibrosing alveolitis, or even to one with an acute and self-limiting condition which produces pain and suffering. However, the spirit that has captured the world in the past 30 years, since the establishment of St Christopher's Hospice in London and the Royal Victoria Hospital palliative care unit in Montreal – the two pioneers of hospice, home-, and hospital-based care – is the care of people dying from cancer. In the following discussion I will explore the nature of this concentration of emotion, energy, and resources for end-of-life care, and I will construct an argument that life **before** it comes to the end, with either chronic or curable distressing illnesses, is also worthy of equally energetic dedication from the healthcare professions. This is the basis of the notion of **supportive care**, which is in the title of this volume and the series of books in which it lies.

In summary, rehabilitation, palliation, and end-of-life care – together with the underlying principle of always giving comfort – are important in the field of respiratory disease. To justify

Table 1.3 Curability, possibility of prolonging life, and ability to palliate in various pulmonary diseases

Condition	Cure?	Prolong life?	Palliate?
Infections			
Acute bronchitis	++	++	++
Pneumonia	+	++	+
TB	±	++	+
HIV	–	++	++
Chronic disorders			
COPD	–	++	+
Cystic fibrosis	±	+	+
Pneumoconiosis and industrial lung diseases	–	±	±
Malignancy			
Primary lung cancer	±	++	++
Mesothelioma	–	±	+
Metastatic cancer	–	±	+

–, never; ±, sometimes; +, frequently; ++, always.

this one needs only to look at the 'curability' of pulmonary diseases, or even when they cannot be cured, at the realistic prospect of prolonging life. Naturally the possibilities of cure or increased survival depend not only on our current knowledge and treatments, but on social and economic variations in the general health of a nation, as well as on the physiological and psychosocial resistance of the individual patient. Table 1.3 shows how powerless medicine really is in halting the deadly progress of so many pulmonary diseases, which highlights the enormous possibilities for relieving suffering.

Models of palliative care

Let us now consider a healthcare approach which incorporates elements from the preceding discussions about symptom perception, medical palliation, and the need to consider incurable and fatal diseases. This approach has come to be known as **palliative care**. The historical reason for this new use of 'palliative' is the reluctance of the newly developing terminal care services in French-speaking Canada in the 1970s to use the term 'hospice', which had already been accepted in Britain. To the francophones in Montreal, the word 'hospice' implied a residential system for elderly people, with strongly negative connotations. It is said that Mount, a surgeon working in the Royal Victoria Hospital who had been inspired by Dame Cicely Saunders to establish the first terminal care service in Canada, started to use the term 'palliative care' as an alternative to both hospice and terminal care. This new usage rapidly gained currency on both sides of the Atlantic and is now the favoured expression worldwide to describe what are essentially end-of-life healthcare services. It is, however, somewhat regrettable that the same term 'palliative' has been used to describe the healthcare system as is used for the relief of symptoms, since this has only added to the confusion about what the former is.

What actually is palliative care? A common starting point for understanding this is the WHO view which was first published in its landmark 1986 booklet *Cancer pain relief and palliative care*. The second edition (1990) gives the following definition:[23]

> Palliative care is the active total care of patients whose disease is not responsive to curative treatment. Control of pain, of other symptoms and of psychological, social and spiritual problems is paramount. The goal of palliative care is achievement of the best possible quality of life for patients and their families.

WHO expanded and tried to clarify its definition with the following statements from the same publication:

> Many aspects of palliative care are also applicable earlier in the course of the illness, in conjunction with anticancer treatment.

Palliative care:

◆ affirms life and regards dying as a normal process;
◆ neither hastens nor postpones death;
◆ provides relief from pain and other distressing symptoms;
◆ integrates the psychological and spiritual aspects of patient care;
◆ offers a support system to help patients live as actively as possible until death;
◆ offers a support system to help the family cope during the patient's illness and in their own bereavement.

These statements have been extremely influential, just as the pain relief programme which accompanied it in the WHO booklet has been. But has this definition stood the test of time? In one way it clearly has, as so many other organizations and publications refer to and borrow from it. Also, these sentences have clearly been powerful in opening the minds of clinicians, and perhaps more importantly, of policymakers to release the resources needed to improve the care of cancer patients at the end of life. Who could argue with the need to control pain, breathlessness, and other symptoms, to achieve the 'best quality of life' for patients and families, and to offer a support system to help patients live as actively as possible?

But the premise on which all these statements were based is that the patient has to have an incurable and fatal cancer. How can we reconcile that with the humane need to offer care to people who have potentially curable cancer; or those with cancer whose life may be still extended; and to all those whose primary disease is not cancer? The WHO definition makes reference to 'many aspects of palliative care' being applicable to earlier stages of disease. However, this only underlines the perception that palliative care itself is confined to terminally ill patients. Further evidence that these are linked in the WHO approach is given by their diagram of how resources in cancer care should be allocated, which is reproduced in Figure 1.2.[23]

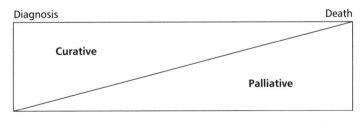

Fig. 1.2 The WHO model of resource allocation in cancer care.

This model has been influential in advising policy-makers on allocating resources for palliative care for cancer patients who are incurable. Unfortunately, it has also unavoidably been seen as a clinical model, encouraging surgeons and oncologists to practice their interventions in separate compartments of the healthcare system from the palliative care services. This may be efficient and convenient for the services, but it leads to discontinuity from the point of view of the recipients. The WHO model also imposes an additional, unnecessary trauma for patients who need to be transferred at a vulnerable time from what is often loosely called 'active' to palliative care. Furthermore, a too literal reading of the WHO resource model implies that curative treatment is superior to palliative care, and has to take precedence over it. Leaving aside the question of how 'curable' many cancers really are at the outset, this view gives individual clinicians involved in curative treatments (and also in primary care) the discretion to withhold referral to palliative care until it is thought that the 'time is right'.

In 1987 a group of doctors in the UK convened a new association for those working in the newly emerging field of medical practice in hospices and community- or hospital-based palliative care services. Forming what is now called the Association for Palliative Medicine of Great Britain and Ireland, they adopted a new definition of what shortly afterwards became recognized by the Royal Colleges of Physicians in the UK as the specialty of palliative medicine. The definition is:

> Palliative medicine is the study and management of patients with active, progressive, far-advanced disease for whom the prognosis is limited and the focus of care is the quality of life.

This definition has no doubt helped medical colleagues in other established specialties to understand and accept what palliative medicine is trying to do. But again, we can see that there is an unmistakable emphasis on the end of life. The definition also uses terms which are not themselves clear. To take the elements separately:

- **Active, progressive**: How does one determine this, even in malignant disease? We may know when a cancer is actively progressing, from biochemical markers, radiological and perhaps clinical signs, but how can we be sure when it is not active, but stable? Are symptoms and other problems from stable disease not worthy of attention? Patients who have come through devastating disease and invasive treatments may be medically 'stable', but they may well have major need for rehabilitation: whose task is it to provide that? And how much 'progression' needs to occur before palliative medicine becomes relevant? Should cancer patients be referred at the time when the first metastasis is detected; or should they wait until the oncologist or surgeon has exhausted second-, or third-line therapies?

- **Far-advanced disease**: What does this evocative term actually mean? Does 'far' imply distance, in other words, metastatic disease in the case of cancer? And if a disease is only locally advanced, e.g. lung cancer which is causing pain through intercostal nerve infiltration or breathlessness through bronchial obstruction, then does palliative medicine have no part to play? If, on the other hand, 'far-advanced' is another way of saying 'end-stage' regardless of metastatic status, perhaps it would be better to use plainer language. If we consider non-malignant diseases, does the concept of 'far-advanced' still have currency and a measurable threshold – for example, when does it start in COPD, musculoskeletal disorders, or tuberculosis? Furthermore, if the specialty of palliative medicine does not consider that it should study and manage symptoms and problems in disease which are not 'far-advanced', whose responsibility should this be?

◆ **The prognosis is limited**: This is more helpful than the original WHO statement 'not responsive to curative treatment', because it implies that some patients may be eligible for palliative medicine right from the time of diagnosis, regardless of how successful 'curative' treatment may be for them. It would be helpful if there were consensus about what constitutes 'limited prognosis' – common sense suggests that it should apply if the probability of cure (i.e. not dying from this disease) is less than 50%. Seen this way, the large majority of solid malignancies at diagnosis, with the exception of basal cell carcinomas of skin, carry a 'limited prognosis'. How limited does the prognosis need to be in order for palliative medicine to be involved? Should it be measured in terms of chance of survival, e.g. less than 10%; or does 'limited' mean that the actual survival time is now estimated to be short, e.g. months rather than years? These are not facile questions, because they have everyday implications for the referral criteria to palliative medicine used by doctors and hospice services in general. All too often one hears regret that a patient was referred 'too late'. Paradoxically, the public's observation that services such as hospices and specialist palliative care nurses and doctors are usually activated when the prognosis is poor, often turns into a reason for them to resist referral for themselves or a relative, until 'it is really necessary'. The definition therefore both requires a limited prognosis and ensures it.

◆ **The focus of care is quality of life**: It is hard to disagree with this element of the definition. In practice, quality of life is not routinely measured from the patient's point of view, and so it is difficult to verify if this goal is actually being achieved. Several studies have shown that physicians and nurses do not reliably estimate patients' quality of life, or even the symptoms and other concerns which contribute to it.[24] There is also increasing evidence that improved symptom control by itself does not necessarily lead to a measurable improvement in quality of life, even when validated quality-of-life instruments are employed.[25,26] This is in contrast to, say, increased survival being the 'focus' of oncology or improved exercise capacity being the 'focus' of pulmonary rehabilitation – i.e. routinely measured and objectively auditable goals.

What is the purpose of dissecting and challenging these definitions? Why should a physician working in palliative medicine question the very basis of his own profession? My purpose is to show that palliative care (if it wishes to retain this convenient but euphemistic name) has a duty to be crystal clear in its objectives and its sphere of influence. If palliative medicine is concerned not only with incurable, malignant disease and with care at the end of life, then these references should be stripped from the definition.

From this discussion of the meaning and scope of palliative care, three strands emerge. First, there is the question of the purpose and importance of the definition of palliative care. Does it really matter exactly what is meant by this term? What harm does it do if different countries and different professional disciplines hold the words to mean different types of healthcare? The answer to these questions has two parts, semantic and practical. It seems to be a retrograde step to allow ambiguity and contradictions into the very words which we use to describe a clinical discipline or healthcare policy. It would not be helpful if 'oncology' meant to some people a discipline covering all neoplastic disease and its consequences, but other people restricted it to only the metastatic stage of cancer, whereas others chose to include some benign growths which did not display malignant changes. At the practical level, would it be considered reasonable if a country's professional association for pulmonary medicine declared that it would henceforth only concentrate on diseases which ultimately cause death, but not on acute or chronic conditions which would need to be picked up by other healthcare agencies? (Another reason for seeking a robust definition of palliative care is that this discipline is crucially important within the emerging field of supportive care – as will be discussed in detail below.)

The second issue is: is there enough consensus at present to offer a new definition? Sadly, there is little evidence of this, or even of the mechanism which is required to propose one. One promising compromise (rather than true consensus!) that this author is aware of has recently emerged from a working group of 24 palliative care, cancer and pain specialists which was convened by the European School of Oncology in late 2000.[27] The purpose of this workshop was to propose a new European programme of activities and priorities for harmonizing and improving palliative care across the European Union. The workshop has proposed the following new definition which builds on the previous ones and tries to clarify the problems noted above:

> Palliative care is the person-centred attention to physical symptoms, psychological, social and existential[1] distress and cultural needs in patients with limited prognosis, in order to optimize the quality of life for the patients and their families or friends.

The workshop also agreed that it is essential to separate palliative care interventions which can and should be undertaken by any healthcare professional, and those which should fall within the responsibility of specialists with postgraduate training. This view gave rise to the following further definitions of how palliative care could be implemented:

> **Basic palliative care** is palliative care which should be provided by all healthcare professionals, in primary or secondary care, within their duties to patients with life-limiting disease.

> **Specialized palliative care** is palliative care provided at the expert level, by a trained multiprofessional team, who must continually update their skills and knowledge, in order to manage persisting and more severe or complex problems and to provide specialized educational and practical resources to other non-specialized members of the primary or secondary care teams.

It is immediately apparent that these definitions, which were submitted in early 2001 to the Council of Healthcare Ministers of the European Union, are not watertight. That is, they still allow some ambiguity about how seriously ill and near to death patients need to be before they are considered to fall within the purview of palliative care. The term 'specialized' was used in preference to 'specialist', as in most European countries palliative care is not yet recognized as a specialty within medicine or nursing. However, given the history of the field and the existing large variations between the 12 countries contributing to these statements, these definitions represent useful starting points for further work.

This leads to the last issue, which is that if there should be uniformity in how palliative care is defined, across both geographical and professional boundaries, then how should that standardization be reached? Does it need international ratification, like the definition of 'pain' which has been adopted by the International Association for the Study of Pain, and serves as a reference point for studies and policies? It would seem appropriate that the WHO, which launched the first helpful but now outdated definition, should take on the responsibility of coordinating a new universal statement of what palliative care is. A good starting point would be the joint European statements presented above, together with the current definitions used by governments and the national palliative care organizations which have chosen to develop

---

[1] 'existential' here includes 'spiritual' and 'religious' but is not confined to people with established faiths.

their own definitions. It would also be wise to agree that a review of any new definition should be made within at least 5 years, so that it is updated in the light of further global changes in theory and practice.

Palliative medicine as a specialty

The specialty of palliative medicine has been mentioned above, but it is worth emphasizing that it is still recognized in only a very few countries – currently the UK, Ireland, Poland, Australia, and Canada. In the UK, entry is based on general professional training, resulting in the post-graduate membership of either the Royal College of Physicians or the Royal College of General Practitioners, and there is then a 4-year training programme leading to accreditation as a consultant physician in palliative medicine. Even in the UK, where the specialty has been officially recognized since 1987, there is not universal acceptance of its place alongside other hospital-based specialities, or vis-à-vis general practice. Thus in 1999 a vigorous correspondence followed a polemical paper in the *Journal of the Royal Society of Medicine*, which again questioned the need for this new specialty and suggested that its work could be done (as the authors believed it had been done in the past) by general practitioners.[28]

The lack of recognition of palliative medicine as a separate medical specialty might be only a matter for professional pride, were it not for the lost opportunities that result from denying its existence. McIllmurray, a senior UK medical oncologist, has argued that all trainees for oncology should have a period of enforced training in palliative medicine.[29] MacDonald, a Canadian haematology oncologist, has asserted that colleagues in his discipline, even with training in symptom control, will never reach the level of knowledge and skills as those of a palliative medicine doctor.[30] He has further stated that:

> Palliative medicine should be recognized as an integral component of an overall cancer programme. The benefits of liaison are obvious: continuity of care, ready access for patients to all therapies, better coordination between cancer centres, the home, and community institutions, and increased emphasis on symptom control research and education.[31]

The scope of this volume goes far beyond cancer, and the question which arises is: how could the emergence of a specialty of palliative medicine help improve the medical care of patients with non-malignant diseases, as it is believed to have done for cancer? The answer is not clear – most palliative care services still concentrate their efforts on cancer patients. In the UK, the 4-year postgraduate training programme for doctors includes compulsory time in chronic (i.e. non-malignant) pain clinics and in HIV/AIDS services, and requires trainees to keep informed of palliative care issues in other disciplines. However, there is no corresponding compulsory time for palliative medicine trainees to learn in respiratory medicine or cardiology units, even though it is increasingly recognized that palliative care could be usefully be extended to patients with advanced respiratory and cardiac disease.[32,33] This could make specialists in these latter subjects understandably nervous and even sceptical about the competence and usefulness of the palliative contribution that 'specialists' in palliative medicine can offer to them.

The comments above have referred to palliative medicine. So far other professions have been lagging behind in declaring specialisms in palliative care, except that nursing appears to have embraced the concept and often has sections of palliative care nursing within national associations or international oncology societies. In the UK, nurses may train as specialist practitioners in palliative care, and practice their skills in hospices, home care, or hospital teams, alongside – and often outnumbering – specialist doctors. Other members of the multidisciplinary palliative care (which will be discussed below) are typically 'borrowed' from generic services and are not currently required to undergo postgraduate training in their fields.

Why do we need a new concept of supportive care?

From the preceding section, it should be clear that the scope of palliative care – and the goals of medical and nursing specialties which practice it – are based on an uncertain premise. This is the notion of incurable and soon to be fatal disease, which is usually but not always cancer. The emphasis of palliative care on symptom control and quality of life is admirable, but it seems to promote these to the exclusion of prolonging life. Is this in the best interests of patients and their families? What of the large numbers of patients who are hovering between being potentially curable and having frankly incurable disease? Who should look after the symptoms, psychological concerns, and quality of life of patients who are undergoing curative or life-prolonging therapies, with either cancer or any other life-threatening disease? Clearly the specialists who work with these diseases cannot be expected also to be experts in all aspects of palliation, as their technical knowledge and practical skills need to encompass prevention, accurate diagnosis, and attempts to cure or prolong life. To whom can they turn for help? This is where the concept of supportive care has to be invoked.

For many years, supportive care has been spoken of within oncology as a set of specific interventions and manoeuvres aimed at reducing the toxicity of anticancer treatments. For example, antiemetic therapy for nausea and vomiting induced by cytotoxic and radiation therapy took a great stride forward with the introduction of the serotonin or 5HT-3 antagonist drugs, and this also gave a boost to supportive care in oncology services.[34] Similarly, the more recent introduction of bone marrow growth factors, which enable faster recovery of white blood counts after cytotoxic drugs, and erythropoetin[35] which protects against anaemia, have been important elements of support for some cancer patients undergoing aggressive chemotherapy.[36] Antifungal therapies and improved antibiotic regimens, nutritional advice, and supplementation – sometimes with parenteral feeding[37] – are further examples of advances in the last two decades of cancer supportive care.[38,39]

Undoubtedly these forms of support are helpful and reassuring to the patients, who benefit from reduced morbidity and mortality from anticancer treatments. Their oncologists also naturally feel relieved that the interventions can be both less toxic and moreover, because anticancer treatments can be maximized, often more effective. But is supportive care more than this? I will argue that supportive care in the future can indeed be more comprehensive and inclusive, in terms of the benefits to patients and professionals, and also in terms of the diseases and the stages of disease that it covers.

First, supportive care need not be restricted to the end of life. Indeed, oncological supportive interventions were originally not deployed at the end, but rather in the earlier stages of disease, to allow patients to tolerate more aggressive curative treatments. Similar technologies and interventions can be useful in patients with more advanced cancer, and in some cases they can be transferred to other diseases. Supportive care interventions which are directed at symptom control may be palliative by virtue of using type 1 (preventive), type 2 (primary disease-directed), type 3 (distant effects-directed) or type 4 (symptom perception) palliation, as described above (Table 1.2). As such, they are therefore not confined to use only in early-stage disease. If we broaden our view of what constitutes a supportive care intervention, then the possibility of a truly humane, holistic, and respectful system of care becomes possible for patients at any stage of disease, with any serious illness.

Talking of supportive care rather than palliative care may also avoid the situation that has now arisen, in that the word 'palliative' which was introduced as a euphemism for terminal or hospice care has been 'found out' by patients, who are suspicious when it is mentioned. It is unlikely that 'supportive care', even if it were only used cynically as a new euphemism for 'palliative care', would ever in turn be regarded with the same suspicion for two reasons. First, the terms 'support' and 'supportive' are commonplace words with a real vernacular meaning, unlike 'palliative'. Second, if supportive care is deployed from the outset at the beginning of illness as well as at later stages, then the public (and healthcare professionals) should not categorize it as an end-of-life intervention.

How can supportive care be elevated to this new role? Klastersky, one of the pioneers of supportive care in oncology, believes that the process has already begun and that supportive care is a real entity in modern cancer services:

> Basic supportive care is part of any general practitioner's, and at least practising oncologist's, medical armamentarium . . . Supportive care consists of many subspecialties of the traditional medical and nursing care system and encompasses a broad and highly interesting variety of facets.'[40]

He feels that supportive care is a generic set of skills and knowledge, rather than being a distinct specialty, such as palliative medicine:

> Such a definition carries many practical difficulties because it brings under a 'common hat' many different subspecialties that differ considerably in approach, technique and healthcare personnel . . . A common – interdisciplinary and multiprofessional – forum is thus necessary to bridge these various aspects, all of which have one common aim: comprehensive supportive care in cancer.[40]

The driving force behind this concept lies in its emphasis on multidisciplinary team-working, which is fundamental to many branches of healthcare today. But this type of teamwork goes beyond the scope of the typical groupings which operate in cancer and respiratory medicine. Typically, multidisciplinary (or interdisciplinary, or multiprofessional) teams operating in cancer, rehabilitation, or similar services arrange to meet physically in a room on a regular – usually weekly – basis, to discuss patients and plan their investigations or care. In contrast, comprehensive supportive care invokes the concept of a **virtual team**, composed of collaborating professionals (and in some circumstances, volunteers) from different disciplines, and representatives from relevant discrete multidisciplinary teams, making complementary contributions at all stages of illness – without their all having to be present in the same room, building, or even healthcare sector. Thus, comprehensive supportive care is in reality delivered by a network of individuals, teams, and resources.

Implementing a comprehensive supportive care network

How can this idea be implemented? A model has been proposed which describes how supportive care fits in with other aspects of healthcare during a serious illness, and which also gives a legitimate place to palliative care in cancer and other diseases.[41] The 'Sheffield model' is composed of two components: an explanatory step and a logistical step. The former (Figure 1.3) first identifies and separates the elements of care into three streams: (1) those interventions which are directed at the disease process (e.g., COPD, cancer, HIV); (2) care directed towards helping the person who has that disease; (3) support for the family (or other significant carers) of the person who is experiencing the disease. The model uses the term 'therapy' for these elements, as they are more than just medical treatments – they should include holistic assessments

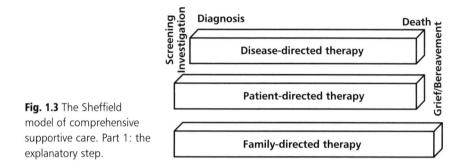

Fig. 1.3 The Sheffield model of comprehensive supportive care. Part 1: the explanatory step.

of the aims of interventions at each stage in the disease progression, and contributions for care can come from a variety of clinical or non-clinical sources.

Note that this model allows for the patient's and family's needs to be recognized and met even before a formal diagnosis is made, i.e. during the screening and investigation phases. This will be increasingly important in the future, as genetic screening programmes and other forms of early disease detection, e.g. by imaging or screening campaigns for biochemical markers, become more widely applied. Potential 'patients' in these programmes often have special fears and information needs, which can lead to anxiety and other consequences within the family. Moreover, many patients, especially if they are elderly, have co-morbidity with a variety of other longstanding or intercurrent illnesses or mental concerns, and these also need support and practical help. In the acute phases of investigation and diagnosis-making, it is easy for hard-pressed professionals to miss or disregard these concerns. If ignored, co-morbidity may become the reason for some patients to refuse or withdraw prematurely from potentially helpful or life-prolonging treatments. In their turn, family members also need support to ease their concerns and – if patients have to give up work or household duties – financial worries. Note also in Figure 1.3 that the family's support needs go on after the patient may die, as some family members (or close friends) could have abnormally disturbed grief reactions.

Note that the explanatory model illustrated in Figure 1.3 does not show a temporal relationship between the stream of disease-directed therapies, and the therapies aimed at supporting the patient and family. This is because supportive care needs may arise at any point in the disease trajectory: they certainly do not only surface when 'the disease is no longer curable'. Providing supportive care for patients' and families' needs at the earliest possible stage should be just as desirable as the current concentration on starting disease-directed therapies as early as possible. In cancer, an earlier start with anticancer treatments may mean the difference between cure or life-prolongation; in COPD, early education and lifestyle modifications may have a better impact on functioning and quality of life. Similarly, many supportive care therapies, whether they are directed at symptoms, psychological concerns, socio-economic difficulties, or existential fears, are probably more useful if they are started early.

The evidence for this statement is naturally lacking, as so far no formal trials have been conducted with comprehensive supportive care starting at the onset of a life-threatening disease. However, a potential example of this principle comes from our recent understanding of the mechanisms of chronic pain syndromes. Common to many of these long-term conditions (which can arise in cancer or AIDS, and after surgery or trauma) is the induction of 'plastic' changes which accompany chronic pain signal transmission in the dorsal horn of the spinal cord.[42] These changes are complex, but a significant element is mediated by the *N*-methyl-D-aspartate (NMDA) receptor channel, the opening of which induces cellular changes that in turn produce a lower threshold for subsequent pain perception.[43] This leads to the so-called 'wind-up' phenomenon, which can be elegantly demonstrated in laboratory studies. NMDA activation also leads to the development of tolerance to opioids, which can cause problems in chronic pain management.

Although it is possible to block the NMDA channel with agents such as ketamine, the results are not uniformly successful. It makes sense theoretically to prevent or attenuate NMDA activation at the onset of the chronic painful stimulus. Thus, so-called **preemptive analgesia** is designed to prevent or reduce the activation of NMDA receptor. This approach has been shown to reduce postoperative pain in animal models and some human studies.[44–46] Referring to the taxonomy of palliation proposed above (Table 1.2), preemptive analgesia falls into the type 1 (preventive) category. Although there is less evidence of preemptive or preventive control for other symptoms, it seems logical to assume that many interventions may best be applied at the earliest opportunity.

It is not necessary to invoke cellular mechanisms of chronic symptom perpetuation to justify earlier intervention: prevention of psychological distress and conditioning could also be a legitimate target. Thus, at the psychosocial level, Vachon[47] has argued that earlier psychological intervention with cancer patients and their relatives may help to prevent or mitigate later family stresses, which include depression, anger, and conflict between patients and family members.[48] With COPD, it has been shown that physical restrictions induced by dyspnoea and reduced exercise tolerance induce a vicious circle of reducing physical and social functioning, which then lead to physical muscle deconditioning that aggravates the dyspnoea[32] (see also Chapter 6). The logical response to this finding is educational and motivational exercise training programmes for COPD patients, offering type I palliation of dyspnoea.

The second part of the Sheffield model aims to clarify the logistics of delivering care to the patient and family. It does this by aggregating the three elements of care from the explanatory step (Figure 1.3) into an integrated clinical and organizational scenario, represented in Figure 1.4. The author acknowledges that this diagram is based on the highly influential WHO resource model for organizing cancer services, which has been discussed above (Figure 1.2). However, a major problem with the WHO diagram was that in practice the resource model became easily seen as a clinical guideline, suggesting that 'curative' therapies should be tried, and seen to fail, before palliative care could be introduced. This has led to the common situation of patients with cancer

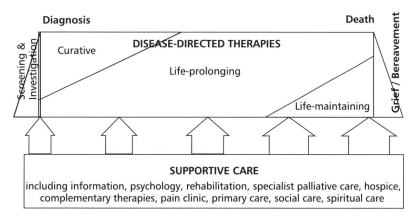

Fig. 1.4 The Sheffield model of comprehensive supportive care. Part 2: the logistical step.

being initially cared for mostly by surgeons and oncologists, who rightly offer and try disease-directed therapies. Often in this phase the presenting symptoms and psychological needs of the patient are overlooked, or managed ineffectively by clinicians who are not trained in palliation and who have rudimentary communication skills. (Primary care teams, which may have both to offer, are frequently unable to help the patient because the focus of care is at the hospital, and they may receive little information about the patient's status.) Co-morbidity issues and family needs are also frequently overlooked. On the day when the patient attends the clinic and is told that the disease has 'failed to respond (or has progressed/recurred)' and that 'there is nothing more that the oncologist can do', they receive two severe psychological blows. They are devastated first by the news itself, and secondly by being recommended to be looked after by another service – the primary care team or the local palliative care team (if indeed, one exists). Patients and families find this period of sudden transition very traumatic, and many of them turn down the offer of palliative care at this time because of this shock and because of the previously mentioned fears that palliative care is synonymous with terminal care.

The Sheffield model handles this area somewhat differently. Whereas the WHO approach was designed to advise governments and oncologists on how to allocate resources in cancer control programmes, the Sheffield logistical model is primarily aimed at advising clinicians and local services planners on how to make the support of patients with chronic disease and their family carers as comprehensive, integrated and 'shock-free' as humanely possible. It encourages the involvement of some supportive services even during the screening and diagnostic stages. In genetic screening for certain cancers, for example, whole families may need information and reassurance. During lung cancer diagnostic work-up, presenting symptoms of cough, haemoptysis, pain, and dyspnoea have to be palliated. In lung cancer it is not unusual for a patient to die from metastatic disease even before a tissue diagnosis is confirmed. If the WHO model is applied too literally, that patient may not be offered palliative care. Should such patients be denied the benefits of good support, just because they do not possess the requisite clinical label?

The Sheffield logistical model (Figure 1.4) has two main sectors of healthcare – those which are directed at the primary disease process (disease-directed therapies) and those which are aimed at patient's and families' needs (supportive therapies). The upper block, which represents disease-directed therapies, looks superficially like the block of cancer therapies in the WHO resource allocation model, but there are three main differences.

◆ First and foremost, the Sheffield model has dissociated the patient- and family-directed needs and therapies from the management of the primary disease. Put another way, palliative care does not need to follow after curative treatments.

◆ Second, the disease-directed therapies now can be focused on any chronic life-threatening disease, not just cancer.

◆ Third, the sequence of treatments within the block of disease-directed therapies are more realistically (one could say more honestly) represented. 'Curative' therapies should of course be applied first. With many chronic inflammatory, degenerative, and also neoplastic diseases, this part of the sequence may be very limited. For them a larger part of the time may be spent with offering the patient 'life-prolonging' treatments. In small-cell cancer, these include chemotherapy which can usefully provide years of extra survival. In HIV/AIDS, modern combination antiviral therapies fall into this category. It is not helpful for clinicians to talk to the patient and family about this phase of treatment in terms of 'chances of cure'; rather, there should be honest discussion about how many extra years, months, or possibly weeks may be gained. Most patients would feel less disillusioned and cheated by their professional advisers if they were aware at the outset that the disease will not be cured – i.e. they will eventually succumb to the disease or its effects, regardless of how dramatically successful the initial treatment may be.

The final part of the sequence within disease-directed therapies is a relatively new concept, that of 'life-maintaining' therapies. By this is meant those interventions that are required to keep a patient alive and functioning to a level that is acceptable to them. The period of time that life may be maintained can vary from days to months. The interventions include regular blood transfusions in a patient with widespread malignancy and bone marrow replacement, as occurs in myeloma or advanced breast cancer. Other examples are assisted ventilation for patients with MND/ALS who have total respiratory muscle paralysis; or artificial hydration in a patient with malignant oesophageal obstruction and who would otherwise die within days of dehydration. Note that in these examples patients will inevitably die anyway, even with the life-maintaining therapies, from the systemic complications of advanced disease – the situation being discussed here is not analogous to long-term artificial ventilation and total nutrition in a patient with coma after head injury. Life-maintaining therapies are respectful and humane if they reflect the wishes of the patient (and ideally also the family, although there are often conflicts at this stage of illness). They are disrespectful and become unethical if they are imposed by medical teams to keep a patient living who would otherwise die, and who has not sought longer survival.

Who could benefit from comprehensive supportive care?

Clearly not all supportive interventions are necessary for patients or family members at each stage of the disease. Early in a serious illness, information and psychological counselling may be more important than symptom control. Before there is a confirmed histological diagnosis, symptom palliation will be predominantly of types 3 and 4, i.e. modifying the distant effects of a disease or relieving the subjective distress arising from it, without tackling the primary cause. Once the diagnosis is made, it is important that alongside initial disease-directed therapies aimed at cure or prolonging life, patients are honestly and realistically informed about the goals of treatment. Their symptoms, co-morbidity, and treatment-related toxicities can then be managed using all of the appropriate types of palliation. As discussed above, this is the phase when 'traditional' oncology-based supportive care, using antiemetics, antimicrobials, and latterly growth factors, have become a routine part of cancer management using chemotherapy. Currently, however, patients are not routinely offered the broader elements of the Sheffield model of supportive care which are directed to the patient's and family's well-being.

If the patient does fail to respond to disease-directed therapy, then the responsibility of care should pass gradually – rather than as at present, suddenly on the day of 'bad news' – to the supportive care virtual team. In some centres, this will involve the patient being discharged to the coordinating umbrella of the primary care team, which will in turn negotiate and obtain specialist help from palliative medicine and nursing, and other relevant services such as dietetics, physiotherapy, social work, and perhaps clergyman, depending on the patient's and family's needs. In order to do this effectively, primary care teams need education and training. It has been suggested by some general practitioners that specialist palliative care teams can 'de-skill' the primary care team by developing a separate knowledge base.[28] This could happen if specialist teams operated exclusively in a different healthcare sector without sharing patients' care. In some cases, the specialist palliative care team may for a variable period have to 'take over' the care of a difficult problem, and occasionally the patient may never return to the primary care team if the problem warrants long-term admission. On the other hand, in many cases staff within primary care teams have never had the requisite skills for giving 'specialized' palliative care. Patients have a right to access specialists either in the community or in centres such as hospices or hospital-based teams, who can then make a trained assessment, initiate appropriate treatment and refer back to the general practitioner or family doctor and community nursing services for continuity.

It must be stressed that it is not only palliative care services which have expertise in the broader interdisciplinary network of supportive care. Some patients may benefit more from the attention of an occupational therapist, dietitian, or art therapist than from any medical or nursing professional. In many places, these professionals will not be found in the local palliative care service. Information resources are becoming more widely available, both through an actual presence in hospitals and hospices, but also via booklets and telephone advice from national help lines, and increasingly, via the internet. Cancer has been well served in this respect: for example, in the UK, the major information resources for cancer include CancerBACUP, CancerLink, and Macmillan Cancer Relief. However, non-cancer patients are also now being served by support groups and national organizations such as the British Lung Foundation, which offers the 'Breathe Easy' programme for patients with COPD and other chronic non-malignant chest diseases. Just as oncologists have come to realize and accept that palliative care can have a positive contribution for their patients, so must palliative care professionals open up their minds to the possibility that, for certain patients with specific needs, other disciplines may have an even more important role than they do.

The UK government has initiated a major review of cancer services, in the form of a 'national service framework', in which it is envisaged that supportive care will be offered by right to cancer patients and their families throughout the disease. (It has also recently published service guidelines for supportive and palliative care.[49] However the guidance is only for cancer patients and it does not cover specific clinical interventions. It has also not clarified what the boundaries are between supportive and palliative care. The Sheffield model aims to fill this vacuum by providing a working structure for this implementation.) The UK government is also announcing other national service frameworks to cover heart failure, care of elderly people, and other chronically ill groups. The pressure will be increasing on specialist palliative care to broaden its base to assist in these other disease areas, and also to share its knowledge and skills with clinicians in those disciplines. Specialist palliative care attempts to respond to non-malignant disease suffering, but in practice after three decades 95% of its users in the UK still have cancer.[50] In 2001–2002 only 9% of the 5% of non-cancer patients in UK palliative care services had a respiratory diagnosis. In the new government perspective, will these services readily move away from this concentration on the end-of-life care in cancer? It is unclear how large the non-cancer workload could eventually be for palliative care services. One estimate of the possible impact of opening specialist palliative care to non-cancer terminal illnesses has suggested that an increase in resources of around 79% will be necessary.[51] It is therefore likely that education and skills training programmes for the relevant specialties will be very important in this work, perhaps even more so than the physical expansion of existing palliative care teams. Existing palliative care teams could be a major source of expertise for this educational programme. They may also act as consultants for difficult cases. An important contribution that academic palliative care could make to this process is broadening research programmes in non-cancer diseases to include studies of palliation and support, as well as their current emphasis on better diagnosis and genomically driven 'curative' therapies.

What is a supportive care network composed of?

We have seen that the modern supportive care 'virtual team' operates as a network of different individuals, teams and resources. What are the actual constituents of this network? Table 1.4 shows one concept of how existing services can be configured to form the network. In this diagram, there are three groups of professionals (and in some sectors, volunteers) operating. Group A is recognizable as having the typical composition of a specialist palliative care service, at least within the UK and other developed countries. The key members of this group are: physicians (preferably trained to a postgraduate level in this subject), nurses (also with post-basic training), social workers, chaplains or religious advisers, and physiotherapists. In many services volunteers assist these professionals, e.g. in providing diversional and social activities in hospices and at day centres. Within these settings, and increasingly in hospitals, staff in group A physically meet on a regular basis to discuss individual patients and overall strategy.

Group A could be regarded as a core element of supportive care, at least where palliative care services are well established. It has already been acknowledged that these staff are most familiar with caring for cancer patients and their families towards the end of life. They are frequently supplemented by a second group which is composed of professionals who are usually based in other departments and who do not have specific palliative care training. This group B includes psychologists, dietitians, occupational therapists, speech and language therapists, pharmacists, and complementary therapists. Many of these will be known as the core elements of a rehabilitation programme. A newly emerging discipline within this group is the creative arts therapists, who may bring painting, other practical arts, writing, or music into the clinical setting.[52,53] (In many UK palliative care services, especially the independent hospices, arts therapy and complementary therapies are provided, but they cannot be regarded as 'essential' to group A.)

A third group of disciplines shown in Table 1.4 consists of teams from other settings which have an impact on the patient's and family's care. Of course, for cancer patients these would include the oncology team. For chronic respiratory disease patients, the pulmonary service is included in group C. The key point is that group C services are included not for their investigative and 'disease-directed' activities, but for their supportive care interventions. Thus, these services may include nurses who specialize in respiratory care; or psychologists, dietitians, and

Table 1.4 Composition of comprehensive supportive care network

Group	Professionals	Health or social care sector
A	Palliative care physicians and nurses; social workers; chaplains/priests; physiotherapists; volunteers	Hospice; day care; hospital-based team; community-based team
B	Psychologists; dieticians; occupational therapists; speech and language therapists; pharmacists; complementary therapists; art therapists; volunteers	Hospital services; community services; some hospices; free-standing agencies; private services
C	Respiratory department; oncology service; pain clinic; breathlessness clinic; lymphoedema service; primary care team; information resource	Hospital services; community; some hospices; telephone or internet-based resource

physiotherapists of their own. Moreover, individual physicians working in group C services may also be interested and have received training in aspects of specialist palliation and psychological support. During the times when the patient is receiving active input from the oncology or respiratory unit, these staff may be the main source of supportive care. A useful function of an oncology unit or respiratory unit is to be the hub of coordination where members of group A or group B can telephone for liaison or physically attend meetings to discuss shared patients.

Other group C elements include hospital-based pain clinics, which may provide both ward and outpatient (ambulatory) support for chronic pain management. Often their main workload consists of chronic non-malignant pain, but they work closely with palliative care teams to provide specialist advice and practical procedures for certain types of pain (see Chapter 29 for examples). Teams and clinics specializing in other symptoms are less common, but a recent development has been the hospital-based breathlessness clinics.[54] These were initially entirely staffed by nurses, which seems contradictory to the current trend towards multidisciplinary team-working. As their skills mature and other practitioners recognize their value, which has been demonstrated in at least one randomized clinical trial,[55] one hopes that they will become multiprofessional resources like pain clinics and will offer help to patients other than cancer. (For a fuller description of what such a service offers, see Chapter 13.) A third example of a specialist supportive care service which has already made significant impact in non-malignant disease is the lymphoedema clinic which some palliative care services offer for patients with breast, pelvic, or genital cancers that cause limb swelling. The specialized clinics are increasingly supporting patients with chronic 'benign' lymphoedema – often still within a palliative care setting.[56]

It is relevant to include the primary care team in group C, as it operates away from either the acute hospital setting of the disease-directed therapies and from the specialist palliative care service. Many general practitioners and community nurses have undergone postgraduate training in aspects of palliation, and can provide the bulk of symptom control and psychological support for their patients. Until now, however, the training has been very much modelled on palliative care, i.e. cancer-focused, programmes. In the future, resources such as information centres which guide patients towards better understanding of their predicament and help them make more informed choices, will increasingly figure within group C supportive care. Some of these resources are simply racks of leaflets in a clinic, whereas others are fully established as staffed information points in hospital departments. Increasingly, patients are turning to the internet for information and guidance and specific resources are being set up: the monitoring of their quality is vital for patients' choices to be rational.[57] Examples of websites which have been designed for patients and carers to access directly are given at the end of the chapter.[58]

Table 1.5 demonstrates the crucial times in the illness process, from screening to possible death, where different elements of the new supportive care virtual teams or networks could have an input. Although this table has been based on the author's experience primarily with cancer, it should be possible for other specialties to adapt this skeleton of a supportive care framework. Thus Table 1.5 attempts to show how staff from all three supportive care groups could also be involved in the stages of diagnosis and progress of COPD and of MND/ALS. For the future of respiratory supportive care, it will be important for experts from within respiratory medicine itself and supportive care professionals within groups A and B to develop these strategies together.

A delicate question is often raised concerning the 'leadership' of the team. This is even more problematic for a virtual team or network than it is for a physical hospital or hospice team that meets regularly. In the early stages of a chronic disease, it is reasonable for group C services to

Table 1.5 Opportunities for supportive care interventions

	Cancer	COPD	MND/ALS
Screening and investigation	C, B	C	C, B
Breaking bad news	C, B	C, B	C, B
Initial disease-directed treatment	C, B	C, B	N/A
Recurrence	C, B, A	N/A	N/A
Progression	A, B, C	C, B, A	B, A, C
Terminal care	A, B, C	C, B, A	A, C, B
Bereavement support	A, C	C	A, C
Information at all stages	C, B, A + internet	C, B + internet	A, C + internet

The resources for offering patients and families supportive at each stage in the three diseases are summarized using the taxonomy of health and social care sectors presented in Table 1.4. The order in which they are presented here is in decreasing likelihood of the sector being relevant for each need.

A, typical palliative care team; hospice; B, other supportive care services; C, hospital-based specialties; pain clinic; information resources; primary care; N/A, not applicable.

take the lead and coordinate other services as needed. With advanced disease, in countries where palliative care is recognized and well resourced, it is customary for the specialist palliative care teams of group A to form the nucleus and hub of the network. One problem with this is that even in the UK, where hospice units have flourished for 30 years, there is still great variation between different services, often in the same city or region. A survey of the facilities and interventions offered by UK palliative care services showed that they are far from homogeneous in terms of their staffing structures and what they can offer patients and families.[59] In general, some European countries, Canada, Australia, and New Zealand will be more likely to have sufficient numbers of well-structured palliative care services for them to take a leadership role in the individual clinical scenarios, and at a national planning level for cancer care. In non malignant disease services, it is quite reasonable – and probably desirable – for teams operating outside palliative care structures to take the leading role for individual patients. For example, physiotherapy and nursing teams, ideally operating from a pulmonary disease service, may be the lead agencies for COPD or MND/ALS.

Towards the end of life, for some patients the key input will come again from the acute hospital-based services or from the primary care teams within group C. Within the field of cancer, oncologists in developed countries have learnt to be accommodating so that patients gradually move their own view of leadership from themselves to the palliative care team. Once there has been greater collaboration between pulmonary services and other supportive care professionals, the same could follow for chronic respiratory disease.

It is crucial, as discussed above, that patients are not 'handed over' suddenly and without warning from the primary hospital unit to the local palliative care unit, or back to the primary care team, on the day that the news of failure to respond to curative therapy, or of recurrence, has been broken. This is likely to happen with cancer patients, because of how recurrence or progression is diagnosed. It should theoretically be less likely to occur with chronic lung disease, as the decision to move over to a palliative care programme could be discussed over several admissions for acute respiratory failure. However, the problem here is that respiratory units do not have the years of experience of working alongside group A or B services. On the other hand, with MND/ALS, at least in the UK, there has been longstanding collaboration between group C and palliative care services, so that as the patient progresses, respite admissions to a hospice may be seen as routine intervention, and final admission for terminal care could be at the hospice or respiratory unit. (See Chapters 18 and 19 for discussions of management of neuromuscular disorders.)

Relationship between supportive care and palliative care

It may be helpful at this point to emphasize the differences and overlaps between traditional palliative care and the new model of supportive care. In essence, the Sheffield model attempts to provide a comprehensive framework, so that palliative care (and its subspecialist field of hospice care) should be seen as components of supportive care. In some diseases such as lung cancer, and for individual patients, palliative care, could be the most important element of supportive care. For other diseases such as COPD or HIV/AIDS, present-day palliative care may have little practical to offer. However, it may still help by sharing its knowledge base with clinicians attending to these diseases. The management of pain, for example, is essentially the same in cancer, COPD or MND/ALS, so long as logical means of palliation (of types 3 or 4) are employed according to their known or putative modes of action. The differences in approach arise in the implications for, say, respiratory depression if opioids are used in these three situations. The use of cytotoxic chemotherapy is obviously one example of a type 2 treatment which is relevant only for oncology. Ventilatory support is used in both COPD and MND/ALS, but is not useful in cancer. There are few other areas of symptom control – and probably even fewer in psychological, social, or spiritual support – which are unique to a disease.

Several possible problems may arise if palliative care philosophy is to dominate in the setting up of comprehensive supportive care networks. First, they may bring their 'traditional' models and ways of working, which have been largely tested and refined in hospices, into situations where such methods are inappropriate or even unhelpful. An example was the early response of the hospice movement to incorporate HIV/AIDS patients: often these patients were much younger, and from a different social background from the usual older hospice cancer patients, and this model was rejected and gradually superseded by separate units being established for AIDS.[60] Because COPD and some other chronic lung disease patients are demographically more similar to cancer patients (especially lung cancer), perhaps this particular problem may be less acute with these illnesses. Indeed, more palliative care units in the UK are reporting that they admit COPD as well as heart failure patients, and although no series have been published, it appears that this approach could be feasible.

However, another problem arises, which is that cancer-based palliative care services are equipped to deal with patients whose prognosis is relatively short and fairly certain. A frequently voiced concern in palliative care circles is how they can then cope with diagnostic groups in which there is far greater uncertainty. Respiratory physicians could also feel ambiguous about referring patients to hospice-based care, where facilities for radiography and even pulse oximetry are limited or absent. These physicians and also the patients could understandably feel nervous about palliative care policies which might deny patients intravenous antibiotics and other interventions which can be useful to maintain life, and even for symptom control. Patients being admitted to most palliative care units are currently not offered the choice of cardiopulmonary resuscitation (CPR) in the event of a respiratory or cardiac arrest.[61,62] Many have argued that CPR is futile for patients with advanced terminal disease, but could hospices, which may in future take patients at an earlier stage, have the skills to determine whether resuscitation or other forms of life support (e.g. temporary assisted ventilation) could be appropriate?[63,64] It is clear that if palliative care services are to incorporate more patients with non-malignant illnesses such as COPD or interstitial lung diseases, then there would have to be a large educational programme for staff in those units, ideally led from acute respiratory care services.

A perceived 'risk' to patients is the cancer-oriented palliative care teams' attitudes to the use of opioids in symptom control, which could be seen by untrained respiratory or cardiological specialists as being 'too casual'. There generally are no doubts about the benefits of morphine or its newer substitutes for pain control in cancer patients. As discussed by Davis in Chapter 9, there is convincing evidence for opioids in the relief of dyspnoea, in both cancer and COPD. However, in reality many patients with advanced non-malignant diseases who are very distressed by breathlessness are denied the benefits of opioids by respiratory physicians, neurologists, and general practitioners. The problem here is actually a tension between the knowledge base and expertise of palliative care, and the doubts over opioids of other clinicians. The usual reasons expressed for the latter are fear of respiratory depression (which need not happen if the opioid is titrated upwards gently); fear of addiction in patients with a relatively uncertain prognosis (although physical dependence may occur temporarily when opioids are withdrawn, antisocial addictive behaviour is hardly ever seen in palliative care); and general reluctance to use the newer opioids if the physician is not familiar with them.[65] All of these reasons should be an indication for seeking advice from palliative care physicians, and not to deny the potential benefits to chronic lung disease patients. The point about including them here as potential 'problems' of instilling a palliative care culture within supportive care is that they represent more of an educational challenge than a true organizational one.

Supportive care needs at earlier stages of illness

If comprehensive supportive care is meant to be more than a new euphemism for palliative care, then what elements of it are distinctive? It is difficult to be precise about this, because both supportive care and palliative care are implemented so variably in different places. However, a good example of what supportive care can offer, beyond the normal scope of palliative care services, lies in the support that is needed by patients and families in the earlier stages of disease. As the diagram of the Sheffield logistical model (Figure 1.4) shows, such elements include information services and rehabilitation.

Considerable research has been conducted in recent years on the information needs of patients with serious life-threatening illnesses, particular cancer.[66,67] It is acknowledged that patients and families need information as early as possible in the illness, and many specialized services for cancer, HIV, and conditions such as MND/ALS have developed written, audio, video, and latterly internet-based information packs. The informational needs of patients with cancer change during the first weeks and months of illness: they shift from a desire for information about the disease process and its causes, to information about support services.[68,69] It should be remembered that the need for information can start even before the illness is formally 'diagnosed', e.g. during the work-up for cancer or interstitial or industrial lung disease.

In the UK, organizations such as Macmillan Cancer Relief and CancerLink produce not only their own information material but also directories of local services. Also in the UK, the charity CancerBACUP provides a telephone helpline with trained nurses who can answer patients' and relatives' questions, backed up by their own leaflets. The Breathe Easy charity provides a similar service for chronic lung disease. Many diseases such as MND/ALS also have dedicated charities that provide information and guidance for anxious and bewildered patients who have just been given the diagnosis. Similar organizations exist in other countries, and indeed international bodies such as the UICC promote cancer information as a major priority. It is tempting to ask why the clinical services which make the diagnoses and arrange primary treatments do not also provide this information. Indeed, some specific services have started to produce their own literature packs. However, the design and wording of such packs is critical and much locally produced material is often written in language that is too technical or unreadable for the average lay person.[70,71] In the future, internet-based information will be increasingly popular and clinicians should know of suitable websites to advise their patients to turn to. Ideally, patients should be able to access websites from the hospital department, hospice, or community health centre, with help at hand for those who are not familiar with this technology.[58]

Rehabilitation is now so well established in many services aimed at COPD and cancer patients following surgery that it may be regarded by those teams to be integral to their package of care. That is of course how supportive care should be seen, but rehabilitation is essentially person- and family-directed, rather than disease-directed. Seen this way, it does not need to be provided by the same service which is making the diagnosis and arranging disease-directed therapy. In Germany there is a very well-developed model of rehabilitation for cancer, which allows all patients to receive one or two weeks of funded rehabilitation in specialist rehabilitation centres (sometimes located in beautiful old spa towns). The packages of rehabilitation in such centres attend to physical, psychological, and social needs. In the UK, most cancer patients do not receive a formal programme of rehabilitation, even after curative but debilitating surgery for lung cancer. By contrast, many UK respiratory units are developing pulmonary rehabilitation programmes for COPD and other lung diseases, such as have been successfully established in the USA.

Another kind of supportive care which is relevant in earlier stages of illness is occupational therapy, which is included within a full rehabilitation programme, but can also be offered for other patients. Psychosexual counselling for people of all ages who have to adapt to genital surgery and other disfiguring neoplastic changes is a relatively rare facility, even within cancer services. They may also be helpful for patients with lung disease who are too breathless to have a normal sex life, or for patients with musculoskeletal disorders with partners who need help to adjust to paralysis. Referring other patients to social workers and financial benefits advisers can be helpful at the outset with a chronic disease, especially if the patient has to make complicated claims for industrial compensation. Palliative care services usually have access to these professionals, but it is unnecessary to refer a patient to palliative care just for this advice. Complementary therapies are another form of supportive care, to which patients are increasingly turning in addition to conventional disease-directed treatments from healthcare services (see Chapter 4). Clinical care providers need to know how to direct patients towards reputable and preferably validated therapies and local therapists, rather than leaving them to learn by trial and error. There needs to be a clear distinction between complementary therapies which are taken up by the patients alongside conventional care – sometimes provided in the same unit, and which may help them to complete disease-directed therapies – and alternative therapies, which in a disease like cancer can lead to patients opting out of potentially beneficial conventional treatments, often at great personal expense. In Britain many palliative care services, in particular hospices, themselves provide a range of complementary therapies ranging from acupuncture, hypnotherapy, and guided relaxation to aromatherapy and reflexology.[72–74] However, it could be a problem for patients at early stage of cancer disease to access these, if it means referral to palliative care.

End-of-life care

An exploration of the management of supportive and palliative care would be incomplete without a discussion of end-of-life care. This is often also called 'terminal care', although many patients and professionals feel uncomfortable with the harshness of the word 'terminal', at least in English. In UK palliative care circles, the expression 'terminal care' is indeed used, but it then refers to comfort measures which dominate in the last few hours, days, or possibly weeks of life. Because these phrases will continue to be used more or less idiosyncratically by different people in different countries, it is difficult to make rigid definitions. In terms of the Sheffield model of supportive care (Figure 1.4), it may be helpful to conceive of end-of-life care as beginning for a particular individual at the point when the aims of disease-directed therapy move from life-prolonging to life-maintaining; and of terminal care starting when the decision is made to withdraw even life-maintaining treatments. Unfortunately, these movements across phases are not always easy to distinguish, especially for a professional who is very close to the day-to-day decision-making for that individual. (The corollary of this is that it is all too easy to see, in retrospect, when the changing aims of management failed to keep step with the actual deterioration in the patient's condition.)

What is special about this phase of chronic disease management? One answer to this is that, for many, how a society takes care of its dying members is a good judge of its civilization. Another response is that dying is still seen as one of the greatest spiritual challenges for humanity, both in religious societies and in increasingly secular cultures. A third, pragmatic response is that there is only one chance to get it right with the dying – the dead do not complain! Finally, there is the pedagogic view that if we 'get it right' with one patient's end-of-life care, this may have an educational effect on other members of that patient's family, who may thus develop a more positive attitude to death and dying. The opposite of this is frequently seen when a bad experience in watching a loved one die in physical, psychological, and spiritual distress can heighten a relative's anxieties and mistrust of the medical profession.

There are numerous excellent textbooks and journals devoted to improving end-of-life care, so only a few points need to be made here, to add to the specific aspects of symptom control covered in other chapters in this volume.[75–79] These points will mainly relate to how supportive care needs to be different at the end of life, if indeed it needs to differ from other stages of disease management.

Physical symptom management

- The pharmacology of some drugs requires more careful monitoring of doses and their timing, e.g. if the patient is developing liver or renal failure.

- As patients become physically weaker and also slip into unconsciousness, the oral route for medication becomes less reliable or even impossible – in this situation, the common alternatives include transdermal, rectal, and parenteral routes.[80–83]

- With parenteral medication, subcutaneous injections are usually preferred by patients to intravenous or deep intramuscular injections, and many of the drugs used in the terminal stage are suitable for this route.[84,85]

- In the terminal stage, some patients may become distressed, severely and constantly, by refractory symptoms (pain, dyspnoea, and nausea amongst others). There is a growing literature on the use of planned and controlled 'palliative sedation' for the relief of this situation, which also distresses those watching and caring for the patient.[86–89] The drugs which can be used to achieve reversible sedation include benzodiazepines (especially rectal diazepam and parenteral midazolam); opioids; and neuroleptics (e.g. haloperidol or levomepromazine). It is important that the sedation is openly declared to have the goal of symptom palliation and for it not to be perceived as a half-hearted euthanasia (see discussion below).

Psychological aspects of management

- ◆ As patients deteriorate they frequently become cognitively impaired. Together with later lapses into unconsciousness, this mean that opportunities for discussing details of management with patients are reduced and so more reliance must be placed on communication with relatives or other carers.

- ◆ The implication of this is clearly that discussions are better held earlier, when patients are mentally clear and participating in decision-making, about their wishes for specific interventions. Increasingly in developed countries, older people and patients with life-threatening illnesses are being encouraged to prepare advance directives or 'living wills' in which their preferences for more or less active interventions at the end of life are explicitly stated.

- ◆ Experience has shown that patients' views about these interventions change as disease progresses, so they should be advised to review and update these directives, preferably in discussion with family carers.[90–93]

Social aspects of the patients' and families' lives

In developed countries it is normal for patients to try to retain social independence for as long as possible, but in some cultures it is accepted for dying people to play a 'sick role' and become dependent on family and healthcare staff. However, many individuals vary from these societal norms and it is important for the multidisciplinary care team to be as accommodating as possible to allow patients their dignity in performing as many activities of daily living as their condition permits.

Spiritual and cultural aspects of care

- ◆ Existential or spiritual fears may dominate some individuals, not only at the end of life but throughout a life-threatening illness. However, these may certainly become more acute in the terminal stage, especially if the patient becomes aware of impending death and has not had the chance to prepare themselves in advance. This is an argument for earlier and open discussion of existential doubts – not for the denial of prognosis to patients!

- ◆ In many cultures and for specific patients, the answer to existential doubts will be found in spiritual or religious doctrines. Such patients should be allowed full access to their religious advisers in the latter stages of disease, when being admitted to a hospital could prevent them from attending their own place of worship.

- ◆ Even for 'non-religious' people or those who have weaker faiths, there should be access to staff members who have special training in discussing existential issues.

- ◆ When a person is dying in hospital or in a hospice, attention must be paid to cultural imperatives with respect to the preparation of the body after death and means of disposal. This may mean that family members, rather than staff from other religions, should be allowed to take over these tasks.

Needs of the family and other carers

Caring for a patient who is approaching death imposes special difficulties for relatives and close friends. The supportive care teams should be aware of the needs of those who are involved with the care:

- There may be, apart from the expected 'anticipatory grieving' for any terminally ill person, a disproportionate fear of impending loss and future helplessness, especially for those who have been dependent on the dying person. Such individuals may need extra support from social workers and nurses to help them prepare for life alone, and for elderly people this may mean facing the possibility of receiving formal care themselves, perhaps by admission to a care institution.

- At the time of death and for some weeks or months afterwards, some individuals may need extra bereavement counselling. The supportive care team may possess such skills, or it may need to refer the relative to a psychological service, if the primary care team or community nursing services are unable to respond to this.

- Some carers may need financial advice and support from the state, especially if the patient had been the wage-earner and the illness had been relatively short. For this reason, it is advisable that all patients who have a life-threatening illness diagnosed should be assessed for future financial needs at an early stage, by a social worker or specialist nurse trained in social benefits.

Needs of healthcare professionals

Healthcare professionals themselves have special needs with respect to the care of patients approaching the end of life, which may not have been covered in the basic education or post-graduate training in their specialty. This is more likely to be a problem for medical staff in, say, oncology or respiratory medicine and surgery, than for specialist nurses or physicians in palliative medicine where these issues are part of the training. Some areas which cause most concern for staff, when dealing with terminally ill patients, include:

- Lack of confidence in communicating openly with dying people about prognosis and the changing aims of treatment. This is particularly likely to cause distress for patients or families who can see that the disease is progressing although the physician cannot or prefers not to acknowledge this.

- As a result of this, the physician may strive – beyond what is 'reasonable' – to prolong life with inappropriate disease-directed therapies, or to maintain it with artificial nutrition and hydration, blood transfusions and other supportive measures. Even if they acknowledge that the patient is deteriorating, physicians may still be so concerned with pursuing disease-directed investigations and therapy that person- and family-directed therapies are overlooked or overruled. In some cultures, where the decision of the attending physician is paramount and cannot be questioned, this may be socially condoned. Increasingly in developed countries this attitude is actively challenged, even by other professional team members. The adage that 'death should not be seen as a failure' is most helpful to those who can see the limitations of modern medicine, or who can recognize their own fallibility. Of course there will be times when death comes unexpectedly soon, or as a result of an adverse effect of a therapy, or because some potentially preventable complication was not anticipated – in these cases, the circumstances and timing of the death may indeed be seen as technically a 'failure' of medicine and its current resources. But it is pointless and harmful for the physician to see it as a personal failure or – unconsciously – to blame the patient or family, or even professional colleagues, for 'giving up'.

◆ Repeated exposure to witnessing deaths which are inexpertly managed, from the point of view of physical symptoms and psychological or spiritual distress, can lead to professionals themselves becoming worn down. In some cases, this can lead to 'burn-out', when the job is made into a routine and there is little personal engagement and no satisfaction.[92,93] The best prevention for this is to work in a supportive team – giving support to fellow professionals as well as patients. This can only work, however, if professionals admit to their fallibility and their need to share their distress at witnessing patients and families suffering.

◆ There are special dilemmas for staff who work in acute healthcare settings where diseases can be cured or at least where patients' lives may be substantially prolonged. Compared to this setting, working in a hospice where all patients have a uniformly terminal prognosis is relatively easy. One solution for this is for patients' progress to be monitored and discussed in a multidisciplinary team, so that it is easier to acknowledge when the chances of cure are receding and later, when it becomes clear that life can no longer be prolonged. Sometimes if the patient is very well known to the hospital unit over a long time, it may be difficult for the team members to confront the fact that the patient is deteriorating. Where there is a well-established and trusted palliative care service, it may be helpful to call in a member from this to see the patient and family separately. This colleague can then act as the patient's advocate, tactfully advising the respiratory or oncology team that the goal of therapy needs to be changed.

Assisted suicide and euthanasia

This chapter would be incomplete without reference to the growing worldwide debate on assisted suicide and euthanasia. The debate is relevant to supportive care in respiratory disease, because the chapters in this volume demonstrate that the potential for suffering and for premature death from pulmonary diseases is great. As these illnesses come to the terminal stage, is there a place for hastening death in a positive way to ease the patient out of extreme distress?

The traditional response of palliative care – and especially of the hospice movement – worldwide has been to totally reject these interventions on grounds of clinical need as well as morality.[96] It is often said that if palliative care were to be more widely available, then people would ask less for assistance with death.[97] Recently these views have been increasingly challenged. It is argued that some patients are still left in an unacceptable physical, psychological, and existential distress even after receiving the best that palliation can offer.[98] Others may live in countries where palliative care just cannot be offered. It is also argued that it is a fundamental human right to have control over one's death, as it is over most aspects of life.[99–101] The recent changes in legislation in the Netherlands and Belgium to decriminalize euthanasia, and the law in Oregon, USA which allows physicians to assist patients to commit suicide, are quoted as examples of an inexorable secular trend globally towards the acceptance of these views.

This has to be countered with the following arguments. First, it is the duty of healthcare systems constantly to find ways of preventing and curing disease, and if that is not possible, then to prolong and maintain life when it is humane to do so, and always to relieve distress. It has never been a recognized function of healthcare to hasten deaths, even if society wishes this facility. (The anecdotal assertion that 'in the past' kindly physicians used to help patients into death with doses of opium is an unsafe ground on which to base future explicit policy.) Recently, carefully conducted surveys have shown that many physicians, e.g. geriatricians who are in regular contact with frail and terminally ill people, feel on the whole uncomfortable with the notion that they may be called upon to assist in hastening death.[102–104]

Occasionally clinicians are faced with a terrible situation, e.g. massive haemoptysis. To give sedation in order to stop the patient's awareness of dying from this almost certain agonal event is quite reasonable, and if the patient dies in a few minutes or hours earlier than without such sedation, that is excusable in most legal systems in developed countries. In the UK this is referred to as the 'doctrine of double effect', in which it is legitimate for a physician to administer a medicine which could cause extreme harm (i.e. death), if the primary purpose of it was to alleviate terrible suffering.[105] However, it is a betrayal of this humane doctrine if physicians hide behind the uncertainty of the response to potent drugs in sick patients, in order deliberately to shorten life – even if the patient requests it.

Ultimately, the response to extreme suffering is not a medical issue, but one in which societies have to make general statements, and specific judgements in particular cases. It is not necessary, or advisable, for healthcare workers with access to potent drugs to take it on themselves to step beyond the law of their country. There cannot be a 'final' solution to this debate, as long as different societies and cultures hold life to be more or less 'sacred' to different degrees. For the purposes of supportive care for patients with respiratory diseases and their families, it should again be emphasized once again that the goal should be to establish a network of professionals from various disciplines, each contributing to relieving suffering as far as is humanly possible and then staying quietly with the patient and family. That will always be preferable to the spectre of the lone doctor or nurse, standing by the bed of a sick patient and making unilateral decisions that involve the taking of a life.

Keypoints

♦ The modern approach to medicine now holistically embraces the subjective needs of patients and their carers

♦ Palliation of symptoms should be considered analytically, and treatment applied using modern scientific principles

♦ Hospices and the modern palliative care movement have made major progress in the care of dying people

♦ Supportive care has to be seen as a comprehensive multidisciplinary approach for patients throughout the course of an illness.

References

1 Clark, D., and Seymour, J. Policy development and palliative care. Chapter 7 in: D. Clark, and J. Seymour (eds) *Reflections on palliative care*. Buckingham: Open University Press, 1999; 131–150.

2 MacDonald, N. The interface between oncology and palliative medicine. Chapter 2.1 in: D. Doyle, G.W.C. Hanks, and N. Macdonald (eds) *Oxford textbook of palliative medicine*. Oxford: Oxford University Press, 1998; 11–17.

3 Moinpour, C.M., Feigl, P., Metch, B., *et al*. Quality of life endpoints in cancer clinical trials: review and recommendations. *J Natl Cancer Inst* 1989; **81**(7): 485–95.

4 Ahmedzai, S. Palliative care in oncology: making quality the endpoint. *Ann Oncol* 1990; **1**: 396–8.

5 MacDonald, N. A proposed matrix for organisational changes to improve quality of life in oncology. *Eur J Cancer* 1995; **31A**(Suppl 6): S18–21.

6 Coleman, R.E. Uses and abuses of bisphosphonates. *Ann Oncol* 2000; **11** (Suppl 3): 179–84.

7 Krajnik, M., Zylicz, Z., Finlay, I., Luczak, J., and van Sorge, A.A. Potential uses of topical opioids in palliative care – report of 6 cases. *Pain* 1999; **80**: 121–5.

8 Christensen, O., Christensen, P., Sonnenschein, C., Nielsen, P.R., and Jacobsen, S. Analgesic effect of intraarticular morphine. A controlled, randomised and double-blind study. *Acta Anaesthesiol Scand* 1996; **40**: 842–6.

9 Inouye, S.K., *et al.* A multicomponent intervention to prevent delirium in hospitalized older patients. *N Engl J Med* 1999; **340**(9): 669–76.

10 Hopwood, P., and Stephens, R.J. on behalf of the MRC Lung Cancer Working Party. Symptoms at presentation for treatment in patients with lung cancer: implications for the evaluation of palliative treatment. *Br J Cancer* 1995; **71**: 633–6.

11 Donnelly, S., and Walsh, D. The symptoms of advanced cancer: identification of clinical and research priorities by assessment of prevalence and severity. *J Palliat Care* 1995; **11**(1): 27–32.

12 Keogh, E., and Herdenfeldt, M. Gender, coping and the perception of pain. *Pain* 2002; **97**(3): 195–201.

13 Zacny, J.P. Morphine responses in humans: a retrospective analysis of sex differences. *Drug Alcohol Depend* 2001; **63**: 23–8.

14 Hyland, M.E. A reformulation of Quality of Life for medical science. *QoL Res* 1992; **1**: 267–72.

15 Ingham, J., and Portenoy, R.K. The measurement of pain and other symptoms. Chapter 6 in: D. Doyle, G.W.C. Hanks, and N. MacDonald (eds) *Oxford textbook of palliative medicine*, 2nd edn. Oxford : Oxford Medical Publications, 1998; 203–19.

16 Clark, D., and Seymour, J. History and development. Chapter 4 in: D. Clark, and J. Seymour, *Reflections on palliative care*. Buckingham: Open University Press, 1999; 65–78.

17 Clark, D., and Seymour, J. Routinization and medicalization, Chapter 6 in: D. Clark, and J. Seymour, *Reflections on palliative care*. Buckingham: Open University Press, 1999; 151–72.

18 Giddens, A. *Modernity and self-identity: self and society in the late modern age.* Cambridge: Polity Press, 1991.

19 Seale, C. Demographic change and the care of the dying: 1969–1987. In: D. Dickenson, and M. Johnson (eds) *Death, dying and bereavement.* London: Sage Publications, 1993; 45–54.

20 Hinton, J. Which patients with terminal cancer are admitted from home care? *Palliat Med* 1994; **8**: 197–210.

21 Rajagopal, M.R., and Suresh, K. Global exchange. A model for delivery of palliative care in India – The Calicut experiment. *J Palliat Care* 1999; **15**(1): 44–9.

22 The Poznan Declaration (1998). *Eur J Palliat Care* 1999; **6**(2): 61–3.

23 WHO. *Cancer pain relief and palliative care: report of a WHO expert committee.* Technical Report Series No. 804. WHO, Geneva; 1990.

24 Heaven, C.M., and Maguire, P. Disclosure of concerns by hospice patients and their identification by nurses. *Palliat Med* 1997; **11**(4): 283–90.

25 Ahmedzai, S., and Brooks, D. Transdermal fentanyl versus sustained-release oral morphine in cancer pain: preference, efficacy, and quality of life. *J Pain Symptom Manage* 1997; **13**(5): 254–61.

26 Cohen, R.S., Boston, P., Mount, B.M., and Porterfield, P. Changes in quality of life following admission to palliative care units. *Palliat Med* 2001; **15**: 363–71.

27 Ahmedzai, S. H., Costa, A., Blengini, C., Bosch, A., *et al.* A New international framework for palliative care. *Eur J Cancer* 2004; **40**: 2192–200.

28 Fordham, S., Dowrick, C., and May, C. Palliative medicine: is it really specialist territory? *J Roy Soc Med* 1998; **91**: 568–72.

29 Bennett, M.I., Alison, D.L., O'Neill, W.M., and McIllmurray, M. Questions of training – choice or force? *Palliat Med* 1996; **10**(1): 43–7.

30 MacDonald, N. The interface between oncology and palliative medicine. Chapter 2.1 in: D. Doyle, G.W.C. Hanks, and N. MacDonald (eds) *Oxford textbook of palliative medicine*, 2nd edn. Oxford: Oxford University Press, 1999; 11–17.

31 MacDonald, N. Oncology and palliative care: the case for co-ordination. *Cancer Treat Rev* 1993; **19**(Suppl A): 29–41.

32 Skilbeck, J., Mott, L., and Page, H., *et al.* Palliative care in chronic obstructive airways disease: a needs assessment. *Palliat Med* 1998; **12**: 245–54.

33 Gibbs, L.M.E., Addington-Hall, J., and Gibbs, J.S.R. Dying from heart failure: lessons from palliative care: Many patients would benefit from palliative care at the end of their lives (editorial). *BMJ* 1998; **317**: 961–2.

34 Gralla, R.J. Antiemetic therapy. *Semin Oncol* 1998; **25**(5): 577–83.

35 Littlewood, T.J., Bajetta, E., Nortier, J.W.R., *et al.* Effects of epoetin alfa on hematologic parameters and quality of life in cancer patients receiving nonplatinum chemotherapy: results of a randomized, double-blind, placebo-controlled trial. *J Clin Oncol* 2001; **19**(11): 2865–74.

36 Berghmans, T., *et al.* Therapeutic use of granulocyte and granulocyte-macrophage colony-stimulating factors in febrile neutropenic cancer patients. A systematic review of the literature with meta-analysis. *Support Care Cancer* 2002; **10**: 181–8.

37 Body, J.J. The syndrome of anorexia-cachexia. *Curr Opin Oncol* 1999; **11**: 255–60.

38 Klastersky, J. Therapy of infections in cancer patients. Chapter 1 in: J. Klastersky, S.C. Schimpff, and H.J. Senn (eds) *Supportive care in cancer. a handbook for oncologists*, 2nd edn. New York: Marcel Dekker, 1999; 1–47.

39 De Pauw, B.E. Fungal infections. In: J. Klastersky, S.C. Schimpff, and H.J. Senn (eds) *Supportive care in cancer. a handbook for oncologists*, 2nd edn. New York: Marcel Dekker, 1999; 49–85.

40 Klastersky, J. Supportive care in cancer. *Curr Opin Oncol* 1997; **9**: 313.

41 Ahmedzai, S.H., and Walsh, D. Palliative medicine and modern cancer care. *Semin Oncol* 2000; **27**(1): 1–6.

42 Willis, W.D., Jr. Central plastic responses to pain. In: G.F. Gebhart, D.L. Hammond, and T.S. Jenson (eds) *Proceedings of the 7th World Congress on Pain. Progress in Pain Research and Management*, Vol. 2. Seattle: IASP Press, 1994; 301–24.

43 Payne, R., and Gonzales, G.R. Pathophysiology of pain in cancer and other terminal diseases. In: D. Doyle, G.W.C. Hanks, and N. MacDonald, (eds) *Oxford textbook of palliative medicine*, 2nd edn. Oxford: Oxford University Press, 1998; 299–310.

44 Fisher, K., Coderre, T.J., and Hagen, N.A. Targeting the *N*-methyl-D-aspartate receptor for chronic pain management: preclinical animal studies, recent clinical experience and future research directions. *J Pain Symptom Manage* 2000; **20**(5): 358–73.

45 Burton, A.W., Lee, D.H., Saab, C., and Chung, J.M. Pre-emptive intrathecal ketamine injection produces a long-lasting decrease in neuropathic pain behaviours in a rat model. *Reg Anaesth Pain Med* 1999; **24**(3): 208–13.

46 DeKock, M., Lavand'homme, P., and Waterloos, H. 'Balanced analgesia' in the perioperative period: is there a place for ketamine? *Pain* 2001; **92**(3): 373–80.

47 Vachon, M.L.S. The emotional problems of the patient. Chapter 14.1 in: D. Doyle, G.W.C. Hanks, and N. MacDonald (eds) *Oxford textbook of palliative medicine*, 2nd edn. Oxford: Oxford University Press, 1999; 883–907.

48 Kissane, D.W., Bloch, S., Burns, W., McKenzies, D., and Posternino, M. Psychological morbidity in the families of patients with cancer. *Psycho-Oncology* 1994; **3**: 47–56.

49 National Institute for Clinical Excellance (NICE). *Improving supportive and palliative care for adults with cancer* NICE: London, 2004. Website: www.nice.org.uk

50 St Christopher's Hospice. Information. www.hospiceinformation.info

51 Field, D., and Addington-Hall, J. Extending specialist palliative care to all? *Soc Sci Med* 1999; **48**(9): 1271–80.

52 C. Malchiodi (ed.). *Medical art therapy with adults.* London: Jessica Kingsley Publishers, 1999.

53 Pratt, M., and Wood, M.J.M. (eds). *Art therapy in palliative care. The creative response.* London: Routledge, 1998.

54 Corner, J., Plant, H., A'Hern, R., and Bailey, C. Non-pharmacological intervention for breathlessness in lung cancer. *Comment Palliat Med* 1997; **11**(2): 170.

55 Bredin, M., Corner, J., Krishnasamy, M., *et al.* Multicentre randomised controlled trial of nursing intervention for breathlessness in patients with lung cancer. *BMJ* 1999; **318**(7188): 901–4.

56 Keeley, V. Oedema in advanced cancer. In: R. Twycross, K. Jenns, and J. Todd (eds) *Lymphoedema.* Abingdon: Radcliffe Medical Press, 2000; 338–58.

57 Ferguson, T. From patients to end users. Quality of online patient networks needs more attention than quality of online health information (editorial). *BMJ* 2002; **324**(9): 555–6.

58 CancerBacup website, www.CancerBACUP.org.uk; PIES. website, www.PIESforCancer.info; NIH website, www.nih.gov; Breathe Easy website, www.lunguk.org

59 Johnson, I.S., Rogers, C., Biswas, B., and Ahmedzai, S. What do hospices do? A survey of hospices in the United Kingdom and Republic of Ireland. *BMJ* 1990; **300**: 791–3.

60 Small, N. HIV/AIDS: Lessons for policy and practice. In: D. Clark (ed.) *The future for palliative care.* Buckingham: Open University Press, 1993; 80–97.

61 Joint Working Party between the National Council for Hospice and Specialist Palliative Care Services and the Ethics Committee of the Association of Palliative Medicine. *Ethical decision making in palliative care: cardiopulmonary resuscitation (CPR) for people who are terminally ill.* London: Association of Palliative Medicine, 2002.

62 Meystre, C.J.N., Burley, N.M.J., and Ahmedzai, S. What investigations and procedures do patients in hospices want? Interview based survey of patients and their nurses. *BMJ* 1997; **315**: 1202–3.

63 Alison, D.L. Resuscitation and non-resuscitation orders. Correspondence. *Palliat Med* 1994; **8**: 79.

64 Willard, C. Cardiopulmonary resuscitation for palliative care patients: a discussion of ethical issues. *Palliat Med* 2000; **14**: 308–12.

65 Paice, I., Toy, C., and Shott, S. Barriers to cancer pain relief: fear of tolerance and addiction. *J Pain Symptom Manage* 1998; **16**: 1–9.

66 Ahmedzai, S. The other information revolution (editorial). *Ann Oncol* 1997; **8**: 821–4.

67 Fallowfield, L., Ford, S., and Lewis, S. No news is not good news: information preferences of patients with cancer. *Psycho-Oncology* 1995; **4**: 197–202.

68 Butow, P.N., Maclean, M., Dunn, S.M., Tattersall, M.H., and Boyer, M.J. The dynamics of change: cancer patients' preferences for information, involvement and support. *Ann Oncol* 1997; **8**(9): 857–63.

69 Jenkins, V., Fallowfield, L., and Saul, J. Information needs of patients with cancer: results from a large study in UK cancer centres. *Br J Cancer* 2001; **84**(1): 48–51.

70 Payne, S., Large, S., Jarrett, N., and Turner, P. Written information given to patients and families by palliative care units: a national survey. *Lancet* 2000; **355**: 1792.

71 NHS IA information packs website: www.doh.gov.uk/research/rd3/ibnformation/infoindex.htm

72 Thompson, E.A., and Reilly, D. The homeopathic approach to symptom control in the cancer patient: a prospective observational study. *Palliat Med* 2002; **16**(3): 227–33.

73 Wilkinson, S., Aldridge, J., Salmon, I., Cain, E., and Wilson, B. An evaluation of aromatherapy massage in palliative care. *Palliat Med* 1999; **13**: 409–17.

74 Filshie, J., Penn, K., Ashley, S., and Davis, C.L. Acupuncture for the relief of cancer-related breathlessness. *Palliat Med* 1996; **10**: 145–50.

75 Doyle, D., Hanks, G.W.C. *Oxford textbook of palliative medicine*, 3rd edn. Oxford: Oxford University Press, 2004.

76 Twycross, R., and Wilcock, A. *Symptom management in advanced cancer*, 3rd edn. Abingdon: Radcliffe Medical Press, 2001.

77 Twycross, R. Wilcock, A., and Thorp, S. *PCF1 palliative care formulary*. Radcliffe Medical Press: Abingdon, 1999.

78 Faull, C., Carter, Y., and Woof, R. *Handbook of palliative care*. Oxford: Blackwell Science, 1998.

79 Woodruff, R. *Palliative medicine*, 2nd edn. Melbourne: Asperula, 1996.

80 Nugent, M., Davis, C., Brooks, D., and Ahmedzai, S.H. Long-term observations of patients receiving transdermal fentanyl after a randomized trial. *J Pain Symptom Manage* 2001; **21**(5): 385–91.

81 Davis, M.P., Walsh, D., LeGrand, S.B., and Naughton, M. Symptom control in cancer patients: the clinical pharmacology and therapeutic role of suppositories and rectal suspensions. *Supportive Care Cancer* 2002; **10**(2): 117–38.

82 Moolenaar, F., Meijlet, W.J., Frijlink, H.W., Visser, J., and Proost, J.H. Clinical efficacy, safety and pharmacokinetics of a newly developed controlled release morphine sulphate suppository in patients with cancer pain. *Eur J Clin Pharmacol* 2000; **56**(3): 219–23.

83 Davis, C. A new 24-hour morphine hydrogel suppository. *Eur J Palliat Care* 2000; **7**(5): 165–7.

84 Stuart-Harris, R., Joel, S.P., McDonald, P., Currow, D., and Slevin, M.L. The pharmacokinetics of morphine and morphine glucuronides metalbolites after subcutaneous bolus injection and subcutaneous infusion of morphine. *Br J Clin Pharmacol* 2000; **49**(3): 207–14.

85 Paul, G. Problems with opiates in cancer pain: parenteral opioids. Review article. *Supportive Care Cancer* 1997; **5**(6): 445–50.

86 Ventafridda, V., Ripamonti, C., De Conno, F., Tamburini, M., and Cassileth, B.R. Symptom prevalence and control during cancer patients' last days of life. Comment. *J Palliat Care* 1991; **7**(2): 50–1.

87 Stone, P., Phillips, C., Spruyt, O., and Waight, C. A comparison of the use of sedatives in a hospital support team and in a hospice. *Palliat Med* 1997; **11**: 140–4.

88 Fainsinger, R.L., *et al.* A multicentre international study of sedation for uncontrolled symptoms in terminally ill patients. *Palliat Med* 2000; **14**(4): 257–65.

89 Hardy, J. Sedation in terminally ill patients. *Lancet* 2000; **356**(9245): 1866–7.

90 Ahmedzai, S. Euthanasia, physician-assisted suicide and the living will. *CME* 1997; **15**(10): 1339–49.

91 Chochinov, H.M., Tataryn, D., Clinch, J.J., and Dudgeon, D. Will to live in the terminally ill. *Lancet* 1999; **354**(9181): 816–19.

92 Doig, J. Living wills: studying the Dutch experience. *Eur J Palliat Care* 1996; **3**(4): 164–6.

93 Waddell, C., Clarnette, R.M., Smith, M., and Oldham, L. Advance directives affecting medical treatment choices. *J Palliat Care* 1997; **13**(2): 5–8.

94 Vachon, M.L.S. The stress of professional caregivers. Chapter 14.3 in: D. Doyle, G.W.C. Hanks, N. MacDonald (eds) *Oxford textbook of palliative medicine*, 2nd edn. Oxford: Oxford University Press, 1999; 919–29.

95 Kissane, D.W., Bloch, S., Burns, W.I., McKenzies, D., and Posterino, M. Psychological morbidity in the families of patients with cancer. *Psycho-Oncology* 1994; **3**: 47–56.

96 Cherny, N.I., Coyle, N., and Foley, K.M. The treatment of suffering when patients request elective death. *J Palliat Care* 1994; **10**(2): 71–9.

97 Foley, K.M. Competent care for the dying instead of physician-assisted suicide. *New Engl J Med* 1997; **336**(1).

98 Wilson, K.G., *et al.* Attitudes of terminally ill patients toward euthanasia and physician assisted suicide. *Arch Intern Med* 2000; **160**(16): 2454–60.

99 Doyal, L., and Doyal, L. Why active euthanasia and physician assisted suicide should be legalised. If death is in a patient's best interest then death constitutes a moral good. *BMJ* 2001; **323**: 1079–80.

100 Farsides, C. Euthanasia: failure or autonomy? *Int J Palliat Nurs* 1996; **2**(2): 102–5.

101 Seale, C., and Addington-Hall, J. Euthanasia: the role of good care. *Soc Sci Med* 1995; **40**(5): 581–7.

102 Clark, D., Dickinson, G., Lancaster, C.J., *et al.* UK geriatricians' attitudes to active voluntary euthanasia and physician-assisted death. *Age Ageing* 2001; **30**: 395–8.

103 Waddell, C., Clarnette, R.M., Smith, M., Oldham, L., and Kellehear, A. Treatment decision-making at the end of life: a survey of Australian doctors' attitudes towards patients' wishes and euthanasia. *Med J Aust* 1996; **165**(18): 540–4.

104 Grassi, L., Magnani, K., and Ercolani, M. Attitudes toward euthanasia and physician-assisted suicide among Italian primary care physicians. *J Pain Symptom Manage* 1999; **17**(3): 188–96.

105 House of Lords Select Committee on Medical Ethics. Report. HL Paper 21–1. HMSO, London; 1994.

Chapter 2

Anatomy and physiology

Martin F. Muers

This account of the anatomy and physiology of the respiratory system is intended to be an aide-memoir for the reader who wishes to be reminded of the normal state before considering a particular symptom or condition. It is not intended to be comprehensive, and readers who wish to have more complete accounts should consult the works listed under Further Reading. Descriptions refer principally to the adult lung. The basic features apply to children, but the dimensions and normal values are different. More detailed accounts of the mechanisms of some common respiratory symptoms, e.g. cough, are given in the relevant chapters elsewhere in this book.

Ribcage, respiratory muscles, and respiratory 'pump'

The basic arrangements for the 12 vertebrae and ribs, the manubrium and sternum, which together comprise the ribcage, are best appreciated by looking at the accompanying diagram and chest radiographs (Figures 2.1–2.3). Movement of the ribs and diaphragm together cause an increase in the volume of the thorax and hence inspiration. The ribs articulate by means of facet (flat) joints on each of two adjoining vertebral bodies, and with another facet joint of a vertebral spine. As the neck of the rib rotates, the rib shaft moves outwards and forwards increasing thoracic diameter. The anterior ends of ribs 1–10 are attached by costal cartilages to the manubrium and sternum. The lower two are shorter and free at their anterior ends.

Diaphragm

This consists of a fibrous central disk-like tendon and peripheral skeletal muscles innervated by the phrenic nerves (C3–5), and is attached to the first three lumbar vertebrae behind and to the xiphisternum and the upper margins of the bottom six ribs laterally and anteriorly. The physiology of diaphragmatic contraction is complex. Essentially, muscle contraction causes the dome to move downwards. The abdomen is a fluid-filled bag, and this downward movement of the diaphragm has to be balanced by an outward movement of the anterior abdominal wall – because the abdomen and contents are fixed in volume. The lower ribs move outwards (inspiration) (1) because of the way the diaphragm muscles are attached and (2) because abdominal pressure pushes them out. Diaphragm paralysis causes 'paradoxical' inward movement of the abdominal wall in inspiration. A hyperinflated chest cannot expand further and sometimes diaphragmatic contraction causes inward movement of the lower ribs – Harrison's sulcus in children, and seen often in adults with severe chronic obstructive pulmonary disease (COPD).

Intercostal muscles

These are two sheets of muscles between adjacent ribs. The external intercostals are predominantly inspiratory and the internal sheet predominantly expiratory, as they have opposing

Fig. 2.1 Rib joints and their movement. This rib is attached to two adjacent upper thoracic vertebrae (A and B) by facet joints on both bodies and on the spinous process of B. The intercostal muscles rotate the neck of the rib, and therefore the shaft moves upwards and forwards (inspiration) increasing the size of the thorax ('pump handle' motion). Lower ribs move more outwards ('bucket handle' motion).

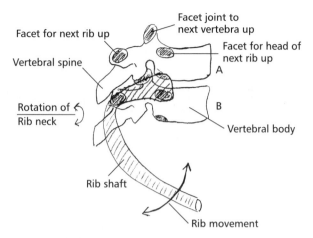

Facet for next rib up

Facet joint to next vertebra up

Facet for head of next rib up

A

Vertebral spine

Rotation of Rib neck

B

Vertebral body

Rib shaft

Rib movement

Fig. 2.2 A posteroanterior (PA) chest radiograph of a normal woman. Conventionally, X-rays are taken on full inspiration, and therefore the diaphragms are contracted and are flatter than in expiration. The natural lung markings are the bronchovascular bundles particularly the pulmonary arteries and adjacent bronchi.

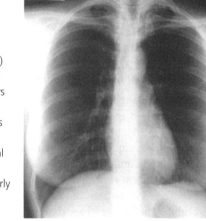

Fig. 2.3 A lateral chest radiograph of the same subject as Figure 2.2. The vertebral bodies can be seen, as can the manubrium and sternum anteriorly.

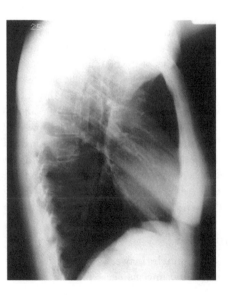

effects on rib movement. Their contribution to this in quiet breathing is small. Innervation is by segmental T1–12 intercostal nerves running along the inferior border of each rib.

The three scalene muscles run from the cervical vertebrae to the anterior first and second ribs and are primary muscles of inspiration moving these outwards. The abdominal muscles (rectus abdominis, external and internal transverse abdominis) connect the lower ribs and the pelvis. Contraction increases abdominal pressure and this forces the lower ribs outwards (inspiration) where the diaphragm is opposed to them. Additionally, because of their insertions to the lower ribs, these muscles assist in expiration as well. The balance of their activity is therefore between the rise in abdominal pressure causing inspiration and direct muscle tension on the lower ribs causing expiration. Their principal activity, however, is in expiration, particularly during activity such as coughing and speaking.

Pleura, pleural space, and pleural fluid

The pleural membrane consists of a layer of mesothelial (pavement cells) on a thin basement membrane and loose connective tissue. The visceral (lung) and parietal (chest wall, diaphragm, and mediastinal) pleura are similar. For the most part the 'pleural space' in health is a potential one as there is a continuous flow of pleural fluid from capillaries below the parietal (i.e. chest wall) pleura into the pleural space where it passes to visceral (i.e. lung) subpleural lymphatics. The volume of this fluid is only a few millilitres. The practical effects of pleural disease are that a pleural effusion compresses lung tissue. Pleural inflammation or tumour may be painful because the intercostal nerves are subjacent to the visceral pleura on the chest wall, and diffuse pleural thickening can both decrease the compliance of the chest wall and restrict lung expansion, causing breathlessness.

Airways

The upper airways are defined as the nasal passages, pharynx, and larynx (Figure 2.4). The lower airways consist of the trachea and all bronchi and bronchioles.

The motor and sensory innervation of the upper airway is via the vagus. The upper airway has no rigid wall, being bounded by muscle and connective tissue. The means that when the pressures within it drops during inspiration as air is drawn into the lungs, it tends to collapse. Reflex muscular tone prevents this. However, if the airway is narrow (as in obesity) or the muscle tension is reduced (as in during sleep), closure can occur – and this is the cause of obstructive sleep apnoea. The anatomy of the aryepiglottic fold, the false cords, and cough reflexes involving the true cords are powerful protective mechanisms preventing inhalation of oral contents, particularly during eating and drinking. These are decreased after, for example, denervation of the larynx as by thoracic tumour causing recurrent laryngeal nerve palsy or bilateral strokes causing pseudo-bulbar palsy.

The trachea is about 10 cm long in an adult, with its bifurcation at the level of the fifth thoracic vertebrae behind and the manubriosternal junction in the front. It consists of a series of anterior horseshoe-shaped cartilaginous rings, connecting to an elastic and muscular membrane posteriorly. Inside these, there is connective tissue, a web of spiral smooth muscle which can narrow the airway, a submucosa which is vascular and contains bronchial glands, and in contact with the air a complex pseudo-stratified ciliated epithelium (the mucus membrane) (Figure 2.5a). The trachea is mobile, shortening and becoming crescent shaped during cough. Bronchi have a similar structure (Figure 2.5b). They divide 'dichotomously', i.e. always into two (although the division may be asymmetrical) into 2 main, 5 lobar, and 19 segmental ones. The cartilage support dwindles to occasional plates with progressive

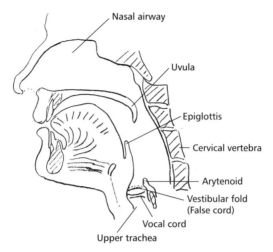

Fig. 2.4 Sagittal section through the nose, pharynx, and larynx. The upper airway extends from the nares to the vocal folds. Because it is bounded by muscles and connective tissues it acts as a partially collapsible tube. During inspiration the airway narrows slightly, and on expiration it widens. Muscular contraction during swallowing moves the epiglottis backwards and the arytenoids upwards and forwards to close off the glottis and prevent aspiration of contents passing to the oesophagus, behind the trachea.

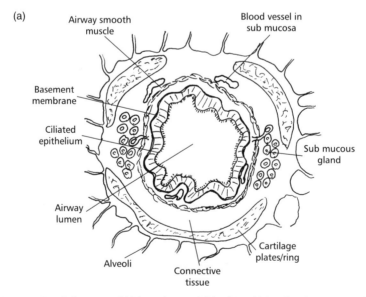

Fig. 2.5 Cross-sectional diagrams of (a) bronchus and (b) a bronchiole. The airways smooth muscle is arranged in a spiral fashion around the submucosa and epithelium and causes narrowing of the airway when it constricts. Bronchial submucous glands are complex tubular stuctures below the smooth muscle and secrete mucus in to the airways. The rigidity of the airway is ensured by the cartilage rings which diminish to separate plates as the airways narrow. By contrast, the bronchiole is a simpler structure lacking cartilage, submucous glands and lymphatics. Smooth muscle is present, but the alveoli are much more closely applied to the bronchiole wall and exert tension on it, keeping the airway open.

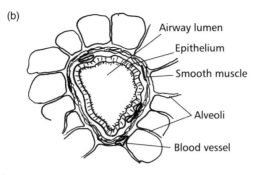

(b)

Airway lumen

Epithelium

Smooth muscle

Alveoli

Blood vessel

Fig. 2.5 *(Continued)*

subdivisions as the bronchi reduce in size. Bronchioles, which have no cartilage at all and depend upon alveolar attachments to keep them open, begin at about 1 mm diameter.

The terminology of the finer anatomy of the lung is confusing (see Box 2.1 for some simple definitions). **Terminal bronchioles** (0.5 mm diameter) are the smallest which act purely to conduct air. These branch to **'respiratory' bronchioles** which have alveolar ducts and alveoli in their walls and participate in gas exchange. There about 300 million **alveoli**, each approximately 250 μm in diameter. These are lined by a very thin epithelium (type I alveolar cells) continuous with the epithelium of the bronchioles. A basement membrane separates this from the attached capillary endothelial walls. Parts of each alveolus have an **interstitium** where there is a bigger gap between the epithelia which is filled by connective tissue and interstitial cells such as fibroblasts, lymphocytes, macrophages, and nerve fibres (Figure 2.6). Type II alveolar cells are found in the corners of alveoli and secrete surfactant. This is essential to reduce surface tension within the alveoli and without this the lung would not be expandable. Alveoli contain a few cells, notably pulmonary alveolar macrophages (PAMS), which are phagocytic and metabolically active. A small quantity of fluid containing proteases regularly extravasates from the capillaries into the alveoli and this moves with PAMS up the bronchial tree.

The **acinus** is conventionally regarded as the smallest functional unit of the lung. This is a portion of lung approximately 7 mm across containing a terminal bronchiole and its associated

Box 2.1 Lung structure: simple definitions

Lobe: Separate bits of each lung, e.g. R upper
Segment: Subdivision of lobe (usually 2–5)
Bronchi: Tubes with cartilage
Bronchioles: Small tubes without cartilage
Terminal bronchiole: Last one, 0.5 mm in diameter
Respiratory bronchiole: Where alveoli and gas exchange begin
Alveoli: Gas-exchanging sacs (parenchyma)
Secondary lobule: Smallest bit of lung surrounded by connective tissue (fibrous) (Kerley B), about 1–2.5 cm in diameter; contains about five terminal bronchioles and the alveoli connected to them, the **acinus** (7 mm diameter)
Primary lobule: One eighth of an acinus; one respiratory bronchiole + alveoli

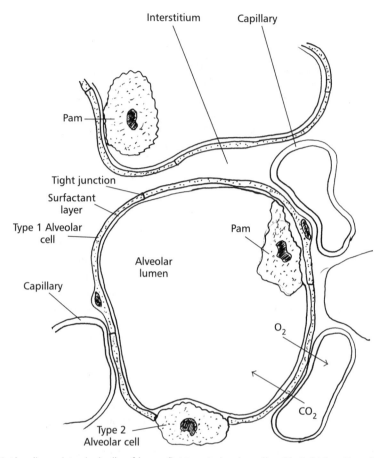

Fig. 2.6 Alveoli consist principally of large, flat type I alveolar cells with tight junctions between them. Type II cells are secretory, forming surfactant which is present as a film lining the alveolar surface. Pulmonary alveolar macrophages (PAMs) migrate from the blood, to the insterstium, into the aveoli. They are scavenger cells. Below the type I cells is a basement membrane (not shown) and a thin loose interstitium, which may contain occasional inflammatory cells such as neutrophils and eosinophils. There are tight junctions between the adjacent walls of alveoli and of capillaries. Gas exchange between the alveolar lumen and the capillaries occurs by diffusion.

respiratory bronchioles and alveoli. Although this is a convenient concept from the functional point of view, a more practically useful subunit is the **secondary lobule**. This is larger, contains a bronchiole and arteriole at its centre and is bounded by loose connective tissue septa. It has pulmonary venules and lymphatics at the edges (Figure 2.7). These lobules are about 1–2.5 cm in diameter and are easily seen on a bronchogram or on CT scanning, particularly when lymphatics are enlarged (Figure 2.8). Bronchioles depend upon the tension of alveolar wall attachments to keep them patent during respiration. Alveolar damage as in emphysema reduces the elasticity ('elastic recoil') of the lung and tension is lost. These small airways then readily collapse in expiration, and this is the major cause of respiratory airflow limitation and hence breathlessness in COPD.

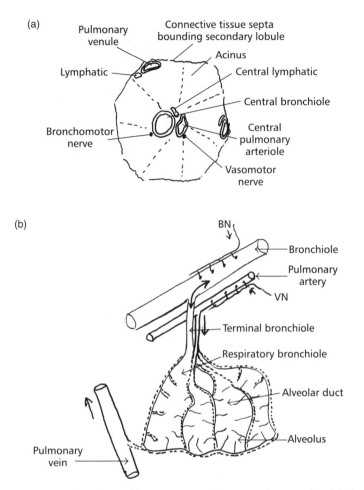

Fig. 2.7 Fine structure of the lungs: (a) Cross-sectional diagram of a secondary lobule. This has a pulmonary arteriole and a bronchiole at its centre together with small lymphatics, nerves, and bronchial vessels (not shown). It is about 1–2 cm across, bounded by loose connective tissue septa, and contains a number of acini. Pulmonary venules (veins) are at the edge of the second-ary lobules with accompanying lymphatics. In conditions such as heart failure and lymphangitis carcinomatosa, the lympatics at the edge of the lobules become distended and are easily seen, for example on CT scanning, when they delineate the edges of the lobules. (b) The anatomy of an acinus. A terminal bronchiole with an accompanying arteriole divides into a number of respiratory bronchioles and then alveolar ducts off which the alveoli open.

By contrast, an increase in the thickness of alveolar walls as in alveolar fibrosis, makes the lungs stiffer, elastic recoil is increased, and expiratory airflow limitation is low.

Lymph

Lymphatics draining the pleura accompany the pulmonary venules and veins at the edges of the secondary lobules. Lymph from acini run within the lobules alongside the centrally placed arterioles and bronchioles (see Figure 2.7). Proximally, the channels converge on perihilar and

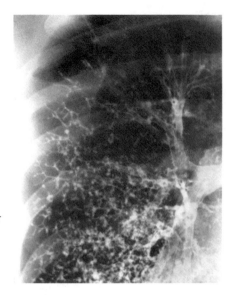

Fig. 2.8 Bronchogram showing the way in which the larger airways divide; the small bronchioles at the centre of secondary lobules can easily be seen.

then mediastinal nodes, eventually forming the thoracic duct which runs posteriorly in the mediastinum and enters the left subclavian vein. Engorgement of subpleural lymphatics and hence interlobular lymphatics, as in left ventricular failure or lymphangitis carcinomatosa, allows these structures to be very clearly seen on CT. Lymph channels are the principal means whereby the lung is kept dry.

Pulmonary vessels

The gross anatomy of these vessels is demonstrated in an angiogram (Figures 2.9). Pulmonary arteries course and branch with bronchi so that they accompany each other down to the alveoli and are at the centres of secondary lobules. Pulmonary veins form at the periphery of acini and interlobular septa, and run separately, to drain via the four main pulmonary veins, two from the upper lobes and the right middle lobe and two from the lower lobes, into the left atrium.

Bronchial circulation

Bronchial arteries provide oxygenated blood to lung structures. From the aorta on the left and from an intercostal artery on the right, the main bronchial arteries accompany the bronchi as they divide within the lungs. There is a very rich vascular network within airway walls. Peripherally small bronchiolar arterioles may drain into pulmonary veins or via small bronchiolar veins. The bronchial circulation supplies abnormal tissue too, such as tumours, and bronchiectatic segments. In the latter condition the bronchial arteries may enlarge and severe haemoptysis may require bronchial artery embolization (block) to control it.

Innervation

The lung is innervated by the vagi (parasympathetic) and sympathetic nerves from the paravertebral sympathetic chain and the stellate ganglia at the lung apices. There are no

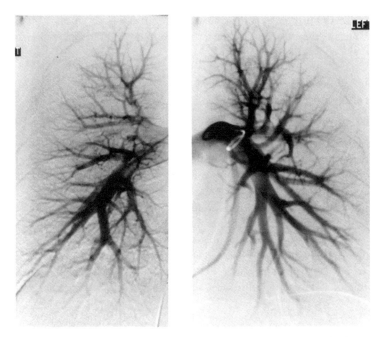

Fig. 2.9 (a) An arteriogram showing the anatomy of the pulmonary arteries, which accompany the bronchi as they subdivide in the lung tissue. (b) Venous phase of a pulmonary arteriogram. The venules run from the edges of the secondary lobules and coalesce to form larger vessels which enter the left atrium.

somatic nerves, and thus no localization of lung sensation is possible. The parasympathetic motor supply innervates airway smooth muscle (causing cholinergic bronchoconstriction), and bronchial submucus glands, (stimulating secretion) and subepithelial blood vessels (causing constriction).

Afferent fibres come from three types of nerve endings: rapidly adapting type I receptors instigating cough and irritant reflexes; slowly adapting nerve endings (type II) giving rise to the Hering–Breuer reflex (inhibition of inspiration at high lung volume) and lastly type III receptors (J-receptors) which are found in the lung periphery and are sensitive both to mechanical distortion and chemical stimuli. Sympathetic and purinergic (non-adrenergic, non-cholinergic) nerves also supply the airways smooth muscle, the submucosa and vessels. The sympathetic nerves have an opposite effect to the parasympathetic supply. Cough receptors (type I) are concentrated at branching points within the airways and particularly around the larynx.

Integration

Ventilation

The motive power for ventilation is provided by the primary inspiratory muscles, which act to increase the volume of the chest. Because of this a negative pressure relative to the atmosphere develops in the pleural space. It is typically –10 to 20 cmH_2O (1–2 kPa) at the bases and -5 cmH$_2$O (0.49 kPa) at the apices. The negative pressure encourages movement of air into the lungs as they expand. The force required to expand them must overcome:

◆ resistance to airflow in the airways
◆ stiffness or compliance of the lung tissue
◆ stiffness of the chest wall and abdomen
◆ inertia of the whole system.

At rest, the lungs tend to collapse. A complete pneumothorax shows this. This tendency to collapse is counter-acted by the tendency of the chest wall to move outwards. The point where these two forces are equal is at 'resting' lung volume, i.e. the **functional residual capacity** (FRC) (Figure 2.10, Table 2.1).

Work is needed to increase thoracic gas volume above this, for example to total lung capacity (TLC), or to expel air out further (to residual volume). The physical properties of the lung mean that more work is needed to inflate them at both high and low lung volume. Consequently relatively more work has to be done by the muscles to achieve a tidal volume when they are already hyperinflated as in COPD. An abnormally stiff chest wall, as in ankylosing spondylitis, or as a result of diffuse pleural thickening, or distortion of the chest wall (as in

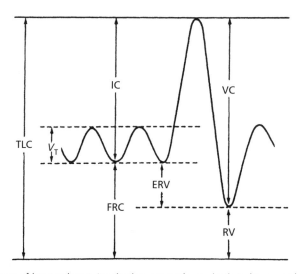

Fig. 2.10 Subdivisions of lung volume. Inspiration upwards, expiration downwards. The volume of air breathed in and out during quiet respiration (tidal volume, V_T) is shown on the left. At the end of quiet expiration, the forces of the chest wall tending to move the lungs outwards, and the stretching of the lung itself tending to move the lungs inwards, are balanced and this volume is known as the functional residual capacity (FRC). IC = inspiratory capacity. If a maximal inspiration is taken from FRC and then a full forced expiration is taken, this is known as the vital capacity (VC). At the end of a forced expiration, the volume of air in the lungs which still remains is called the residual volume (RV). The combination of the vital capacity and the residual volume gives the total lung capacity (TLC). The expiratory reserve volume (ERV) is similar to the inspiratory capacity and simply represents the volume in reserve after a tidal expiration. These lung volumes can change with chronic disease (see Table 2.1).

Table 2.1 Differing effects of obstructive versus restrictive chronic lung disease on pulmonary function. (A) Changes in lung function in a 60-year-old woman with COPD: predicted values for a person of her age and height, then her observed value and then her values expressed as a percentage of the predicted value. It can be seen that her total lung capacity (TLC) is increased, as are her functional reserve capacity (FRC) and residual volume (RV), showing gas trapping in the lungs. The FEV_1 is low, at 36% of predicted, as is the FEV_1/FVC ratio. The transfer factor and coefficient are low because of emphysema which reduces the area of alveolar wall available for gas exchange. (B) By contrast, this shows the percentage predicted values of a 47-year-old man with severe fibrosing alveolitis (restrictive lung disease). The lung volumes are reduced, but the FEV_1/FVC ratio is better than predicted. The transfer factor and coefficient are reduced because of inflammation and scarring of the alveolar walls, which diminishes gas exchange

	A			B	
	Predicted	**Observed**	**%Predicted**	**% Predicted**	
Lung volumes (L)					
Vital capacity	2.8	3.3	115	42	!
TLC	4.9	6.0	123	! 52	!
FRC	2.7	5.8	216	! 78	!
RV	2.1	4.6	220	! 87	!
Mechanics					
FEV_1	2.3	0.83	36	! 51	!
FVC	2.7	2.8	103	42	!
Ratio FEV_1/VC	77	29	37	97	
Carbon monoxide diffusion *(mmol* min^{-1} kPa^{-1}*)*					
Transfer factor	7.5	3.8	50	! 25	!
Transfer coefficient	1.5	0.64	41	! 47	!

! denotes an abnormal value (>2 SD below predicted).

kyphoscoliosis) also can cause an increased work of ventilation. Expiration is a passive relaxation using stored energy in which the elasticity of the chest wall and lungs, stretched during inspiration, returns then to resting dimensions, and air is therefore expelled when this happens.

Airway resistance

This is by far the most important resistance to ventilation. It derives from the need to cause gas to flow within the airways. In quiet breathing, surprisingly, the major resistance to airflow is in the nose, and in mouth breathing the larynx. Resistance within healthy small airways contributes only about 25% to total airway resistance because there are so many of them and their total cross-sectional area is very high. The airway resistance of the lungs is affected by many things, including airway smooth muscle and oedema or mucus in small airways. In some diseases these factors, and airway collapse in expiration due to alveolar destruction, can increase the resistance to expiration hugely. Likewise, a tumour narrowing a major airway can increase resistance throughout the breathing cycle. The physiology of forced expiration is described in Figure 2.11.

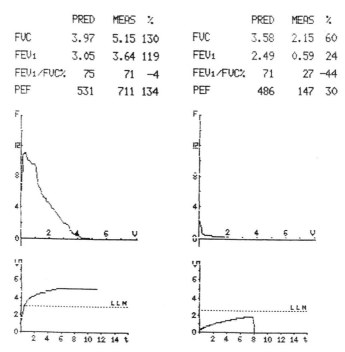

	PRED	MEAS	%		PRED	MEAS	%
FVC	3.97	5.15	130	FVC	3.58	2.15	60
FEV1	3.05	3.64	119	FEV1	2.49	0.59	24
FEV1/FVC%	75	71	−4	FEV1/FVC%	71	27	−44
PEF	531	711	134	PEF	486	147	30

Fig. 2.11 Physiology of forced expiration. This shows spirometer readings from, on the left, a healthy 45-year-old man, and on the right a 70-year-old man with severe COPD. Upper panels are flow–volume plots (F–V) and the lower plots are spirograms plotting volume against time (t). The healthy man rapidly reaches a high peak flow of about 11 L/s, and as expiration continues flow rate declines in a straight line towards residual volume which is reached at about 5 L. The spirogram shows that the FEV$_1$ is approximately 3.5 L. The vital capacity is reached in about 5 s. By contrast, the patient has a lower peak flow rate of about 3 L/s and the flow rate is reduced very abruptly. It continues at a very low rate thereafter. Similarly, the spirogram shows the FEV$_1$ is approximately 0.8 L and even at 8 s expiration is still continuing, although at a very low rate. The abrupt decline in peak flow rate during a forced expiration in these patients occurs because of a loss of lung elasticity which allows the small airways to shut off; this is known as **pressure-dependent airway collapse**. In asthma the pattern of expiratory flow is similar to normal, although at a much lower level **(volume-dependent airway narrowing)**.

Pulmonary gas exchange

The purpose of ventilation is to achieve gas exchange. Oxygen enters the alveoli by convection (bulk flow) and there diffuses down a molecular concentration gradient from alveolar gas across the alveolar membrane, to attach to haemoglobin in the capillary red cells. Carbon dioxide conversely diffuses from the capillary plasma down a concentration gradient to the alveoli and is expelled by ventilation. Efficient exchange between alveolar gas and pulmonary capillary blood needs 'matching' between air and blood, i.e. there needs to be an appropriate supply of each in all alveoli. Even in health this does not happen, with alveoli being relatively over-perfused at the lung bases (gravitational effect) and over-ventilated at the lung apices. Major changes in alveolar perfusion, to improve matching, probably occur in health as a result of local regulation of arteriolar tone and hence flow in pulmonary arterioles as a result of hypoxic vasoconstriction, which is mediated by nitric oxide. A crude clinical estimate of the inhomogeneity is the alveolar-arterial oxygen gradient measure of the lungs' efficiency at gas exchange. Lung damage increases this, and the use of multiple inert gases (MIGET techniques) in the laboratory can show that the lung in disease can be thought of as a mixture of 'compartments' in which the alveoli are relatively over- or under-perfused and ventilated.

An increase in alveolar ventilation helps to correct any consequent hypoxaemia (because this increases the oxygen uptake in the alveoli with low ventilation) and there is a concomitant reduction in alveolar PCO_2 as more than the physiologically required carbon dioxide is expelled.

The clinical measure of alveolar gas exchange is the transfer coefficient for carbon monoxide (a marker gas) or TL_{CO} (sometimes called the diffusing capacity, DL_{CO}) (Table 2.1). Typically this might be reduced in disease where there is alveolar inflammation and fibrosis as in fibrosing alveolitis, or alveolar damage as an emphysema. It is usually normal in pure airway diseases such as asthma.

Carbon dioxide is carried in the blood principally as a dissolved bicarbonate:

$$CO_2 + H_2O \leftrightarrows H_2CO_3 \leftrightarrows HCO_3 + H^+$$

The blood has a high capacity for bicarbonate and this acts as a buffer against big changes of pH. In health ventilation is regulated to maintain the PCO_2 at 40 mmHg (5.32 kPa) and the pH of blood at 7.4. Lung damage can result in an inability to ventilate alveoli sufficiently to remove the body's carbon dioxide load. The PCO_2 of the blood rises as a consequence and the bicarbonate rises too. This combination is seen typically in the type II hypercapnic respiratory failure of COPD, where although the pH of blood is in a stable state is normal, the PCO_2 may for example be 60 mmHg (7.98 kPa) and the bicarbonate 40 mmol rather than 24 mmol.

Regulation of breathing

Breathing is regulated by an exquisite but incompletely understood neuronal control system. Fundamentally, peripheral aortic and carotid chemoreceptors provide hypoxic 'drive' to ventilation and these and medullary chemoreceptors regulate ventilation in response to changes in PCO_2, in the case of the latter as a result of subsequent changes in cerebrospinal fluid pH. Short-term changes in ventilation usually occur in response to the need to control PCO_2 and hence blood pH (Figure 2.12).

It appears that the drive of inspiratory neurones in the medulla is modulated by a variety of inputs (e.g. nerve traffic from pharyngeal and chest wall stretch receptors) which not only set the overall level of ventilation (PCO_2) but also determine the length and depth of each breath. Expiration timing is regulated and it can be an active rather than a passive process depending upon the ventilation requirements. This automatic control of breathing is susceptible to many changes that reduce the drive, for example hypnotics. One or two drugs are known which can increase ventilation drive, for example doxapram, which increases the sensitivity of peripheral chemoreceptors. Central conscious respiratory drive can override the usually medullary automatic control. The resultant breathing pattern is usually less regular and the blood PCO_2 is often reduced in hyperventilation, which is the usual pattern (see Chapter 6).

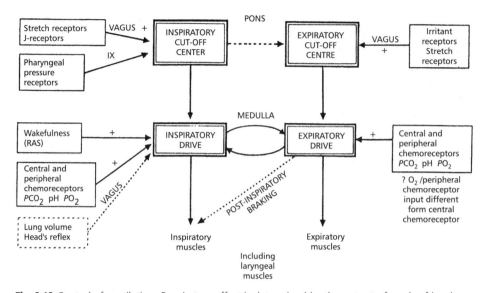

Fig. 2.12 Control of ventilation. Respiratory effort is determined by the output of pools of inspiratory and expiratory neurones in the medulla which are mutually inhibitory. These integrate factors tending to increase and decrease ventilation deriving from, for example, the central and peripheral chemoreceptors in the lung via the vagus, and (not shown) afferents from the chest wall muscles and joints. The influence of cortical and other factors is shown in a similar diagram in Chapter 12. From J. Stradling, in *Respiratory Medicine*, 2nd edn, W.B. Saunders Philadelphia, 1995, with permission.

Breathing during exercise

Ventilation is increased in steady-state exercise because muscles require additional oxygen to generate the ATP for muscle contraction from carbohydrate fuel and ADP. The associated increase in carbon dioxide production stimulates the medullary and peripheral chemoreceptors. If anaerobic metabolism occurs it generates lactate and hydrogen ions (reducing blood pH) and again stimulates chemoreceptors. The components of drive at the onset of sudden exercise are not understood, although they probably include important inputs from active muscles. As the intensity of exercise increases, tidal volume also increases so that the rapidity and depth of breathing approaches 75% of the maximal flow–volume loop (Figure 2.13). In disease states, the limits of expiratory flow may be reached far more quickly.

The factors limiting exercise are not fully understood in detail. However, there is usually a component of peripheral muscle discomfort sensed as fatigue, and respiratory muscles may contribute to this. The work of breathing is hugely increased in exercise; for example, the measured intrapleural pressure changes may rise to +20 cm H_2O (1.99 kPa) compared with 5 cm H_2O (0.49 kPa) at rest. The sensation of dyspnoea is complex (see Chapter 6) but may be present even at rest in very disabled people. Measures of exercise capacity in the laboratory range between bicycle or treadmill tests enabling accurate plots of tidal volume, frequency, oxygen consumption and carbon dioxide production, or less formal tests of capacity such as the 6-minute walking distance, or the shuttle walk test. The latter are, however, perfectly suitable for clinical work in patients with respiratory disease.

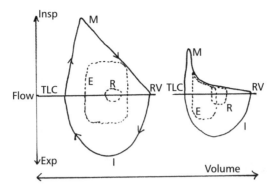

Fig. 2.13 Flow–volume loops at rest and exercise. On the left a normal subject, on the right a patient with COPD. In the normal flow–volume loop, done in the laboratory, the subject takes a maximum breath in to TLC, then breathes out as hard and fast as possible. Expiratory flow rate rises rapidly (M), then declines to residual volume. A maximum inspiration (I) is shown below the zero flow line. At rest (R) the normal subject breathes well away from his maximum flow–volume envelope. During exercise, lung volume used is less than the maximum flow–volume loop, and expiratory flow is limited only during a short portion of the respiratory cycle (E). By contrast, the patient with COPD is flow-limited during quiet breathing (R). During exercise the patient has to inflate his lungs to increase ventilation, and most of the expiratory flow is limited and occurs at his maximum rate (E). Dynamic hyperinflation is often accompanied by feelings of discomfort in such patients.

Lung defence mechanisms

The lungs are open to the air, and we inhale 10 000 L of air with its contained particles every day. The lungs need protection against inhaled dusts, fumes, and microorganisms as well as oral fluids and solids. Their defences are physical (airflow patterns, mucociliary and alveolar clearance, cough) cellular, and humoral.

The nose acts as a crude particulate filter, and turbulence and changes of flow direction here cause particles to impact on the mucus membrane. The same occurs in the mouth and in the larynx where narrowing of the airways generates turbulence and increases impaction. Within the lung vortices occur at bifurcations of large airways, but gas flow becomes so slow here, as the cross-sectional of the airways increases, that fine particles of <2.5 μm diameter can only leave the inspired air by sedimentation.

Particles are removed from the lung by means of the mucociliary escalator. Airway lining fluid (ALF) is secreted predominantly by submucous glands, which occur about every square millimetre of mucus membrane. Approximately 10 mL/24 h is produced in health and the upwards flow rate is about 5 mm/min. Fluid is swallowed or expectorated when it reaches the larynx.

Additional fluid is secreted by the goblet cells of the airway (Figure 2.14). Respiratory mucus is a highly complex liquid containing macromolecules and proteins which give it physical properties suitable for its function as a protective layer over the underlying cells. The cilia of the epithelial cells beat in a coordinated fashion in a sol of fluid and the mucus is thicker above them (gel phase). The water and ion content of ALF is regulated by cellular protein pumps on the apical and basal surface of airway epithelial cells. There is a movement of sodium ions, chloride ions, and water, determined by an ATPase pump at the base of the epithelial cells. Active

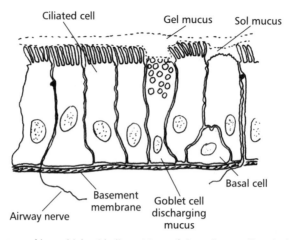

Fig. 2.14 Ultrastructure of bronchial epithelium. Most of the cells are ciliated; the cilia beat in a coordinated fashion in a sol of bronchial fluid with the more tenacious gel phase at their tips. Bronchial mucus is secreted by goblet cells and also by submucus bronchial glands (not shown). The mucus membrane regenerates from basal cells. Airway nerves penetrate the tight junctions between adjacent epithelial cells. Below the basement membrane is the submucosa where there are blood vessels, fibroblasts and neutrophils, and eosinophils (not shown).

secretion of chloride ions can, however, increase the water content of ALF. Genetic defects of this chloride pump (CFTR or cystic fibrosis transmembrane regulator) are the primary lesion in cystic fibrosis where the airway mucus is characteristically extremely thick and tenacious. Genetic defects in ciliary structure (primary ciliary dyskinesias), e.g. Kartagener's syndrome, are associated with mucus retention, secondary infection and resulting bronchiectasis.

Particles deposited in alveoli are cleared differently. The majority are phagocytosed by PAMs (Figure 2.6), which subsequently pass upwards. However, the lining cells of the alveoli can 'unzip', allowing cells and particles to pass across the membrane, and PAMs can migrate in this way through the epithelium and to lymphatics. Other particles are caught in surfactant and removed up the mucociliary escalator and others may enter epithelial cells (type I alveolar cells) which subsequently die and are phagocytosed. Pulmonary clearance of particle loads may take many days, and some fibrous particles defy clearance. Asbestos is the prime example: asbestos fibres may be detected 50 or more years after inhalation. Coal dust may similarly accumulate over years in peribronchial areas (causing emphysema) and in submucosal lymphoid tissue. Some soluble inhaled substances can pass directly across the pulmonary epithelium and enter the circulation – which is the basis of systemic effects of some inhaled drugs.

In addition to physical clearance mechanisms, the lungs are protected by airway proteins present there either as a result of diffusion through the mucus membrane (for example α_1-antiprotease or albumin) or as a result of secretion by airway cells, for example complement components. Examples of proteins with protective effects are lyzozyme and immunoglobulins. These are particularly important for neutralizing bacterial pathogens. Congenital lack of surfactant IgA, for example, causes bronchiectasis. Cytokines are involved in the exceedingly complex activation of IgE-dependent reactions in response to some inhaled molecules. This may be physiologically appropriate, as for parasite control, or inappropriate, as in allergy to house dust mite particles.

Airway cells (PAMs, lymphocytes, neutrophils, and eosinophils) have two roles in lung defence. They may initiate an immune response (afferent limb) or function as 'effector' cells contributing to an inflammatory response once an immune response has been elicited. In addition, PAMs and neutrophils act as airway scavengers ingesting particles, microbes, and proteins. Defects in cell function (for example, T-cell defects in HIV) allow lung infection with 'opportunist' organisms that are usually prevented from lung colonization by immune and cellular surveillance.

Lung inflammation

Inflammation is a 'normal' host defence response to persistent antigens in lung tissue. It is stimulated either directly by foreign proteins or by cytokines deriving from antigen–macrophage interaction (e.g. IL-8 or TNF). Neutrophils adhere to pulmonary capillary endothelium and migrate into lung tissue. They release a large array of cytokines and proteins which recruit more cells and alter vessel permeability, leading to protein and fluid accumulation in the inflamed area. The mechanisms underlying inflammatory response are very complex and incompletely understood. We do not understand, either, why the results of inflammation vary. In some cases it terminates and resolves with lung repair, leaving normal tissue – as after a streptococcal pneumonia. In other cases lung destruction occurs, for example *Klebsiella* pneumonia or tuberculosis, and this leads to permanent scarring. In others, inflammation itself continues chronically, as in fibrosing alveolitis. Much lung disease is the result of persistent chronic inflammation – COPD, chronic severe asthma, ARDS, cystic fibrosis, and the alveolitis of systemic vasculitis, for example. Thus, a chronically ill patient may have lung tissue which is scarred, secondary infected, or persistently inflamed as a result of an initial event. Few, if any of these processes can be modulated by therapy, a lone example being steroid treatment for the inflammation of allergic asthma.

Keypoints

- An adult breathes 10 000 L of air in 24 h
- The primary inspiratory muscles are the diaphragm and the intercostals (mainly internal)
- Expiration is mainly a passive act during tidal breathing
- Forced expiration uses external intercostals, abdominal muscles, and others
- The bronchial tree branches dichotomously to about 30 000 terminal bronchioles 0.5 mm in diameter
- Alveoli are lined by type I 'pavement' cells with type II secretory-surfactant cells at intervals
- The interstitium of the lung consists of basement membranes, little connective tissue with protein matrix and inflammatory cells
- Neurological control of respiration depends upon modulation of two reciprocally firing neurone pools in the medulla
- Important changes in the airways of obstructive lung disease are hyper-reactive muscle, inflammation of the bronchial walls, and loss of alveolar wall tension, so that small bronchioles collapse in expiration. This leads to 'trapping' of gas in the lung
- Gas exchange in emphysema and diffuse parenchymal lung diseases is poor, because of abnormal ventilation–perfusion matching in the alveoli

Further reading

Bates, D.V. *Respiratory function and disease*, 3rd edn. Philadelphia: W.B. Saunders; 1989. Classic account of the perturbations of pulmonary physiology as a result of disease. Includes basic accounts of airways structure, function, and pulmonary physiology.

Fraser, R.S., Muller, N.L., Colman, N., and Pare, P.D., *Diagnosis of diseases of the chest*, 4th edn. Philadelphia: W.B. Saunders; 1999. Volume 1, Part 1, The normal chest (pp. 1–297). An account of the anatomy and physiology of the lung. There is an emphasis on radiological anatomy.

Gibson, G.J., Geddes, D.M., Costabel, U., Sterk, P.J., and Corrin, B. *Respiratory Medicine*, 3rd edn. London. W.B. Saunders; 2003. Part A, Structure and function contains 12 chapters on the anatomy and physiology of the lungs and chest.

Chapter 3

Quality of life – models and measures of quality of life

Michael E. Hyland and Samantha C. Sodergren

The term quality of life (QoL) refers to the patient's subjective experience of life, but beyond that there are a wide variety of interpretations.

Table 3.1 provides a list of several different kinds of definition. Broadly speaking, definitions vary in terms of perspective. According to some definitions [1-3] QoL is defined in terms of content or theory by researchers. Other definitions, however,[4-6] suggest that quality of life is something that is defined entirely by the patient. This difference is by no means trivial, because it has an impact on those aspects of life which, by definition, fall within the remit of QoL. In this chapter we compare scales in terms of their content. Each scale is valid from the perspective of the researchers' definition of QoL, but because different researchers have different perspectives on QoL, their scales are by no means identical, and particular scales may be more suited to particular purposes than others.

There are three purposes of QoL assessment: resource allocation between diseases, treatment selection for a single disease, and clinical management. In this chapter we focus on the last two of these aims: the aim of comparing QoL gain between two treatments, and the aim of using QoL as part of decision making for patient management.

Table 3.2 shows the increase in the amount of time and effort devoted to the topic of QoL during the last 15 years. The increased emphasis on QoL reflects an important shift in medical thinking. Whereas traditionally health outcome was considered in terms of mortality and morbidity, nowadays QoL is also considered. More importantly, where there is conflict between QoL versus mortality/morbidity outcomes, it is no longer accepted that the former should play a less important role. That is, there may be circumstances when maintaining the patient's QoL takes priority over prolonging life or reducing morbidity, and this is particularly true for terminally ill patients.[7] The judgement of the relative importance of mortality, morbidity, and QoL is always a subjective one, and different conclusions may be drawn about patients who have identical medical conditions. Thus, understanding the patient's QoL and what the patient wants to attain in terms of QoL is crucial to optimal patient management.

As a general rule, patients value the quality of life much more than its quantity, and place little value on physiological measures of morbidity. Thus the shift in focus of medicine towards QoL parallels the way patients would like to be treated. This shift reflects the consumerization of medicine, where the method of treatment is decided not just by the doctor but by a negotiated agreement between the doctor and the patient, bearing in mind that the patient's own views may change with time. One of the problems with the 'living will' concept is that patients' views about how they should be treated can change as the level of illness deepens. Patients who feel that a particular health state is 'not worth living' when they are well may have a very

Table 3.1 Proposed definitions of quality of life

Definition	Authors
Having as much money as possible left over after taking care of basic necessities, and having the necessary time and opportunities for spending it in a pleasant way	Singer[1]
The more or less 'good' or 'satisfactory' character of people's life	Szalai[2]
The quality of life measures the difference or the gap at a particular period of time between the hopes and expectations of an individual and the individual's present experiences	Calman[3]
An overall evaluation of the subjective experience of life	DeHaes and van Knippenberg[4]
Patients' performance in four areas: physical and occupational function, psychologic state, social interaction, and somatic sensation	Schipper et al.[5]
The quality, or value of an individual's life is no more and no less than what she considers it to be	Hayry[6]

Table 3.2 Citations of 'quality of life' in titles, keywords or abstracts

	Database	
Year	Medline	Psychlit
1983	273	84
1984	284	94
1985	331	125
1986	407	153
1987	483	191
1988	489	208
1989	790	229
1990	903	264
1991	928	282
1992	1104	326
1993	1395	309
1994	1700	456
1995	2536	456
1996	2915	539
1997	2219	580
1998	1932	462

different view of the matter when they are ill. Thus negotiations between the doctor and patient must take into account the fact that patients are in a vulnerable state and that this vulnerability extends to decision-making about QoL.

It is important to emphasize that good clinicians have always treated patients as people first and foremost, and hence been sensitive to QoL. The original definition of health given by the World Health Organization in 1947 was: '. . . a state of complete physical, mental and social well-being and not merely the absence of disease and infirmity'.[8] Good clinicians have always balanced the physiological needs of the patient against the psychological consequences of different kinds of treatment. However, what we have now at the beginning of the 21st century is a formalization of the process of caring for patients as people. Like treatment guidelines, the definitions, the measures, and all the paraphernalia that go with the QoL approach, all have the aim of providing a more consistent service for the patient.

Measuring quality of life

Information about the patient's QoL can be obtained in many different ways. Talking to the patient and history-taking all provide relevant information. However, questionnaires provide a more structured form of assessment and these can be either self-completed or interviewer administered, depending on the scale and the patient's ability. In addition, if patients are capable of completing a questionnaire, they can be asked to do this before the clinical interview and guide the kind of questions asked by the clinician, thereby achieving a more patient-focused interview.

There are a wide range of QoL questionnaires, which broadly fall into three categories: disease-specific, which are designed for a specific disease; generic scales, designed for any disease; and idiographic scales which, in effect, provide a different scale for each patient.

Disease-specific scales

Disease-specific scales are designed to include items that distinguish patients with the disease from healthy controls (see Table 3.3). Unlike generic scales, disease-specific scales do not include items which are irrelevant to the disease (e.g., an asthmatic is not given questions about eating problems) and so they often have a high degree of user acceptability. However, either explicitly or otherwise, such scales are also designed for a particular purpose and so the content of the scale also reflects that purpose. Most of these scales (for example, the Chronic Respiratory Disease Questionnaire,[9] the St George's Respiratory Questionnaire,[10] and the Asthma Quality of Life Questionnaire,[11] have been designed for clinical trials where a tool is needed to assess outcome in drug treatment. Such scales include a range of items (see sub-scales in Table 3.3). However, they do not include items that are irrelevant to a clinical trial, for example, they do not include items about the inconvenience or cost of inhaler, as this is irrelevant to a clinical trial. One scale (the Asthma Bother Profile[12]) is designed for clinical use and so does include items about convenience and cost of inhalers, as well as items concerning perceived care. Items include: 'How much does the cost of your asthma medicines bother you?' and 'My doctor/nurse has carefully explained how I should manage my asthma'. However, a scale designed for clinical use may be less sensitive as a clinical trial tool. Another scale (a shortened version of the Breathing Problems Questionnaire[13]) was designed for evaluating the outcome of pulmonary rehabilitation, and so may be less sensitive to outcome changes produced by other means. Thus, the different disease-specific scales are by no means equivalent in terms of item content, because they have been designed for different purposes. In addition, one scale (the St George's Respiratory Questionnaire[10]) was designed for asthma and

Table 3.3 Disease-specific scales

Measure and	Authors	Mode of administration	Number of items and subscales, target population	Subscales
Asthma Bother Profile	Hyland et al.[12]	Self-complete	22 items 2 sub-scales Adult asthma	(a) Bother (b) Management
Asthma Quality of Life Questionnaire	Juniper et al.[11]	Self-complete or interviewer administered	32 items 4 sub-scales Adult asthma	(a) Activity limitations (b) Symptoms (c) Emotional function (d) Exposure to environmental stimuli
Breathing Problems Questionnaire-Long version	Hyland et al.[16]	Self-complete	33 items 13 or 2 sub-scales COPD	(a) Walking (b) Bending or reaching (c) Washing and bathing (d) Household chores (e) Social interactions (f) Effects of weather or temperature (g) Effects of smells and fumes (h) Effects of colds (i) Sleeping (j) Medicine (k) Dysphoric states (l) Eating (m) Excretion urgency
Breathing Problems Questionnaire-Short version	Hyland et al.[13]	Self-complete	10 items No sub-scales COPD	(a) Problems (b) Evaluations
Childhood Asthma Questionnaires	French and Christie[14]			None
Form A (4–7 years)		Completed by the child with assistance	14 items (also 10 questions for parents) 2 sub-scales	(a) Distress (b) Quality of living
Form B (8–11 years)		Completed independently by the child	Child asthma 38 items (also 6 questions to be completed by parents) 3 sub-scales	(a) Distress (b) Severity (c) Active quality of living
Form C (12–16 years)		Completed independently by the child	Child asthma 46 items 5 sub-scales	(a) Distress (b) Severity (c) Reactivity (d) Active quality of

Table 3.3 (continued)

Measure and	Authors	Mode of administration	Number of items and subscales, target population	Subscales
			Child asthma	living (e) Teenage quality of living
Chronic Respiratory Disease Questionnaire	Guyatt et al.[9]	Interviewer administered	20 items 4 sub-scales Chronic obstructive pulmonary disease	(a) Dyspnoea (b) Fatigue (c) Emotional function (d) Mastery
European Organisation for Research and Treatment of Cancer QLQ-C30	EORTC[19]	Self-complete or interviewer administered	30 items 6 sub-scales and 3 symptom scales Cancer	(a) Physical (b) Role (c) Cognitive (d) Emotional (e) Social (f) Global QOL (g) Fatigue (h) Nausea and vomiting
Living with Asthma Questionnaire	Hyland[20]	Self-complete	68 items 11 or 4 sub-scales Adult asthma	(a) Social or leisure (b) Sport (c) Holidays (d) Sleep (e) Work and other activities (f) Colds (g) Mobility (h) Effects on others (i) Medication use (k) Sex (l) Dysphoric states and attitudes (m) Activities (n) Avoidance (o) Preoccupation (p) Distress
Paediatric Quality of Life Questionnaire	Juniper et al.[17]	Interviewer administered	23 items 3 sub-scales Child asthma	(a) Activity limitation (b) Symptoms (c) Emotional function
Paediatric Asthma Caregiver's Quality of Life Questionnaire	Juniper et al.[18]	Self-complete	13 items 2 sub-scales Asthma caregiver	(a) Activity limitations (b) Emotional function
St George's Respiratory Questionnaire	Jones et al.[10]	Self-complete	76 items 3 sub-scales Adult asthma or COPD	(a) Symptoms (b) Activity (c) Impact

chronic obstructive pulmonary disease (COPD), whereas the other scales have been designed for either asthma or COPD, and again, this is reflected in item content.

Finally, scales for children require very different items compared to those for adults, and in one case, different scales are used for children of different ages (Childhood Asthma Questionnaire[14]). Young children are asked to respond to questions using smiley faces, with questions such as: 'Which picture describes how you feel about running around at playtimes?' and 'Which picture describes how you feel when you cough?'.

Generic scales

Generic scales are designed for any disease and may therefore contain items that are irrelevant to a particular patient group. This fact, coupled with their weaker sensitivity to change, may lead some to conclude that generic scales have little clinical use. This, however, is not the case as some generic scales include items which, for one reason or another, are missing from disease-specific scales. Thus, one questionnaire appropriate for advanced illness (the McGill Quality of Life Questionnaire[21]) measures the existential or spiritual domain of life quality that is neglected in the disease-specific scales. Items include: 'My personal existence is utterly meaningless and without purpose'; 'In achieving life goals I have made no progress whatsoever'; and 'I feel good about myself as a person'. Another palliative care questionnaire applicable to any illness (the Missoula-VITAS quality of life index[22]) includes items describing positive experiences in a number of dimensions including transcendence which are not measured in disease-specific questionnaires, simply because the disease-specific questionnaires are not designed to assess QoL in palliative care. For example, items in this questionnaire include: 'I have a greater sense of connection to all things now than I did before my illness'; 'I have a better sense of meaning in my life now than I have had in the past'; and 'I am more satisfied with myself as a person now than I was before my illness'. Finally, the Silver Lining Questionnaire[23] also includes items that measure the extent to which illness has been a positive experience (rather than being less of a negative experience) and thus provides an entirely different perspective on QoL, but one which may be very relevant to the patient. Items include: 'I appreciate life more because of my illness'; 'My illness made me a better person'; and 'My illness helped me find myself'. Thus, although not all generic scales provide a more sensitive measure of QoL than disease-specific scales in respiratory disease, some undoubtedly do (see Table 3.4).

Idiographic scales

The Schedule for the Evaluation of Individual Quality of Life (SEIQoL)[27] is the best-known example of an idiographic questionnaire. Patients are asked to describe five aspects of their life which best characterizes their quality of life to them. Then patients are asked to rate each of those five aspects in terms of how good or bad they are. The result of this procedure is that there is a unique scale of QoL for each patient, because the meaning of QoL differs between patients. That is, the measurement of QoL is individualized rather than normative.

Critics of the individualized approach suggest that a scale which differs between patients is not particularly useful in making the between-patient comparisons needed for clinical trials, though certainly this approach has value as a clinical tool. Critics of the more conventional normative approach, however, argue that although the same questionnaire is given to different patients, in practice different patients interpret that same questionnaire differently so in practical terms the patients are actually receiving different questionnaires.[28] These different views are currently unresolved. Perhaps there is room for both approaches.

Table 3.4 Generic scales

Measure administration	Authors	Mode of administration	Number of items and subscales	Subscales
McGill Quality of Life Questionnaire	Cohen et al.[21]	Self-complete	16 core items, 2 additional questions 5 sub-scales	(a) Physical symptoms (b) Physical well-being (c) Psychological (d) Existential (e) Support
Missoula-VITAS quality of life index	Byock and Merriman[22]		25 items 5 sub-scales	(a) Symptom (b) Function (c) Interpersonal (d) Well-being (e) Transcendent
Nottingham Health Profile	Hunt et al.[26]	Self-complete	38 items in Part I 7 items in Part II 6 sub-scales in Part I	(a) Physical mobility (b) Pain (c) Energy level (d) Emotional reactions (e) Sleep (f) Social isolation
SF-36 Health Survey	Ware and Sherbourne[24]	Self-complete or interviewer administered	36 items 8 sub-scales	(a) Physical functioning (b) Role limitation – physical (c) Bodily pain (d) General health (e) Vitality (f) Social functioning (g) Role limitation – emotional (h) Mental health
Silver Lining Questionnaire	Sodergren and Hyland[23]	Self-complete	38 items No sub-scales	None
Sickness Impact Profile	Bergner et al.[25]	Self-complete or interviewer administered	136 items 12 sub-scales	(a) Sleep and rest (b) Body care and movement (c) Home management (d) Mobility (e) Ambulation (f) Work (g) Recreation and pastime activities (h) Feeding (i) Emotional behaviour (j) Alertness/intellectual behaviour (k) Communication (l) Social interaction

Response options

All three kinds of QoL questionnaire – generic, disease specific, and idiographic – require the patient to respond on a scale of response options. For example, the Asthma Bother Profile uses scales of varying levels of bother: 'No bother at all'; 'Minor irritation'; 'Slight bother'; 'Moderate bother'; 'A lot of bother'; 'Makes my life a misery', but for some scales the type of response option varies between items. As a general rule, increasing response options up to about seven increases the discriminability of that item, so items with more rather than less (e.g. two) response options have some advantages. The disadvantage of having more response options is that the item takes longer to complete. Hence, there is a balance between number of items and response options for an equivalent length of questionnaire completion time. If many items are required, then a simpler form of response option is needed to prevent questionnaire completion becoming over-burdensome.

Response options can consist of numbers with end-point descriptions, multiple verbal descriptors (sometimes added to numbers), and visual analogue scales (VAS). Early research which has later been confirmed[20] shows that VAS are the least reliable, whereas scales which include multiple verbal descriptors are most reliable.

Statistical matters

One of the difficulties encountered by QoL researchers is that questionnaires are sometimes returned partly completed. The researcher then has the option of including data from the partially completed questionnaire in the eventual analysis or excluding it. Of course, some questionnaires are poorly constructed and this encourages missing data, but as a general rule missing data indicate poor competence in questionnaire completion. A good rule of thumb is to include as valid data questionnaires that miss less than 10% of data. Others may be considered unreliable. Test constructors should, however, examine missing responses to items in the process of test development to ensure that, where missing items occur, it is fault of the patient and not of the test.

Responses to many scales are normally distributed, leading to the inference that parametric tests can be employed. However, QoL scales are ordinal scales rather than ratio scales. Even with scales using weighted items, there is no clear evidence that the scale has equal interval properties. Although parametric statistics are often used, it is worth bearing in mind that the underlying assumption of the scale is that it is non-parametric.

Implications of QoL for treatment selection and patient management: the individualized perspective

Whether it is measured by a normative scale or an individualized scale, QoL is something which is highly individual. What is important for one patient may not be important for another. This means that in order to optimize QoL for an individual patient, the clinician needs to individualize treatment rather than to select treatment on a routine basis.

Individualization of treatment is recommended for two reasons, physiological and psychological. Clinical experience shows that some patients show a better physiological response to one drug than to another. The reason for patient specificity to drug treatment is not well understood. For example, sometimes a patient will respond better to one inhaled steroid rather than another, whereas another patient may respond best to a different one. The effect of long-acting β_2-agonists also tends to vary between patients. These individual differences in response mean that conclusions drawn from clinical trials should be treated with caution. Although one drug may be, on average, better than another, this does not mean that it will always be better.

A second reason for individualization of treatment is psychological. Aggressive treatment is more burdensome for some patients than for others. Indeed, intentional non-compliance can be the consequence of patients judging that the burden of treatment outweighs its benefit. For some patients, improvement in physiology has little benefit in terms of QoL. If a patient wishes only to watch television, then improved asthma control may make little difference. However, if a patient wishes to engage in sport, small physiological gains can have substantial QoL advantages. The 'minimal significant clinical gain' may vary substantially between patients.

Keypoints

◆ Management of a patient's QoL requires an individualized approach to treatment. This approach can be assisted by questionnaire, of which there are many kinds

◆ There is no substitute for careful, humane understanding of the patient

◆ The clinician needs to find a way of managing the patient where multiple objectives are affected differently by different courses of action

◆ Good QoL is just one objective, albeit an important one, in the clinical management of patients

References

1 Singer, cited in *The quality of life concept*. United States Environmental Protection Agency Office of Research and Monitoring Environmental Studies Division, 1974.

2 Szalai, A. The meaning of comparative research on the quality of life. In: A. Szalai, and F.M. Andrews (eds) *The quality of life, comparative studies*. London: Sage Publications, 1980; 7–21.

3 Schipper, H., Clinch, J., and Powell, V. Definitions and conceptual issues. In: B. Spilker (ed.) *Quality of life assessments in clinical trials*. New York: Raven Press, 1990; 11–24.

4 Calman, K.C. Quality of life in cancer patients – an hypothesis. *J Med Ethics* 1984; **10**: 124–7.

5 DeHaes, J.C.J.M., and van Knippenberg, F.C.E. The quality of life of cancer patients: a review of the literature. *Soc Sci Med* 1985; **20**: 809–17.

6 Hayry, M. Measuring the quality of life: Why, how and what? *Theoret Med* 1991; **12**: 97–116.

7 Clinch, J.J., and Schipper, H. Quality of life assessment in palliative care. In: D. Doyle, G.W.C. Hanks, and N. MacDonald (eds) *Oxford textbook of palliative medicine*. Oxford: Oxford University Press, 1993; 61–9.

8 World Health Organization. The constitution of the World Health Organization. *WHO Chron* 1947; **1**: 29.

9 Guyatt, G.H., Berman, L.B., Townsend, M., Pugsley, S.O., and Chambers, L.W. A measure of quality of life for clinical trials in chronic lung disease. *Thorax* 1987; **42**: 773–8.

10 Jones, P.W., Quirk, F.H., and Baveystock, C.M. The St. George's Respiratory Questionnaire. *Respir Med* 1991; **85**(suppl B): 25–31.

11 Juniper, E.F., Guyatt, G.H., Epstein, R.S., *et al*. Evaluation of impairment of health related quality of life in asthma: Development of a questionnaire for use in clinical trials. *Thorax* 1992; **47**: 76–83.

12 Hyland, M.E., Ley, A., Fisher, D.W., and Woodward, V. Measurement of psychological distress in asthma and asthma management programmes. *Br J Clin Psychol* 1995; **34**: 601–11.

13 Hyland, M.E., Singh, S.J., Sodergren, S.C., and Morgan, M.P.L. Development of a shortened version of the breathing problems questionnaire suitable for use in a pulmonary rehabilitation clinic: a purpose-specific, disease-specific questionnaire. *Qual Life Res* 1998; **7**: 227–33.

14 French, D.J., and Christie, M.J. Developing outcome measures for children: the example of 'Quality of Life' assessment for paediatric asthma. In: A. Hutchinson, E. McColl, M.J. Christie, and C.L. Riccalton (eds) *Health outcomes in primary and outpatient care.* Chur, Switzerland: Harwood Academic, 1995.

15 Hyland, M.E., Finnis, S., and Irvine, S.H. A scale for assessing quality of life in adult asthma sufferers. *J Psychosom Res* 1991; **35**: 99–110.

16 Hyland, M.E., Bott, J., Singh, S., and Kenyon, C.A.P. Domains, constructs and the development of the breathing problems questionnaire. *Qual Life Res* 1994; **3**: 245–56.

17 Juniper, E.F., Guyatt, G.H., Feeny, D.H., *et al.* Measuring quality of life in children with asthma. *Qual Life Res* 1996; **5**: 35–46.

18 Juniper, E.F., Guyatt, G.H., Feeny, D.H., *et al.* Measuring quality of life in the parents of children with asthma. *Qual Life Res* 1996; **5**: 27–34.

19 EORTC. The European Organisation for Research and Treatment of Cancer QLQ-C30: a quality of life instrument for use in international clinical trials in oncology. *J Natl Cancer Inst* 1993; **85**: 365–76.

20 Hyland, M.E. The Living with Asthma Questionnaire. *Respir Med* 1991; **85**(suppl B): 13–16.

21 Cohen, S.R., Mount, B.M., Strobel, M.G., and Bui, F. The McGill Quality of Life Questionnaire: a measure of quality of life appropriate for people with advanced disease. A preliminary study of validity and acceptability. *Palliative Med* 1995; **9**: 207–19.

22 Byock, I.R., and Merriman, M.P. Measuring the quality of life for patients with terminal illness: the Missoula-VITAS ® quality of life index. *Palliative Med* 1998; **12**: 231–44.

23 Sodergren, S.C., and Hyland, M.E. What are the positive consequences of illness? *Psychol Health* (in press).

24 Ware, J.E., and Sherbourne, C.D. The MOS 36 item Short-Form Health Survey. *Med Care* 1992; **30**: 473–83.

25 Bergner, M., Bobbit, R.A., Carter, W.B., and Gilson, B.S. The Sickness Impact Profile: Development and final revision of a health status measure. *Med Care* 1981; **19**: 787–805.

26 Hunt, S., McEwen, J., and McKenna, S. *Measuring health status.* London: Croom Helm, 1986.

27 O'Boyle, C.A., McGee, H., and Joyce, C.R.B. Quality of life: assessing the individual. In: R. Fitzpatrick (ed.) *Advances in medical sociology.* Greenwich, CT: JAI Press, 1994; 159–80.

28 Hyland, M.E. Defining and measuring quality of life in medicine. *JAMA* 1998; **279**: 430–1.

29 Hyland, M.E., and Sodergren, S.C. Development of a new type of global quality of life scale, and comparison of performance and preference for 12 global scales. *Qual Life Res* 1996; **5**: 469–80.

Chapter 4

Complementary medicine for respiratory diseases

Jacqueline Filshie and Adrian White

Currently there is unprecedented worldwide interest in non-drug treatments for a whole range of conditions. In financial terms, the out-of-pocket expenses for complementary medicine in the USA are greater than those for hospitalization.[1] Some patients look for alternatives to orthodox medicine in order to avoid side effects: one study has shown that drugs appear to be between the fourth and sixth largest cause of death in the USA.[2] Complementary medicine is also popular in its own right for a variety of reasons, including the perception that it is natural and therefore safe, and the fact that patients are frequently offered long consultations. On the other hand, complementary medicine has its drawbacks: its evidence base is often sparse, it offers the opportunity for exploitation in unscrupulous hands, and particular therapies may produce adverse psychological effects such as guilt and false memory syndrome. Moreover, although the side-effect profile may be less than that of drugs, it is not necessarily negligible.

Ernst *et al.*[3] defined complementary medicine as 'diagnosis, treatment and/or prevention which complements mainstream medicine by contributing to a common whole, by satisfying a demand not met by orthodoxy, or by diversifying the conceptual frameworks of medicine'. In effect, unconventional medicine includes therapies which range from **alternative** via **complementary** to **integrated** as the amount of supporting evidence, and acceptance by the medical profession, increases. Acupuncture, for example, is generally regarded as complementary but in fact is already highly integrated into some aspects of health care in the UK, being used in 84% of pain clinics[4] and 86% chronic pain services sampled.[5] The evidence for its neurophysiological mechanisms is considerable, and for its clinical efficacy moderate.[6] It is even taught in some British medical schools.

Space permits the inclusion of only a number of commonly used complementary therapies here (Table 4.1), in the management of asthma, chronic obstructive airways disease and advanced cancer-related breathlessness.

Asthma

Surveys of use of complementary therapies

Complementary medicine in its widest sense, i.e. including self-management and over-the counter products, is very widely used by patients with asthma. For example, out of 4741 adult asthmatics who responded to a questionnaire survey sent to 17 000 members of the National Asthma Campaign, 60% of those with moderate asthma, and 70% of those with severe asthma, have used complementary therapies to treat their condition.[7] This result can only be seen as a guide to prevalence of complementary medicine because of the survey's low response rate of

Table 4.1 Complementary medicine therapies used in respiratory disease

Acupuncture Chiropractic and osteopathy Healing	Massage (including aromatherapy and reflexology)
Herbalism Homoeopathy	Mind–body techniques (including hypnosis meditation, relaxation, and yoga)

28%. In response to the question, 'Which complementary therapies have you used to treat your asthma?', the most popular responses among adults were breathing techniques (30%), followed by homoeopathy (12%), herbal medicine (11%), yoga (9%), acupuncture (7%), and osteopathy (3%). Other therapies were used by 1% or less. Between 40 and 45% of respondents claimed to have benefited at least moderately from their treatment. Over 50% had spent less than £50 on complementary medicine, but about 1% had spent more than £500.

The National Asthma Campaign survey was also analysed for the use of complementary therapies by children: 33% had tried one or more therapies, the most popular being homoeopathy (15%), breathing techniques (15%), herbalism (6%), and osteopathy (2%).[8] Another survey of 55 children aged 1–6 years attending an asthma clinic in Australia found that a higher proportion (55%) had used complementary therapies, in some cases several.[9] In this instance, the most popular therapies were relaxation/meditation (28%) and massage (20%). Other commonly used therapies were diets (18%), positive therapy (16%), and vitamins (12%).

In spite of the frequency with which asthmatic patients use complementary medicine, it cannot be assumed that practitioners are necessarily skilled or experienced in treating asthma: in a survey of 101 complementary therapists, respiratory problems accounted for less than 2% of all presenting complaints.[10]

An effective non-drug treatment for asthma is appealing, especially in view of the concern whether current treatment is contributing to the morbidity and mortality of the disease.[11] As 15% of patients with methacholine-induced breathlessness could not identify their own airway obstruction even when it was marked,[12] objective measurements of lung function are recommended. The placebo effect can be important in asthmatics; Butler and Steptoe[13] induced asthma with a sham bronchoconstrictor and then demonstrated that it could be prevented by pretreatment with a placebo that had been described as a powerful new drug. The placebo or non-specific component of any complementary medicine may be powerful, in addition to any specific effect of therapy.

There are numerous aetiological factors associated with asthma – for example, allergens, exercise, stress, and more recently pollution – but this subject is covered elsewhere.

Acupuncture

Evidence for the efficacy for acupuncture for asthma has been reviewed by several authors.[14–19] Acupuncture has been shown to release endogenous opioids, and steroids, and to affect autonomic function.[20–23] It also releases oxytocin which has powerful sedating actions[24] and has effects on the immune system.[25] Most conventional drugs stimulate only one receptor, whereas acupuncture may affect multiple sites. In addition drugs are less likely to have as perfect agonist receptor matching as endogenously generated substances released by acupuncture.

There are more than a dozen randomized controlled trials (RCTs) of acupuncture for asthma, using a variety of regimens and number of treatments for different forms of asthma; their conclusions are conflicting. This is partly because there is no consensus on an ideal needle-free placebo, and needles used as a control placed superficially or away from acupuncture sites do exert an effect. Choice of control is particularly complex.[26,27] Some negative studies have been criticized for using as the control procedure genuine acupuncture points that other workers have argued could well have a positive effect on the condition. In other words the comparisons involved two different forms or 'doses' of acupuncture rather than acupuncture versus a placebo treatment. Jobst attempted to address this problem in his review on the subject and concluded that 14 out of 16 studies had a positive outcome when both real and sham needling results were compared with the original baseline levels.[18]

Linde *et al.* reviewed the acupuncture literature for treatment of asthma for a Cochrane Review.[28] They included RCTs with an observation period of at least a week. In 59 publications they found 15 RCTs. They chose to exclude five trials of experimentally induced asthma, one trial on spontaneous asthma, and two on short-term effects on lung function. This left seven for analysis. They included trials where objective and subjective parameters were measured. Five of these trials included adults, only one covered children, and one included both children and adults. The methodology varied greatly between trials; five involved needle insertion and two lasers. Six trials used a formula approach and only one individualized treatments. This is in contrast with clinical practice when treatments are frequently modified, on the basis of individual response, throughout a course of therapy. All used some form of 'dummy acupuncture': in four trials stimulation was given at a non-point, but in three trials, true acupuncture points were used, by no means a true 'inert' placebo.

Their main results showed two acupuncture studies to be superior to 'dummy' treatment. No significant difference was found between treatment and sham groups for the remaining five. Data on lung function tests was inconsistently presented and peak expiratory flow rate in three studies was not statistically significantly different between groups. In the remaining four trials no marked effect compared with sham was found.

It was disappointing that only 7 RCTs were included in the review, with only 174 patients in total, and no consistency of sample, design, intervention, and outcome measures. The conclusion was that it is not yet possible to make any recommendations to patients or physicians/acupuncturists about the practice of acupuncture for asthma, given the existing data. Linde *et al.*[29] highlighted the need for quality research and recommend the inclusion of a third 'no treatment' control group in any further studies. Patients should be matched for age, duration of asthma, and severity of lung function abnormalities. The mode of therapy – individualized or not – should be very carefully addressed, so that the treatment regimen is not as artificially prescriptive as most trials are to date. The challenge to acupuncture is particularly complex as there are so many variables to include such as needle depth, sites, duration of insertion, mode of stimulation, etc.

Nevertheless, in view of the wide-ranging effects acupuncture has on neurophysiological function, which can modulate respiratory function, it merits further serious consideration.

Chiropractic and osteopathy

Chiropractic treatment aims to improve the function of the lungs by freeing the movement of the spine and reducing muscle tension in the intercostal muscles. However, two RCTs of chiropractic compared with simulated chiropractic showed no demonstrable effect.[30,31]

Healing

Unfortunately there are no reports on controlled studies on the use of healing for asthma to date.

Herbalism and dietary treatments

No herbal treatments for asthma are included in one modern book of rational phytotherapy,[32] and no clinical trials are described. Ginkgo has been used in Chinese herbal medicine for some years, and there is evidence that ginkgolides may reduce the platelet-activating factor (PAF), an inflammatory mediator. In one randomized controlled crossover study in 21 children, Hsieh[33] found that the ginkgolide inhibited bronchoconstriction induced by PAF and allergen, but not by methacholine. Other Chinese herbal remedies may provide a source of ephedrine which may be effective (though not clinically reliable unless prepared in standardized dosage). A systematic review of Chinese herbal remedies could not make firm recommendations, largely because of inadequate trial methodology.[34]

Dietary approaches to the treatment of asthma are steeped in controversy and emotion. Clearly atopy can be very important in precipitating asthma attacks, but care should be taken to distinguish between the roles of proven inhaled allergens, known ingested major allergens such as peanut, and the often unfounded diagnosis of 'food allergy' and subsequent dietary manipulation. Various complementary approaches to investigation and treatment of allergy have been proposed.

Conventional management with desensitization by serial injections of known allergens may be effective, although a recent rigorous study in which children were randomized to receive a course of injections of either a mixture of up to seven aeroallergens or placebo found no difference in use of medication over the subsequent 2 years.[35] Partial remission of asthma was noted in about 30% of both groups. A recent meta-analysis of current methods of house dust-mite eradication concluded that they seem to be ineffective at improving the symptoms of asthma.[36] Methods of identifying allergens in which unorthodox laboratories test various body samples have been convincingly shown to be very unreliable.[37]

Exclusion diets often improve patients' symptoms at least temporarily, which may be a non-specific effect seen with many conditions. Rigorous tests with randomized double-blind placebo-controlled challenges demonstrate that 2–6% of asthmatic patients have genuine food sensitivity.[38] It is reasonable to exclude these known allergens from the diet of this small group of patients. Another hypothesis, that avoiding common allergens in late pregnancy would reduce the incidence of atopy including asthma in the children, was not supported in a long-term RCT.[39]

The role of vitamins, or vitamin depletion, in the management of asthma is still not established; Baker *et al.* found reduced dietary intake of vitamins A, C, and E, as well as selenium and magnesium, in children with brittle asthma:[40] Cohen *et al.* found vitamin C to be protective against exercise-induced asthma,[41] and some children have been shown to obtain a reduction in the severity of exercise-induced asthma with vitamin C. Hasselmark *et al.* found that selenium supplements in children produced an improvement in symptoms that did not reach statistical significance.[42] The role of the ratio of ingested essential fatty acids has also been discussed: omega-3 fatty acids are potentially beneficial since they compete against the formation of an important inflammatory mediator, arachidonic acid, from omega-6 fatty acids. It has been suggested that the increase in omega-6 fatty acids in the diet over recent years may have contributed to increased symptoms of asthma.[43] It is therefore plausible that fish oil (high in omega-3 fatty acids) may be protective for asthma. This hypothesis was not supported by a survey of young adults in Norway.[44] However the situation may be extremely complex, involving not only the ratio of n–3 to n–6 fatty acids but also individual responsiveness. One study found that some patients with asthma responded positively to increased fish oil in the diet, but others were made worse.[45] The question must be regarded as still unresolved. An RCT of evening primrose oil showed no benefit in asthma.[46]

Homoeopathy

Homoeopathy for asthma has been the subject of rather few studies, but that of Reilly *et al.* counts as one of the most rigorous trials of this therapy.[47] In this study 28 patients with allergic asthma were skin-tested to identify the particular allergen they were sensitive to. This allergen was then prepared homoeopathically. Patients were randomized to receive either the genuine remedy or an identical placebo and were measured for 4 weeks. A significant difference in symptom scores appeared, in favour of homoeopathy, and was accompanied by favourable (but not statistically significant) trends in peak flow and forced vital capacity. This study was included with two others in a Cochrane Review.[29] Of the other two trials, one showed positive changes in lung function tests and medication use, the other found an improvement in both homoeopathy and placebo groups, with no difference between them. The homoeopathy employed in these trials was not typical of standard practice (they used either immunotherapy or standardized medication for all participants) and therefore the results could not be combined quantitatively. The authors concluded that 'Evidence was insufficient to assess the possible role of homoeopathy in the treatment of asthma'.[29] More relevant studies are required, involving rigorous design with homoeopathic management individualized for each subject, randomization to a control group who receive identical placebo, and measurement of both clinical and quality of life outcomes over a prolonged time period.

Massage, aromatherapy, and reflexology

Massage is calming and of potential benefit, but has not been the subject of many RCTs. In one recent study, children were randomized to receive 20 min of either massage or relaxation instruction from their parents, every night before going to bed.[48] The children were stratified by age at the start of the study. Those aged 6–8 years had improvements in short-term anxiety and lung function at 30 days, which was significantly better than the relaxation controls. In the older children, aged 9–11, there was no difference between the groups. If these results are confirmed, massage could prove to be an easy and valuable therapy for young children. Parents also reported that their own anxiety was lessened, possibly through being able to take an active part in treatment.

Mind/body techniques

Asthma is clearly of multiple origins, but in many cases attacks are triggered by emotional events; highly anxious subjects also appear more likely to suffer asthma and be perhaps more difficult to manage therapeutically. Therefore, procedures that aim to calm the mind have been extensively used, mainly progressive relaxation, or transcendental meditation. A systematic review has located five such RCTs for asthma prevention, spanning the years from 1975 to 1995.[49] Two early studies showed a small effect, but the three remaining, more rigorous, studies showed no sustained effect on either symptoms or lung function. In the subgroup of children in whom anxiety was high and attacks were triggered by emotion, there was no effect.

The acute beneficial effects of relaxation on asthma have been demonstrated in two RCTs,[50,51] but another study found a reduction of lung function, possibly by reduction of sympathetic drive.[52]

It appears, then, that relaxation may have short-term effects but is of no proven long-term benefit in asthma. It may seem somewhat surprising that the benefit is not sustained. One reason might be that simple muscle relaxation methods soon lose their novelty, so that subjects fail to continue practising them. The enthusiasm that can be associated with particular, special techniques may provide the necessary sustained motivation, and two studies have suggested that this may be the case. Autogenic training was found to be superior to supportive psychotherapy in improving lung function;[53] and biofeedback was superior to sham biofeedback in improving lung function, though not symptoms.[54]

Hypnotherapy combines mental relaxation with a psychological technique that can include suggestion (for example, dealing with stressful situations more calmly) and sometimes psychotherapy (such as identifying previously unrecognized stress). Four RCTs have shown the benefit of hypnosis and autohypnosis, with improvement either in lung function, symptoms, or emergency hospital attendance for asthma crises.[55–58] Hypnosis can induce a feeling of calm that could make the patient underestimate the severity of symptoms, and patients should be warned.

Buteyko breathing technique

Breathing techniques in general are regarded as conventional, but a new method, known as the Buteyko breathing technique (BBT), has been widely publicized. It is based on the theory that people with asthma hyperventilate, and the resultant hypocapnia increases bronchoconstriction. The hypocapnia is thought to increase the oxygen-binding of the haemoglobin, so reducing oxygenation of the tissues. It is also believed to increase bronchoconstriction, although there is not general agreement among respiratory physiologists that this actually happens. The aim of BBT is to train asthma patients to breath more slowly and thereby raise the blood carbon dioxide levels to normal. One study with 39 volunteers compared a course of BBT to conventional breathing exercises.[59] It confirmed the hypocapnia and hyperventilation of people with asthma. A 3-month course of BBT, compared to conventional breathing exercises combined with education, reduced the minute volume, but did not change the concentration of carbon dioxide in the blood. There was no change in peak flow rates or use of inhaled steroids, but β_2-agonist use was significantly reduced and quality of life significantly improved. No firm conclusions can be drawn because of possible confounding factors such as the increased contact with the patients of the Buteyko trainer, and further studies are in progress.

A breathing training apparatus, known as the Pink City Lung Exerciser, has been compared with a placebo version in two crossover studies.[60,61] The apparatus is designed to slow the rate of breathing so that expiration takes twice as long as inspiration, and therefore has much in common with BBT. In the first study, an improvement in peak flow was found, but the second study showed only a trend towards improvement of lung function tests. Both sample sizes were small.

The practice of yoga combines the potential benefits of muscle relaxation through postures and mental relaxation through meditation, together with the slowing down of the breathing rate mentioned above. Formal yoga training for asthma has produced equivocal results. Nagarathna and Nagendra[62] randomized 106 asthma patients to an intensive yoga training programme or no extra therapy; those who continued to use yoga regularly, on at least alternate days, during the follow-up period of 4.5 years showed a significant reduction in asthma drug use, number of asthma attacks, and increase in peak flow rate, compared with the matched controls. This result is marred by the fact that nearly half of the treatment group failed to continue to practice yoga. Fluge *et al.*[63] found that 3 weeks' yoga training, followed by regular practice, improved the mental state of asthma patients but had no effect on lung function. On the other hand, conventional breathing exercises both improved the mental state and lung function, significantly. A smaller RCT of yoga practice three times a week for 16 weeks, compared with no additional treatment, found no effect on pulmonary function although the yoga group did record a significant degree of relaxation and positive attitude.[64] This negative result may be due to the short study period or small sample size, and larger studies of the effect of yoga on asthma are justified.

Chronic obstructive airways disease (COPD)

One RCT on acupuncture for COPD showed significant benefit of traditional acupuncture over the control group for 6-min walking distance and subjective breathlessness scores, but not for pulmonary function tests.[65] Maa *et al.* showed that real acupressure reduced dyspnoea measured on a visual analogue scale (VAS), as compared to sham acupressure;[66] however, real acupressure exacerbated peripheral sensory symptoms. An RCT with COPD showed yogic breathing exercises to be superior to physiotherapy breathing exercises for exercise tolerance, recovery following exercise, and control over acute attacks of shortness of breath.[67]

Advanced cancer-related breathlessness

A pilot study explored the use of acupuncture for advanced cancer-related breathlessness which was refractory to conventional treatment.[68] Twenty patients who were breathless at rest due to primary or secondary malignancy received treatment with four fine needles, two over the upper sternum and one in each hand. Needles were not stimulated and were left for 10 min, and assessments were performed over the following 90 min. There was a significant ($p < 0.005$) reduction in the mean breathlessness as measured by VAS and Borg score, improvement relaxation and anxiety levels measured by the HAD score, and an objective reduction in respiratory rate. Fourteen of the patients (70%) reported marked global improvement in symptoms. Semi-permanent indwelling studs were used to prolong the control of dyspnoea, being massaged before exercise or during panic attacks (Figure 4.1). Semi-permanent studs are being

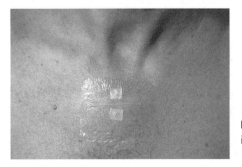

Fig. 4.1 Semi-permanent indwelling studs.

used widely for up to 4 weeks at a time, using a clear plastic dressing in the upper sternal position. Their use in a within-patient crossover trial is currently being formally tested, but results are not available. The patient must be able to massage the studs comfortably in the clinic before they are sent home with the studs in situ.

It is particularly important that complementary practitioners should not attempt extreme measures (such as severe dietary restriction) in terminally ill patients without any evidence of effectiveness.

Conclusion

A large number of studies have been performed with different forms of complementary medicine for patients with asthma and, not surprisingly, the results have been mixed. Funding for RCTs is a problem, since drug companies have little interest in funding non-drug treatments and many orthodox doctors have dismissed most forms of complementary medicine as quackery. Now that experienced research teams are becoming interested in studying these therapies, we hope for more definitive and comprehensive answers than we can present today.

Keypoints

- ◆ The public are increasingly seeking more natural alternatives to conventional medicine
- ◆ Evidence from RCTs is accumulating: acupuncture, homoeopathy and yoga look promising
- ◆ Early observational work on acupuncture for chronic obstructive airways disease and advanced cancer related breathlessness show promise for future research
- ◆ Complementary therapies should be rigorously testing, so that patients can be better informed about which treatments will benefit them most
- ◆ Side-effects of complementary therapies do occur, though rarely; more information is needed about the benefit to risk profile of each therapy

References

1 Eisenberg, D.M., Kessler, R.C., Foster, C., *et al.* Unconventional medicine in the United States. Prevalence, costs, and patterns of use. *N Engl J Med* 1993; **328**(4): 246–52.

2 Lazarou, J., Pomeranz, B.H., and Corey, P.N. Incidence of adverse drug reactions in hospitalized patients. A meta analysis of prospective studies. *JAMA* 1998; **279**(15): 1200–5.

3 Ernst, E., Resch, K-L., Mills, S., *et al.* Complementary medicine – a definition. *Br J Gen Pr* 1995; **45**: 506.

4 Woollam, C.H.M., and Jackson, A.O. Acupuncture in the management of chronic pain. *Anaesthesia* 1998; **53**: 589–603.

5 Clinical Standards Advisory Group (CSAG). *Services for patients with pain.* London: Department of Health; 2000. Report obtainable from: Department of Health, PO Box 777, London SE1 6XH.

6 Filshie, J., and White, A. *Medical acupuncture: a western scientific approach.* Edinburgh: Churchill Livingstone, 1998.

7 Ernst, E. Complementary therapies for asthma: what patients use. *J Asthma* 1998; **35**: 667–71.

8 Ernst, E. Use of complementary therapies in childhood asthma. *Pediatr Asthma Allergy Immunol* 1998; **12**: 29–32.

9 Andrews, L., Lokuge, S., Sawyer, M., *et al.* The use of alternative therapies by children with asthma: a brief report. *J Paediatr Child Health* 1998; **34**: 131–4.

10 Thomas, K.J., Carr, J., Westlake, L., and Williams, B.T. Use of non-orthodox and conventional health care in Great Britain. *BMJ* 1991; **302**: 207–10.

11 Barnes, P.J., and Chung, K.F. Difficult asthma. *BMJ* 1989; **299**: 695–8.

12 Rubinfeld, A.R., and Pain, M.C.F. Perception of asthma. *Lancet* 1976; **1**: 882–4.

13 Butler, C., and Steptoe, A. Placebo responses: an experimental study of psychophysiological processes in asthmatic volunteers. *Br J Clin Psychol* 1986; **25**: 173–83.

14 Vincent, C.A., and Richardson, P.H. Acupuncture for some common disorders: a review of evaluative research. *J R Coll Gen Pract* 1987; **37**: 77–81.

15 Aldridge, D., and Pietroni, P.C. Clinical assessment of acupuncture in asthma therapy: discussion paper. *J R Soc Med* 1987; **80**: 222–4.

16 Kleijnen, J., Ter Riet, G., and Knipschild, P. Acupuncture and asthma: a review of controlled trials. *Thorax* 1991; **46**: 799–802.

17 Lane, D.J., and Lane, T.V. Alternative and complementary medicine for asthma. *Thorax* 1991; **46**: 787–97.

18 Jobst, K.A. A critical analysis of acupuncture in pulmonary disease: efficacy and safety of the acupuncture needle. *J Alternative Complementary Med* 1995; **1**(1): 57–85.

19 Lewith, G.T., and Watkins, A.D. Unconventional therapies in asthma: an overview. *Allergy* 1996; **51**: 761–9.

20 Stux, G., and Pomeranz, B. *Basics of acupuncture*, 4th edn. Berlin: Springer, 1998.

21 Bowsher, D. Mechanisms of acupuncture. In: J. Filshie, and A. White (eds) *Medical acupuncture – a western scientific approach*. Edinburgh: Churchill Livingstone, 1998; 69–82.

22 White, A. Neurophysiology of acupuncture analgesia. In: E. Ernst, and A. White, (eds) *Acupuncture – a scientific appraisal*. Oxford: Butterworth-Heinemann, 1999; 60–92.

23 Lundeberg, T. Effects of sensory stimulation (acupuncture) on circulatory and immune systems. In: E. Ernst, and A. White, (eds) *Acupuncture – a scientific appraisal*. Oxford: Butterworth-Heinemann, 1999; 93–106.

24 Uvnas-Moberg, K. Physiological and endocrine effects of social contact. *Ann N Y Acad Sci* 1997; **807**: 146–63.

25 Jonsdottir, I.H. Physical exercise, acupuncture and immune function. *Acupunct Med* 1999; **17**(1): 50–3.

26 Hammerschlag, R. Methodological and ethical issues in clinical trials of acupuncture. *J Alternative Complementary Med* 1998; **4**(2): 159–71.

27 Filshie, J., and Cummings, T.M. Western medical acupuncture. In: E. Ernst, and A. White (eds) *Acupuncture – a scientific appraisal*. Oxford: Butterworth-Heinemann, 1999; 31–59.

28 Linde, K., and Jobst, K.A. Homoeopathy for chronic asthma (Cochrane Review). *Cochrane Library* 1998; Issue 2.

29 Linde, K., Jobst, K., and Panton, J. Acupuncture for the treatment of asthma bronchiale. *Cochrane Database of Systematic Reviews* 1997; Issue 2.

30 Balon, J., Aker, P.D., Crowther, E.R., *et al.* A comparison of active and simulated chiropractic manipulation as adjunctive treatment for childhood asthma. *N Engl J Med* 1998; **339**: 1013–20.

31 Nielsen, N.H., Bronfort, G., Bendix, T., Madsen, F., and Weeke, B. Chronic asthma and chiropractic spinal manipulation: a randomised clinical trial. *Clin Exp Allergy* 1995; **25**: 80–8.

32 Schulz, V., Haensel, R., and Tyler, V.E. *Rational phytotherapy*. Berlin: Springer, 1998.

33 Hsieh, K-H. Effects of PAF antagonist, BN52021, on the PAF-, methacholine-, and allergen-induced bronchoconstriction in asthmatic children. *Chest* 1991; **99**: 877–82.

34 Liu, C., and Douglas, R.M. Chinese herbal medicines in the treatment of acute respiratory infections: a review of randomised controlled clinical trials. *Med J Aust* 1998; **169**: 579–82.

35 Adkinson, N.F., Eggleston, P.A., Eney, D., *et al.* A controlled trial of immunotherapy for asthma in allergic children. *N Engl J Med* 1997; **336**: 324–31.

36 Gotzsche, P.C., Hammarquist, C., and Burr, M. House dust mite control measures in the management of asthma: meta-analysis. *BMJ* 1998; **317**: 1105–10.

37 *Which way to health.* London: Consumers' Association, 1998.

38 Monteleone, C.A., and Sherman, A.R. Nutrition and asthma. *Arch Intern Med* 1997; **157**: 23–34.

39 Falth-Magnusson, K., and Kjellman, N.I. Allergy prevention by maternal elimination diet during late pregnancy – a 5-year follow-up of a randomized study. *J Allergy Clin Immunol* 1992; **89**: 709–13.

40 Baker, J.C., Tunnicliffe, W.S., Duncanson, R.C., and Ayres, J.G. Reduced dietray intakes of magnesium, selenium and vitamins A, C and E in patients with brittle asthma. *Thorax* 1995; **50** (Suppl 2): A75.

41 Cohen, H.A., Neuman, I., and Nahum, H. Blocking effect of vitamin C in exercise-induced asthma. *Arch Pediatr Adolesc Med* 1997; **151**: 367–70.

42 Hasselmark, L., Malmgren, R., Zetterstrom, O., and Unge, G. Selenium supplementation in intrinsic asthma. *Allergy* 1993; **48**: 30–6.

43 Hackman, R.M., Stern, J.S., and Gershwin, M.E. Complementary and alternative medicine and asthma. *Clin Rev Allergy Immunol* 1996; **14**: 321–36.

44 Fluge, O., Omenaas, E., Eide, G.E., and Gulsvik, A. Fish consumption and respiratory symptoms among young adults in a Norwegian community. *Eur Respir J* 1998; **12**: 336–40.

45 Broughton, K.S., Johnson, C.S., Pace, B.K., Liebman, M., and Kleppinger, K.M. Reduced asthma symptoms with n-3 fatty acid ingestion are related to 5-series leukotriene production. *Am J Clin Nutr* 1997; **65**: 1011–17.

46 Hederos, C.A., and Berg, A. Epogam evening primrose oil treatment in atopic dermatitis and asthma. *Arch Dis Child* 1996; **75**: 494–7.

47 Reilly, D., Taylor, M., Beattie, N.G.M., *et al.* Is evidence for homoeopathy reproducible? *Lancet* 1994; **344**: 1601–6.

48 Field, T., Henteleff, T., Hernandez-Reif, M., *et al.* Children with asthma have improved pulmonary functions after massage therapy. *J Paediatr* 1998; **132**: 854–8.

49 Huntley, A., White, A.R., and Ernst, E. Relaxation therapies for asthma: a systematic review. *Thorax* 2002; **57**(2): 127–31.

50 Alexander, A.B., Miklich, D.R., and Hershkoff, H. The immediate effects of systematic relaxation training on peak expiratory flow rates in asthmatic children. *Psychosom Med* 1972; **34**: 388–94.

51 Loew, T.H., Martus, P., Rosner, F., and Zimmermann, T. Wirkung von funktioneller entspannung im vergleich mit salbutamol und einem plazeboentspannungsverfahren bei akutem asthma bronchiale. *Monatsschr Kinderheilkd* 1996; **144**: 1357–63.

52 Lehrer, P.M., Hochron, S.M., Mayne, T., *et al.* Relaxation and music therapies for asthma among patients prestabilized on asthma medication. *J Behav Med* 1994; **17**(1): 1–24.

53 Henry, M., de Rivera, J.L.G., Gonzalez-Martin, I.J., and Abreu, J. Improvement of respiratory function in chronic asthmatic patients with autogenic therapy. *J Psychosom Res* 1993; **37**: 265–70.

54 Kotses, H., Harver, A., Segreto, J., *et al.* Long-term effects of biofeedback-induced facial relaxation on measures of asthma severity in children. *Biofeedback Self Regul* 1991; **16**: 1–21.

55 British Tuberculosis Association. Hypnosis for asthma – a controlled trial. *BMJ* 1968; **4**: 71–6.

56 Ewer, T.C., and Stewart, D.E. Improvement in bronchial hyper-responsiveness in patients with moderate asthma after treatment with a hypnotic technique: a randomised controlled trial. *BMJ* 1986; **293**: 1129–32.

57 Kohen, D.P. Relaxation/mental imagery (self-hypnosis) for childhood asthma: behavioral outcomes in a prospective, controlled study. *Hypnosis* 1995; **22**: 132–44.

58 Maher-Loughnan, G.P., Mason, A.A., Macdonald, N., and Fry, L. Controlled trial of hypnosis in the symptomatic treatment of asthma. *Br Med J* 1962; **11**: 371–6.

59 Bowler, S.D., Green, A., and Mitchell, C.A. Buteyko breathing techniques in asthma: a blinded randomised controlled trial. *Med J Aust* 1998; **169**: 575–8.

60 Singh, V. Effect of respiratory exercises on asthma. *J Asthma* 1987; **24**: 355–9.

61 Singh, V., Wisniewski, A., Britton, J., and Tattersfield, A. Effect of yoga breathing exercises (pranayama) on airway reactivity in subjects with asthma. *Lancet* 1990; **335**: 1381–3.

62 Nagarathna, R., and Nagendra, H.R. Yoga for bronchial asthma: a controlled study. *BMJ* 1985; **291**: 1077–9.

63 Fluge, T., Richter, J., Fabel, H., *et al*. Langzeiteffekte von atemgumnastik und Yoga bei Patienten mit Asthma bronchiale. *Pneumologie* 1994; **48**: 484–90.

64 Vedanthan, P.K., Kesavalu, L.N., Murthy, K.C., *et al*. Clinical study of yoga techniques in university students with asthma: a controlled study. *Allergy Asthma Proc* 1998; **19**: 3–9.

65 Jobst, K., Chen, J.H., McPherson, K., *et al*. Controlled trial of acupuncture for disabling breathlessness. *Lancet* 1986; **ii**: 1416–19.

66 Maa, S., Gauthier, D., and Turner, M. Acupressure as an adjunct to a pulmonary rehabilitation program. *J Cardiopulmonary Rehab* 1997; **17**: 268–76.

67 Tandon, M.K. Adjunct treatment with yoga in chronic severe airways obstruction. *Thorax* 1978; **33**: 514–17.

68 Filshie, J., Penn, K., Ashley, S., and Davis, C.L. Acupuncture for the relief of cancer-related breathlessness. *Palliative Med* 1996; **10**: 145–50.

Chapter 5

Economics applied to respiratory supportive care

Niels Neymark

Containment of healthcare costs is an item high on the agenda in almost all countries, and most clinicians know how it feels to have some of their options constrained by cost considerations. Attempts at assessing the costs of particular treatments are therefore frequently met with suspicion, and expectations that the results will be used to constrain the clinical options even further.

For analysts working with economic assessment of healthcare interventions it is therefore of utmost importance to stress that economics is not about cost containment or reductions. Economics, as a scientific discipline, is based on the insight that means are scarce in relation to the desired ends. The resources committed to achieve a certain aim are not available for other uses, so there is inevitably a trade-off between seeking a particular objective and sacrificing others in the process. Economists view this sacrifice of other objectives as the real costs of using resources for one particular purpose, and call this the **opportunity costs**.

The purpose of applying the methods of economic analysis to healthcare interventions is, accordingly, to determine the relation between the outcome in terms of beneficial effects on the patients' health and the costs in terms of resources used to obtain this health benefit. The analysis attaches equal importance to the expected health benefits and to the costs of obtaining them. The ultimate aim of applying economic analysis to healthcare options is to ensure that the available resources are used in such a way that the health benefits of the treatments provided are the best possible given the resources. In practical analyses, two or more competing treatment options for a particular patient group are compared in a so-called **economic evaluation** in order to determine the consequences in terms of both costs and benefits of changing from one option to the other.

This chapter defines briefly the notion and purpose of an economic evaluation and sets out the essential steps of carrying out the analysis in practice. These principles are not dependent on the particular field of medicine to which they are applied, and, although fundamental for the proper interpretation of published economic studies, they are still relatively unknown to clinicians. Their significance for an appropriate understanding of economic evaluations make it worthwhile reiterating them.

There are still relatively few published studies of economic evaluations of the various choices that must be made in relation to providing supportive care in respiratory disease. One example that illustrates the formulation of the question to address in an economic evaluation is the title of a recent study by Regueiro et al.:[1] 'A comparison of generalist and pulmonologist care for patients hospitalized with severe chronic obstructive pulmonary disease: resource intensity, hospital costs, and survival'. A number of other recent studies of some interest are mentioned in the list of references.[2–9] A brief survey of the literature on the economics of COPD and respiratory supportive care is provided later in the chapter.

Economic evaluation: defining the term

Economic evaluation is a general methodological approach to assess the relative worth of various activities, in cases where such assessments are not performed by the normal market mechanisms. This approach is not confined to healthcare; it is widely used in other areas, notably in assessing regulatory interventions to protect the environment. An economic evaluation should always compare two or more alternative ways of achieving a particular objective, while taking both costs and benefits of each alternative into account. The information about each alternative in the comparison must be collected, treated and assessed according to **uniform, systematic and consistent criteria**. The basic tasks in any economic evaluation are therefore to systematically identify, measure and value all the costs and effects of the alternatives. These tasks will be elaborated further below.

There are four different important types of economic evaluation in healthcare, which basically differs in their valuation of treatment outcomes, while costs are assessed in the same way. These are summarized in Table 5.1.

- In **cost-effectiveness analysis**, by far the most commonly used method, the treatment outcomes are measured by means of a single natural physical unit, such as reduction in the number of episodes of serious dyspnoea.

- In **cost-utility analysis**, outcome is valued by estimating the impact of the treatments on the patients' quality of life, thereby trying to overcome the problems in cost-effectiveness analysis engendered by the fact that outcome assessment is restricted to one single dimension.

Table 5.1 The four principal forms of economic evaluation

Type of study	Measurement/ valuation of costs	Identification of consequences	Measurement/valuation of consequences
Cost-minimization analysis	Particular currency, preferably the relevant one for the study site	Identical in all relevant respects (assumes that differences are irrelevant)	None
Cost-effectiveness analysis	As above	Single effect of interest, common to both alternatives, but achieved to different extent	Natural units (e. g. life years gained, number of episodes of severe dyspnoea avoided)
Cost-utility analysis	As above	Single or multiple effects, not necessarily common to both alternatives	Utility of health states or quality-adjusted life-years
Cost-benefit analysis	As above	Single or multiple effects, not necessarily common to both alternatives	Particular currency, based on estimates of the willingness-to-pay of people concerned by the treatment options

Source: Adapted from Drummond et al.[10]

- In **cost-minimization analysis**, it is assumed that outcomes of the treatment alternatives are identical, so that only the costs need to be assessed.
- In **cost-benefit analysis**, which has been rather rare until now but is enjoying increasing interest, treatment outcomes are valued in pecuniary terms. In this way, costs and benefits become commensurate, and the net benefits of a treatment may be determined as total benefits minus total costs. Only treatments with positive net benefits should be implemented.

Cost-effectiveness analysis, step by step

In this section, the basic steps of a cost-effectiveness analysis are outlined and briefly discussed. The other types of economic evaluations follow essentially the same steps, with the appropriate modifications concerning the valuation of outcomes.

1 Define the clinical objective to be achieved

This part of the task is often relatively neglected, but it is fundamental for any evaluation. Without an explicit and clear formulation of the clinical objective, it is impossible to determine to what degree it has been achieved, or to identify all the possible ways of achieving it.

2 Identify all the ways of achieving the principal clinical objective

This difficult but important step is indispensable in carrying out the most relevant evaluation possible.[11] Unfortunately, it is most often ignored in practical evaluations, which are usually limited to comparing two treatments of immediate interest, such as a standard and an experimental treatment. If the control treatment has not been evaluated in relation to possible alternatives, the evaluation can only be considered as partial, as it is perhaps not the most relevant in relation to the ultimate objective of the treatments.

3 Determine the viewpoint of the cost-effectiveness analysis

The viewpoint or perspective of the analysis determines what is to be considered as costs and therefore which elements should be included in the analysis and how they should be valued. The classical example of the importance of the viewpoint is the question of inpatient treatment versus home care. Several recent studies (e.g. the one by Shepherd *et al.*[12]) show that, from a societal perspective which includes all costs, home care does not result in a significant reduction in costs compared to inpatient care, but there is a significant shifting of costs from the hospital to the patients, their relatives, and the social services of the patients' local area.

Conventionally, it is recommended that the analysis should be carried out from the societal viewpoint, because this ensures that all costs are taken into account, no matter who has to bear them in the end. However, most evaluations are carried out from a narrower viewpoint, typically that of the provider (hospital) or the health insurance system that usually bears most of the financial costs.

4 Identify and quantify all types of resources used and health benefits obtained

To ensure a comprehensive and systematic evaluation it is important to identify all the resources used in the treatments and all the consequences for the patients' health, including adverse events in the short or longer term. At the later stages of the analysis, it may be decided to leave certain of these factors out of account, if they are considered to be of minor importance, but they should at least be recognized. For example, in a cost-effectiveness analysis, one outcome such as length of survival may be considered to have overriding importance and the effectiveness of the treatments is only assessed and compared in this dimension; any differences in adverse events and patterns of disease progression are ignored in the quantitative analysis.

The factors to include in the analysis must also be measured as accurately as possible, in appropriate physical units, such as days of hospital stays; number of blood transfusions; incidence, severity, and duration of adverse events. In recent years there have been many attempts to integrate economic evaluations in randomized clinical trials, so that resource utilization data are collected prospectively alongside the clinical data for the patients in the trial. In principle, all the necessary data for resource use and clinical events may in this way be collected at the individual patient level. However, the superiority of this way of collecting data is far from being uncontested (as Neymark et al.[13] have argued), and this discussion must be considered to be as yet undecided. Other possible sources of relevant data should always be considered, and in most analyses some data must in any case be collected outside the trial context, particularly because the time horizon of interest for an economic evaluation is usually longer than that for a clinical trial.

5 Valuation of resources used and of consequences

To enable determination and comparisons of costs, quantities of resources used must be converted into costs in pecuniary terms. This requires identification of appropriate unit prices for all the resources used, and these will again depend on the perspective chosen for the analysis. For example, it is well known that the charges for clinical services reimbursed by a public or private health insurer have no necessary relation to the cost for the provider of the service.

Identifying appropriate unit prices for the resources used is one of the principal problems of carrying out valid economic evaluations. The least problematic solution is to carry out the analysis from the perspective of the health insurance system in a country such as Belgium, where the providers are remunerated on a fee-for-service basis. A comprehensive and detailed list of tariffs for the various services is established after negotiation, and the hospital has an obvious incentive to register very accurately all the services provided to the individual patient.

At the opposite end of the spectrum of difficulty are hospitals in a system with global hospital budgets funded by general tax revenues. The accounting principles conventionally used do not provide the kind of cost figures ideally needed for an economic evaluation, and there are very few incentives for the decision-makers to determine the real opportunity costs of the various services and procedures. In most cases, the analyst will have to make do with the figures provided by the accountancy departments, while being aware of the limitations of these data.

On the health effect side, no additional valuation is necessary in a cost-effectiveness analysis, because the health outcome of interest is measured in natural physical units, such as survival time in months or years.

6 Calculation and comparison of costs and effects

The main issue of interest is to calculate the mean total cost per patient for each treatment option and relate these mean costs to the expected health outcome for the typical or average patient. Cost data are usually right-skewed because some patients have very high costs, so the mean is higher than the median. Cost analyses focus on the mean costs, because the expected total costs of selecting a treatment option are most relevant for decision-making.[14]

In comparing two or more treatment options, the variable of primary interest is the relation between changes in costs and in outcomes when switching from one treatment to the other. Provided the outcomes of the treatments differ significantly, the analytical task is to determine the **incremental** costs of obtaining the observed change in outcome. If the experimental treatment is more effective and less costly than the control, the incremental costs will be negative and the experimental treatment will be said to be the **dominant solution**. If the experimental arm is more effective and also more costly, which is the most frequent situation, the analyst must present the decision-makers with data on the trade-off between better treatment results and the higher costs engendered. Figure 5.1 represents this process of decision-making graphically.

7 Presentation and interpretation of results

If a dominant solution exists, choosing this treatment is clearly indicated, unless other considerations are decisive in determining the choice. In the usual case in which there is no dominant solution, the result of the analysis is normally presented as an **incremental cost-effectiveness ratio** (ICER). This is a way of standardizing the presentation of results, which makes it easier to compare the results of several evaluations. With survival as the principal outcome, the results are then presented as the ICER per life year gained. If, for instance, the experimental treatment results in an improvement in mean survival of 3 months, the difference in costs between the treatments is multiplied by four to find the ICER per life-year gained.

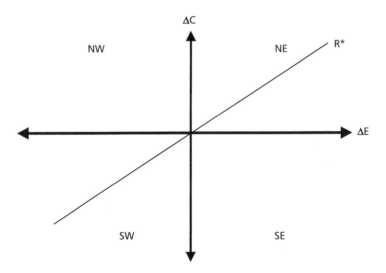

Fig. 5.1 The cost-effectiveness plane. The results of comparing two treatments, A (experimental) and B (control), may be expressed in the cost-effectiveness plane. ΔC indicates the difference in cost, say with ΔC > 0 indicating higher costs for A, and ΔE measuring the difference in effectiveness, with ΔE > 0 indicating a benefit with A. If the result of the analysis is in quadrant SE, A is a dominant solution, with higher effectiveness and lower costs. In quadrant NW the situation is reversed, B being the dominant solution. Results in quadrants NE and SW indicate a trade-off situation, where a treatment benefit can be obtained, but only at the expense of a cost increase (or a cost reduction can be obtained at the expense of reduced effectiveness). R* indicates a hypothetical threshold value for society's willingness-to-pay for a gain in effectiveness.

The ICER is a relative measure, which can not be interpreted without being related to some external standard. Just presenting an ICER per gain in health outcome does not allow one to determine whether this gain is actually worth obtaining, taking the opportunity costs into consideration. Ideally, it would be possible to determine a societal trade-off, i.e. the increase in costs that society is willing to accept for a particular gain in outcome. Without such a standard having been firmly established, results are usually presented in relation to certain reference values, that, although rarely well founded, have achieved a certain status as signposts. For a long time, the ICER per life year gained after kidney transplantation served as such a signpost, as this treatment was costly but also quite frequent and apparently widely accepted in most communities. The relationship between cost-effectiveness and society's willingness to pay can be graphically represented in the **cost-effectiveness acceptability curve** (Figure 5.2).

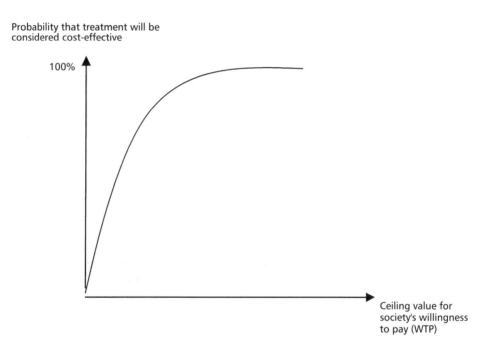

Fig. 5.2 The cost-effectiveness acceptability curve was introduced recently by Briggs and Fenn[15] as a potentially fruitful way of stating the results of cost-effectiveness analyses, given that the threshold value for society's willingness to pay for a gain in effectiveness is normally not known. Expressing the results of a cost-effectiveness analysis in the standard way, as an incremental cost-effectiveness ratio (ICER) may not be very helpful, if this cannot be related to a known threshold value (cf. the line R* in Figure 5.1). It may be more useful for decision-makers if the results of an analysis are presented as the probability that the new treatment should be considered cost-effective. This probability will normally be an increasing function of the unknown critical value for society's willingness to pay for a gain in effectiveness. The cost-effectiveness acceptability curve in the figure illustrates that when the threshold value for society's willingness to pay for an improved outcome is increased, the probability that the new treatment is cost-effective rises. The curve converges to a value determined by the likelihood that the new treatment is more effective than the standard (here indicated as 100%, but in most cases less).

8 Analysing the impact of uncertainty

No matter how data for an economic evaluation are collected, they will be surrounded by significant uncertainty. No analysis can be considered complete without an analysis of how sensitive the results are to plausible changes in the values of the variables of the analysis, particularly in variables of major importance for the total costs or for the measure of effectiveness. If the results are very sensitive, the analysis will probably have little impact on decision-making and an effort at finding improved data with less uncertainty would be indicated. If the results are robust to such changes, the analysis will appear more convincing and probably have greater impact.

The development of principles for the conduct of sensitivity analysis has received far too little attention until recently. But, as economic evaluations are increasingly integrated into clinical trials, making available data on the level of the individual patient, so the possibility of analysing the impact of uncertainty by appropriate statistical methods has opened up. An important part of the methodological discussion in recent years has been concerned with developing statistical methods for analysis of uncertainty, which has been well described by Briggs and Fenn.[15] This has also had an impact on the conduct of sensitivity analysis of studies that do not have individual patient data for all the variables and have to rely on more aggregate data.

The economics of COPD and respiratory supportive care

The following brief account of the economics of COPD and respiratory supportive care is essentially based on two recently published reviews by Ruchlin and Dasbach[17] and Friedman and Hilleman.[18]

The worldwide information generated in the Global Burden of Disease Study[19] indicated that chronic obstructive pulmonary disease (COPD) ranked sixth among the leading causes of death. The incidence, morbidity, and mortality of COPD is increasing throughout the world, and it is projected to be the third leading cause of death by the year 2020. Finding that in 1994 COPD-related research funding only amounted to 1.3% of the total research funding of the US National Institutes of Health, Gross et al.[20] claim that COPD was the most underfunded disease relative to its burden and cost of illness.

Assistance in setting research priorities is one of the possible uses of the numerous cost-of-illness studies now being performed and published. In such studies, an attempt is made to determine all the medical and non-medical costs associated with a specific disease and to assess its total burden on society. The most important non-medical cost is usually the loss of production and utility-providing leisure time caused by illness, and non-medical costs often account for roughly half of the estimated cost of illness. By relating the estimated costs of a disease such as COPD to corresponding cost estimates for other diseases or for the overall costs to society of illness, an estimate of the relative burden of this particular disease can be obtained.

Wilson et al.[21] estimated the direct medical costs of COPD in the US in 1996 to have been US$ 16.6 billion (in year 2000 values), with 57% accounted for by inpatient care and the rest by outpatient care. Similar cost-of-illness studies have been carried out in other countries and relating to other time periods. There is general agreement that the major cost factors are inpatient care, medications, and oxygen therapy, but the estimated costs per patient per year differ widely. Expressed in year 2000 values, Sullivan et al.[22] found a yearly cost per patient in the UK of US $2631, while a Swedish patient was estimated to cost much less, about US$ 930 per year.[23]

Differences in medical practice patterns, but also in the absolute and relative prices of medical care resources, account for such differences.

Treatment costs have been shown to be directly and highly correlated with disease severity. Hilleman *et al.*[24] found a stage III patient (stages defined by the criteria established by the American Thoracic Society) to cost around US$ 14 000 per year, seven times more than a stage I patient (about US$ 2200). An even greater difference was found in a French study by Pannier,[25] with US$ 350 for a stage I patient and US$ 11 500 for a stage III patient. Other correlates of costs found in the literature are patient age, physician specialty, geographic location, and type of insurance coverage.

The major problem with cost-of-illness studies and other analyses identifying and determining costs is that they completely ignore the outcome of the healthcare interventions considered. From the economic point of view, which stresses that economic value can only be properly assessed by relating outcomes obtained with the costs of obtaining them, it is clear that cost analyses should be considered as only a preliminary step, which in itself is therefore only of strictly limited information value. Only by performing a full economic evaluation, which attaches as much importance to the assessment of the outcomes of healthcare interventions as to the determination of their costs, can economic analysis provide the kind of information, which is valuable for making decisions about healthcare interventions.

Ruchlin and Dasbach[17] identified 34 actual economic evaluations for their review. These covered six types of interventions: pharmacotherapy, oxygen therapy, home care, surgery, exercise and rehabilitation, and health education. Of the 15 studies concerned with pharmacotherapy, 6 evaluated various antimicrobial agents used in case of acute exacerbations. The others were mainly evaluations of various bronchodilators (such as salbutamol, theophylline, and ipratropium bromide) and other agents such as α_1-antitrypsin replacement or the immunoactive bacterial extract OM-85 BV as prevention of acute exacerbations in patients with chronic bronchitis. Five evaluations focused on the use of oxygen therapy and four addressed the use of different types of home care (e.g. specialized versus regular nurses). Three studies evaluated different surgical techniques, and seven addressed types of interventions such as exercise and rehabilitation or education of the patients.

The findings of the economic evaluations reviewed cannot easily be summarized, because they are quite heterogeneous with regard to the study questions posed, the analytical techniques applied, and the way that outcomes of the interventions were assessed. A meta-analysis of randomized controlled trials of antimicrobial agents indicated that there was not much difference between the costs (per patient who received successful treatment in case of exacerbation) of first-line agents such as amoxicillin (US$ 136) and third-line agents such as ciprofloxacin (US$ 157), but a second-line agent such as cefaclor was more costly (US$ 208). With treatment outcomes measured as quality-adjusted life years (QALYs) gained, two studies found a cost per QALY of about US$ 16 700.

Friedman *et al.*[4] evaluated the most commonly used bronchodilators and showed that total healthcare costs can be significantly influenced by the choice of drug for the initial drug therapy. The use of ipratropium bromide, alone or in combination with salbutamol, was compared with salbutamol alone in patients with moderate to severe COPD, based on two randomized controlled trials involving 1067 patients (>40 years old) and running over a 85-day period. Outcome was measured as FEV_1AUC_{0-4} (the mean area under the FEV_1 response–time curve from 0 to 4 h). The cost assessment comprised the acquisition cost of the drugs, both initial and add-on therapy, and of hospitalizations.

The drug acquisition cost was lowest in the salbutamol-alone group (US$ 63 per patient); for ipratropium bromide it was US$ 94, and for combination therapy US$ 106. However, the patients in the salbutamol-alone group had significantly more exacerbations, and these were associated with an increase in hospital days and the use of antibacterials and corticosteroids. As a result of this, the mean total costs per patient over the 85 days were US$ 269 for salbutamol alone, US$ 156 for ipratropium bromide, and US$ 197 for ipratropium bromide plus salbutamol. Similar results have been found in other studies, such as that by Hilleman et al.[24]

Evaluations of the cost-effectiveness of α_1-antitrypsin replacement indicated that this was less attractive than pharmacotherapy, as the ICERs determined were generally more than US$ 50 000. As stated earlier, the threshold for society's willingness to accept a cost increase for a better health outcome is not known, but a threshold value of US$ 50 000 is often invoked as a benchmark. Interventions with an ICER of less than US$ 50 000 per QALY are thus claimed to pass the 'value for money' test without problems.

One study evaluating lung transplantations resulted in an estimate of US$ 231 000 per QALY, another US$ 450 000 per QALY. Comparisons of alternative surgical techniques for reduction of lung volume have indicated similar outcomes and costs (about US$ 36 000). Mechanical ventilation of patients with acute respiratory failure has been estimated to have a cost per QALY of between US$ 26 000 and US$ 58 000 in best- and worst-case scenarios respectively.[17]

Studies of various types of home care have not assessed any measure of the possible differences in benefits or outcomes, and as this intervention cannot be shown to be associated with reductions in the use of any other type of medical resources, it engenders an increase in costs of US$ 10 000–15 000 per patient per year.[17] Studies evaluating exercise and rehabilitation programmes used various effect measures, notably the number and duration of hospital stays in a pre–post design, with or without control group, but the power of these studies is generally considered too weak for them to be of value for the evaluation of such interventions.

Concluding remarks

This brief account of the published studies on the economics of COPD and respiratory supportive care obviously cannot do more than give an overview of the types of questions

Table 5.2 Outcomes associated with the treatment of COPD over 85 days

Outcome	Salbutamol	Ipratropium bromide	Ipratropium bromide + salbutamol
n	357	362	358
Patients with exacerbations	62 (18%)*	45 (12%)	44 (12%)
Total patient days with exacerbations	770*	504	554
Total hospital days	103*	28	46
Total patient days with increased corticosteroid use	222*	171	162
Patient days with increased antibacterial use	429	281	304

* Indicates statistical significance at $p < 0.05$ level.

addressed by the research carried out so far. One of the major challenges for future research in this area is to obtain reliable and valid estimates of the long-term effects of various clinical interventions on patients' quality-adjusted survival. So far, published studies have mainly used improvement in lung function, e.g. measured by changes in FEV_1, as the measure of effectiveness. This may be a necessary first step, but there is no clear economic methodology for valuing such gains, unless one posits a critical threshold value for society's willingness to accept an increase in healthcare costs for a given increase in FEV_1. To avoid having to elicit such threshold values for a large number of diverse proxy measures, it is preferable to focus on the estimation of quality-adjusted survival, which will also broaden the domain of diseases across which comparisons can be made. Such a move would also be in keeping with the emphasis on quality of life which is at the heart of supportive care.

Summary

It is unfortunate that, in the perception of many, if not most, clinicians, economics continues to be associated with cost reduction or containment. This is not surprising, as the methods of economic evaluation have largely been introduced and developed in the field of healthcare during a period marked by increasing pressure on healthcare budgets all around the world. With a proper understanding of the objectives of carrying out economic evaluations of healthcare interventions and of the methods used and their limitations, clinicians might take a much more enthusiastic interest in using and developing these types of analysis. The active interest of clinicians and their close collaboration with economic analysts is a precondition for the relevance and validity of economic evaluations, so it is essential to arouse the clinicians' interest in taking part in such work.

The methods of economic evaluation are applicable to all types of clinical issues, indeed to all assessments of the relation between the efforts and sacrifices involved in obtaining certain desired results. In principle, any analytical approach to a clinical question in order to base clinical decisions on the best available evidence would benefit from the inclusion of cost considerations. Many clinical issues in respiratory supportive care, such as the appropriate role of oxygen therapy in different patient groups or the use of mechanical ventilation in critically ill cancer patients,[16] may have important cost consequences. A systematic assessment of the 'value for money' of the various clinical options for the patients concerned would provide medical decision-makers with an important supplement to the other types of information used for decision-making.

Keypoints

- ◆ Economic analyses attach equal importance to the expected benefits on the patients' health as to the costs of achieving them
- ◆ The basic tasks of an economic evaluation are to systematically identify, measure and value all the costs and beneficial effects of alternative healthcare options
- ◆ In assessing costs of interventions, the quantities of resources used and their unit prices should be reported separately to enhance the transparency of the analysis
- ◆ Cost assessments focus on mean costs per patient, because the total expected costs of choosing an intervention are important for decision-making
- ◆ The final result of an economic evaluation is an assessment of the expected changes in costs and health outcomes of selecting a new treatment instead of the standard

References

1 Regueiro, C.R., Hamel, M.B., Davis, R.B., *et al.* A comparison of generalist and pulmonologist care for patients hospitalized with severe chronic obstructive pulmonary disease: resource intensity, hospital costs, and survival. SUPPORT investigators. Study to understand prognoses and preferences for outcomes and risks of treatment. *Am J Med* 1998; **105**: 366–72.

2 Andersson, F., *et al.* The costs and effects of adding formoterol to budesonide – results from the FACET study. *Am J Respir Crit Care Med* 1999; **159** (Suppl): 762.

3 Hurrell, C., *et al.* Cost-effectiveness of inhaled fluticasone propionate in the treatment of patients with chronic obstructive pulmonary disease. *Am J Respir Crit Care Med* 1999; **159** (Suppl): 797

4 Friedman, M., Witek, T.J. Serby, C.W., *et al.* Pharmacoeconomic evaluation of a combination of ipratropium plus albuterol compared with ipratropium alone and albuterol alone in COPD. *Chest* 1999; **115**: 635–41.

5 Skilbeck, J., Mott, L., Page, H., *et al.* Palliative care in chronic obstructive airways disease: a needs assessment. *Palliative Med* 1998; **12**: 245–54.

6 Reina-Rosenbaum, R., Bach, J.R., and Penek, J. The cost/benefits of outpatient-based pulmonary rehabilitation. *Arch Phys Med Rehabil* 1997; **78**: 240–4.

7 Limberg, T.M. How does pulmonary rehabilitation survive in a managed care market? *Respir Care Clin N Am* 1998; **4**: 129–48.

8 Smith, K.J., and Pesce, R.R. Pulmonary artery catherization in exacerbations of COPD requiring mechanical ventilation: a cost-effectiveness analysis. *Respir Care* 1994; **39**: 961–7.

9 Schapira, D.V., Studnicki, J., Bradham, D.D., Wollf, P., and Jarrett, A. Intensive care, survival and expenses of treating critically ill cancer patients. *JAMA* 1993; **269**: 783–86.

10 Drummond, M.E., O'Brien, B., Stoddart, G.L., and Torrance, G.W. *Methods for the economic evaluation of health care programmes.* Oxford: Oxford University Press, 1997.

11 Tiggelen, O. Van., Storme, G., Torfs, K., and Van den Berge, D. Using appropriate comparisons in economic evaluations. An exercise in Belgium. *Int J Technol Assess Health Care* 1999; **15**: 243–63.

12 Shepperd, S., Harwood, D., Gray, A., Vessey, M., and Morgan, P. Randomised controlled trial comparing hospital at home care with inpatient hospital care. II: cost minimisation analysis. *BMJ* 1998; **316**: 1791–6.

13 Neymark, N., *et al.* Methodological and statistical issues of quality of life (QoL) and economic evaluation in cancer clinical trials: Report of a workshop. *Eur J Cancer* 1998; **34**: 1317–33.

14 Briggs, A., and Gray, A. The distribution of health care costs and their statistical analysis for economic evaluation. *J Health Serv Res Policy* 1998; **3**: 233–45.

15 Briggs, A., and Fenn, P. Confidence intervals or surfaces? Uncertainty on the cost-effectiveness plane. *Health Econ* 1998; **7**: 723–40.

16 Kongsgaard, U.E., and Meidell, N.K. Mechanical ventilation in critically ill cancer patients: outcome and utilization of resources. *Support Care Cancer* 1999; **7**: 95–9.

17 Ruchlin, H.S., and Dasbach, E.J. An economic overview of chronic obstructive pulmonary disease. *PharmacoEconomics* 2001; **19**: 623–42.

18 Friedman, M., and Hilleman, D.E. Economic burden of chronic obstructive pulmonary disease. *PharmacoEconomics* 2001; **19**: 245–54.

19 Murray, C.J.L., and Lopez, A.D. Mortality by cause for eight regions of the world: global burden of disease study. *Lancet* 1997; **349**: 1269–76.

20 Gross, C.P., Anderson, G.F., and Powe, N.R. The relationship between funding by the National Institutes of Health and the burden of disease. *N Engl J Med* 1999; **340**: 1881–7.

21 Wilson, L., Devine, E.B., and So, K. Direct medical costs of chronic obstructive pulmonary disease: chronic bronchitis and emphysema. *Respir Med* 2000; **94**: 204–13.

22 Sullivan, S.D., Ramsey, S.D., and Lee, T.A. The economic burden of COPD. *Chest* 2000; **117**(2 suppl): 5–9s.

23 Jacobson, L., Hertzman, P. Lofdahl, C.G., *et al.* The economic impact of asthma and chronic obstructive pulmonary disease (COPD) in Sweden in 1980 and 1991. *Respir Med* 2000; **94**: 247–55.

24 Hilleman, D.E., Dewan, N., Malcker, M., *et al.* Pharmacoeconomic evaluation of COPD. *Chest* 2000; **118**: 1278–85.

25 Pannier, R. Socio-economic causes and consequenses of chronic bronchitis and emphysema: an overview. *Eur J Respir Dis* 1986; **69**(Suppl 146): 77–85.

Part II

Mechanisms and assessment of dyspnoea

Chapter 6

Mechanisms of dyspnoea

Michael A. Gillette and Richard M. Schwartzstein

The term 'dyspnoea' means 'difficult breathing,' and derives from the Greek *duspnoos,* meaning 'short of breath'. It has never been a part of common English parlance. In medicine it has been used rather imprecisely as a term for patients' subjective difficulty or discomfort in breathing. Even if the word has never entered into popular usage, however, the condition it describes is all too common. Diseases typically associated with dyspnoea include chronic obstructive pulmonary disease (COPD), asthma, and congestive heart failure (CHF) among many others; these conditions affect tens of millions of people in the United States alone, with associated healthcare costs in the tens of billions of dollars[1,2] and immeasurable costs in human disability. In advanced cancer patients dyspnoea is a major palliative care issue, affecting between 20% and 80% of that population.[3]

As dyspnoea has become a subject of intensive study, efforts have been made to define the term more closely. This has proved to be a significant challenge, for most definitions of suitable conciseness and clarity are neither sufficiently comprehensive nor sufficiently exclusive.[4] A healthy individual breathing through a tube of middling diameter, for instance, might agree breathing was difficult (effortful) but not be dyspnoeic; the same individual at the end of a 200-m sprint might be dyspnoeic but not feel that breathing was especially difficult. Among a myriad of abridged definitions, 'uncomfortable breathing' is perhaps most satisfactory, though it too is imperfect: if our sprinter strained intercostal muscles in his exertions he might later note uncomfortable (painful) breathing but deny dyspnoea. In its 1998 Consensus Statement on dyspnoea, the American Thoracic Society explicitly acknowledged the limitations of existing concise definitions, opting for breadth and comprehensiveness:

> Dyspnoea is a term used to characterize a subjective experience of breathing discomfort that consists of qualitatively distinct sensations that vary in intensity. The experience derives from interactions among multiple physiological, psychological, social, and environmental factors, and may induce secondary physiological and behavioral responses.[5]

Difficulties in precise definition often imply underlying complexity. If dyspnoea is indeed not a discrete experience but a set of related sensations corresponding to various states of disordered breathing, some of the variability might emerge from an array of different mechanisms underlying the sensation of dyspnoea. Additionally, differential cerebral processing of those sensations might promote a range of dyspnoeic experiences. A practical assumption is that an individual's experience of dyspnoea has a one-to-one correlation with a theoretically definable neuroelectrical/chemical/humoral 'brain state', which is itself a product of receptor signals and their processing within the current overall biological context of the organism. A further assumption, contested more philosophically (e.g. are two people's experience of red the same?) than scientifically, is that individuals with similar receptor input and signal processing will have similar experiences. This line of reasoning, together with the observation that common language descriptions of the dyspnoeic state are numerous and varied, has prompted some investigators to scrutinize the language of dyspnoea.[6–9] Data are accumulating that people indeed experience dyspnoea in different ways, that they can communicate those differences, and that those differences depend in large measure upon the underlying physiological or pathophysiological state tempered by idiosyncrasies of cognitive processing. Attention to descriptors may thus help discriminate the particular causes of a patient's dyspnoea.

This chapter considers the mechanisms of dyspnoea. It begins with a review of the known physiology of respiratory system receptors and their relation to uncomfortable breathing. There follows a discussion of theories pertaining to the primary and secondary processing of respiratory receptor signals. Finally, we briefly consider how receptor signals and processing can be used to explain dyspnoea in particular disease states, and the importance of language in disease-specific diagnosis and management.

The nature of dyspnoea

Dyspnoea is essentially a conscious phenomenon. Like pain, to which it is often compared, the individual experiencing it is in a unique position with respect to the experience. Someone manifesting clinical or biochemical signs typically associated with dyspnoea, such as rapid, shallow, or laboured breathing or hypercapnia, who nevertheless denies any attendant discomfort, cannot accurately be said to be dyspnoeic.

Like pain, dyspnoea tends to elicit psychological and behavioural responses. A patient with obstructive pulmonary disease experiencing dyspnoea might for instance be distressed, might alter his activity in such a way as to minimize the dyspnoea, and might take a bronchodilator for relief or contact his physician.

Dyspnoea, then, is a conscious state positioned somewhere along the pathway between the eliciting stimulus and the response. Since effective and clinically important interventions might be made at any point along the pathway, it is useful to elaborate the stages in the generation of dyspnoea and response. Numerous efforts have been made in this direction. Figure 6.1, modified from Ripamonti and Bruera,[3] attempts such a comprehensive model.

In this analysis, a **sensation** is taken to be a primary sensory event. As such, it is not thought to be accessible to consciousness, which deals with information that has already undergone some degree of processing and integration. Sensations processed in this way are referred to as **perceptions**. Vision provides a convenient example. The activation of photoreceptors constitutes the sensation, while the perception might be one of a small, lightly coloured, rounded object on the ground. **Interpretation** takes this processing a step further, and is generally the level informing more complex behaviours. Thus, depending upon individual experience, circumstances, available environmental clues, and so forth, the object might be 'seen' (i.e. interpreted) to be a golf ball, a mushroom, or a stone. However fundamental the conscious experience, it does not impinge at the sensory level. Thus 'bright' might be fundamental at the perceptual level, but retains the sensory underpinnings of intense photoreceptor excitation and signalling.

The situation with dyspnoea is still more complicated. The sensory apparatus subserving vision is known and the processing pathways leading to visual perception have become well characterized, but there is no 'dyspnoea receptor' nor are there, to date, clearly defined neural pathways leading to the perception. Indeed, the lack of a discrete receptor and pathway is implicit in the nature of the stimulus: whereas the visual system responds (essentially) only

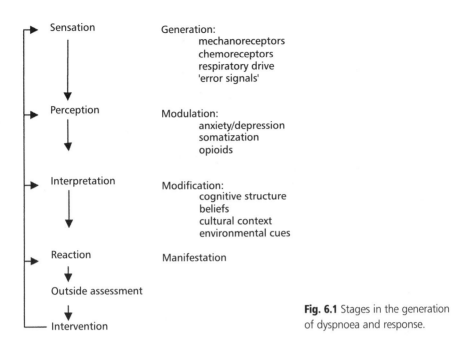

Sensation   Generation:
                         mechanoreceptors
                         chemoreceptors
                         respiratory drive
                         'error signals'

Perception   Modulation:
                         anxiety/depression
                         somatization
                         opioids

Interpretation   Modification:
                         cognitive structure
                         beliefs
                         cultural context
                         environmental cues

Reaction   Manifestation

Outside assessment

Intervention

Fig. 6.1 Stages in the generation of dyspnoea and response.

to light, dyspnogenic stimuli include acid–base disturbances, respiratory system pressures, hypoxia, chemical irritants, and others. Many years of research in anatomy, neurophysiology, and respiratory physiology have, however, illuminated portions of the sensory and perceptual apparatus, and have collectively contributed to a growing understanding of the nature of dyspnoea.

Basic physiology

To say that a dyspnoea receptor has not been identified is not merely to make the point that dyspnoea does not have a discrete stimulus in the manner of light or sound. Pain is not something that is primarily transduced, but the activation of C-fibres by sufficient degrees of pressure or heat constitutes an effective pain receptor. By contrast, there is no specific receptor that when activated directly and consistently produces an experience of dyspnoea. There are, however, numerous receptors, stimulation of which has been found to be reliably associated with dyspnoea. These fall into two principal classes, chemoreceptors and mechanoreceptors; a further class, the ergoreceptors, has recently also been implicated (see Box 6.1).

Chemoreceptors

Respiration is the process by which an organism assimilates oxygen and releases carbon dioxide and other products of oxidation. It is therefore unsurprising in teleological terms that there are receptors sensitive to the partial pressures of these gases. Central chemoreceptors within the medulla are exquisitely responsive to changes in the PCO_2 of blood, probably through associated changes in pH. Peripheral chemoreceptors on the carotid and aortic bodies respond to changes in the ambient PO_2, though their sensitivity is less.

Box 6.1 Receptors involved with dyspnoea

Chemoreceptors

- ◆ hypercapnia
- ◆ hypoxia

Mechanoreceptors

- ◆ airway and pulmonary parenchymal receptors

Ergoreceptors (metaboreceptors)

- ◆ skeletal muscle tissues

Acute hypercapnia

Elevations in PCO_2 have long been known to be potent stimulators of ventilation,[10] and strongly associated with dyspnoea. For many years it was believed that the increased ventilation was the exclusive proximal cause of hypercapnic dyspnoea. Other data have accrued to suggest, however, that elevated PCO_2 makes an independent contribution to the sensation.

Experimental increases in PCO_2 have been used since the early 20th century to study dyspnoea and the control of respiration.[4,11–13] Campbell and associates measured breath holding time and associated hypercapnia in a normal male volunteer, and repeated the experiment after muscular paralysis with D-tubocurarine.[14] Communications were maintained with the subject via finger signals from an arm, perfusion of which was occluded by an inflatable cuff. With paralysis, breath holding was terminated only by impending loss of consciousness; the subject did not report dyspnoea. This seminal experiment was interpreted as demonstrating that hypercapnia without attendant ventilatory response was not associated with 'the distressing sensation normally experienced in the chest'.

Campbell's conclusions conflicted with both earlier and later studies. An experimentally paralysed subject had previously noted 'shortness of breath' after brief termination of ventilatory support.[15] Patients with respiratory paralysis from polio had complained of respiratory discomfort either with brief termination of ventilation or with administration of inspired carbon dioxide.[16] Similarly, experiments in which ventilation was voluntarily targeted at levels below those the subjects had spontaneously attained for a given PCO_2 consistently produced increased breathlessness.[17,18] This hypercapnic dyspnoea was out of proportion to even careful and detailed measures of respiratory effort.[19] Chonan and colleagues subsequently took the opposite tack, driving subjects to similar levels of hyperventilation by progressive hypercapnia, incremental exercise, or isocapnic voluntary hyperventilation. Dyspnoea was greatest in the hypercapnic condition.[20] Demediuk and colleagues extended Chonan's findings in a very compelling effort to dissociate dyspnoea from a sense of respiratory effort. Subjects maintained high (50–60 L/min) ventilation with help of a visual feedback system. After a eucapnic control period with end-tidal PCO_2 ($P_{ET}CO_2$) of 40 mmHg (5.32 kPa), subjects were exposed to a test period of either 40 or 50 mmHg (5.32 or 6.65 kPa) $P_{ET}CO_2$ and asked to independently rate the unpleasant urge to breathe and the perceived respiratory effort. Although dyspnoea was significantly greater in the hypercapnic group, the sense of respiratory effort was less.[13]

Banzett and colleagues perhaps most definitively addressed the issues raised by Campbell in another series of experiments. They reasoned that only breathlessness occurring despite complete absence of input from respiratory muscle afferents would eliminate the possibility that changes in muscle function exclusively drove hypercapnic dyspnoea. To test this, they first subjected three tracheostomized high-level quadriplegic patients to increasing levels of inspired PCO_2. In blinded, forced-choice trials these subjects were able to detect changes in PCO_2 of 7–11 Torr (0.93–1.47 kPa), and reported perceptions of 'air hunger' or uncomfortable breathing.[21] They went on to paralyse four normal volunteers (themselves) and modulate $P_{ET}CO_2$ in a blinded fashion, sustaining communication in a manner similar to that in Campbell's earlier experiments. Subjects were markedly sensitive to increases in $P_{ET}CO_2$, feeling 'air hunger' or 'shortness of breath' like that of breath holding at a median 44 Torr (5.87 kPa), the same levels that induced a like perception before paralysis. There was no essential difference in the quality of dyspnoea between the normal and paralysed state.[4]

The above discussion focuses on dyspnoea related to peripherally measurable changes in PCO_2 or $P_{ET}CO_2$, but it should be remembered that the principal chemoreception of carbon dioxide is medullary. Adams *et al.* observed that dyspnoea and hyperventilation became damped as the frequency of an oscillating hypercarbic stimulus was increased, presumably reflecting delay in full equilibration with central chemoreceptors across the blood–brain barrier.[22] Similarly, it is a common clinical observation that symptomatic resolution of hypercarbic dyspnoea or lethargy lags behind improvements in $PaCO_2$ and pH.

Collectively, these data overwhelmingly demonstrate that acute hypercapnia can be dyspnogenic independently of its effects on ventilation. These experiments document the effects of acute hypercapnia; patients with chronic hypercapnia and compensated respiratory acidosis do not manifest the same degree of dyspnoea for a given PCO_2, consistent with the idea that the chemoreceptors respond to carbon dioxide changes principally as mediated through changes in pH. Chronically hypercapnic individuals may also demonstrate reduced ventilatory sensitivity to changes in PCO_2.[22] The neural mechanisms underlying the dyspnoeic response to hypercapnia are unknown. A direct connection from chemoreceptor to forebrain has been proposed, but the possibility that the cerebral stimulus is corollary (i.e. parallel nervous discharge) from the medullary respiratory neurons to the sensory cortex, seems equally compelling.

Hypoxia

The belief that low oxygen levels are the principal cause of dyspnoea is commonly held, and seems to have great intuitive appeal. Manifestations of the belief are legion: dyspnoeic patients frequently report that they 'need more oxygen;' competitive athletes often inhale oxygen during pauses in the contest; healthcare providers habitually reach for oxygen when presented with a person complaining of uncomfortable breathing.

Within the scientific community, hypoxia is accorded much lower status as a dyspnogenic stimulus. In a study of normal subjects undertaking heavy exercise, Chronos and colleagues found that breathlessness was worse with hypoxic gas mixtures than with air; 100% oxygen reduced the breathlessness.[23] Breath holding in normal subjects is prolonged by increases of FiO_2.[24] Hypoxia may not be a consistent cause of dyspnoea, however: Mak and associates, studying a population of patients with advanced chronic obstructive pulmonary disease (COPD), found no correlation between visual analogue scale ratings of breathlessness and either mean oxygen saturation or mean exertional oxygen desaturation.[25] Furthermore, improvements in dyspnoea by supplemental oxygen in COPD patients may not be entirely explained by improvement in hypoxemia.[26] In a randomized double-blind crossover trial in patients with COPD, dyspnoea and exertional tolerance were significantly improved when 40% oxygen was substituted for compressed air, even in patients without evidence of oxyhaemoglobin desaturation.[26] Increased airflow proved as effective as oxygen in alleviating dyspnoea in a population of advanced cancer patients, including those with lung disease and baseline hypoxia.[27]

Although it is a less potent stimulus than hypercapnia, hypoxia is thought to generate dyspnoea principally because of the consequent increase in ventilation. Patients with severe COPD experienced less breathlessness during exercise when 60% oxygen was substituted for air, but the correlation between breathlessness and ventilation was unaffected.[28] Lane and colleagues found that the addition of hypoxia to exercise did not increase breathlessness in subjects at matched levels of ventilation.[29] Nevertheless, numerous studies subtly suggest that a decreased PO_2 may be a weak independent contributor to breathlessness. In the early 1980s, Adams and colleagues reported that breathlessness preceded increases in ventilation in exercising subjects exposed to hypoxic gas mixtures.[30] Conversely, in their study of exercising normal subjects they later found that improvements in dyspnoea with oxygen administration preceded reductions in ventilation.[23] Dean and colleagues argued that reductions in ventilation were at most only partially responsible for COPD patients' improved exercise tolerance with supplemental oxygen.[26]

Despite the popular correlation between low oxygen levels and breathlessness, the data supporting hypoxia as a central dyspnogenic stimulus remain less compelling than those for hypercarbia. This academic uncertainty has a practical parallel. As noted by Manning and Schwartzstein,[31] it is a common clinical observation that hypoxaemic patients may not be dyspnoeic, and dyspnoeic patients may not be hypoxaemic.[32] Correction of hypoxemia may leave dyspnoea unabated.[31]

Mechanoreceptors

Mechanoreceptors (capable of transducing mechanical stimuli) are positioned throughout the human body, providing information to the central nervous system on local pressure, stretch, flow, and position. The respiratory system is replete with them, within the airways, the pulmonary parenchyma, and the chest wall. These mechanoreceptors appear to contribute to a sensation of breathlessness, and can in some cases be the principal stimulus for dyspnoea.

Airway and pulmonary parenchymal receptors

Receptors important to dyspnoea in humans may be found throughout the respiratory system. Breath holding time is increased when cold air is blown across a subject's face.[33] Normal subjects made breathless by hypercapnia or inspiratory resistive loading experience symptomatic relief when cold air is blown across their faces.[34] In subjects with elevated end-tidal PCO_2 in whom inspiratory load, breathing pattern, and total ventilation were fixed, dyspnoea was worsened when a mouthpiece was added to a tight-fitting face mask.[35,36] This effect was abolished by topical anaesthesia of the oral mucosa or by inhalation of warm humidified air. These data support the existence of flow receptors in the oral mucosa or the face, which decreases the intensity of breathlessness when activated. A related observation was that in breathless cancer patients, the sensation of dyspnoea was reduced when either air or oxygen was administered via nasal cannulae.[27]

Electrophysiological studies in animals have suggested there are several subtypes of pressure receptors throughout the tracheobronchial tree.[37] Some saturate within the range of normal airway pressures, but sustain their output during prolonged stimulation; others have a more linear response to increasing pressures. Some respond to longitudinal stretch but most are sensitive principally to circumferential stretch. These receptors are topographically distinct. Somewhat similar classes of receptor exist in human airways. Increases in airway wall tension stimulate pulmonary stretch receptors in large central airways. These slowly adapting receptors (SARs) mediate the Hering–Breuer reflex, described in 1868, in which lung inflation promotes expiration and deflation promotes inspiration. Irritant receptors are rapidly adapting receptors (RARs) that respond to inhaled irritants, histamine, direct mechanical stimulation, and large changes in lung volume. Juxtacapillary (J-) receptors and C-fibres occur in small airways and throughout the pulmonary parenchyma near alveolar capillaries, responding to mechanical stimuli and vasoactive agents including bradykinin, prostaglandins, histamine, and serotonin. Afferent inputs from these various receptors are conducted through the vagus nerve, known since the early 19th century to be involved in respiration.[38]

There are varying degrees of support for the roles of each of these receptor subtypes, and generally for vagal afferents in the generation of dyspnoea. Because they have lost structural support through damage to surrounding lung tissue, small- and medium-sized airways in COPD patients are prone to collapse during expiration when pleural pressure exceeds airway pressure. Pursed-lip breathing, which increases airway pressures, can reduce dyspnoea in this setting, while negative pressure applied at the mouth exacerbates discomfort.[39] These effects are likely to be caused by airway wall receptors responding to changes in transmural pressures. Similar mechanisms probably underlie the observation that passively ventilated C1–C3 quadriplegics experience increased air hunger for a given end-tidal carbon dioxide level when their tidal volumes are decreased.[40] Because of their high cervical lesions, these patients had little if any input from the chest wall; relevant afferent input can therefore only have been via vagal or parenchymal receptors.[38]

Irritant receptors may be pivotal in the breathlessness associated with allergic bronchoconstriction. Dyspnoea is worse after histamine-induced bronchoconstriction than with an external resistive load causing the same total airway resistance.[41] Dyspnoea due to the former but not the latter was relieved by inhaled lignocaine (lidocaine), and this result is consistent with the contention that histamine acts via epithelial receptors. Furthermore, the quality of the dyspnoeic sensations is markedly different in the two situations; with bronchoconstriction but not external resistance the predominant sensation was one of chest tightness or constriction.[42]

C-fibres in the lung are stimulated by pulmonary congestion, and lead to a rapid shallow breathing pattern similar to that seen in patients with pulmonary oedema.[43] When lobeline, a C-fibre stimulant, was injected into normal subjects, all experienced a choking sensation in the throat, and almost half noted constriction or heaviness in the upper chest.[44]

As vagal stimulation is known to affect respiratory pattern, and several classes of receptor thought to be important to the sensation of dyspnoea are vagally mediated, it is reasonable to imagine that vagotomy might significantly affect breathlessness. However, studies are inconclusive. Temporary vagal block increases breath holding time in normal subjects,[45] and several case reports describe relief of dyspnoea of various aetiologies by temporary vagal interruption. Controlled studies are lacking and systematic efforts to control breathlessness by vagotomy have only demonstrated an inconsistent benefit.[46]

Central (cortical) projections are known to exist from respiratory muscle spindles and costovertebral joints in the chest wall.[47] These could mediate the sensation of breathlessness. Chest wall receptors are also involved in spinal and supraspinal reflexes, which are not directly involved in breathlessness. When these receptors are studied, it is difficult to ensure that stimuli are localized to the chest wall. Thus, though it is known that normal subjects have an increased tolerance of fixed levels of hypercapnia when they are allowed to increase their tidal volume,[48] the studies in high cervical quadriplegics cited above[40] point to localization of the relevant receptors to the airways. However, numerous studies have suggested that the subjective assessment of changes in inspired volume, which is quite accurate in humans, utilizes afferent information from chest wall receptors, particularly those signalling muscle tension.[49–51] After finding that the accuracy and resolution of sensation of inspired volumes did not differ significantly between normal subjects and quadriplegics, Altose and colleagues suggested that inputs from ribcage receptors were not essential for that discrimination.[49] However, lack of change after inhalation of aerosolized 2% lignocaine (lidocaine) also argued against an exclusive role for upper airway receptors.

Stronger support for a modulatory role of chest wall receptors on dyspnoea comes from a variety of studies using muscular vibration as a local stimulus. In normal subjects made dyspnoeic by hypercapnia and resistive loading, vibration over parasternal intercostal muscles reduced dyspnoea.[52] In patients with chronic lung disease and dyspnoea at rest, vibration of inspiratory intercostals during inspiration and expiratory intercostals during expiration decreased dyspnoea, while out-of-phase vibration increased dyspnoea.[53] These data are of considerable interest for their therapeutic implications, but their mechanistic significance is tempered by uncertainty that vibrations are restricted to the intercostal musculature. Nevertheless, it is possible that there is redundancy in the system, and that information from either the lungs or the chest wall may allow the central nervous system to monitor volume changes and modify the intensity of dyspnoea.

Ergoreceptors

A fascinating class of receptors that may contribute importantly to dyspnoea in some clinical settings is the ergoreceptors (metaboreceptors). In the ergoreflex (metaboreflex), which these receptors subserve, metabolic changes in exercising skeletal muscle lead to increases in ventilation. It is believed that lactic acid is important for this, but certain other metabolites may also have a role. Since the reflex is augmented, not reduced, when blood from the exercising limb is prevented from returning centrally by an occlusion cuff, it is thought to be neurally mediated and reflects local, peripheral metabolic change.[54] Currently the subject of much investigation, the ergoreflex may help to explain the rapid increase in exercise ventilation which occurs before such 'error signals' as an increased PCO_2 can be detected. In some pathophysiological states, such as chronic congestive heart failure, abnormalities in skeletal muscle may augment the ergoreflex and so exacerbate exertional dyspnoea.[55] This may also help to explain the observation that in cardiac transplant patients dyspnoea may remain limiting despite marked improvement in haemodynamics.

Central processing

The preceding section has described several types of peripheral receptors which may contribute to generating sensation of dyspnoea. However, activation of these receptors alone may not be sufficient to activate dyspnoea sensation, in much the same way that photoreceptor stimulation is necessary, but not sufficient by itself, for vision. As described in the introduction, the experiential nature of dyspnoea implies its correlation to certain sorts of central nervous system activity. It is convenient to imagine that each type and intensity of dyspnoea corresponds to a particular 'brain state'. For the purposes of this discussion, it is also useful to postulate a 'dyspnoea centre' comprising those areas involved in the dyspnoeic brain state – although to date, no neuroanatomical region has been convincingly identified which could correspond to a discrete dyspnoea centre (cf. ref. 56). Within this model, any condition of the dyspnoea centre's activation in which dyspnoea was experienced by the subject represents a 'dyspnoea state'.

Broadly speaking, three sorts of central mechanisms have been proposed to effect such dyspnoea states. Because dyspnoea emerges essentially from pathways involved in control of breathing, it is reasonable to borrow from the familiar terminology of regulatory systems and refer to feedback, feedforward, and error signal mechanisms.

- In **feedback processing**, dyspnoea states emerge from the input of peripheral or central receptors to the dyspnoea centre. For example, excessive input from carbon dioxide receptors, insufficient input from flow receptors, or static input from stretch receptors, might lead to dyspnoea states.

- In **feedforward processing**, dyspnoea states might emerge from corollary output of the respiratory motor command neurones. The term 'corollary' here refers to the discharge of neurones from one part of the brain to another, e.g. from the motor to the sensory cortex, simultaneously with the discharge from the motor cortex to the ventilatory muscles. This is conceived as a mechanism by which the brain may monitor motor output. If respiratory motor output were for instance sufficiently intense or sufficiently prolonged, corollary discharge to the dyspnoea centre might achieve a dyspnoea state. Of course, the relationship between the motor output and the corollary discharge need not be linear; input to the dyspnoea centre might for instance be a logarithmic function of motor output, or might occur only after a certain threshold level. Furthermore, corollary discharge might be different depending on whether the motor output was voluntary or automatic; Plum reported that patients with brainstem lesions who had voluntary but not automatic ventilatory control did not experience breathlessness.[57] It is also noteworthy that the relationship between respiratory motor output and overall respiratory system function is complex: the respiratory motor output of a trained athlete sprinting up a flight of stairs might for instance be similar to that of a chronic lung disease patient at rest, suggesting that the two conditions could yield similar dyspnoea states.

- In **error signal** processing, dyspnoea states emerge from incongruity between the corollary discharge from the motor centre and feedback information from peripheral receptors (possibly deriving from incongruity between different sets of peripheral receptor – see below). An 'inadequate' increment in feedback from stretch receptors or decrement in feedback from carbon dioxide receptors for a given increment in corollary motor discharge might thus constitute a dyspnoea state. Whichever conditions constituted the dyspnoea state, it would also be subject to modulation by inputs relating to the general physiological, emotional, and environmental context in which it occurs. although many additional subtleties and complexities are involved, these three basic mechanisms, rendered at the centre of the schema shown in Figure 6.2, provide a framework in which to understand leading theories on the central processing of dyspnoea.

The concept of feedback processing underlies the preceding discussion of receptors which are potentially important in generating dyspnoea. Feedforward signal processing warrants further explanation. Dyspnoea has commonly been hypothesized to represent one manifestation of the subjective sensation of respiratory muscle effort. This hypothesis provides an account of breathlessness in the setting of either increased load or increased ventilation: respiratory effort would be greater for a given rate and extent of muscle shortening if the impedance increased, and greater for a given impedance if the rate or extent of shortening increased. Theoretically, this sense of effort could derive from either afferent inputs from the respiratory musculature or corollary discharge from the respiratory motor centre. Using psychophysical experiments in normal volunteers, Gandevia found that subjects could discriminate between the tension developed in their respiratory muscles and the motor command ('effort') required to accomplish this. When muscles became fatigued (or weakened with partial-dose paralytics), subjects

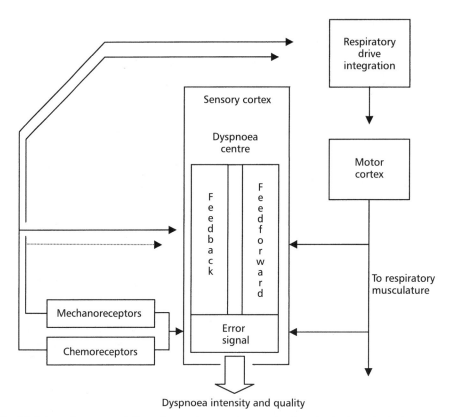

Fig. 6.2 Schematic representation of central processing mechanisms in the hypothetical 'dyspnoea centre'. See text for details.

overestimated muscle tension, suggesting that conscious awareness of the motor command, and not input from muscle or other peripheral receptors, was the dominant reference for load and effort.[58] These findings paralleled and extended those from work in other skeletal muscle.[59]

Some investigators have therefore hypothesized that feedforward and feedback components may make distinct contributions to the experience of dyspnoea. In normal subjects undergoing graded exercise loads and external inspiratory resistances, El-Manshawi and colleagues showed that breathlessness was significantly and independently correlated with estimated inspiratory pressure, flow rate, and tidal volume, which were interpreted as surrogates for muscle tension, rate of shortening, and extent of shortening, respectively.[60] Peripheral mechanoreceptor feedback (signalling 'force') or central corollary motor discharge (signalling 'effort') could both generate such a correlation. Under fixed conditions force and effort are proportional, but only until force-generating capacity or mechanical conditions are altered; the authors suggest that in the setting of such alterations effort appears the better correlate of dyspnoea (as shown by Gandevia[61]). They note, however, that while the intensity of breathlessness was comparable between the conditions of high ventilation with low impedance and low ventilation with high impedance, the quality was not. This qualitative nature of breathlessness they ascribe to modulatory input from respiratory muscle sensors. Table 6.1 shows how the three

Table 6.1 Possible mechanisms of dyspnoea in selected disorders

Processing	Mechanism	Asthma	COPD	Chronic CHF	ILD	Neuromuscular	PE
FF/ES	↑ Motor output (effort)	X	X	X	X	X	±
ES	Afferent mismatch	X	X	X	X	X	
FB/ES	Hypercapnia		±		±*		
FB/ES	Hypoxia	±*	±	?	±	±*	±
FB/ES	Stretch receptor	?	?				?
FB/ES	Irritant receptor	X					?
FB/ES	J-receptor		?	?			?

COPD, chronic obstructive pulmonary disease; CHF, congestive heart failure; ES, error-signal; FB, feedback; FF, feedforward; ILD, interstitial lung disease; PE, pulmonary embolism. 'X' indicates a major, '±' a minor, and '?' a possible contribution to dyspnoea; '*' suggests relevance only in advanced or severe disease. See text for details.

Modified from Schwartzstein.[8]

elements of feedforward, feedback, and error signal are hypothesized to cause dyspnoea in different disease states.

The feedforward model has specific limitations. Although in certain cases motor command (feedforward) or receptor-driven (feedback) mechanisms may predominate in producing dyspnoea, an 'error signal' is probably more frequently implicated. There is considerable teleological appeal to the idea of dyspnoea being due not so much to the correlation of substantial respiratory motor output or intense respiratory work, as to a discrepancy between the effort and the result. It is when the need to respond to increases in load or metabolic derangement cannot be met, or can barely be met, that respiration – and hence the organism itself – is imperilled. In an early formulation of this concept, Campbell and Howell proposed that dyspnoea developed when the change in respiratory muscle length and lung volume was disproportionately low for the force applied. This 'length–tension inappropriateness' is closely related to other theories including 'efferent–reafferent dissociation'[62] (cf. ref. 63) and 'neuroventilatory dissociation';[64] all postulate types of error signal mechanisms.

Studies of dyspnoea ratings by subjects exposed to various levels of ventilation and PCO_2 provide some of the clearest support for this type of processing. Chonan and colleagues found that normal subjects experienced less dyspnoea for a given PCO_2 if they set their own ventilatory level than if ventilation was targeted to a fixed level.[17] Results were similar when PCO_2 was held constant but ventilation was voluntarily reduced. They suggested that hypercapnia was the initial dyspnoeic stimulus, leading to increased respiratory motor output, but that the sensation of dyspnoea was amplified by diminished feedback from mechanoreceptors to brainstem or cortical centres. In an important extension of this work, Demediuk and colleagues examined both breathlessness and sense of respiratory effort in normal subjects who maintained a high, fixed level of ventilation in both eucapnic and hypercapnic conditions. Dyspnoea increased with hypercapnia, but the sense of effort to breathe decreased. Since hypercapnia would be expected to increase automatic motor output, less voluntary effort would then be required to maintain a given level of ventilation. The authors interpreted these results to suggest that sense of effort might be more closely dependent upon corollary output from voluntary than automatic respiratory centres. Most significant, however, was the demonstration of dissociation between respiratory effort and dyspnoea, which would not be easily explicable under a purely feedforward model of dyspnogenesis.[13]

In the complex interplay between respiratory motor command and receptor feedback, different error signals may have different relative potencies. Using regression analysis in data from 50 patients with chronic obstructive pulmonary disease, Cloosterman and colleagues found that the mechanical load on respiratory muscles and length–tension inappropriateness emerging from dynamic hyperinflation were the principal determinants of exertional dyspnoea during eucapnia. In patients in whom hypercapnia occurred, however, it appeared to override the mechanical stimuli for dyspnoea.[65] The therapeutic implications of error signal mechanisms of generating dyspnoea were demonstrated in a study of the effects of bronchodilator therapy in patients with chronic obstructive pulmonary disease.[66] By reducing dynamic hyperinflation and so improving neuroventilatory coupling (decreasing length–tension inappropriateness), bronchodilator use decreased exertional dyspnoea.

Receptors and pathways identified in the search for mechanisms of dyspnoea are largely those implicated in the control of breathing (see Figure 6.3). Efforts to identify a 'dyspnoea centre' have drawn attention to brain regions not commonly cited in respiratory control. Using PET scanning in normal subjects, Corfield and associates found that hypercapnia with attendant dyspnoea was associated with increased activation in the upper brainstem and throughout the limbic system. No activation was seen in primary motor cortex at sites previously demonstrated

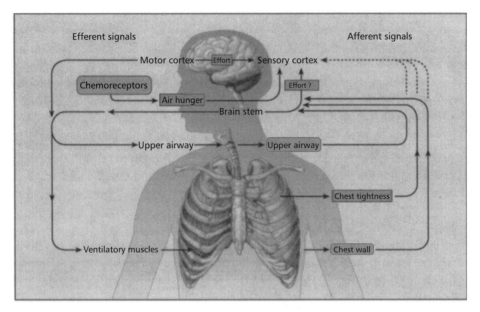

Fig. 6.3 Schematic representation of neurological signalling in perception of dyspnoea 'While all perception ultimately occurs in the sensory cortex, the information that is processed to produce these perceptions arises from a variety of neurological signals. Corollary discharge from motor cortex to sensory cortex is thought to account for the perception of respiratory effort. Brainstem activity may contribute to this. In the setting of chemoreceptor stimulation the brainstem may also mediate the sensation of air hunger. Vagally mediated irritant receptors from the chest wall probably mediate chest tightness. Airway, lung, and chest-wall afferent information is transmitted to the brainstem, and may also be relayed directly to sensory cortex. See text for details. Modified from Manning and Schwartzstein.[31]

to be associated with voluntary breathing.[56] Furthermore, the precise relationship between a dyspnoea state and respiratory control is unclear. In particular, a dyspnoea state may be integral to, or merely derivative of, mechanisms involved in the control of breathing. By analogy, consider a thermostat in which activation of the heating element is achieved by closing an electrical contact, and signalled by illumination of a light. Both contact closure and light illumination may be visible to the observer, but they are not equally relevant to the function of the thermostat. Both are avoided if the temperature is already at the set point. Similarly, dyspnoea is avoided in the absence of hypercapnia, hypoxia, airway irritation, neuromechanical dissociation, and so forth. If the dyspnoea state is ancillary, like the light, however, it may become possible to suppress it directly without impairing respiratory control; if integral, direct suppression may always come at a cost to control. As neuromodulatory drugs become more refined, the therapeutic implications of this distinction may become substantial.

Clinico-pathological links

Respiration is the process by which an organism assimilates oxygen and releases carbon dioxide and other products of oxidation. This complex process is subserved by the respiratory system *per se*, and also the cardiovascular and circulatory systems, and the peripheral tissues.

These systems each include a pump (to move gas in and out of the lungs; to circulate blood from heart to metabolically active tissue and back again) and a region in which diffusion occurs (oxygen and carbon dioxide exchange in the lung and in the systemic capillaries). Disturbances anywhere in these systems can reduce the effectiveness or efficiency of respiration, and so can alter local and systemic levels of oxygen or carbon dioxide, local and regional mechanical properties, or the work required to maintain respiratory homeostasis. Thus despite a popular tendency to think of dyspnoea as a sensation related specifically to problems with breathing, it is diagnostically and therapeutically essential to recall that a wide range of physiologic abnormalities can generate dyspnoea. While it is somewhat artificial to treat components of a complex system separately, it is clinically and heuristically useful to consider cardiovascular, respiratory, and other systemic causes of chemical and mechanical derangement associated with dyspnoea, as summarized in Box 6.2.

Cardiovascular system dyspnoea

From the standpoint of respiratory homeostasis, the function of the cardiovascular system is to circulate blood carrying oxygen and carbon dioxide in various states between the tissues and the lungs. Abnormalities in the pump (heart), the conduits (blood vessels), or the fluid (blood) can lead to dyspnoea.

Cardiac disease

Although a detailed description of cardiac physiology or pathophysiology is well beyond the scope of this chapter, a limited discussion is necessary for a practical understanding of mechanisms of dyspnoea. The heart is essentially two interdependent pumps in series, the right heart perfusing the pulmonary circulation and the left heart perfusing the systemic circulation. As with any hydraulic pump, normal cardiac function requires that the chambers fill and empty properly, maintain forward flow, and provide adequate driving pressure to circulate fluid at the required rate. Optimum cardiovascular function also requires that the pulmonary and systemic circulations remain in series, without direct mixing. Abnormalities in function occur when these requirements are not met. Because the cardiovascular system is essentially closed, local

Box 6.2 Pathophysiological causes of dyspnoea

Cardiovascular

- ◆ cardiac disease
- ◆ vascular disease (systemic, pulmonary)
- ◆ deconditioning
- ◆ anaemia

Respiratory

- ◆ respiratory controller
- ◆ ventilatory pump
- ◆ gas exchanger

disturbances tend to have repercussions throughout the system. If pumping weakens or a valve narrows, higher pressures tend to develop upstream and lower pressures develop downstream of the abnormality. These simplified concepts are helpful in understanding cardiogenic dyspnoea.

Most cardiac-derived dyspnoea ultimately involves elevation of pulmonary venous and capillary pressure. Often this results from increased left ventricular end-diastolic pressure (LVEDP), communicated in retrograde fashion to the pulmonary venous system. Whatever the aetiology of the venous pressure elevation, the disturbance of the Starling equilibrium can lead to transudation of fluid into the pulmonary interstitial space, which decreases lung compliance. Interstitial oedema stimulates the J-receptors.[67,68] If pulmonary venous hypertension is prolonged, pulmonary venous and perivascular tissue reaction can further decrease compliance. In both acute and chronic situations, the congested interstitium crowds small airways, leading to an increase in airflow resistance. This may be exacerbated by bronchospasm induced by airway receptor stimulation,[69,70] although this has not been uniformly demonstrated.[71] The combination of decreased lung compliance and increased airways resistance means that for any given level of ventilation more work (and hence more effort) is required. Respiratory muscles can become fatigued,[72] and in chronic heart failure, can weaken.[73,74] Skeletal muscle abnormalities resulting in increased ergoreflex activity may contribute to dyspnoea, and may be the sentinel causes of dyspnoea in chronic heart failure.[75] Increased metabolic demands of the respiratory musculature require a greater fraction of the cardiac output and produce more carbon dioxide, which results in ventilation in people with chronic heart failure being more steeply dependent on PCO_2 than in normal individuals.[76]

Gas exchange is further compromised as local changes lead to increased ventilation–perfusion inequalities. Frank hypoxaemia may develop, potentially exacerbating respiratory fatigue while worsening ventricular contractility and compliance and so increasing pulmonary venous congestion. Mechanisms of cardiac-derived dyspnoea due to pulmonary venous congestion thus may include input from chemoreceptors, mechanoreceptors, and ergoreceptors; augmented corollary respiratory motor output and increased sense of effort; and neuroventilatory dissociation in the setting of respiratory muscle fatigue and weakness. In conditions where anatomical connections and pressure gradients lead to parallel connections from the pulmonary to the systemic circulations (right-to-left shunt), severe hypoxia can generate dyspnoea which is resistant to oxygen therapy.

Vascular disease

Abnormalities in the vascular conduits can be involved in the generation of dyspnoea. The commonest of these, systemic hypertension, is principally important only in its contribution to cardiac disease as outlined above. Pulmonary vascular diseases, including pulmonary venous thromboembolism (pulmonary embolism), primary and secondary pulmonary artery hypertension, and pulmonary veno-occlusive disease, are much more directly associated with dyspnoea, which is thus a prominent part of the clinical manifestation of each of these conditions.

The rare condition of pulmonary veno-occlusive disease leads to pulmonary venous congestion similar to that seen in congestive heart failure, and may trigger many of the same mechanisms of dyspnoea. Pulmonary embolism, if massive, can lead to cardiogenic shock and so to cardiogenic dyspnoea. Most pulmonary emboli do not, however, have such devastating haemodynamic consequences. The redirection of blood flow away from the embolic obstruction alters ventilation–perfusion relationships in such a way that both hypercapnia and hypoxia may occur, though dyspnoea in pulmonary embolism is often more severe than would be predicted solely on the basis of these gas exchange abnormalities (cf. ref. 31).

Since vascular pressure increases due to embolism lead to J-capillary receptor C-fibre activation,[77] it is likely that these C-fibres at least are involved in producing dyspnoea in pulmonary embolism. The rapid shallow breathing pattern induced in part by C-fibre stimulation and in part by pleuritic chest pain may alter inputs from pulmonary stretch receptors and so contribute to the sensation of dyspnoea. An additional contribution may come from irritant receptors being mechanically or chemically activated.

If the mechanisms of dyspnoea in pulmonary embolism are incompletely understood, those relevant to primary pulmonary hypertension are even more obscure. The hypoxia and heart failure of advanced disease may contribute, but dyspnoea is likely to be due principally to a constellation of mechano- and chemoreceptors which are yet to be defined. In pulmonary artery hypertension secondary to cardiopulmonary disease, the underlying disease may contribute to the nature and severity of dyspnoea.

Deconditioning

In practical terms, deconditioning is one of the most common clinical conditions promoting dyspnoea. It is of particular importance as it offers an opportunity for therapeutic intervention. Deconditioning can complicate pulmonary and cardiovascular disease, chronic illnesses of all causes, obesity, and a sedentary lifestyle. In patients with severe obstructive pulmonary disease, as well as in exquisitely conditioned athletes, ventilatory limitations to exertion may be critical, and in pulmonary hypertension, pulmonary vascular limits may contribute. Cardiopulmonary exercise testing shows, however, that even in these populations the usual boundaries to exercise tolerance are cardiovascular in nature, based upon limited augmentation of cardiac output and oxygen uptake by exercising muscle. In patients with chronic congestive heart failure, skeletal muscle abnormalities are thought to account for much of the severity of exertional dyspnoea. Data are accruing to suggest that physical deconditioning of any sort, including sedentary lifestyle in otherwise healthy individuals, may lead to similar skeletal muscle impairments,[78] and hence similar mechanisms of dyspnoea. With training, muscle changes including increased capillary density, mitochondrial number, and aerobic enzyme concentration facilitate aerobic metabolism.[79] The consequent delay in anaerobic metabolism and lactic acidosis[80] may decrease ergoreceptor stimulation, postpone the compensatory increase in ventilation associated with the onset of metabolic acidosis, and prevent attendant dyspnoea. Even in patients with markedly reduced ventilatory reserve, such as those with advanced obstructive lung disease, suitable cardiovascular conditioning can improve exertional dyspnoea and exercise tolerance.[81]

Anaemia

In anaemia, especially with haemoglobin concentration <7 g/dL, exertional dyspnoea can be marked. Though numerous plausible explanations have been advanced, the mechanism is unknown. As oxygen delivery to the tissues is a function of oxygen content (reduced in anaemia) and cardiac output, augmentation of the latter is the principal initial physiologic response. In addition to tachycardia, ventricular contractility may be increased, leading to higher LVEDP and so potentially activating J-receptors. Decreased oxygen delivery to skeletal muscle may provide a stimulus to ergoreceptors, with consequent dyspnoea and increased ventilation.

Respiratory system dyspnoea

An appreciation of the aetiology of dyspnoea in lung disease is facilitated by a mechanistic view of respiration. The respiratory system itself can be viewed as having three components: the respiratory controller, the ventilatory pump, and the gas exchanger.[82] (See Chapter 2 for further discussion of this topic.) For the purpose of this discussion, the controller comprises the network of peripheral receptors and central mechanisms that establish ventilatory drive. The ventilatory pump includes the entire bellows mechanism responsible for circulating air between the environment and the lungs. The gas exchanger is the alveolar-capillary interface across which gas diffusion occurs. Table 6.2 gives a summary of disease states in which these mechanisms may play a part in the generation of dyspnoea.

Respiratory controller

Most of the elements described in the section on basic physiology of dyspnoea, including chemoreceptors, mechanoreceptors, and central mechanisms, are appropriately considered as parts of the respiratory controller. Thus the activity of the respiratory controller is important to virtually all respiratory-system-induced dyspnoea. Indeed, although derangement of controller function can be dyspnogenic, the controller differs from the pump and the gas exchanger in that its normal physiological function as a homeostatic mechanism can lead to dyspnoea. The nature of stimuli that affect respiratory control and promote dyspnoea will not be reiterated here, but it is useful to relate these to causal mechanisms from respiratory disease.

Chemoreceptor stimulation is likely to be a seminal factor in dyspnoea in all causes of acute or decompensated hypercapnic respiratory failure. In neuromuscular disease with pneumonia,

Table 6.2 Diseases causing dyspnoea. Disorders of the respiratory system are categorized on the basis of the major mechanisms by which they produce dyspnoea. Any of these conditions, if they are associated with hypoxia and/or hypercapnia, may also lead to breathing discomfort via stimulation of the respiratory controller

Respiratory controller	Asthma Pulmonary vascular disease Interstitial lung disease High altitude Increased progesterone in pregnancy
Ventilatory pump	COPD/asthma – hyperinflation Kyphoscoliosis Neuromuscular disease Pleural disease Morbid obesity Interstitial lung disease
Gas exchanger	Pneumonia Pulmonary oedema Obliterative bronchiolitis Emphysema Interstitial lung disease

or acute respiratory decompensation in COPD, rapid accumulation of carbon dioxide and respiratory acidosis are potent promoters of ventilation and dyspnoea. Because the chronic compensated hypercapnia often seen with advanced obstructive lung disease is usually not associated with dyspnoea, it is likely that acidosis is the relevant chemical abnormality. Further support for this comes from the dyspnoea experienced in acute metabolic acidoses (such as diabetic ketoacidosis) in patients with normal respiratory mechanics, in which compensatory hyperventilation can lead to very low PCO_2 without resolution of breathlessness. Clinically, this group of patients may be less dyspnoeic for a given degree of acidaemia than others with primary respiratory acidosis. This is likely to represent the independent contribution of precipitating respiratory abnormalities to the dyspnoeic state. Though typically a less robust stimulus, hypoxia may contribute to dyspnoea in pulmonary vascular disease, interstitial lung disease, and COPD.[26] It is, however, probably the primary derangement leading to exertional dyspnoea at high altitudes. In pregnancy, increased ventilation due to increased levels of progesterone may lead to dyspnoea.[83] Some pregnant women may moreover, also have a higher sensitivity to hypoxia and hypercapnia and they may increase ventilation excessively to meet metabolic demand.[84]

Mechanoreceptor stimulation is a primary cause of dyspnoea in a variety of respiratory diseases. As noted above, irritant receptors may contribute to breathlessness in asthma. Dyspnoea is worse with histamine-induced bronchoconstriction than with a matched external resistive load, and bronchoconstrictive but not external resistive dyspnoea is relieved by inhaled lignocaine (lidocaine).[41] J-receptors or other mechanoreceptors may also contribute to dyspnoea in interstitial lung disease. Some animal models support this possibility,[85] though early efforts to control dyspnoea in restrictive lung disease with vagal blockade had mixed results.[46] In normal subjects with mechanically induced hyperinflation, dyspnoea may persist even when ventilatory work is markedly reduced by continuous positive airway pressure,[86] though this has not been consistently shown.[39] This finding raises the possibility that dyspnoea in hyperinflated lungs is mediated in part by mechanoreceptors. A similar mechanism might then contribute to dyspnoea in asthmatic hyperinflation.

Combinations of feedforward and error-signal central processing provide probably the most ubiquitous connection between the respiratory controller and dyspnoea. The various sorts of mechanical disadvantage and respiratory muscle weakness seen in obstructive pulmonary disease, interstitial lung disease, and neuromuscular disease (see below and Chapter 18) lead to high levels of respiratory effort and to neuroventilatory dissociation. These are all associated with breathlessness.[60,61,64]

Not all disturbances in the respiratory controller cause dyspnoea. An important example is the hypercapnic tolerance manifest by a subset of patients with COPD, the so-called 'blue bloaters'. In this population the ventilatory response to CO_2 is markedly blunted. PCO_2 rises, usually leading to compensatory metabolic alkalosis and a new steady state. The mechanism of this alteration is incompletely understood. Teleologically, however, it may represent an adaptation which reduces both work of breathing and dyspnoea, since a chronically elevated PCO_2 allows the individual to eliminate the daily product CO_2 of metabolism with a reduced alveolar ventilation.

Ventilatory pump

The effectiveness of the ventilatory pump is determined by the mechanical work required for movement of air into and out of the lungs and the force-generating capacity of the respiratory muscles. When respiratory mechanics are poor or respiratory muscles are weak, respiratory effort and neuroventilatory dissociation lead to dyspnoea. If hypoventilatory failure ensues, hypercapnia and eventually hypoxia may exacerbate breathlessness.

Abnormalities in the ventilatory pump occur in many of the commonest respiratory diseases and play a prominent role in the pathophysiology of dyspnoea. In asthma and COPD, resistance to airflow is high; in COPD, airway compliance is also increased. Negative pleural pressures on inspiration promote airway patency, whereas positive pressures on expiration can lead to dynamic airway compression in COPD. Severe obstructive lung disease thus leads to progressive air trapping and thoracic hyperinflation, which can worsen during exacerbations. Hyperinflation shifts the chest wall to a flatter part of its compliance curve, meaning that more work is required for any given volume of expansion. Hyperinflation also leads to loss of diaphragmatic curvature; this muscular shortening decreases its ability to generate tension and places the diaphragm at 'mechanical disadvantage'. Thus airway resistance and hyperinflation conspire to increase work of breathing for a diaphragm that is already compromised. Oxygen uptake by the muscles of respiration increases dramatically, especially with exertion; the fraction of cardiac output delivered to the respiratory muscles rises accordingly. If uptake outstrips delivery, diaphragmatic fatigue ensues, exacerbating dyspnoea and heralding respiratory failure.

In restrictive diseases, the airway resistances may be normal and lung and thoracic volumes normal or small. Work of breathing is nevertheless increased due to decreased respiratory system compliance. This 'stiffening' can be extrinsic to the lung, as in kyphoscoliosis, pleural thickening, and morbid obesity, or intrinsic to the lung, as in interstitial lung disease. Problems with the gas exchanger often complicate these conditions. High minute ventilation must be maintained; tidal volumes are limited by compliance, and a pattern of rapid shallow breathing is characteristic. Dyspnoea can be severe, especially with exertion.

Dyspnoea is a hallmark of advanced neuromuscular disease. Although respiratory muscle weakness and fatigue can further compromise ventilatory pump function in any patient with altered respiratory mechanics, severe primary neuromuscular weakness can lead to ventilatory failure despite essentially normal respiratory mechanics. In myasthenia gravis,[87] muscular dystrophy,[88] or amyotrophic lateral sclerosis,[89] respiratory failure can be fatal unless mechanical ventilatory support is initiated. In each of these conditions, measures of respiratory drive are elevated at rest. As with other abnormalities of the ventilatory pump, dyspnoea derives from an increased sense of respiratory effort, neuroventilatory dissociation, or both. Ventilation–perfusion mismatch and atelectasis due to hypoventilation can worsen dyspnoea through respiratory controller mechanisms as outlined above. Atelectasis may additionally promote dyspnoea through J-receptor stimulation (see Chapters 18 and 19 for further details of dyspnoea in neuromuscular disease).

Gas exchanger

Abnormalities of the gas exchanger are common in respiratory disease. Alveolar gas and capillary blood need to be aligned across the semipermeable alveolar capillary membranes in suitable ratios and over sufficient time for exchange of oxygen and carbon dioxide to occur. By definition, a failure of the gas exchanger leads to hypoxia, hypercapnia, or both, and the mechanisms of dyspnoea are those mediated by the relevant chemoreceptors. Derangement of the gas exchanger rarely exists in isolation from other respiratory abnormalities, and associated dyspnoea is virtually always multifactorial.

Gas can be prevented from reaching the membranes by mechanical obstruction of the alveoli or small airways. This can be acute, as in pneumonia or pulmonary oedema, or sub-acute/chronic, as in obliterative bronchiolitis. Blood flow to the interface can be altered by vascular occlusion, as with pulmonary thromboembolism, by vascular constrictive changes, as with pulmonary artery hypertension, or by interstitial pressure changes, as with interstitial oedema or increased alveolar pressure. The area of interface can be reduced by parenchymal destruction in emphysema, pulmonary fibrosis, or suppurative infection. Compensatory mechanisms including hyperventilation and hypoxic vasoconstriction may be partially corrective, but are overwhelmed if the area of effective exchange is sufficiently reduced.

In addition to these abnormalities of the gas exchanger, the alveolar–capillary interface can be altered in such a way that specific diffusion is reduced. This impairment is particularly marked in interstitial lung disease. Oxygen exchange is more compromised than carbon dioxide exchange, in part because of its lower diffusion coefficient. Although it can be an important cause of exertional hypoxia, a diffusion limitation is rarely the cause of clinically important hypoxia at rest. In the normal lung, the interplay of alveolar–capillary oxygen gradient, rate of oxygen diffusion, rate of capillary blood flow, and oxyhaemoglobin saturation characteristics, is such that haemoglobin is completely saturated during the first third of its transit along the pulmonary capillaries. Interstitial changes alone are rarely sufficient to prevent saturation. With exertion, however, the decrease in mixed venous oxygen saturation, and particularly the decreased transit time of capillary blood, can lead to significantly reduced saturation in the setting of preexisting diffusion limitations.

Language of dyspnoea

An emerging understanding of the clinical physiology of dyspnoea depends upon the elucidation of specific arrays of mechanisms leading to dyspnoea which are active in particular disease states. If the perception of dyspnoea (via a central 'dyspnoea state') differs from one mechanism to another, (for example, if stretch receptors, irritant receptors, and carbon dioxide receptors each engender a different perceptual experience), then it is highly plausible that these different combinations of activation are also discernible, i.e. are perceived as being different. If they may be so discriminated, the particular qualities of dyspnoea associated with particular disease states may be verbally communicable. Careful use of language might then provide both a powerful diagnostic tool and an instrument with which to dissect the mechanisms underlying dyspnoea in different disease states.

There are daunting challenges to this approach. For many decades, cognitive psychologists studying colour perception have known that individuals from different cultures speaking different languages show both striking similarities and important differences in how they name and organize colours. Arguments persist about the relative importance of concordant physiology and discordant culture and linguistics in the human experience of colour. Dyspnoea is still more complicated, and its physiological substrate is much less well understood than the physiology of colour discrimination.

Colour is a universal human experience, but at least certain types of dyspnoea are much more sporadic. Despite some variability in number and scope of the terms, every language has dedicated words for colours, whereas many of the descriptors of dyspnoea are borrowed ('heaviness', 'tightness', 'hunger'). In these respects, the contemporary study of the language of dyspnoea more closely parallels that of the language of pain, which indeed is its scientific progenitor.[7,8]

Early work on the language of dyspnoea attempted to identify elemental attributes of dyspnoea, somewhat akin to the attributes of hue, brightness, and saturation which are ascribed to colour perception. Following the work in pain perception, current investigations of the language of dyspnoea have developed through three stages: elaboration of descriptors of dyspnoea; identification of clusters of descriptors associated with defined respiratory tasks; and correlation between those clusters and the experiences of patients with known cardiovascular or respiratory system disease.

Simon and colleagues surveyed dyspnoeic patients with a variety of cardiopulmonary conditions and developed a list of phrases describing their qualitative sensation of respiratory discomfort (Box 6.3).

The descriptors reflected perceptions suggestive of limitations to flow or volume ('breath does not go in' or 'out all the way'), of abnormal respiratory system mechanics ('chest is constricted' or 'tight'), of increased effort, of a visceral desire to augment ventilation ('hunger for more air') and of a global sense of inadequate ventilation ('suffocating'). Normal subjects

Box 6.3 Qualitative descriptors of dyspnoea

- My breath does not go in all the way
- My breathing requires effort
- I feel that I am smothering
- I feel a hunger for more air
- My breathing is heavy
- I cannot take a deep breath
- I feel out of breath
- My chest feels tight
- My breathing requires more work
- I feel that I am suffocating
- I feel that my breathing stops
- I am gasping for breath
- My chest is constricted
- I feel that my breathing is rapid
- My breathing is shallow
- I feel that I am breathing more
- I cannot get enough air
- My breath does not go out all the way
- My breathing requires more concentration

From Simon *et al.*[6]

made dyspnoeic by a variety of chemical and mechanical stimuli, as well as by the performance of physical and respiratory tasks, were then asked to select from the list the most apt descriptors of their experience. Not surprisingly, cluster analysis revealed that subsets of descriptors were intrinsically linked. More importantly, dyspnoea elicited by different tasks was associated with different profiles of descriptor clusters, supporting subjective claims that the experiences were distinctive. For instance, breathing against a resistive load yielded descriptions of increased 'work of breathing' and 'air hunger', while breathing with decreased tidal volume was associated with descriptions of 'rapid', 'shallow' breathing requiring 'increased concentration'.[6]

In a follow-up study, 53 patients experiencing dyspnoea in the context of pregnancy or because of cardiopulmonary disease selected from the established list of descriptors those that best captured the quality of their breathlessness. As had been the case with dyspnoea induced in normal subjects, each pathophysiological condition was associated with a particular profile of descriptor clusters.[12] Elliot and colleagues conducted a similar study on 208 patients in the UK with an array of cardiopulmonary disorders, providing them with an expanded questionnaire including 45 descriptors of 'troubled breathing' during exertion.[90] There was substantial overlap in the groups' identification of descriptor clusters and their assignment of those clusters to disease states (Table 6.3). Skevington et al.[91] investigated the quality and intensity of dyspnoea in a sample of 80 patients drawn largely from cardiopulmonary and oncology wards. Using an open-ended, unstructured format, the authors solicited spontaneous descriptions of breathlessness from their patients. Following a sorting of these responses by experienced healthcare providers, a clustering algorithm revealed four categories. The 'physical sensations' category closely approximated the clusters derived by Simon et al.[12] In addition, a second major category that included phrases representing affective and evaluative components of breathlessness was noted.

The pattern of relationship between descriptors and pathophysiological states in the study of Simon and colleagues is noteworthy. Each disease state was characterized by a unique combination of multiple clusters, while each cluster was represented in multiple disease states. This suggests that dyspnoea in any particular disease is a complex entity, and supports the idea of shared dyspnoea mechanisms in different conditions.

Table 6.3 Descriptor clusters associated with common cardiopulmonary diseases

Descriptor cluster	COPD	CHF	ILD	Asthma	NM/CW	PVD
Rapid breathing		×				×
Incomplete exhalation			×			
Shallow breathing				×		
Increased work or effort	×		×	×	×	
Feeling of suffocation		×				
Air hunger	×	×				
Chest tightness			×			
Heavy breathing			×			

CHF, congestive heart failure; COPD, chronic obstructive pulmonary disease; ILD, interstitial lung disease; NM/CW, neuromuscular and chest wall disease; PVD, pulmonary vascular disease.

Modified from Schwartzstein.[6]

However, despite these studies, it has not been possible to demonstrate comprehensive and compelling linguistic links between particular experiences of dyspnoea and their underlying mechanisms. Descriptor clusters are imprecise, and may not permit full resolution of dyspnoeic perceptions. Existing descriptors may not include the whole range of dyspnoeic experience. Primary perceptions of dyspnoea may themselves not have a strict one-to-one correlation with causative mechanisms. Differences in language, culture, emotional state, and circumstance may lead to differences between groups and individuals in descriptions of dyspnoea quality despite there being similar underlying mechanisms. Yet, despite these practical and theoretical limitations, scrutiny of language usage is emerging as a powerful tool in the diagnosis and management of conditions causing dyspnoea.

Descriptions of chest tightness in the dyspnoeic patient are strongly suggestive of reactive airways disease, and amelioration of that tightness provides insight into the efficacy of bronchodilator and other therapies.[92] Prominence of air hunger in any cardiopulmonary disease appropriately prompts evaluation for hypoxia or hypercapnia, and a sense of inability to draw a full breath often indicates hyperinflation. As associations between descriptors, disease states, and dyspnogenic mechanisms are further elaborated, language is likely to become an increasingly important ally to patient, clinician, and investigator alike.

Therapeutic implications

Investigation into the mechanisms of dyspnoea has promoted understanding of respiratory physiology, control of breathing, and the pathophysiology of cardiopulmonary disease. Ultimately, however, the goal of research is the amelioration of a common, troublesome, and often disabling condition. As represented in Figure 6.1 above, important interventions can be made at any stage in the generation of dyspnoea, or in the patient's consequent reaction and response. A detailed and accurate analysis of the genesis of dyspnoea in particular diseases, or better still, in individual patients, may facilitate the design of effective and appropriate treatments.

There are hierarchies of intervention in dyspnoea. In a patient in whom the substrate for dyspnoea is established, it is preferable to interrupt the mechanism at the fundamental, sensory level, than merely to modulate it by blunting the perception. Such blunting may, however, be essential in acute or intractable dyspnoea (see Chapter 1 for discussion of the different types of symptom palliation). In some instances, modifying the emotional or behavioural sequelae of dyspnoea may be critical, as in teaching stoic asthmatics not to ignore worsening breathlessness, encouraging badly deconditioned patients to tolerate a measure of dyspnoea during a programme of cardiopulmonary rehabilitation, or helping patients with severe COPD to achieve a sense of control over their breathing and so avoid the precipitation of acute anxiety or panic attacks (see Chapter 11 for more on this issue).

Table 6.4 gives a summary of how a better understanding of the mechanisms underlying dyspnoea can lead to more specific and, it is hoped, more successful therapy. For fuller discussions of these approaches, see the appropriate chapters elsewhere in this volume.

Table 6.4 Therapeutic interventions targeted to mechanisms of dyspnoea

Target mechanism	Therapeutic intervention
1. Modify chemoreceptor activity	
Hypoxia	Supplemental oxygen: nasal cannula, transtracheal
	Correct hypoventilation: non-invasive mechanical ventilatory support
	Improve conditioning
Hypercapnia (acute)	Improve ventilatory mechanics:
	bronchodilators
	anti-inflammatory agents
	treat pneumonia/pulmonary oedema
	treat abdominal distension
	Non-invasive mechanical ventilatory support
	? Suppress ventilatory drive (opiates)
Hypercapnia (chronic)	Optimize ventilatory mechanics
	Avoid respiratory stimulants
	? Intermittent non-invasive mechanical ventilatory support
	? High-calorie, low-carbohydrate diet
2. Modify mechanoreceptor activity	
Stimulate flow receptors	Fan
	Supplemental oxygen
	Compressed air
Suppress irritant receptors	Avoid irritants
	? Inhaled topical anesthetics
Suppress J-receptors	Diuresis in congestive heart failure
Stimulate chest wall receptors	In-phase chest wall vibration
3. Modify central processing	
Feedforward (decrease effort)	Improve ventilatory mechanics
	Non-invasive mechanical ventilatory support
Feedback	Improve conditioning (decrease effort / workload)
4. Modify receptor activity	As for '2', +
Error-signal	Improve neuroventilatory equilibrium: feedforward and select feedback mechanisms
5. Modify perception and interpretation	
	Opiates
	? Non-sedating anxiolytics
	Serotonergic medications
	Cognitive-behavioural therapy
	relaxation techniques
	breathing retraining
	symptom control
	Psychotherapy

Keypoints

♦ Consideration of the mechanisms of dyspnoea promotes a focused diagnostic approach and refinement of therapeutic interventions

♦ The patient's verbal descriptions of the dyspnoeic experience can help to make a diagnostic evaluation

♦ If the specific chemoreceptor, mechanoreceptor or central processing elements causing breathlessness can be identified for a given patient, a tailored therapeutic regimen can be devised

♦ Ultimately, a more detailed subtler understanding of the nature of and interplay between the mechanisms of dyspnoea holds the promise of more appropriate and effective therapies for the amelioration of this major cause of distress

References

1 Higgins, M. Epidemiology of obstructive pulmonary disease. In: R. Cassaburi, and T.L. Petty (eds) *Principles and practice of pulmonary rehabilitation.* Philadelphia, Pa.: W.B. Saunders, 1993.

2 American Thoracic Society. Standards for the diagnosis and care of patients with chronic obstructive pulmonary disease. *J Respir Crit Care Med* 1995; **152**: S77–120.

3 Ripamonti, C., and Bruera, E. Dyspnea: Pathophysiology and assessment. *J Pain Symptom Manage* 1997; **13**(4): 220–32.

4 Banzett, R.B., Lansing, R.W., *et al.* 'Air hunger' from increased PCO_2 persists after complete neuromuscular block in humans. *Respir Physiol* 1990; **81**: 1–8.

5 American Thoracic Society. Dyspnea. *J Respir Crit Care Med* 1999; **159**: 321–40.

6 Simon, P.M., Schwartzstein, R.M., *et al.* Distinguishable sensations of breathlessness induced in normal volunteers. *Am Rev Respir Dis* 1989; **140**: 1021–7.

7 Schwartzstein, R.M., and Cristiano, L.M. Qualities of respiratory sensation. In: L. Adams, and A. Guz (eds) *Respiratory sensation.* New York: Marcel Dekker, 1996; 125–54.

8 Schwartzstein, R.M. The language of dyspnea. In: D.A. Mahler (ed.) *Dyspnea.* New York: Marcel Dekker, 1998; 35–62.

9 Schwartzstein, R.M. The 'language' of dyspnea: Using verbal clues to the diagnosis. *J Crit Illness* 1999; **14**(8): 435–41.

10 Clark, F.J., and von Euler, C. On the regulation of depth and rate of breathing. *J Physiol* 1972; **222**: 267–95.

11 Hill, L., and Flack, F. The effect of excess carbon dioxide and want of oxygen upon the respiration and the circulation. *J Physiol* 1908; **37**: 77.

12 Simon, P.M., Schwartzstein, R.M., *et al.* Distinguishable types of dyspnea in patients with shortness of breath. *Am Rev Respir Dis* 1990; **142**: 1009–14.

13 Demediuk, B.H., Manning, H., *et al.* Dissociation between dyspnea and respiratory effort. *Am Rev Respir Dis* 1992; **146**: 1222–5.

14 Campbell, E.J.M., Godfrey, S., *et al.* The effect of muscular paralysis induced by tubocurarine on the duration and sensation of breath-holding during hypercapnea. *Clin Sci* 1969; **36**: 323–328.

15 Smith, S.M., Brown, H.O., *et al.* The lack of cerebral effects of d-tubocurarine. *Anesthesiology* 1947; **8**: 1–14.

16 Opie, L.H., Smith, A.C., *et al.* Conscious appreciation of the effects produced by independent changes of ventilation volume and of end-tidal PCO2 in paralysed patients. *J Physiol (London)* 1959; **149**: 494–9.

17 Chonan, T., Mulholland, M.B., *et al.* Effects of voluntary constraining of thoracic displacement during hypercapnia. *J Appl Physiol* 1987; **63**(5): 1822–8.

18 Schwartzstein, R.M., LaHive, K., *et al.* Detection of hypercapnia by normal subjects. *Clin Sci* 1987; **73**: 333–5.

19 Schwartzstein, R.M., Simon, P.M., *et al.* Breathlessness induced by dissociation between ventilation and chemical drive. *Am Rev Respir Dis* 1989; **139**: 1231–7.

20 Chonan, T., Mulholland, M.B., *et al.* Sensation of dyspnea during hypercapnia, exercise, and voluntary hyperventilation. *J Appl Physiol* 1990; **68**(5): 2100–6.

21 Banzett, R.B., Lansing, R.W., *et al.* 'Air hunger' arising from increased PCO_2 in mechanically ventilated quadriplegics. *Respir Physiol* 1989; **76**: 53–68.

22 Fahey, P.J., and Hyde, R.W. 'Won't breathe' vs 'can't breathe': Detection of depressed ventilatory drive in patients with obstrructive pulmonary disease. *Chest* 1983; **84**: 19–25.

23 Chronos, N., Adams, L., *et al.* Effect of hyperoxia and hypoxia on exercise-induced breathlessness in normal subjects. *Clin Sci* 1988; **74**: 531–7.

24 Davidson, J.T., Whipp, B.J., *et al.* Role of the carotid bodies in breath-holding. *N Engl J Med* 1974; **290**: 819–22.

25 Mak, V.H.F., Bugler, J.R., *et al.* Effect of arterial oxygen desaturation on six minute walk distance, perceived effort, and perceived breathlessness in patients with airflow limitation. *Thorax* 1993; **48**: 33–8.

26 Dean, N.C., Brown, J.K., *et al.* Oxygen may improve dyspnea and endurance in patients with chronic obstructive pulmonary disease and only mild hypoxemia. *Am Rev Respir Dis* 1992; **146**: 941–5.

27 Booth, S., Kelly, M.J., *et al.* Does oxygen help dyspnea in patients with cancer? *Am J Respir Crit Care Med* 1996; **153**: 1515–8.

28 Swinburn, C.R., Wakefield, J.M., *et al.* Relationship between ventilation and breathlessness during exercise in chronic obstructive airways disease is not altered by the prevention of hypoxia. *Clin Sci* 1984; **67**: 515–19.

29 Lane, R., Adams, L., *et al.* The effects of hypoxia and hypercapnia on perceived breathlessness during exercise in humans. *J Physiol* 1990; **428**: 579–93.

30 Adams, L., Chronos, N., *et al.* The dyspnogenic effect of hypoxia – dissociation from ventilatory response. *Clin Sci* 1982; **63**: 17P.

31 Manning, H.L., and Schwartzstein, R.M. Mechanisms of dyspnea. In: D.A. Mahler (ed.) *Dyspnea*. New York: Marcel Dekker, 1998; 63–95.

32 Woodcock, A.A., Gross, E.R., *et al.* Oxygen relieves breathlessness in 'pink puffers.' *Lancet* 1981; **I**: 907–909.

33 McBride, B., and Whitelaw, W.A. A physiological stimulus to upper airway receptors in humans. *J Appl Physiol* 1981; **51**: 1189–97.

34 Schwartzstein, R.M., Lahive, K., *et al.* Cold facial stimulation reduces breathlessness induced in normal subjects. *Am Rev Respir Dis* 1987; **136**: 58–61.

35 Rodenstein, D.O., Mercenier, C., *et al.* Influence of the respiratory route on the resting breathing pattern in humans. *Am Rev Respir Dis* 1985; **131**: 163–6.

36 Simon, P.M., Basner, R.C., *et al.* Oral mucosal stimulation modulates intensity of breathlessness induced in normal subjects. *Am Rev Respir Dis* 1991; **144**: 419–22.

37 Miserocchi, G., and Sant'Ambrogio, G. Responses of pulmonary stretch receptors to static pressure inflations. *Respir Physiol* 1974; **21**: 77–85.

38 von Euler, C. Brain-stem mechanisms for generation and control of breathing pattern. In: N.S. Cherniack, and J.G. Widdicombe (eds) *Handbook of Physiology*. Section 3: *The Respiratory System, Volume II: Control of Breathing. Part 1.* Bethesda, MD: American Physiologic Society, 1986; 1–68.

39 O'Donnell, D.E., Sanii, R., *et al.* Effect of dynamic airway compression on breathing pattern and respiratory sensation in severe chronic obstructive pulmonary disease. *Am Rev Respir Dis* 1987; **135**: 912–18.

40 Manning, H.L., Shea, S.A., *et al.* Reduced tidal volume increases 'air hunger' at fixed PCO_2 in ventilated quadriplegics. *Respir Physiol* 1992; **90**: 19–30.

41 Taguchi, O., Kikuchi, Y., *et al.* Effects of bronchoconstriction and external resistive loading on the sensation of dyspnea. *J Appl Physiol* 1991; **71**: 2183–90.

42 Moy, M.L., Weiss, J.W., Sparrow, D., Israel, E., and Schwartzstein, R.M. Quality of dyspnea in bronchoconstriction differs from external resistive loads. *Am J Respir Crit Care Med* 2000; **162**: 451–5.

43 Green, J.F., Schmidt, N.D., *et al.* Pulmonary C-fibres evoke both apnea and tachypnea of pulmonary chemoreflex. *J Appl Physiol* 1984; **57**: 562–7.

44 Raj, H., Singh, V.K., *et al.* Sensory origin of lobeline-induced sensations: a correlative study in man and cat. *J Physiol* 1995; **482**: 235–46.

45 Noble, M.I.M., Eisele, J.H., *et al.* Effect of selective peripheral nerve blocks on respiratory sensations. In: R. Porter (ed.) *Breathing: Hering–Breuer centenary symposium.* London: J. & A. Churchill, 1970; 233–51.

46 Guz, A., Noble, M.I.M., *et al.* Experimental results of vagal block in cardiopulmonary disease. In: R. Porter (ed.) *Breathing: Hering–Breuer centenary symposium.* London: J. & A. Churchill, 1970; 315–29.

47 Shannon, R. Reflexes from respiratory muscles and costovertebral joints. In: N.S. Cherniack, and J.G. Widdicombe (eds) *Handbook of Physiology.* Section 3: *The Respiratory System, Volume II: Control of Breathing. Part 1.* Bethesda, MD: American Physiologic Society, 1986; 431–47.

48 Remmers, J.E., Brooks, J.G., *et al.* Effect of controlled ventilation on the tolerable limit of hypercapnia. *Respir Physiol* 1968; **4**: 78–90.

49 Altose, M.D., DiMarco, A.F., *et al.* The sensation of respiratory muscle force. *Am Rev Respir Dis* 1982; **126**: 807–11.

50 Stubbing, D.G., Killian, K.J., *et al.* The quantification of respiratory sensations by normal subjects. *Respir Physiol* 1981; **44**: 251–60.

51 McCloskey, D.I., Ebeling, P., *et al.* Estimation of weights and tensions and apparent involvement of a 'sense of effort'. *Exp Neurol* 1974; **42**: 220–32.

52 Manning, H.L., Basner, R., *et al.* Effect of chest wall vibration on breathlessness in normal subjects. *J Appl Physiol* 1991; **71**: 175–81.

53 Sibuya, M., Yamada, M., *et al.* Effect of chest wall vibration on dyspnea in patients with chronic respiratory disease. *Am J Respir Crit Care Med* 1994; **149**: 1235–40.

54 Piepoli, M., Ponikowski, P., *et al.* A neural link to explain the 'muscle hypothesis' of exercise intolerance in chronic heart failure. *American Heart Journal* 1999; **137**: 1050–1056.

55 Grieve, D.A., Clark, A.L., *et al.* The ergoreflex in patients with chronic stable heart failure. *Int J Cardiol* 1999; **68**: 157–64.

56 Corfield, D.R., Fink, G.R., *et al.* Evidence for limbic system activation during CO_2-stimulated breathing in man. *J Physiol* 1995; **488**(1): 77–84.

57 Plum, F. Breathlessness in neurological disease: the effects of neurological disease on the act of breathing. In: J.B.L. Howell, and E.J.M. Campbell (eds) *Breathlessness.* London: Blackwell Scientific, 1966; 203–22.

58 Gandevia, S.C. The perception of motor commands or effort during muscular paralysis. *Brain* 1982; **105**: 151–195.

59 McCloskey, D.I. Kinesthetic sensibility. *Physiol Rev* 1978; **58**(4): 763–820.

60 El-Manshawi, A., Killian, K.J., *et al.* Breathlessness during exercise with and without resistive loading. *J Appl Physiol* 1986; **61**(3): 896–905.

61 Gandevia, S.C. Proprioceptive mechanisms of the respiratory muscles. In: D. Garlick (ed.) *Proprioception, Posture and Emotion.* Sydney: Committee in Postgraduate Medical Education, University of NSW, 1982; 92–102.

62 Schwartzstein, R.M., Manning, H., *et al.* Dyspnea – a sensory experience. *Lung* 1990; **140**: 168–185.

63 McCloskey, D.I., Gandevia, S., *et al.* Muscle sense and effort: motor commands and judgements about muscular contractions. In: J.E. Desmedt (ed.) *Motor control mechanisms in health and disease.* New York: Raven Press, 1983.

64 O'Donnell, D.E., and Webb, K.A. Exertional breathlessness in patients with chronic airflow limitation: The role of lung hyperinflation. *Am Rev Respir Dis* 1993; **148**: 1351–7.

65 Cloosterman, S.G.M., Hofland, I.D., *et al.* Exertional dyspnea in patients with airway obstruction, with and without CO_2 retention. *Thorax* 1998; **53**: 768–74.

66 Belman, M.J., Botnick, W.C., *et al.* Inhaled bronchodilators reduce dynamic hyperinflation during exercise in patients with chronic obstructive pulmonary disease. *Am J Respir Crit Care Med* 1996; **153**: 967–75.

67 Paintal, A.S. Mechanism of stimulation of type J pulmonary receptors. *J Physiol* 1969; **203**: 511–32.

68 Paintal, A.S. Sensations from J receptors. *News Physiol Sci* 1995; **10**: 238–43.

69 Lloyd, T.C. Reflex effects of left heart and pulmonary vascular distension on airways of dogs. *J Appl Physiol* 1980; **49**: 620–6.

70 Cabanes, L.R., Weber, S.N., *et al.* Bronchial hyperresponsiveness to methacholine in patients with impaired left ventricular function. *N Engl J Med* 1989; **320**: 1317–22.

71 Chua, T.P., Lalloo, U.G., *et al.* Airway and cough responsiveness and exhaled nitric oxide in non-smoking patients with stable chronic heart failure. *Heart* 1996; **76**: 144–149.

72 Aubier, M., Trippenback, T., *et al.* Respiratory muscle fatigue during cardiogenic shock. *J Appl Physiol* 1981; **51**: 499–508.

73 Hammond, M.D., Bauer, K.A., *et al.* Respiratory muscle strength in congestive heart failure. *Chest* 1990; **98**: 1091–1094.

74 McParland, C., Krishnan, B., *et al.* Inspiratory muscle weakness and dyspnea in chronic heart failure. *Am Rev Respir Dis* 1992; **146**: 467–72.

75 Clark, A.L. The origin of symptoms in chronic heart failure. *Heart* 1997; **78**: 429–430.

76 Buller, N.P., and Poole-Wilson, P.A. Mechanism of the increased ventilatory response to exercise in patients with chronic heart failure. *Br Heart J* 1990; **63**: 281–3.

77 Armstrong, D.J., Luck, J.C., *et al.* The effect of emboli upon intrapulmonary receptors in the cat. *Respir Physiol* 1976; **26**: 41–54.

78 Chati, Z., Zannad, F., *et al.* Physical deconditioning may be a mechanism for the skeletal muscle energy phosphate metabolism abnormalities in chronic heart failure. *Am Heart J* 1996; **131**: 560–6.

79 Saltin, B., and Gollnick, P.D. Skeletal muscle adaptability: significance for metabolism and performance. In: L.D. Peachey (ed.) *Handbook of physiology: skeletal muscle.* Washington, DC: American Physiological Society, 1983; 555–631.

80 Casaburi, R., Storer, T.W., *et al.* Effect of endurance training on possible determinants of VO_2 during heavy exercise. *J Appl Physiol* 1987; **62**: 199–207.

81 Casaburi, R., Patessio, A., *et al.* Reductions in exercise lactic acidosis and ventilation as a result of exercise training in patients with obstructive lung disease. *Am Rev Respir Dis* 1991; **143**: 9–18.

82 Schwartzstein, R.M., and Manning, H.M. Mechanisms of dyspnea. In: N.S. Cherniack, M.D. Altose, and I. Homma (eds) *Rehabilitation of the patient with respiratory disease.* New York: McGraw-Hill, 1999; 191–203.

83 Field, S.K., Bell, S.G., *et al.* Relationship between inspiratory effort and breathlessness in pregnancy. *J Appl Physiol* 1991; **71**: 1897–902.

84 Garcia-Rio, F., Pino, J.M., *et al.* Regulation of breathing and perception of dyspnea in healthy pregnant women. *Chest* 1996; **110**: 446–453.

85 Phillipson, E.A., Murphy, E., *et al.* Role of vagal stimuli in exercise ventilation in dogs with experimental pneumonitis. *J Appl Physiol* 1975; **39**: 76–84.

86 Fessler, H.E., Brower, R.G., *et al.* CPAP reduces inspiratory work more than dyspnea during hyperinflation with intrinsic PEEP. *Chest* 1995; **108**: 432–40.

87 Zulueta, J.J., and Fanburg, B.L. Respiratory dysfunction in myasthenia gravis. *Clin Chest Med* 1994; **15**: 683–91.

88 Lynn, D.J., Woda, R.P., *et al.* Respiratory dysfunction in muscular dystrophy and other myopathies. *Clin Chest Med* 1994; **15**: 661–74.

89 Kaplan, L.M., and Hollander, D. Respiratory dysfunction in amyotrophic lateral sclerosis. *Clin Chest Med* 1994; **15**: 675–81.

90 Elliott, M.W., Adams, L., *et al.* The language of breathlessness: use by patients of verbal descriptors. *Am Rev Respir Dis* 1991; **144**: 826–32.

91 Skevington, S.M., Pilaar, M., Routh, D., and MacLeod, R. On the language of breathlessness. *Psychol Health* 1997; **12**(5), 677–89.

92 Moy, M.L., Harver, A., *et al.* Language of dyspnea in assessment of patients with acute asthma treated with nebulized albuterol. *Am J Respir Crit Care Med* 1998; **158**: 749–53.

Chapter 7

Assessment of dyspnoea in research

Helen R. Harty and Lewis Adams

The American Thoracic Society has recently defined dyspnoea as a term used to characterize 'a subjective experience of breathing discomfort that is comprised of qualitatively distinct sensations that vary in intensity.'[1] Quantification and analysis of such a sensation is complex, but is important because assessment of the severity of dyspnoea may guide diagnostic evaluation and aid subsequent treatment. In addition, more objective measures may allow responses to therapeutic interventions to be documented and thereby increase our understanding of the neurophysiological basis of this multifaceted symptom. Many tools are available to aid in the assessment of dyspnoea but currently there is no single method that encompasses all of its features. Therefore, the best tools needed to answer a particular question need to be selected. For example, if we want to measure the impact of dyspnoea on functional limitation, indirect methods such as questionnaires are appropriate and informative. However, if we want to attempt to quantify the perceived intensity of dyspnoea (particularly with respect to an intervention), direct scaling methods are more suitable.

The importance of language

Before deciding whether indirect (e.g. questionnaires) or direct (e.g. 'scales') methods of assessment are the more suitable, the importance of the language of dyspnoea must be acknowledged. As far as we can tell, when patients complain of being 'short of breath' (or 'breathless' or 'out of breath'), they are reporting sensations familiar to them when they were healthy but which have become troublesome, particularly at low levels of exertion. When questioned further, patients may volunteer comments like 'hard to breathe', 'can't get enough air', or 'feeling tight', but beyond that they usually do not have the capacity to describe their discomfort more specifically. This language of dyspnoea has been investigated.[2,3] Using questionnaires modelled on the McGill Pain Questionnaire,[4] individuals without dyspnoea were subjected to varying constraints on their breathing (e.g. external resistance, breath holding, breathing carbon dioxide) and asked to select terms which described their breathing discomfort.[2] A similar approach was used for the study of breathlessness experienced by patients.[3] These studies led to the concept that specific words may be used to identify differing stresses on the respiratory system. In recent studies, both patients and healthy subjects undergoing exercise testing reported increased 'effort' and 'heaviness' in breathing, but patients with either chronic obstructive or interstitial lung disease were more likely to choose 'increased inspiratory difficulty' and 'unsatisfied inspiratory effort'. Obstructed patients further identified 'shallow breathing' whereas those with interstitial lung disease reported 'rapid breathing.'[5]

Part of the difficulty in understanding the language of dyspnoea has been the tendency to confuse terms relating to awareness of mechanical events (e.g. shallow or rapid breathing) with terms relating to awareness of the 'discomfort' of breathing (e.g. 'unsatisfying inspiratory effort', 'heaviness'). In general, studies of the language of dyspnoea have shown significant differences between groups of patients, but none of the terms or phrases is unique to a specific disease group and none has yet been shown to be useful in clinical evaluation of an individual patient.

As dyspnoea is so clearly affected by emotions, it has both an intensity and an affective component. This was recognized by Comroe more than three decades ago when he stated that dyspnoea '. . . involves both perception of the sensation by the patient and his reaction to the sensation'.[6] Recently, it has been shown that both normal individuals and patients with respiratory disease can distinguish the intensity of breathlessness from the distress it causes.[7,8] The affective component (i.e. distress) may relate to the psychological profile of individuals or their perception of the significance of the symptom, whereas the sensory component (i.e. intensity) would be better explained by the pathophysiological event and afferent information reaching the central nervous system.[9] This distinction may be important therapeutically, as the affective components may be treatable even when the sensory are not. (See Chapter 6 for further exploration of this theme.)

Indirect methods of assessment

Early attempts to evaluate the severity of dyspnoea involved the use of patients' assessments of their own exercise tolerance, on the assumption that in lung disease dyspnoea was the primary symptom which limited exercise. However, this approach made it difficult to compare the degree of associated dyspnoea between patients, since exercise limitation often depends on many other factors. For this reason a number of questionnaires have been developed to measure quality of life, functional status, and dyspnoea. They are simple to understand, and their wide use over many years has established them as the standard method for the assessment of dyspnoea in the clinical setting in a number of different countries. These scales have been validated and have been shown to be reasonably reproducible, to correlate with each other, and to relate appropriately to physiologic measurements. Recent work has indicated that disease-specific questionnaires in particular are able to monitor improvement in dyspnoea in response to pulmonary rehabilitation programmes[10,11] and to drug therapy in patients with chronic obstructive pulmonary disease (COPD).[12,13] Unfortunately these indirect tools of assessment are limited in their application as most can only be applied to patients with lung disease. A summary outlining the main questionnaires used in common practice today is shown in Table 7.1.

Clinical ratings of dyspnoea: measurement of dyspnoea during activities of daily living

In the clinical setting, the UK **Medical Research Council Scale** (Table 7.2) is the scale most commonly used to assess what physical tasks induce dyspnoea.[14] It is in the form of a five-point scale and is extremely popular as it is useful in characterizing the patient population under investigation and is easy to administer. However, it is not concerned with the intensity of the sensation.

The **Oxygen Cost Diagram** (OCD) (Figure 7.1) is another method used commonly when clinical ratings of dyspnoea are required.[15] It is a scale designed to relate a number of different activities, ranging from sleeping to walking briskly up a hill, to the oxygen required for the

Table 7.1 Indirect methods of assessment of dyspnoea in common usage

Questionnaire	Reference	Summary of key features	Comments on usage
Clinical ratings of dyspnoea: measurement of dyspnoea during activities of daily living			
Medical Research Council scale (MRC)	14	5-point scale ranging from 'no breathlessness on exertion' to 'breathless during dressing'	Interviewer-administered Lacks discrimination but useful in defining or characterization of the patient population
Oxygen cost diagram (OCD)	15	Subjects make ratings using a 100-mm scale for 13 defined activities	Self administered Intermediate reproducibility and validity
Baseline dyspnoea index (BDI)	17	Examines functional impairment, magnitude of task and effort evoking dyspnoea Open-ended questions concerning 3 indices with 4 grades Can be repeated after an intervention to generate a transition dyspnoea index (TDI)	Trained interviewer required Discriminative tool available in several languages Good reproducibility and validity
Non-specific quality-of-life (QoL) questionnaires			
Sickness Impact profile	18	Examines many physical, social and psychosocial functions concerned with QoL	Self administered, 136 items Time consuming (>30 min) Good reproducibility and validity
Medical outcomes study short form 36 (SF36)	19	Examines many physical, social, and psychosocial functions concerned with QoL	Self administered Good reproducibility and validity Straightforward
Disease-specific quality-of-life questionnaires			
St George's respiratory questionnaire	20	Examines symptoms, activity, and impact of disease on daily life	Self administered, 76 items Discriminative tool available in several languages Good reproducibility and validity
Chronic respiratory questionnaire	21	Examines dyspnoea, fatigue, control, and emotional dysfunction	Trained interviewer required Discriminative tool available in several languages Good reproducibility and validity

Table 7.2 MRC breathlessness scale

Grade 1	Are you ever troubled by breathlessness except on strenuous exertion?
Grade 2	If Yes: Are you short of breath when hurrying on the level or walking up a slight hill?
Grade 3	If Yes: Do you have to walk slower than most people on the level? Do you have to stop after a mile or so (or after 30 min) on the level at your own pace?
Grade 4	If Yes to either: Do you have to stop for breath after walking about 100 yards (or after a few minutes) on the level?
Grade 5	If Yes: Are you too breathless to leave the house, or breathless after undressing?

Source: Fletcher *et al.* (1959).[14]

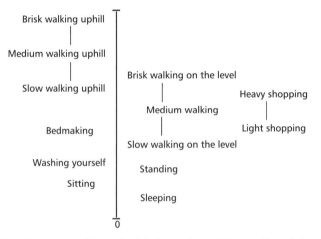

Fig. 7.1 Oxygen Cost Diagram consisting of a list of everyday activities positioned alongside a 100-mm vertical scale proportional to their oxygen cost. Values for oxygen uptake during the activities were taken from Durnin and Passmore.[16] Patients mark a line at the point above which dyspnoea would not allow them to go when at their best, and the result is expressed as the distance of the mark in millimetres above zero.

completion of the task. The values for oxygen uptake during the various activities were taken from Durnin and Passmore.[16] The OCD consists of a 100-mm vertical visual analogue scale and the subject is required to make a mark between the two extremes for 13 specific activities. A disadvantage with the OCD is that not all subjects participate in all of the activities outlined and some patients need more assistance than others in carrying out the rating task.

The **Baseline Dyspnoea Index** (BDI) is an interviewer-administered test which includes measures of functional impairment, magnitude of task, and magnitude of effort as dimensions that provoke a required level of dyspnoea.[17] The interviewer asks open-ended questions concerning these different dimensions and then using specific criteria allocates a value between 0 (severe) and 4 (not impaired). A BDI total score ranging between 0 and 12 is then obtained by adding the scores together, with lower scores indicating more severe dyspnoea. These measurements are made at a baseline state, and can also be repeated after an intervention to generate a **Transition Dyspnoea Index** (TDI). The BDI/TDI is a discriminative instrument which allows the level of reported dyspnoea of the patient to be monitored and is available in a number of different languages including German, Spanish, Italian, and Japanese.[22]

Tanaka et al.[23] have shown that in lung cancer patients three factors could explain the sensation of dyspnoea – sense of effort, sense of anxiety, and sense of discomfort. They have incorporated these elements into a new cancer dyspnoea scale, which could prove promising in cancer treatment research.

Quality of life and dyspnoea

In many studies the level of reported dyspnoea can appear excessive or highly variable in comparison to the levels of underlying pathophysiology, and increasingly a comprehensive assessment of dyspnoea requires a measure of the health-related quality of life.[24] A number of non-specific quality of life/health status questionnaires exist, and the choice of such a measure depends fundamentally on the purpose of the study. Generic measures may be useful, particularly for surveys which attempt to document the range of disability in a general population or patient group, as the general impact can often be overlooked by focusing too specifically on the clinical correlates of a particular disease. A well-designed measure of quality of life should capture the wide variety of consequences of a disease and many result in a single summary score which can help in the design of treatment strategies and cost-effectiveness analyses.

One of the most commonly used quality of life questionnaires used is the **Sickness Impact Profile** (SIP).[18] The SIP includes 136 items that describe the effect of sickness on behavioural function and assesses a broad range of areas including movement, body care, emotional and social behaviour, sleeping, eating, and recreation. The SIP has been used extensively to document the quality of life in patients with COPD and to assess the efficacy of a number of treatments.[25] Although the SIP has been used widely and is well evaluated, it is cumbersome. An alternative is the SF-36, which was developed from the Medical Outcome Study (MOS).[19] This is easier to administer than the SIP and has been well validated.[19,26] More information on generic quality-of-life questionnaires can be found in a number of recent reviews.[27,28]

Valuable information can be gained, too, from disease-specific questionnaires which allow the measure of health-related quality of life to include an assessment of the influences attributable to dyspnoea. These disease-specific questionnaires provide more sensitivity than the generic scales and are therefore more useful when evaluating treatment efficacy in large groups of patients. Several disease-specific questionnaires have been developed to assess the interaction between dyspnoea and quality of life on a short or longer term basis in response to therapeutic interventions. Guyatt developed an interviewer-administered **chronic respiratory disease questionnaire** (CRQ) focusing on four dimensions of illness: dyspnoea, fatigue, emotional function, and the patient's feeling of control over the disease.[21] Unique to Guyatt's questionnaire is the rating of dyspnoea in response to the five most troublesome activities identified by each individual. This makes comparison of individual scores from patients in clinical studies more difficult as a person is asked to report the dyspnoea related to any 5 activities from personal experience and/or a list of 26 activities which include running, lying flat, eating, being angry, and vacuuming. If more than 5 items listed by the interviewer have been identified, the interviewer then helps the subject identify the 5 most important activities in their day-to-day life. A summary of the instructions for the CRQ is provided in Table 7.3. The severity of dyspnoea is graded by the patient using a scale of 1 (extreme) to 7 (none) for each of the activities. The scores are added and the sum is then divided by 5 to obtain the overall score for the CRQ. The questionnaire then

Table 7.3 Summary of instructions for the dyspnoea component of the CRQ

Score	Activity (individual specific)
1–7	A
1–7	B
1–7	C
1–7	D
1–7	E
Sum/5 = mean dyspnoea score	

Source: Guyatt et al. (1987).[21]

asks 15 questions which are identical for each subject. CRQ scores have been shown in several large studies on patients to be quite sensitive to change.

The St George's Respiratory Questionnaire is a self-administered 76-item questionnaire which assesses the impact of dyspnoea on daily life. Dyspnoea is not evaluated specifically, but it is included in the symptom category along with information about other respiratory symptoms.[20] The SGRQ has been shown to be twice as responsive as the generic SIP.

Rutten-van Molken et al.[29] compared the SGRQ and the CRQ and concluded that both questionnaires were similar in terms of reliability, validity, and responsiveness to change. One difference which is important to consider when designing studies is that the SGRQ is self-rated by subjects whereas the CRQ is interviewer-rated (see Chapter 15 for further discussion of these measures) More detailed information on disease-specific quality-of-life questionnaires and how they compared to generic questionnaires is provided in a number of recent reviews.[30–32]

Direct methods of assessment

The discipline of psychophysics originated in the last century and is concerned with the direct scaling of perceived intensity of sensations (e.g. light, sound, touch). This extensive area of research has since been adapted to the field of respiratory physiology and has provided valuable insights into the physiological basis of respiratory perceptions.[33]

Scaling

Scaling relates the relationship between the intensity of the physical stimulus to the resulting perceptual experience and both ratio and, more frequently, category scaling have been adapted for measurement of dyspnoea. In **ratio scaling** the subject assigns a numerical value proportional to the magnitude of the sensation. Studies in which dyspnoea has been scaled in this way have shown that the rate of growth of perception increases as the stimulus increases, a relationship which can be defined by the psychophysical power law, i.e. as the intensity increases linearly, the sensation increases exponentially.[33] A practical problem associated with ratio scaling is that subjects are required to make assessments of the intensity of their sensation relative to a standard intensity, which has to be remembered.

Category scaling is more convenient for the measurement of respiratory sensations in the clinical and experimental setting. In category scaling, the subject assigns a value on a scale which is divided into categories often defined by words to which numerical values can be subsequently assigned. Many category scaling techniques have been validated and are in regular use both clinically and in research. These include the Borg scale, which is the most commonly utilized and was originally developed for rating perceived exertion during exercise[34] when it consisted of 15 grades with numbers ranging from 6 to 20. More recently the Borg scale has been modified and now consists of a vertical scale labelled 0–10 with corresponding verbal expressions of progressively increasing sensation intensity from 'nothing at all' to 'maximal.'[35] This is illustrated in Figure 7.2.

Subjects can select any number or fraction in association with a specific descriptor, and the verbal descriptors included in the Borg scale may assist subjects in rating the intensity of their sensations. The relative proximity of the terms 'slight' and 'severe' in the Borg scale may reduce its sensitivity and discourage subjects from using the whole scale, but this disadvantage may be outweighed by the simplicity of the scale and reproducibility of the results obtained both in the short term[36] and with repeated testing over time.[37] O'Donnell *et al*.[38] used the Borg scale to monitor changes in dyspnoea during exercise in COPD and showed measurements were both highly reproducible and responsive to change. However, they showed that peak ratings were not appropriate in evaluating symptom responses to therapy because ratings were similar before and after interventions despite improvements in exercise endurance, and they suggested that comparisons of sub-maximal rating were more appropriate.

Another common scaling method used in the field of respiratory sensation is the **visual analogue scale** (VAS) which was first used for quantifying the sensation associated with increased airway resistance[39] and later adopted for the quantification of breathlessness.[40] The VAS is depicted as a horizontal or vertical straight line, usually 10 cm long, anchored at either end with words such as 'no respiratory discomfort ' and 'maximal respiratory discomfort' (Figure 7.3). The subject is instructed to make a mark between the two anchor points either using a pen and paper or a linear potentiometer and a computer screen. In response to a question (e.g. 'How short of breath are you?'), the subject marks a point on the line indicating the intensity of the

0	Nothing at all
0.5	Very, very slight (just noticeable)
1	Very slight
2	Slight (light)
3	Moderate
4	Somewhat severe
5	Severe (heavy)
6	
7	Very severe
8	
9	
10	Very, very, severe (almost max)

Fig. 7.2 Borg scale. The 0–10 category-ratio (CR-10) scale modified for use to measure dyspnoea.

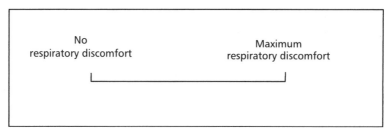

Fig. 7.3 Visual analogue scale (VAS) used to measure dyspnoea. The subject or patient marks a point on the 100-mm line, somewhere between the two anchor points, which corresponds to their level of dyspnoea (in this example, described as 'respiratory discomfort').

sensation. In practice, the rating of respiratory discomfort or breathlessness with a VAS is easily understood by most normal individuals[40] and patients.[41,42] The VAS is now frequently used both in clinical therapeutic studies and in studies of the physiological mechanisms underlying the sensation. VAS dyspnoea measurements have short-term reproducibility, but long-term reproducibility studies are lacking. The VAS has the potential to provide a more reliable and sensitive measure of dyspnoea because it allows greater precision in the measurements than the Borg scale. However, because the intensity of dyspnoea is an extremely subjective experience, the comparison with different populations may be difficult and it may be more convenient to use the Borg scale which has established categories for inter-individual comparisons.

Simple numerical rating scales from 0 to 10 have also been used extensively, and other verbal descriptor scales such as a five-point scale with 'absent', 'mild', 'moderate', 'severe', and 'excruciating' or the seven-point verbal category scales consisting of the descriptors 'no urge to breathe' through 'mild', 'moderate', and 'extreme' with additional points halfway between, are also commonly used.[43,44] The size of the steps between the extremes limits the resolution but allows for clear distinctions between the different categories and is easy to administer.

Multiple scaling

It is important to decide what aspect of respiratory sensation a study will focus on, as increasingly researchers, more aware of the importance of language, are asking subjects to rate different respiratory sensations (for example respiratory effort and shortness of breath) rather than more general respiratory sensations such as respiratory discomfort. Thus, direct comparisons between studies cannot be made. In addition, although it is clear that both normal individuals and respiratory patients can distinguish qualitatively between respiratory effort and shortness of breath, it still remains to be seen whether they can differentiate between these sensations in a quantitative manner at a single session. Preliminary data suggests that normal individuals are unable to do so,[45] and in a study where COPD patients were asked to rate their level of respiratory and leg discomfort in the same exercise test, no significant difference between either sensation was observed even after a bronchodilator which improved respiratory performance was administered.[46]

Any of these scaling techniques can provide valid estimates of this respiratory sensation, and the choice is not crucial. However a problem common to all of them is that they do not allow for the impact of emotional states and personality traits on the sensation of dyspnoea. Measured singly, direct scaling methods are of limited use for collecting clinically useful information about dyspnoea but by providing repeatable quantitative information during experiments (e.g. with exercise), these direct scales can provide valuable information about how the symptom develops and the efficacy (if any) of therapy.

Physiological correlates of dyspnoea

Despite increasing evidence to the contrary, there is a prevailing scepticism about the reliability of measuring the intensity of dyspnoea with subjective scales. Clinicians and researchers have therefore tried to correlate the level of dyspnoea with objective measures such as changes in lung volumes, FEV_1,[38] gas exchange parameters such as diffusion capacity,[47] and, most frequently, with alterations in exercise performance. Another approach has been to relate the maximal level of ventilation attained to the maximum voluntary ventilation. The ratio of the two is known as the **dyspnoeic index**.[48] The intensity of breathlessness has been shown to increase progressively with the level of ventilation during exercise (V_E). Dyspnoea is often expressed as the slope of oxygen consumed (VO_2) on V_E. However, it is not simply the level of ventilation *per se* that determines the intensity of the sensation. For example, external loading during inspiration leads to an increase in breathlessness for any given level of ventilation,[49] and relief of dyspnoea after bronchodilator therapy[50] or volume reduction surgery[51] may occur in the absence of any changes in minute ventilation. These measures are of limited use if they are applied alone, because the sensory experience of dyspnoea derives from interactions between physiological, psychological, social, and environmental factors and these may themselves induce secondary physiological and behavioural responses.

Physical exercise is a stimulus for both physiological and perceptual responses; the sensation of breathlessness with exertion is usually one of the first clinical symptoms patients experience and often precedes significant derangements in pulmonary mechanics or gas exchange. The measurement of dyspnoea on exercise is commonly used both for clinical and research purposes and can provide an objective index of functional impairment. However, exercise tests tend to focus more on physiological limitation than on the symptoms which actually limit exercise. Conventional exercise protocols using predetermined workloads on a bicycle or treadmill, and concomitant ventilatory measurements, generate useful physiological information, but formal exercise testing is complex, expensive, and may be inappropriate for very sick or elderly patients. Because of these concerns, simple 'corridor walk' and 'shuttle' tests have been developed. In the walk test, for example, the patient is simply asked to cover the maximum possible distance (with stops if necessary) in a fixed time, usually 6 or 12 minutes.[52–55]

These tests are simple to perform, are fairly reproducible, and have become popular in the explanatory assessment of dyspnoea. Their results correlate better with questionnaire responses reporting exercise limitation than do objective assessments of static pulmonary function.[56] As exercise tolerance is of more relevance to a patient, assessment of dyspnoea during or after exercise provides a useful approach for research purposes and evaluations of therapy. However, it must be noted that because these tests are performed in a laboratory they may not reflect the frequency, distress, or quality of the respiratory sensations experienced in the subject's usual setting.

Conclusions

An increase in the understanding of the mechanisms which underlie the sensory experience of dyspnoea can be best gained by adopting a disciplined approach to assessment. There are many ways of assessing dyspnoea, and the most appropriate method depends on the study to be undertaken. In research studies it would be advisable to use a combination of different methods designed to obtain a more complete picture.

Keypoints

◆ Assessments of the nature and severity of dyspnoea are essential in research studies involving evaluation of the breathless patient and help to provide useful information during the design of new therapeutic and pulmonary rehabilitation strategies

◆ Patients can distinguish between the **intensity** of breathlessness and the **distress** it causes. This could be important for therapeutic purposes, as the affective components (distress) may be treatable even when the sensory components (intensity) are not

◆ Patients can distinguish between different respiratory sensations, but multiple scaling techniques require further validation

◆ Disease-specific questionnaires such as the chronic respiratory disease questionnaire or the St George's respiratory questionnaire are superior to generic questionnaires

◆ Indirect assessment of dyspnoea can take the form of a generic or disease-specific questionnaire which attempts to measure the impact of dyspnoea on health-related quality of life

◆ Indirect forms of assessment are less sensitive in therapeutic intervention studies and for ease of use, the modified Borg or visual analogue scale should be considered

References

1 American Thoracic Society. Dyspnoea. Mechanisms, assessment and management: A consensus statement. *Am J Respir Crit Care Med* 1999; **159**: 321–40.

2 Simon, P.M., Schwartzstein, R.M., Weiss, J.W., *et al.* Distinguishable sensations of breathlessness induced in normal volunteers. *Am Rev Respir Dis* 1989; **140**: 1021–7.

3 Simon, P.M., Schwartzstein, R.M., Weiss, J.W., *et al.* Distinguishable types of dyspnoea in patients with shortness of breath. *Am Rev Respir Dis* 1990; **142**: 1009–14.

4 Melzack, R., and Katz, J. The McGill Pain Questionnaire: appraisal and current status. In: D.C. Turk, and R. Melzack (eds) *Handbook of pain assessment.* New York: Guilford Press, 1992.

5 Manning, H.L., and Schwartzstein, R.M. Pathophysiology of dyspnoea. *N Engl J Med* 1995; **333**: 1547–53.

6 Comroe, J.H. In: J.B.L. Howell, and E.J.M. Campbell (eds) *Breathlessness.* London: Blackwell Scientific, 1996.

7 Wilson, R.C., and Jones, P.W. Differentiation between the intensity of breathlessness and the distress it evokes in normal subjects during exercise. *Clin Sci* 1991; **80**: 65–70.

8 Carrieri-Kohlman, V., Gormley, J.M., Douglas, M.K., Paul, S.M., and Stulbarg, M.S. Differentiation between dyspnoea and its affective components. *West J Nurs Res* 1996; **18**: 626–42.

9 Gift, A.G., Plaut, S.M., and Jacox, A. Psychological and physiologic factors related to dyspnoea in subjects with chronic obstructive pulmonary disease. *Heart Lung* 1986; **15**: 595–601.

10 Singh, S.J., Sodergren, S.C., Hyland, M.E., Williams, J., and Morgan, M.D. A comparison of three disease-specific and two generic health-status measures to evaluate the outcome of pulmonary rehabilitation in COPD. *Respir Med* 2001; **95**: 71–7.

11 Camp, P.G., Appleton, J., and Reid, W.D. Quality of life after pulmonary rehabilitation: assessing change using quantitative and qualitative methods. *Phys Therapy* 2000; **80**: 986–95.

12 Di Lorenzo, G., Morici, G., Drago, A., *et al.* Efficacy, tolerability, and effects on quality of life of inhaled salmeterol and oral theophylline in patients with mild-to-moderate chronic obstructive pulmonary disease. SLMT02 Italian Study Group. *Clin Therapy* 1998; **20**: 1130–48.

13 Jones, P.W., and Bosh, T.K. Quality of life changes in COPD patients treated with salmeterol. *Am J Respir Crit Care Med* 1997; **155**: 1283–9.

14 Fletcher, C.M., Elmes, P.C., and Wood, C.H. The significance of respiratory symptoms and the diagnosis of chronic bronchitis in a working population. *Br Med J* 1959; **1**: 257–66.

15 McGavin, C.R., Artvinli, M., and Naoe, H. Dyspnoea, disability, and distance walked: comparison of estimates of exercise performance in respiratory disease. *Br Med J* 1978; **2**: 241–3.

16 Durnin, J.G.V.A., and Passmore, R. *Energy, work and leisure.* London: Heinemann, 1967.

17 Mahler, D., Weinberg, D., Wells, C., and Feinstein, A. The measurement of dyspnoea: contents, inter-observer agreement and physiologic correlates of two clinical indexes. *Chest* 1984; **85**: 751–8.

18 Bergner, M., Bobbitt, R.A., Carter, W.B., and Gilson, B.S. The sickness impact profile: development and final revision of a health status measure. *Med Care* 1981; **19**: 787–86.

19 Ware, J.E., and Sherbourne, C.D. The MOS 36-item short-form health survey (SF-36). I. Conceptual framework and item selection. *Med Care* 1992; **30**: 473–83.

20 Jones, P.W., Quirk, F.H., Baveystock, C.M., and LittleJohn, T. A self complete measure of heath status for chronic airflow limitation. *Am Rev Respir Dis* 1992; **145**: 1321–7.

21 Guyatt, G.H., Berman, L.B., Townsend, M., Pugsley, S.O., and Chambers, L.W. A measure of quality of life for clinical trials in chronic lung disease. *Thorax* 1987; **142**: 773–8.

22 Mahler, D.A., Jones, P.W., and Guyatt,G.H. Clinical measurement of dyspnoea. In: D. Mahler (ed.) *Dyspnea.* New York: Marcel Dekker, 1998; 149–98.

23 Tanaka, K., *et al.* Development and validation of the Cancer Dyspnoea Scale: a multidimensional, brief, self-rating scale. *Br J Cancer* 2000; **82**(4): 800–5.

24 Mahler, D.A. How should health-related quality of life be assessed in patients with COPD? *Chest* 2000; **117**: 54–7S.

25 Curtis, J.R., Deyo, R.A., and Hudson, L.D. Pulmonary rehabilitation in chronic respiratory insuffi-ciency. 7. Health-related quality of life among patients with chronic obstructive pulmonary disease. *Thorax* 1994; **49**: 162–70.

26 Ware, J.E., and Gandek, B. Overview of the SF-36 Health Survey and the International Quality of Life Assessment (IQOLA) Project. *J Clin Epidemiol* 1998; **51**: 903–12.

27 Anderson, R.T., Aaronson, N.K., Bullinger, M., and McBee, W.L. A review of the progress towards developing health-related quality-of-life instruments for international clinical studies and outcomes research. *Pharmacoeconomics* 1996; **10**: 336–55.

28 Andresen, E.M., and Meyers, A.R. Health-related quality of life outcomes measures. *Arch Phys Med Rehab* 2000; **81**: S30–45.

29 Rutten-van Molken, M., Roos, B., and Van Noord, J.A. An empirical comparison of the St Georges's respiratory questionnaire (SGRQ) and the chronic Respiratory Disease Questionnaire (CRQ) in a clinical trial setting. *Thorax* 1999; **54**: 995–1003.

30 Cullen, D.L. Measures of functional status and quality of life in chronic obstructive pulmonary disease. *Monaldi Arch Chest Dis* 1999; **54**: 183–5.

31 Nishimura, K., Tsukino, M., and Hajiro, T. Health-related quality of life in patients with chronic obstructive pulmonary disease. *Curr Opin Pulmon Med* 1998; **4**: 107–15.

32 Mahler, D.A., and Jones, P.W. Measurement of dyspnoea and quality of life in advanced lung disease. *Clin Chest Med* 1997; **18**: 457–69.

33 Lansing, R.W., and Banzett, R.B. Psychological methods in the study of respiratory sensation. In: L. Adams, and A. Guz (eds) *Respiratory sensation.* New York: Marcel Dekker, 1996; 69–100.

34 Borg, G. Perceived exertion as an indicator of somatic stress. *Scand J Rehab Med* 1970; **2**: 92–8.

35 Burdon, J.G.W., Junniper, E.F., Killian, K.J., Hargreave, F.E., and Campbell, E.J.M. The perception of breathlessness in asthma. *Am Rev Respir Dis* 1982; **126**: 825–8.

36 Wilson, R.C., and Jones, P.W. A comparison of the visual analogue scale and modified Borg scale for the measurement of dyspnoea during exercise. *Clin Sci* 1989; **76**: 277–82.

37 Wilson, R.C., and Jones, P.W. Long-term reproducibility of Borg scale estimates of breathlessness during exercise. *Clin Sci* 1991; **80**: 309–12.

38 O'Donnell, D.E., Lam, M., and Webb, K.A. Measurement of symptoms, lung hyperinflation, and endurance during exercise in chronic obstructive pulmonary disease. *Am J Respir Crit Care Med* 1998; **158**: 1557–65.

39 Aitken, R.C.B. Measurement of feelings using visual analogue scales. *Proc Roy Soc Med* 1969; **62**: 989–93.

40 Adams, L., Chronos, N., Lane, R., and Guz, A. The measurement of breathlessness induced in normal subjects: validity of two scaling techniques. *Clin Sci* 1985; **69**: 7–16.

41 Muza, S.R., Silverman, M.T., Gilmore, G.C., Hellerstein, H.K., and Kelsen, S.G. Comparison of scales used to quantitate the sense of effort to breathe in patients with chronic obstructive pulmonary disease. *Am Rev Respir Dis* 1990; **141**: 909–13.

42 Mador, M.J., and Kufel, T.J. Reproducibility of visual analogue scale measurement of dyspnoea in patients with chronic obstructive pulmonary disease. *Am Rev Respir Dis* 1992; **146**: 82–7.

43 Guyatt, G.H., Townsend, M., Berman, L.B., and Keller, J.L. A comparison of Likert and visual analogue scales for measuring change in function. *J Chron Dis* 1987; **40**(12): 1129–33.

44 Price, D.D., Bush, F.M., Ling, S., and Harkins, S.W. A comparison of pain measurement characteristics of mechanical visual analogue and simple numerical rating scales. *Pain* 1994; **56**(2): 217–26.

45 Harty, H.R., and Adams, L. Can normal subjects scale different respiratory sensations simultaneously during steady state exercise. *Clin Sci* 1994; **87**: 27P.

46 Killian, K.J. Sense of effort and dyspnoea. *Monaldi Arch Chest Dis* 1998; **153**: 654–60.

47 Mahler, D.A., Harver, A., Rosiello, R., and Daubenspeck, J.A. Measurement of respiratory sensation in interstitial lung disease. Evaluation of clinical dyspnea ratings and magnitude scaling. *Chest* 1989; **96**: 767–71.

48 Cotes, J.E. *Lung function: assessment and application in medicine*, 5th edn. London: Blackwell Scientific, 1993; 392–4.

49 Altose, M.D. Assessment and management of breathlessness. *Chest* 1985; **88**: 77S–83.

50 Belman, M.J., Botnick, W.C., and Shin, J.W. Inhaled bronchodilators reduce dynamic hyperinflation during exercise in patients with chronic obstructive pulmonary disease. *Am J Respir Crit Care Med* 1996; **153**: 967–75.

51 Keller, C.A., Ruppel, G., Hibbett, A., Osterloh, J., and Naunheim, K.S. Thoracoscopic lung volume reduction surgery reduces dyspnea and improves exercise capacity in patients with emphysema. *Am J Respir Crit Care Med* 1997; **156**: 60–7.

52 McGavin, C.R., Gupta, S.P., and McHardy, G.J. Twelve-minute walking test for assessing disability in chronic bronchitis. *Br Med J* 1976; **3**: 822–3.

53 Guyatt, G.H., Thompson, P.J., Berman, L.B., *et al.* How should we measure function in patients with chronic heart and lung disease? *J Chron Dis* 1985; **38**: 517–24.

54 Singh, S.J., Morgan, M.D.L., Scott, S., *et al.* The development of shuttle walking test of disability in patients with chronic airways disease. *Thorax* 1992; **47**: 1019–24.

55 Booth, S., and Adams, L. The shuttle walking test: a reproducible method for evaluating the impact of shortness of breath on functional capacity in patients with advanced cancer. *Thorax* 2001; **56**: 146–50.

56 Cockcroft, A., Adams, L., and Guz, A. Assessment of breathlessness. *Quart J Med* 1989; **72**: 669–76.

Chapter 8

Assessment of dyspnoea in clinical practice and audit

Eduardo Bruera and Catherine M. Neumann

Dyspnoea has been defined as an uncomfortable awareness of breathing.[1] Although everyone has experienced the sensation and has an intuitive understanding of this symptom, there is no universal agreement as to its definition. Dyspnoea is essentially a subjective sensation and cannot be defined by the physical abnormalities that are accompanied by such an unpleasant subjective experience. For the purposes of this chapter, dyspnoea is defined as an unpleasant sensation of difficult, laboured breathing.

The purpose of this chapter is to review the main aspects of the assessment from the perspective of clinical care and audit.

Assessment of the underlying cause

Box 8.1 summarizes the most important abnormalities capable of causing dyspnoea. From the pathophysiological view, dyspnoea can result from three main abnormalities:[2]

- an increase in respiratory effort to overcome a certain load (e.g. obstructive or restrictive lung disease, pleural effusion

- an increase in the proportion of respiratory muscle required to maintain the normal workload (e.g. neuromuscular weakness, cancer cachexia)

- an increase in ventilatory requirements (hypoxemia, hypercapnea, metabolic acidosis, anaemia

In many patients, different proportions of the three abnormalities may coexist, thereby making the pathophysiological interpretation of the intensity of dyspnoea more complex.

Box 8.1 Underlying causes of dyspnoea

- Increased respiratory effort required, e.g. obstructive/restrictive lung disease, pleural effusion

- Decreased respiratory muscle strength, e.g. cancer cachexia, neuromuscular disorders

- Increased ventilatory requirements e.g. hypoxemia, hypercapnia, metabolic acidosis, anemia

- Altered central sensory perception, e.g. anxiety, depression

From a clinical perspective, it is of great importance to establish both the underlying disease capable of causing dyspnoea in a certain patient (e.g. lung cancer) and which of the three mechanisms are involved in causing dyspnoea in a given patient. For example, a patient with lung cancer may have dyspnoea as a result of progressive lung replacement by tumour or pleural effusion, severe cachexia or a paraneoplastic myasthenic syndrome, or the presence of severe hypoxemia. The management of dyspnoea due to lung cancer will, therefore, be quite different depending on the main mechanism involved.

Even in very advanced stages of illness, patients' symptoms can be significantly improved by an appropriate characterization of the mechanisms involved.

In most patients, the assessment of the underlying cause can be established from a simple history and physical examination in addition to a chest radiograph, simple blood tests, and occasionally bedside pulmonary function tests. Modern equipment allows for the bedside determination of forced vital capacity (FVC) and forced expiratory volume in 1 s (FEV_1). These non-invasive tests will assist in the characterization of dyspnoea in patients with lung disease. Oxygen saturation (SaO_2) can easily be obtained at the bedside by pulse oximetry. End-tidal carbon dioxide can be easily measured at the bedside, and this information will make the testing of arterial blood gases unnecessary in most patients; however, this equipment is expensive and not widely available in clinical settings. Finally, the maximal inspiratory pressure (MIP) is a simple bedside measure of the strength of respiratory muscles that can be useful in patients with severe cachexia.

Assessment of intensity

As dyspnoea is a subjective sensation, the main goal of diagnostic and therapeutic interventions is to reduce the perceived distress. Therefore, regular intensity assessments are essential, as they not only allow for appropriate characterization of the results of treatments over time, but these assessments also provide the most useful information for the auditing of clinical programs. Table 8.1 summarizes some of the most common instruments for the intensity of dyspnoea.

There are four main modalities of assessment: repeated assessment of symptom distress, assessment of dyspnoea associated with daily activities, assessment of dyspnoea during exercise, and dyspnoea as part of quality-of-life assessment.

Repeated assessment of symptom distress

These consist of assessments of the intensity of dyspnoea perceived by the patient at the present time, or asking patients to provide a global estimation of dyspnoea during time intervals such as the last 24 h, the last week, etc.

The most frequently used scales for this purpose are the visual analogue scale (VAS) and the Borg scale, as well as numerical scales and verbal ratings.

The VAS consist of a horizontal or vertical line anchored by statements such as 'no shortness of breath' and 'worst possible shortness of breath'. In most cases, the length of this line is 100 mm.

The Borg scale[3,4] was originally developed for rating perceived exertion during exercise. In the currently used modified form, the numbers from 0 to 10 and the verbal descriptors are placed so that doubling the numerical rating corresponds to a twofold increase in sensation intensity.

Most of the scales developed for the assessment of intensity have been validated. The most commonly used scales such as the VAS and the Borg scale have been found to correlate well with each other and with other instruments [5–7]

Table 8.1 Methods for the assessment of dyspnoea

Intensity of symptom distress	Visual analogue scale (VAS)
	Numerical rating
	Verbal rating
	Borg scale
Daily activities	Shortness of breath questionnaire (SOBQ)
	Modified Medical Research Council questionnaire (MRC)
	Oxygen cost diagram (OCD)
	Baseline dyspnoea index (BDI)
Exercise	Treadmill or bicycle
	Speech?
	Breath-holding?
Quality of life	EORTC[a] lung cancer module (LC-13)
	Chronic Respiratory Questionnaire (CRQ)

[a] European Organization for Research and Treatment of Cancer.

One of the main problems associated with the repeated assessment of dyspnoea is the variable intensity of this symptom according to the level of activity and even spontaneously during different moments of the day. A similar problem is well described in patients experiencing pain, where it is known as 'incident pain'. [8,9] The variation in intensity of dyspnoea over time makes pharmacological and non-pharmacological symptomatic interventions difficult to assess. In respiratory and cardiovascular populations, one approach to this problem has been to attempt to assess the intensity of dyspnoea during specific activities, or by relating this intensity of dyspnoea to daily activities performed by the patient.

Assessment of dyspnoea associated with daily activities

These instruments relate the intensity of dyspnoea to specific daily activities that patients are expected to perform, such as 'bed making', 'shopping', 'walking uphill', etc. The most commonly used questionnaires include the Modified Medical Research Council (MRC) scale, the Oxygen Cost Diagram (OCD)'the Baseline Dyspnoea Index (BDI), and the recently developed Shortness of Breath Questionnaire (SOBQ). [10–12]

These instruments vary in length and measure slightly different dimensions of dyspnoea, but a number of studies have found them to correlate well with each other. [10,13–15] A recent study found that the MRC, BDI, and OCD appeared generally to measure similar dimensions of dyspnoea, whereas the Borg scale appeared to evaluate aspects of dyspnoea unrelated to daily activities. [15] Therefore, for a comprehensive assessment of the impact of dyspnoea on function and distress of a patient, it may be preferable to include a combination of scales that assess symptom distress together with scales that relate to daily activity.

One of the main limitations of such scales of daily activities such as the MRC and OCD is that they relate the intensity of dyspnoea with examples of activities performed mostly by ambulatory patients. Most seriously ill and palliative care patients cluster in the upper levels of severe functional limitations. The interpretation of these scales is made even more complex by the fact that, in many patients, the main reason for their limitation in function may be different from dyspnoea, such as pain, cachexia, and asthenia. Therefore, in patients with conditions such as advanced cancer or AIDS in whom dyspnoea is only one of the multiple severe symptom components, these scales are of limited value for clinical assessment.

In a recent study, 142 hospitalized patients were assessed on the same day using four different instruments. The VAS and Borg scale, which detect the intensity of symptom distress, found the frequency of dyspnoea to be 33%, whereas the MRC and OCD, which relate dyspnoea with functional limitations, found a frequency of 76–78%.[14] It is likely that patients did not express dyspnoea on the VAS or Borg scale because they were refraining from performing the symptom-causing manoeuvres described in the MRC or OCD scale. Until there is more knowledge of the complex interaction between these two types of instruments, the ideal clinical assessment will result from a combination of tools from these two groups.

Assessment of dyspnoea during exercise

These assessments take place during progressive exercising on the treadmill or bicycle so that patients or volunteers are subjected to a predictable workload.[16] Dyspnoea is then measured at fixed intervals and expressed in relationship to the workload. Tools such as the VAS, numerical or verbal rating, or the Borg scale are frequently used in combination with exercise in these patients. Unfortunately, one of the main limitations of these assessment methods in normal clinical practice is that many very ill patients are unable to participate in these stress tests.

One potentially less invasive approach to the production of dyspnoea would be breath holding.[17,18] This technique has apparently been successful in volunteers and patients. It requires minimal physical and cognitive ability. Unfortunately, the mechanisms of dyspnoea associated with breath holding are not exactly as those associated with other activities and this manoeuvre might not be an ideal measure of potential response to other therapeutic interventions.

Lee *et al.*[19] have recently emphasized the importance of speech impairment in dyspnoea and developed an assessment tool to quantify this. The assessment of speech-induced dyspnoea might be useful in palliative care patients.

Dyspnoea as part of quality of life assessment

Quality-of-life questionnaires address multiple dimensions affected normally by health and disease. Dyspnoea ratings are incorporated in the Chronic Respiratory Questionnaire (CRQ)[20] (see also Chapter 7). The European Organization for Research and Treatment of Cancer (EORTC) has produced a global quality of instrument, the QLQ-C30, and has designed a specific module for lung cancer (LC-13), which asks detailed questions on dyspnoea and other respiratory symptoms.[21]

The main advantage of these quality-of-life questionnaires is that they provide some integration between the dyspnoea and other symptoms that patients may be experiencing. Their main limitation is that they are usually lengthy and cover many dimensions that may not necessarily be the focus of daily interventions by physicians and nurses. Therefore, while these tools are of great use in research, they are of limited value in daily clinical care and audit.

Directions in dyspnoea assessment

In recent years, there has been generalized consensus that the assessment should be completed, as much as possible, by the patient. Recent studies have shown that there are significant differences in the appreciation of dyspnoea and other symptoms at a given time between physicians, nurses, and patients.[22,23] In some cases, such as after a patient has been discharged or has died, or when there is significant cognitive impairment, patient-based instruments may not be appropriate. In these cases, other instruments such as the STAS,[24] which is completed by trained staff, have been proven to be very useful for the purpose of auditing the quality of care in patients receiving palliative care in different settings.

Some preliminary research has suggested that the descriptors used by patients to describe dyspnoea might be different depending on the underlying clinical condition. For example, words such as 'heavy' or 'suffocating' were associated with congestive heart failure while words such as 'hunger for air' or 'constriction' were more frequently associated with asthma[25,26] (see also Chapter 7). More research is needed in order to establish if specific descriptors are able to predict the mechanisms and intensity of dyspnoea that might respond to different therapeutic interventions, and at present these cannot be relied on in clinical practice.

In the case of pain, specific descriptors have previously been associated with specific pathophysiological syndromes.[27] For example, burning or numb sensation has traditionally been associated with neuropathic pain. In many cases, the descriptor alone is enough to make a diagnosis and suggest the need for specific drug therapy. It is possible that in future questionnaires containing descriptors of breathlessness will help diagnose the underlying cause and identify the specific mechanism of dyspnoea in a given patient.[26]

Multidimensional assessment

There has been variable but generally low correlation between the intensity of subjective dyspnoea and abnormalities both in blood gases and in pulmonary function tests.[15,16,28–30] These findings suggest that factors other than clinically measurable abnormalities have a major influence on the intensity of dyspnoea.

Figure 8.1 summarizes the different stages in the sensation of dyspnoea. Neither the production nor perception of dyspnoea can be measured at present. The amount of afferent input

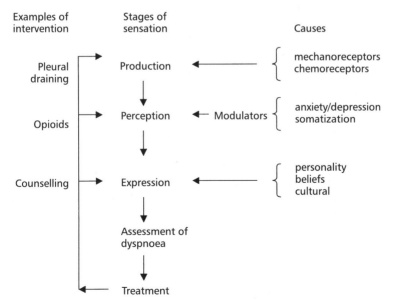

Fig. 8.1 Different stages in the production of the sensation of dyspnoea.

No dyspnoea   0 _____x_____ 100 Worst possible dyspnoea

1   2   3

Fig. 8.2 Components of the dyspnoea compiled in a 38-year-old man with lung cancer. The components of cumulative dyspnoea in this case are (1) locally advanced carcinoma + pleural effusion; (2) a major depression episode leading to somatization, and (3) excessive activity leading to poor energy conservation. Modified and reproduced with permission from Lippincott-Raven Publishers, from Bruera. E., Ripamonti. C. Dyspnoea in patients with advanced cancer. In: A. Berger, *et al.* (eds.) *Principles and practice of supportive oncology.* Philadelphia: Lippincott-Raven, 1998.[32]

from chemoreceptor or mechanoreceptor stimulation at the level of the lung can vary widely from one individual to another. In addition, the level of perception can vary significantly according to different factors capable of amplifying or decreasing the level of the stimulus. Finally, expression of the intensity of dyspnoea can be influenced by a number of factors described in the figure and should not be interpreted as a direct representation of the intensity of production of dyspnoea at the level of mechanoreceptors or chemoreceptors.

Whereas the level of glucose in a diabetic patient or the level of blood pressure in a hypertensive patient is generally assumed to be a direct expression of underlying pathophysiological mechanisms, dyspnoea should be interpreted as a multidimensional construct in which the intensity described by a given patient is a result of the interaction of different factors.

Figure 8.2 summarizes the different components in the intensity of dyspnoea for a 38-year-old man with advanced carcinoma of the lung. This patient had dyspnoea caused by progressive lung disease. The patient's expression of dyspnoea (as expressed in a VAS) summarized the combination of progressive lung cancer and pleural effusion, plus somatization due to clinical depression, and poor use of his energy by continuously trying to be physically active. A unidimensional interpretation of this symptom would have resulted in excessive pharmacological intervention with limited therapeutic success. Instead, a multidimensional assessment identified the need for a combined approach using symptomatic therapy with opioids, antidepressant treatment, and occupational therapy for energy conservation. Determining the relative contribution of each dimension to the overall symptom expression can be estimated only by disciplined assessment that includes all the relative dimensions. At this point, it becomes possible to plan a therapeutic approach for a given patient in a multidimensional manner.

Follow-up during treatment

Once the main underlying causes and mechanisms for dyspnoea have been established, the intensity has been appropriately characterized both by assessment of symptom distress and by relating to daily activities, and the multiple dimensions have been characterized, therapeutic intervention should be expected to modify the intensity of dyspnoea.

Multiple assessments will need to take place. The frequency of such assessments may vary depending on the severity of dyspnoea and the type of interventions. Instruments used for follow-up should, as much as possible, resemble those used during the initial assessment. However, because they have to be administered repeatedly, these tools should be particularly simple. For example, the initial 'diagnostic' workup for a breathless patient may involve a VAS, Borg scale, quality-of-life scale, spirometry, and oxygen saturation. Once treatment has started,

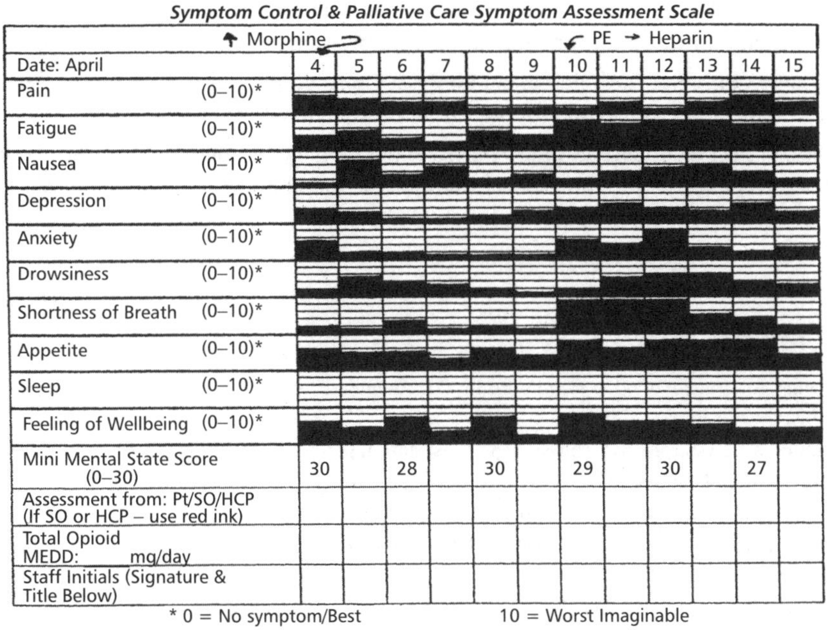

Symptom Control & Palliative Care Symptom Assessment Scale

		4	5	6	7	8	9	10	11	12	13	14	15
Date: April													
Pain	(0–10)*												
Fatigue	(0–10)*												
Nausea	(0–10)*												
Depression	(0–10)*												
Anxiety	(0–10)*												
Drowsiness	(0–10)*												
Shortness of Breath	(0–10)*												
Appetite	(0–10)*												
Sleep	(0–10)*												
Feeling of Wellbeing	(0–10)*												
Mini Mental State Score (0–30)		30		28		30		29		30		27	
Assessment from: Pt/SO/HCP (If SO or HCP – use red ink)													
Total Opioid MEDD: mg/day													
Staff Initials (Signature & Title Below)													

Top markers: ↑ Morphine ⇒   ⌒ PE → Heparin

* 0 = No symptom/Best   10 = Worst Imaginable

Fig. 8.3 Example of ESAS score used at M.D. Anderson Cancer Center. Note the sudden increase in dyspnoea during day 7 due to pulmonary embolism.

it will be appropriate to repeat the VAS weekly and the quality-of-life scale and spirometry/-saturation monthly. However, if the intervention includes a bronchodilator, then weekly or even daily spirometry may be relevant.

In patients in whom dyspnoea is the main symptom, such as patients with congestive heart failure or chronic lung disease, follow-up is quite different from what it is for patients in whom dyspnoea is just one part of the overall symptom distress, such as those with cancer or AIDS. Particularly in the latter group, dyspnoea assessment should not take place in isolation, but should be part of the overall symptom distress assessment. Tools such as the Edmonton Symptom Assessment System (ESAS)[31] allow for the assessment of multiple visual analogue scales that can be displayed graphically on the patient's chart. This provides a simple visual record of changes in intensity of dyspnoea over time and also allows a comparison between dyspnoea and other symptoms that might be present in a given patient (Figure 8.3).

Keypoints

♦ Dyspnoea is a common and devastating symptom. It is often not appropriately assessed in the clinical or audit setting. However, there are many valid and reliable instruments that can be used for its initial assessment and follow-up

♦ An accurate diagnosis of the cause of dyspnoea will help in deciding the symptomatic management, even in terminally ill patients

♦ Ideally, a combination of a tool that assesses symptom distress with a tool that assesses the impact of dyspnoea on daily activities should be used

- Because of the multidimensional nature of this symptom, an attempt should be made to characterize the different components of the expression of dyspnoea in a given patient

- Because of multiple morbidities, and the need for multiple and repeated assessments, it is crucial to utilize simple tools for regular follow-up

- Perhaps the main challenge in the assessment of dyspnoea is not so much the generation of new or better tools, as convincing clinicians of the importance to adopting disciplined assessment as part of the regular care of their patients

References

1 Baines, M. Control of other symptoms. In: C.M. Saunders (ed.) *The management of terminal disease.* Chicago: Year Book, 1978.

2 Tobin, M.J. Dyspnoea: pathophysiologic basis, clinical presentations and management. *Arch Intern Med* 1990; **150**: 1604–13.

3 Borg, G.A.V. Psychophysical bases of perceived exertion. *Med Sci Sports Exerc* 1982; **14**: 377–87.

4 Mador, M.J., Rodis, A., and Magalang, U.J. Reproducibility of Borg scale measurements of dyspnoea during exercise in patients with COPD. *Chest* 1995; **107**: 1590–7.

5 Wilson, R.C., and Jones, P.W. A comparison of the visual analogue scale and modified Borg scale for the measurement of dyspnoea during exercise. *Clin Sci* 1989; **76**: 277–82.

6 Cockcroft, A., Adams, L., and Guz, A. Assessment of breathlessness. *Q J Med* 1989; **72**: 669–76.

7 Aitken, R.C.B. Measurement of feelings using visual analogue scales. *Proc Roy Soc Med* 1969; **62**: 989–93.

8 Portenoy, R.K., and Hagen, N.A. Breakthrough pain: definition, prevalence and characteristics. *Pain* 1990; **41**: 273–81.

9 Bruera, E., Macmillan, K., Hanson, J., and MacDonald, R.N. The Edmonton staging system for cancer pain: preliminary report. *Pain* 1989; **37**: 203–9.

10 Eakin, E.G., Resnikoff, P.M., Prewitt, L.M., Ries, A.L., and Kaplan, R.M. Validation of a new dyspnoea measure. The UCSD shortness of breath questionnaire. *Chest* 1998; **113**: 619–24.

11 McCord, M., and Cronin-Stubbs, D. Operationalizing dyspnoea: focus on management. *Heart Lung* 1992; **21**: 167–79.

12 van der Molen, B. Dyspnoea: a study of measurement instruments for the assessment of dyspnoea and their application for patients with advanced cancer. *J Adv Nurs* 1995; **22**: 948–56.

13 Mahler, D.A., and Harver, A. A factor analysis of dyspnoea ratings, respiratory muscle strength, and lung function in patients with chronic obstructive pulmonary disease. *Am Rev Respir Dis* 1992; **145**: 467–70.

14 Farncombe, M. Dyspnoea: assessment and treatment. *Support Care Cancer* 1997; **5**: 94–9.

15 Hajiro, T., Nishimura, K., Tsukino, M., *et al.* Analysis of clinical methods used to evaluate dyspnoea in patients with chronic obstructive pulmonary disease. *Am J Respir Crit Care Med* 1998; **158**: 1185–9.

16 Mahler, D.A., and Harver, A. Clinical measurement of dyspnoea. In: D.A. Mahler (ed.) *Dyspnoea.* Mount Kisco, NY: Futura, 1990; 75–126.

17 Taskar, V., Clayton, N., Atkins, M., *et al.* Breath-holding time in normal subjects, snorers, and sleep apnea patients. *Chest* 1995; **107**: 959–62.

18 Nunn, J.F. Control of breathing: breathholding. In: *Applied respiratory physiology, 2nd edn.* London: Butterworths, 1977; 95–9.

19 Lee, L., Friesen, M., Lambert, I.R., and Loudon, R.G. Evaluation of dyspnoea during physical and speech activities in patients with pulmonary diseases. *Chest* 1998; **113**: 625–32.

20 Wijkstra, P.J., Ten Vergert, E.M., Van Altena, R., *et al.* Reliability and validity of the chronic respiratory questionnaire. *Thorax* 1994; **49**: 465–67.

21 Bergman, B., Aarouson, N.K., Ahmedzai, S., *et al.* The EORTC QLQ-LC13: a modular supplement to the EORTC Core Quality of Life Questionnaire (QLQ-C30) for use in lung cancer clinical trials. EORTC Study Group on Quality of Life. *Eur J Cancer* 1994; **30A**: 635–42.

22 Nekolaichuk, C.L., Bruera, E., Spachinsky, K., *et al.* A comparison of patient and proxy symptom assessments in advanced cancer patients. *J Pain Symptom Manage* 1998; **15**: S10.

23 Higginson, I.J., and McCarthy, M. Validity of the support team assessment schedule: do staffs' ratings reflect those made by patients or their families? *Palliative Med* 1993; **7**(3): 219–28.

24 Higginson, I. Audit methods: a community schedule. In: *Clinical audit in palliative care*. Abingdon: Radcliffe Medical Press, 1993; 34–47.

25 Simon, P.M., Schwartzstein, R.M., Weiss, J.W., *et al.* Distinguishable types of dyspnoea in patients with shortness of breath. *Am Rev Respir Dis* 1990; **142**: 1009–14.

26 Mahler, D.A., Harver, A., Lentine, T., *et al.* Descriptors of breathlessness in cardiorespiratory diseases. *Am J Respir Crit Care Med* 1996; **154**(5): 1357–63.

27 Foley, K. The treatment of cancer pain. *N Engl J Med* 1985; **313**: 84–95.

28 Mahler, D.A., Rosiello, R.A., Harver, A., *et al.* Comparison of clinical dyspnoea ratings and psychophysical measurements of respiratory sensation in obstructive pulmonary airway disease. *Am Rev Respir Dis* 1987; **135**: 1229–33.

29 Stoller, J.K., Ferranti, R., and Feinstein, A.R. Further specification and evaluation of a new clinical index for dyspnoea. *Am Rev Respir Dis* 1986; **134**: 1129–34.

30 Bruera, E., Schmitz, B., Pither, J., Neumann, C.M., and Hanson, J. The frequency and correlates of dyspnoea in patients with advanced cancer. *Supportive Care Cancer* 1999; **O6**.

31 Bruera, E., Kuehn, N., Miller, M.J., Selmser, P., and Macmillan, K. The Edmonton symptom assessment system (ESAS): a simple method for the assessment of palliative care patients. *J Palliative Care* 1991; **7**(2): 6–9.

32 Bruera, E., Ripamonti, C. Dyspnoea in patients with advanced cancer. In: A. Berger, *et al.* (eds) *Principles and practice of supportive oncology*. Philadelphia: Lippincott-Raven, 1998.

Part III

Management of dyspnoea

Chapter 9

Drug therapies

Carol Davis

Breathlessness is experienced by patients with both malignant and non-malignant diseases. In some cases there will be a mixed aetiology. The underlying pathophysiology will determine the appropriate selection and use of both disease-orientated and palliative interventions. The aetiology of breathlessness (as discussed in Chapter 6) is usually multifactorial and will include psychosocial factors, which may precipitate, exacerbate, and maintain the symptom. Anxiety is a common problem and may require specific therapy. Primary symptomatic measures may be considered irrespective of pathophysiology. Standard practice in this regard is developing from an empirical foundation.[1] Appropriate management requires the judicious and individualized application of both drug and non-drug treatments. Non-pharmacological approaches to care may be preeminent in some clinical situations.[2]

The palliative care approach summarizes a particular orientation to care[3] which may benefit some patients who experience breathlessness. More specifically, a scientific approach to symptom management has been described which places an essential commitment to holism within an explicitly biomedical framework.[4] According to this model, multifunctional evaluation precedes multimodel treatment.

A systematic approach is assisted by classification. Drug therapy, for example, may be classified according to route of administration and putative site of action (systemic or inhaled).

A clinical classification which distinguishes certain characteristics of breathlessness may influence the selection of appropriate drug therapies:

- continuous
- intermittent
- resting
- exertional
- paroxysmal.

Careful assessment at each stage of disease progression is required. The appropriateness of any drug therapy, or indeed intervention, varies not only between individuals but also, in any one individual, it varies over time.

In this chapter we discuss drugs used in the management of breathlessness, by class; in the dying patient; and relevant ethical issues. Throughout, we presume that all appropriate disease-orientated drug and non-drug therapies have been and are being employed. We describe palliative drug therapies which are usually turned to when disease-orientated strategies are exhausted but which could, or perhaps should, be used alongside them. (See comprehensive model of supportive care in Chapter 1.)

Our aim is to describe a practical approach based upon evidence which summarizes current best practice. The symptomatic treatment of breathlessness has in the recent past been described as difficult[5] and unsatisfactory.[6] Is this still the case today?

Phosphodiesterase inhibitors and bronchodilators

Theophylline has been used for the relief of bronchospasm, the primary indication being reversible airway obstruction. It may be used as an adjunct to standard bronchodilator therapy in the management of asthma[7] and chronic obstructive pulmonary disease (COPD).[8] Its effects are complex, however, and involve both intra- and extrapulmonary sites of action. Clinical use may be limited by drug interactions and a narrow therapeutic range.

Lung cancer and COPD may frequently coexist. Treatment of reversible airflow obstruction in patients with recently diagnosed lung cancer with standard inhaled bronchodilator therapy, either by handheld inhaler or by nebulizer, can improve breathlessness.[9] In day-to-day clinical practice a trial of bronchodilator therapy, sometimes including theophylline, can be helpful in this group of patients early in the disease course. In patients with advanced cancer in the lung, however, the relative importance of any reversible airway obstruction is usually minimal. Most clinical research on the relationship between airflow obstruction and breathlessness, and the therapeutic use of phosphodiesterase inhibitors in particular, has been conducted in patients with non-malignant disease. Some of these patients may experience an improvement in breathlessness with theophylline.[10] There is evidence that the site of action may be at the level of the diaphragm, the mechanism being increased diaphragmatic contractility.[11] Theophylline is a weak and non-selective phosphodiesterase inhibitor, which is difficult to use in clinical practice, and newer, more selective phosphodiesterase inhibitors are under clinical development.[12]

Corticosteroids

Corticosteroids are anti-inflammatory agents used as adjuncts in the management of asthma,[7] COPD,[8] and fibrotic lung disease,[13] and to palliate respiratory symptoms including breathlessness in end-of-life care. Evidence to support the latter derives largely from clinical experience. There are some specific, albeit non-licensed, indications in breathless cancer patients:

◆ lymphangitis carcinomatosa

◆ upper airway obstruction causing stridor

◆ pneumonitis related to radiotherapy

◆ early superior vena caval obstruction.

Some suggestions for acute and maintenance drug therapies for breathlessness according to cause are shown in Table 9.1.

Severe upper airway obstruction and superior vena caval obstruction are usually regarded as medical emergencies and need rapid treatment. Unless the patient is dying, it is essential to

Table 9.1 Acute and maintenance drug therapies for breathlessness

Indication	Acute	Maintenance
Diffuse airway obstruction	Corticosteroid Bronchodilator	Corticosteroid Bronchodilator
Upper airway obstruction	Corticosteroid	–
Inflammation (lymphangitis, pneumonitis)	Corticosteroid	Corticosteroid
Superior vena caval obstruction	Corticosteroid	–

consider appropriate palliative interventions. These may include external beam radiotherapy, stenting of the airway or superior vena cava, and endobronchial techniques such as cryoablation, laser, and brachytherapy. These interventions are discussed in Chapter 30.

The choice of corticosteroid seems to be determined by individual clinician preference. The benefits of dexamethasone, which is widely used in the palliative care setting, as compared with prednisolone include reduced mineralocorticoid effects, increased potency, and higher solubility. Disadvantages of all corticosteroids include adrenal insufficiency following abrupt withdrawal and a wide range of well-known adverse effects related to both mineralocorticoid and glucocorticoid actions. Poor understanding on the part of patients about why they are taking steroids and the consequent precautions needed, has been documented.

In principle, a meaningful therapeutic trial implies an explicit indication, adequate starting doses, and appropriate duration of treatment. Close monitoring of treatment outcome is essential, together with a willingness to discontinue the drug if it proves unhelpful. Definitive advice about the details of prescribing corticosteroids is not available from controlled studies.[16] In practice, therefore, an individualized benefit–burden assessment should be made, based on the relevant clinical findings and a careful appraisal of risk factors for steroid adverse effects. Proximal myopathy is a particularly burdensome side effect for patients already weakened by disease. Oropharyngeal candidiasis is common, but easily treated once looked for specifically. A history of either hyperglycaemia or psychiatric illness demand particular caution, the latter because steroids may precipitate depression or acute psychosis in susceptible individuals.

A helpful review about corticosteroid use and peptic ulceration concluded that there is a low incidence of peptic ulceration and other gastrointestinal complications in patients taking corticosteroids alone.[14] There are, however, four particular risk factors which increase this incidence significantly:

+ high cumulative dose of corticosteroid (dexamethasone >140 mg)
+ previous history of peptic ulceration
+ advanced malignant disease
+ co-prescription of a non-steroidal anti-inflammatory drug (NSAID).

The increase in relative risk by 15-fold when steroids and an NSAID are used together is particularly striking and carries particular clinical relevance. Prophylaxis against peptic ulceration should be considered if two or more risk factors are present. If an NSAID is one of the risk factors, misoprostol[15] has been recommended as the prophylactic drug of choice in palliative care. In the treatment of established NSAID-related gastroduodenal injury, however, the use of a proton pump inhibitor is more effective.[16]

In practice, 8 mg dexamethasone per day administered orally in divided doses for 5–7 days is commonly used in cancer related breathlessness.[17] A higher dose is usually employed in patients with superior vena caval obstruction. A longer trial is recommended for patients with COPD,[18] in which setting prednisolone is traditionally the steroid of choice, at a dose of 30 mg daily for 2 weeks. If treatment with steroids is found to improve breathlessness, then the lowest effective dose should be used over time. Iatrogenic insomnia may be avoided by taking steroids in the morning. Dexamethasone may be administered by continuous infusion via a syringe driver, when the patient is unable to take oral medications, for example, if vomiting or unconscious.[19] Important precautions are to use no more than two drugs in a syringe driver containing therapeutic doses of dexamethasone, ensuring as dilute a solution as possible, using 'water-for-injection' as the recommended diluent, and being aware that discolouration of the solution reflects drug incompatibility.[19] Special precautions may need to be taken to avoid the possibility of precipitation with other drugs in the syringe.

In respiratory medicine, inhaled steroids are used for maintenance therapy. No published clinical trials have assessed the therapeutic potential of inhaled steroids in patients with cancer-related breathlessness. However, personal observations suggest that the use of inhaled steroids in patients with diffuse inflammation, such as lymphangiitis and pneumonitis, may be beneficial on occasion.

Whenever possible, patients should be involved in the decision to use steroids, be aware of the reasons why, and be warned of potential side effects. They should be issued with a steroid alert card. The general practitioner must be kept informed when the patient is discharged from hospital.

Respiratory stimulant drugs

Theoretically, pharmacological stimulation of ventilation in some chronically hypoxaemic patients with carbon dioxide retention could improve symptoms, and prevent or delay the development of polycythaemia and pulmonary hypertension.

In laboratory studies, low-dose progestagens,[20] doxapram,[21] almitrine,[22] inhaled cannabis,[23] nabilone,[24] and nebulized local anaesthetics[25,26] have all been shown to stimulate ventilation. With the exception of progestagens, these agents tend to have dose-limiting or potentially severe side effects. The side effects of therapeutically administered cannabis tend to be more pronounced in older people.

In practice respiratory stimulant drugs are hardly ever used. They may have a role in a few patients in whom hypoxia or hypercapnia causes excessive daytime somnolence or night-time sleep disturbance. Currently, interest focuses on mechanically rather than pharmacologically assisted ventilation (see Chapter 10).

Respiratory sedative drugs

Benzodiazepines

The benzodiazepines are respiratory sedative drugs which reduce respiratory drive and may reduce pulmonary ventilation.[27] Their use in cancer-related breathlessness has not been evaluated in clinical trials.

Studies in patients with COPD have produced conflicting results;[28,29] but the doses used previously (diazepam 25 mg per day) are significantly higher than those used in clinical practice today. In a later study, alprazolam was reported to be ineffective in relieving the perception of breathlessness.[30] Despite the lack of scientific evidence of efficacy, this class of drug is widely used in the palliative treatment of breathlessness.

It is possible that the anxiolytic properties of these drugs are therapeutic in some breathless patients. Alternatively, drugs in this class may affect breathlessness through a direct effect on respiration, or by causing relaxation of respiratory muscles, or perhaps more likely, through a combination of factors.

Diazepam is the oral drug of choice in empirical practice.[31] In view of its plasma half-life of 40 h it may be administered as a single night-time dose of 2–5 mg. The dose can be titrated according to efficacy and side effects. Some anxious, breathless patients tolerate doses of up to 30 mg daily.

Lorazepam is preferred for self-administration during respiratory panic attacks, a common manifestation of the breathlessness–anxiety cycle. It is well absorbed sublingually and has a rapid onset of action. The dose is 0.5–1 mg. In the absence of any clinical trials of the use of lorazepam for this indication, one can only speculate on why this treatment seems to work, sometimes dramatically well, in some patients. It seems likely that encouraging the breathless patient to use sublingual lorazepam, after trying non-pharmacological strategies to limit panic, may restore their sense of control and that this, as well as any pharmacological effect may be important.

Midazolam is a useful benzodiazepine for parenteral administration, either intermittently as a bolus injection (2.5–5 mg) or continuously by means of a subcutaneous infusion via a syringe driver (starting dose 10–20 mg over 24 h). Its use for breathlessness in dying patients has been recommended in palliative care textbooks,[32] frequently in combination with a low-dose opioid such as diamorphine. This is discussed further in the section on the dying patient.

In practice, the use of low-dose benzodiazepines in the form of a therapeutic trial may be cautiously recommended, particularly when anxiety is prominent and when breathlessness appears intractable. Unfortunately, there is very little scientific evidence upon which to base clinical decision-making and none to inform the decision as to whether a therapeutic trial of an opioid drug or a benzodiazepine or both may be appropriate.

Opioids

Opioid drugs have been used for centuries for a wide range of indications, including the relief of breathlessness. Most palliative care physicians agree that low-dose systemic opioids have a place in the symptomatic management of breathlessness in patients with both malignant and, probably, non-malignant lung disease. This was not always so. Ever since the recognition of the potential hazard of opioid-induced respiratory depression in the 1950s,[33] caution has been advocated in the prescribing of strong opioid drugs, particularly in the treatment of breathlessness. Opioids can indeed cause respiratory depression, but it is important to remember that this risk varies between patients and appears to be related to a number of factors including the underlying pathophysiology, prior exposure to opioids, route of administration, rate of dose titration, and coexisting pathology. Walsh in 1984 demonstrated no respiratory depression, assessed by arterial blood gases, in most of a group of cancer patients taking more than 100 mg of oral morphine per day for pain.[34]

Surprisingly, perhaps, more clinical trials have addressed the therapeutic potential of opioids in breathless patients with non-malignant disease than in those with malignant disease. The only published studies assessing weak opioid drugs have been conducted in patients with COPD. These trials are summarized in Table 9.2 and the trials of opioids in breathless patients with cancer in Table 9.3. At present, the evidence suggests that low-dose systemic opioids have a role in the management of breathless patients with COPD and those with primary or secondary lung malignancy and that their use is not associated with significant respiratory depression. Weak opioids, e.g. dihydrocodeine, may be underused.

The oral route is preferred for opioids in cancer pain management. The only study of initiating oral opioids for breathlessness in patients with cancer used low-dose controlled-release morphine sulfate and failed to show any effect; in addition, the drug was poorly tolerated.[47] There were similar findings in a separate study in patients with COPD.[42] Anecdotally, controlled-release preparations are often reported as being less efficacious than immediate-release oral preparations for this indication. If this is the case then possible explanations could be that frequent plasma peaks of morphine and/or its metabolites are required for any effect on breathlessness, or that breathless patients are reassured by receiving regular, 4-hourly doses

Table 9.2 Summary of clinical trials of opioids for breathlessness in patients with non-malignant disease

Author	Drug	No. of patients	Placebo controlled	Disease group	Dose/schedule	Route	Outcome Reduction in dyspnoea	Improved exercise tolerance
Woodcock[35,36]	Dihydrocodeine	12	Yes	COPD	1 mg/kg single dose	PO	Yes	Yes
Johnson[37]	Dihydrocodeine	18	Yes	COPD	15 mg PRN pre exercise, 1 week; 15 mg alternate days, 1 week	PO; PO	Yes; No	No; No
Robin[38]	Hydromorphone	1	n of 1	COPD	3 mg 4 × day, 3 days	PR	Yes	N/A
Browning[39]	Hydrocodone	7	Yes	COPD	20 mg/m² per day, 48 h	PO	No	No
Light[40]	Morphine	13	Yes	COPD	0.8 mg/kg, single dose	PO	Yes	Yes
Eiser[41]	Diamorphine	10	Yes	COPD ('pink puffers')	2.5–5 mg 4 × day, 2 weeks	PO; PO	No; No	No; No
Eiser[41]	Diamorphine	8	Yes	COPD	7.5 mg, 2 doses, 4 h apart			
Poole[42]	Morphine	16	Yes	COPD	Dose titrated from 10 mg 1 × day to 20 mg 2 × day over 2 weeks, modified release preparation (MST)	PO	No	No

N/A, not assessed; PO, oral; PR, rectal; PRN, as required.

Table 9.3 Summary of clinical trials of opioids for breathlessness in patients with malignant disease

Author	Drug	No. of patients	Placebo controlled	Dose/schedule	Route	Reduction in dyspnoea
Cohen[43]	Morphine	8	No	Titrated vs. response, continuous infusion, mean dose 5.6 mg/h	IV	Yes
Bruera[44]	Morphine	20	No	4 hourly dose 5 mg or 2.5 × 4- hourly dose	SC	Yes
Bruera[45]	Morphine	10	Yes	Single dose, 50% greater than 4-hourly dose, mean dose 34 ± 12 mg morphine	SC	Yes
Allard[46]	Strong opioids	33	Randomized, continuous sequential trial	15 successive pairs of patients, matched on route of administration, random allocation of 2 opioid doses (25% and 50% of 4-hourly dose)	PO(20) SC(13)	Yes, both dose levels
Boyd[47]	Morphine	15	No	Regular oral preparation, MST 10 mg 2 × day (13) or 30% increase in dose (2)	PO	No

IV, intravenous; SC, subcutaneous

of medication for their breathlessness and this, in itself, makes them less anxious and, perhaps, less breathless. The same arguments can be applied when considering parenterally administered opioids. Further work is required to investigate how opioids relieve breathlessness.

In clinical practice in breathless patients previously naive to opioids, a therapeutic trial of low-dose oral opioids, for example 2.5 mg of immediate release morphine sulfate every 4 h, is often appropriate. The dose can be titrated upwards. There is debate about the choice of opioid dose for breathlessness in patients who are already receiving strong opioid drugs for pain.[46] Most advocate an increase in dose, but the size of this dose increment should probably be decided on an individual patient basis. Allard *et al.*[46] found that dose increases of 25% or 50% of the usual opioid dose gave equally good results. Some clinicians convert the total daily dose of immediate-release morphine sulfate to a once or twice daily controlled-release preparation. Although this may improve patient compliance, we prefer to continue regular 4-hourly immediate release medication for the reasons stated in the last paragraph.

Parenteral opioids (for example 2.5 mg diamorphine as a subcutaneous bolus injection or 10 mg diamorphine as a subcutaneous infusion over 24 h) are used in patients in whom oral drug administration is no longer appropriate, or possible.

There is no research investigating the possibility of using opioid drugs preemptively in patients who become breathlessness on exertion but, in our experience, this strategy seems effective in some patients and may restore a sense of control.

Finally, it must be remembered that breathless patients may be constipated because of their disability or other medication. If opioids are used, the co-prescription of appropriate laxative therapy is particularly important.

Nebulized opioids

Over the past decade, there has been a vogue for the use of nebulized opioids in the symptomatic management of breathlessness. This vogue runs contrary to the scientific evidence. Of eight reported randomized controlled trials (RCTs), only one supports the use of nebulized opioids for this indication. The trials are described in Table 9.4. There are many important methodological differences between them. Most were based on either progressive or endurance exercise tests, but in two purely subjective outcome measures were used.[54,55] All were single-dose studies. It may be that it is not appropriate to extrapolate these results to day-to-day clinical practice, but nevertheless it is a fact that the scientific evidence to date does not support the use of nebulized opioids for the relief of breathlessness.

Several investigators have studied the pharmacokinetics of nebulized opioids. Bioavailability is a term used to indicate the extent to which a drug reaches its sites of action, or reaches a biological fluid from which the drug has access to its site of action. The only study to assess the systemic bioavailability of a nebulized opioid (morphine up to 30 mg), administered through an Acorn nebulizer, relative to the intravenous route showed a very low bioavailability ($<5.1\%$) in normal volunteers.[57] The bioavailability of any nebulized drug can vary considerably, depending on the equipment used and the inspiratory effort of which the patient is capable. Modern nebulizer technology could be used to administer higher doses of drug to the lung and this may be worthy of investigation.

In the UK most clinicians consider a trial of nebulized saline rather than an opioid if a therapeutic trial of any inhaled therapy is deemed appropriate. This is because current evidence, from trials comparing the effects of nebulized opioids[49–56] and nebulized local anaesthetics[58] with nebulized normal saline, suggest that nebulized normal saline is an effective treatment in selected

Table 9.4 Placebo-controlled, randomized controlled trials of nebulized opioids

Study	No. of patients	Disease (patients)	Drug/dose	Subjective assessment	Exercise test	Efficacy of nebulized morphine?
Young[48]	11	COPD (9) Pulmonary fibrosis (2)	Morphine 5 mg	No	Bicycle endurance	Yes
Beauford[49]	8	COPD	Morphine 1 mg, 4 mg, 10 mg	Yes	Bicycle incremental	No
Davis[50]	18	COPD	Morphine 12.5 mg and M6-G 4 mg	Yes	Bicycle endurance 6 MWT	No
Masood[51]	12	COPD	Morphine 10 mg, 25 mg	Yes	Bicycle incremental	No
Harris-Eze[52]	6	Interstitial lung disease	Morphine 2.5 mg, 5 mg	Yes	Bicycle incremental	No
Leung[53]	10	COPD (9) Pulmonary fibrosis (1)	Morphine 5 mg	Yes	Bicycle incremental	No
Davis[54]	79	Primary or secondary lung cancer	Morphine 5–50 mg dose randomized in different patients	Yes	No	No
Noseda[55]	17	Severe lung or cardiac disease, mainly COPD, 3 with primary/secondary lung malignancy	Morphine 10 mg with oxygen Morphine 20 mg with oxygen Morphine 10 mg without oxygen	Yes	No	No
Jankelson[56]	16	COPD	Morphine 20 mg, 40 mg	Yes	6 MWT	No

6 MWT, 6 minute walking test

breathless patients. Unlike nebulized opioids, normal saline carries minimal risk of local or systemic toxicity. Any clinician should be cautious in advocating the use of opioids in an unlicensed way, especially when such use is not supported by current scientific evidence. Furthermore, the problems of drawing up licensed drugs from glass vials in the domiciliary setting should not be underestimated. Nebulized opioids should not be considered part of standard practice.

Other respiratory sedative drugs

Antihistamines

In a placebo-controlled, randomized study of 18 patients with COPD, promethazine (total daily dose 125 mg) caused a significant improvement in breathlessness and exercise tolerance.[29] Drug-induced drowsiness was a problem in 2/18 patients. Only 7/11 patients completed another randomized, cross-over study of promethazine (total daily dose 100 mg) and codeine,[59] and antihistamine-related toxicity (worsening airflow obstruction in 1, drowsiness in 3) prompted early cessation of the study. Perhaps less sedating antihistamines might be useful, but this has not been investigated.

Butyrphenones

The dopamine antagonist haloperidol, used commonly as an antiemetic and, at higher doses, as an antipsychotic drug, might be expected to relieve breathlessness but this has not been studied. If nausea and breathlessness coexist in the same patient, then it seems sensible to consider haloperidol as the antiemetic drug so long as the nausea is thought to be caused by stimulation of the chemoreceptor trigger zone (e.g. by drugs, toxins. or metabolites).

Phenothiazines

Chlorpromazine has been shown to reduce the 'want of air' in healthy subjects after exercise.[60] Surprisingly this suggestion of therapeutic potential has not been submitted to RCTs. In an open study, the combination of morphine and chlorpromazine, at doses of 10 mg and 25 mg respectively, reduced breathlessness caused by massive parenchymal lung metastases.[61] Levomepromazine is used widely in palliative care for sedation, and in lower doses, as an antiemetic. The possibility that it may relieve breathlessness does not appear to have been evaluated. Thus, phenothiazines may relieve breathlessness in some patients but this has been inadequately evaluated. However, use of this class of drugs is likely to be limited by side effects.

Alcohol

There is some evidence that alcohol may decrease the intensity of breathlessness in patients with COPD[35,62] and, in moderation, many patients may prefer to try their own 'favourite tipple' rather than some other medication of unproven efficiency!

Management of breathlessness in the terminal phase

The terminal phase refers to that stage of disease where death appears inevitable and close, usually within days or hours. It usually follows a period of progressive deterioration. It is often less easy to recognize the terminal phase in patients with non-malignant disease than in those with malignant disease.

Breathlessness is common towards the end of life and it is a poor prognostic sign.[63] A study of patients with advanced cancer admitted to a hospice established an inverse relationship between survival and both incidence and severity of breathlessness.[64]

The aim of care is to provide optimum control of symptoms and distress within a broader context of psychological and social support for the patient and family. It has been argued that the control of symptoms, including breathlessness, may depend increasingly upon drug inventions as death approaches, as other methods of therapy become impractical or futile.[19] In our experience, however, selected non-pharmacological interventions such as the use of a freestanding fan, careful attention to positioning, and measures to encourage both muscular and psychological relaxation can be beneficial in some patients very near to death. It is important to emphasize that the primary objective of drug treatment in this context, usually, is to reduce the perception of breathlessness and associated distress and not:

- to hasten death – which is euthanasia
- to prolong life – which may amount to a lingering death
- to induce sedation – although sedation may be a foreseen benefit in selected patients and may be required on occasions, such as in the event of massive haemoptysis.

In practice – the terminal phase

Oral medication may be continued if appropriate. Parenteral drug treatment is administered as either a bolus injection or continuous subcutaneous infusion (CSCI). Bolus injections may be used as an adjunct to oral administration, perhaps for more rapid onset of action. A syringe driver is used for CSCI. The usual indications are:

- nausea and/or vomiting
- dysphagia
- generalized weakness
- coma.

Clearly when a CSCI is started, regular oral administration for those drugs should be discontinued. The doses of opioid and benzodiazepine drugs in terminal care are influenced by the following factors:

- previous requirements
- indication(s)
- estimated body mass
- convention.

There might be multiple indications for both classes of drug. Typical initial doses for diamorphine and midazolam in the naive adult patient are as shown in Table 9.5. It is safer to start with such small doses and titrate rapidly upwards, especially in patients with established pulmonary disease.

Table 9.5 Initial doses in drug-naive patients

	Bolus SC injection	CSCI over 24 h
Diamorphine	2.5 mg	10 mg
Midazolam	2.5 mg	10 mg

Table 9.6 Recommended parenteral drug interventions for breathlessness and associated symptoms during the terminal phase

Problem	Drug class	Drug	Route of administration		
			SC bolus	CSCI	IV titration
Breathlessness	Opioid	Morphine/diamorphine	+	+	+
Tachypnoea	Opioid	Morphine/diamorphine	(+)	−	(+)
Anxiety	Benzodiazepine	Midazolam	+	+	(+)
Noisy breathing (retained intrabronchial secretions)	Anticholinergic	Hyoscine/glycopyrrolate	+	+	−

+, commonly used in palliative care; (+), not commonly used in palliative care; −, not used in palliative care; CSCI, continuous subcutaneous infusion; IV, intravenous; SC, subcutaneous.

In practice patients will often have been taking an opioid by mouth, and a direct conversion to parenteral administration can be undertaken with confidence. There has been some debate about the conversion ratio from oral morphine to subcutaneous diamorphine but, in Europe, a ratio of 3:1 is usually employed.[65] For example, immediate release morphine 10 mg every 4 h by mouth (total dose 60 mg over 24 h) is equivalent to diamorphine 20 mg via CSCI over 24 h.

In the dying patient with both breathlessness and pain the dose of diamorphine is determined empirically on a case-by-case basis by means of careful titration and is guided by observed benefit. The art is to avoid either inappropriate haste or hesitancy, to achieve maximum therapeutic benefit.

The same principles apply in the uncommon case of terminal asphyxia, due perhaps to tumour causing tracheal or bronchial obstruction. In this situation, however, a valid aim of treatment may be the induction of controlled sedation to alleviate the extreme fear of the suffocating patient.

Breathlessness occurring at the end of life may be associated with noisy breathing, sometimes referred to as 'death rattle'. This is due to retention and pooling of bronchial and salivary secretions in the absence of effective cough and swallowing reflexed. In the palliative care setting it is commonly treated with anticholinergic drugs including hyoscine hydrobromide, hyoscine butylbromide, and glycopyrrolate.[66] A recently published comparative study found that hyoscine hydrobromide was as effective as glycopyrrolate at reducing death rattle, but that its speed of onset was more rapid.[67]

In all cases it is important, if possible, to discuss treatment options and aims of care with the patient and relatives in order to reduce the likelihood of misunderstanding. Details of recommended parenteral drug interventions for breathlessness and associated symptoms during the terminal phase are summarized in Table 9.6.

Ethical considerations

Breathlessness can be a challenging symptom for clinicians to palliate and may become intolerable for the patient and family, causing much suffering. Critically, when using pharmacological interventions, the gap between benefit and harm may be narrow.

Under these circumstances, when clinical decision-making is inevitably difficult, the physician may find it helpful to apply an ethical frame of reference. Ethical frameworks are designed to assist and guide clinicians in situations where the definition of appropriate treatment is uncertain.[68]

Difficult and refractory breathlessness

When the symptomatic management of breathlessness with drugs becomes difficult, the physician should continue rigorous clinical evaluation with careful consideration of the following key issues:[69]

◆ the patient's general condition and medical prognosis

◆ the therapeutic aim of each treatment

◆ the potential benefits of treatment from the patient's point of view

◆ the adverse effects of treatment.

Appropriate treatment may vary between different patients experiencing breathlessness, and within the same patient over time.

When breathlessness cannot adequately be controlled despite best treatment it becomes refractory. It is important to distinguish between difficult and refractory symptoms because each is associated with different aims of care. Furthermore, the designation of a symptom as refractory has profound implications for treatment, suggesting that suffering will not be relieved with routine interventions.

Breathlessness is held to be refractory if routine measures are either:

◆ ineffective, or

◆ excessively burdensome to the patient, or

◆ unlikely to provide relief within a tolerable period of time.

Pain, breathlessness, and agitation are the symptoms most often found to be refractory.[70] In the patient experiencing refractory breathlessness at the end of life, sedation may be an appropriate treatment.[71]

The doctrine of double effect

When faced with breathlessness at the end of life which is either difficult or refractory, physicians may experience a conflict between their core responsibilities to preserve life and to relieve suffering. In other words, it may appear that the latter can be achieved only at the possible expense of the former. The doctrine of double effect may be applied in these challenging situations to justify beneficial actions which may hasten death. Justification may be claimed if, and only if, the following five criteria are met:[72]

◆ the intended effect must be a good one – relief of suffering caused by refractory breathlessness, for example

◆ all other interventions are ineffective or futile

◆ the bad effect – such as the patient's death – may be foreseen but must not be intended

◆ the bad effect must not be the means of bringing about the good effect

◆ the good effect must, on balance, outweigh the bad effect.

The doctrine of double effect has been recognized in British law since the 1950s when Lord Justice Devlin stated that 'a doctor who is aiding the dying does not have to calculate in minutes, or even in hours, and perhaps not in days or weeks, the effects upon a patient's life of the medicines he administers or else be in peril of a charge of murder.' (quoted in ref. 73).

In practice:

- The usual aim of management is to ameliorate, not abolish, symptoms. It is important to be realistic about the limitations of care.

- In routine practice, decision-making in individual cases is often difficult. It is rare, however, to involve the doctrine of double effect, as defined above.

Chronic breathlessness before dying

There is no evidence that the correct use of drugs as described in this chapter – especially opioids and benzodiazepines – shortens life. There is some evidence that their cautious use may be beneficial in selected cases.

Acute and severe breathlessness around dying

When the cause is irreversible and death imminent, the appropriate aim of care is relief of suffering. This might arise, for example, in cases of upper airway obstruction. Induction of sedation under these circumstances may be achieved by means of slow intravenous titration of midazolam (10 mg in 10 mL) and morphine or diamorphine (10 mg in 10 mL).

Key points

- Appropriate management of breathlessness requires the careful and individualized use of both non-drug and drug measures

- Benzodiazepines and opioids are the main classes of drugs used in the palliation of breathlessness

- Corticosteroids should only be administered for a specific reason

- Nebulized opioids should not be considered part of standard practice

- It is easy to commence drugs but harder to stop them; a therapeutic trial with preset goals of treatment is recommended

References

1 O'Brien, T., Welsh, J., and Dunn, F.G. Non-malignant conditions. *BMJ* 1998; **316**: 286–9.

2 Bredin, M., Corner, J., Krishnasamy, M., *et al.* Multicentre randomised controlled trial of nursing intervention for breathlessness in patients with lung cancer. *BMJ* 1999; **318**: 901–4.

3 NCHSPCS. *Specialist palliative care: a statement of definitions*. Occasional Paper 8. London: National Council for Hospice and Specialist Palliative Care Services, 1995.

4 Twycross, R. *Symptom management in advanced cancer*. Abingdon: Radcliffe Medical Press, 1997.

5 Davis, C.L. The therapeutics of dyspnoea. In: *Cancer Surveys*, Vol. 21. *Palliative medicine, problem areas in pain and symptom management*. London: Imperial Cancer Research Fund, 1994.

6 Shee, C.D. Palliation in chronic respiratory disease. *Palliative Med* 1995; **9**: 3–12.

7 British Thoracic Society and others. The BTS guidelines on asthma management. *Thorax* 1997; **52**(Suppl 1): 51–21.

8 British Thoracic Society and others. The BTS guidelines for the management of chronic obstructive pulmonary disease. *Thorax* 1997; **52**(5): 51–8.

9 Congleton, J., and Muers, M.F. The incidence of airflow obstruction in bronchial carcinoma, its relation to breathlessness and response to bronchodilator therapy. *Respir Med* 1995; **89**: 291–6.

10 Mahler, D.A., Matthay, R.A., Snyuder, P.E., *et al.* Sustained release theophylline reduced dyspnoea in non-reversible obstructive airway disease. *Am Rev Respir Dis* 1985; **131**: 22–5.

11 Murciano, D., Audier, M., Legocguic, Y., *et al.* Effects of theophylline on diaphragmatic strength and fatigue in patients with chronic obstructive pulmonary disease. *N Engl J Med* 1984; **311**: 349–314.

12 Barnes, P.J. New therapies for chronic obstructive pulmonary disease. *Thorax* 1993; **53**: 437–47.

13 Shee, C.D. Palliation in chronic respiratory disease. *Palliative Med* 1995; **9**: 3–12.

14 Hardy, J. Corticosteroids in palliative care. *Eur J Palliative Care* 1998; **5**(2): 46–50.

15 Ellershaw, J.E., and Kelly, M.J. Corticosteroids and peptic ulceration. *Palliative Med* 1994; **8**: 313–19.

16 Hawkey, C.J., *et al.* Omeprazole compared with Misoprostal for when associated with nonsteroidal anti-inflammatory drugs. *N Engl J Med* 1998; **33**: 727–34.

17 Cowcher, K., and Hanks, G.W. Long term management of respiratory symptoms in advanced cancer. *J Pain Symptom Manage* 1990; **5**: 320–30.

18 Weir, D.C., *et al.* Time course of response to oral and inhaled corticosteroids in non-asthmatic chronic airflow obstruction. *Thorax* 1990; **45**: 118–21.

19 Twycross, R., Wilcock, A., and Thorp, S. *Palliative care formulary*. Abingdon: Radcliffe Medical Press, 1998.

20 Mikami, M., *et al.* Respiration effect of synthetic progestin in small doses in normal men. *Chest* 1989; **96**(5): 1073–5.

21 Burki, N. Ventilatory effects of doxapram in conscious human subjects. *Chest* 1984; **85**: 600–4.

22 Daskalopoulou, E., Patakas, D., Tsara, V., Zoglopitis, F., and Maniki, E. Comparison of almitrine bismesylate and medroxyprogesterone acetate on oxygenation during wakefulness and sleep in patients with chronic obstructive lung disease. *Thorax* 1990; **45**: 666–9.

23 Vachon, L., Fitzgerald, M.X., Solliday, N.H., Gould, I.A., and Gaensler, E.A. Single-dose effect of marihuana smoke. *N Engl J Med* 1973; **288**: 985–9.

24 Ahmedzai, S., Carter, R., Mills, R.J., and Moran, F. Effects of nabilone on pulmonary function. In: *Marihuana '84. Proceedings of the Oxford Symposium on Cannabis*. Oxford: IRL Press, 1984; 371–8.

25 Labaille, T., Clergue, F., Samii, K., Ecoffey, C., and Berdeaux, A. Ventilatory response to CO2 following intravenous and epidural lidocaine. *Anesthiology* 1985; **63**: 179–83.

26 Winning, I., Hamilton, R.D., Shea, S.A., Knott, C., and Guz, A. Effect of airway anaesthesia on the control of breathing and the sensation of breathlessness in man. *Clin Sci* 1985; **68**: 215–25.

27 Ahmedzai, S. Palliation of respiratory symptoms. In: D. Doyle, G.W.C. Hanks, and N. Macdonald (eds) *Oxford textbook of palliative medicine*. Oxford: Oxford University Press, 1993; 361.

28 Mitchell-Heggs, P., Murphy, K., *et al.* Diazepam in the treatment of dyspnoea in the 'pink-puffer' syndrome. *Q J Med* 1980; **44**: 9–20.

29 Woodcock, A., Gross, E.R., and Geddes, D.M. Drug treatment of breathlessness; contrasting effects of diazepam and promethazine in 'pink-puffers'. *BMJ* 1981; **283**: 343–6.

30 Man, G.C., Hsu, K., and Sproule, B.J. Effects of alprazolam on exercise and dyspnoea in patients with chronic obstructive pulmonary disease. *Chest* 1986; **90**(6): 832–6.

31 Davis, C.L. Breathlessness, cough and other respiratory problems. *BMJ* 1997; **315**: 931–4.

32 Wilcock, A. Respiratory symptoms. In: *Tutorials in Palliative Medicine*. Northampton: EPL Publications, 1997.

33 Wilson, R.H., Hoseth, W., and Dempsey, M.E. Respiratory acidosis: effects of decreasing respiratory minute volume in patients with chronic pulmonary emphysema, with specific reference to oxygen, morphine and barbiturates. *Am J Med* 1954; **18**: 464–70.

34 Walsh, T.D. Opiates and respiratory function in advanced cancer. *Recent Results Cancer Res* 1984; **89**: 115–17.

35 Woodcock, A.A., Gross, E.R., Gellert, A., *et al.* Effects of dihydrocodeine, alcohol, and caffeine on breathlessness and exercise tolerance in patients with chronic obstructive lung disease and normal blood gases. *N Engl J Med* 1981; **305**(27): 1611–16.

36 Woodcock, A.A., Johnson, M.A., and Geddes, D.M. Breathlessness, alcohol and opiates. *N Engl J Med* 1982; **306**(22): 1363–4.

37 Johnson, M.A., Woodcock, A.A., and Geddes, D.M. Dihydrocodeine for breathlessness in 'pink puffers'. *Br Med J* 1983; **286**: 675–7.

38 Robin, E.D., and Burke, C.M. Single-patient randomized clinical trial. Opiates for intractable dyspnea. *Chest* 1986; **90**(6): 888–92.

39 Browning, I., D'Alonzo, G.E., and Tobin, M.J. Effects of hydrocodone on dyspnea, respiratory drive and exercise performance in adult patients with cystic fibrosis. abstr 137. *Am Rev Respir Dis* 1988; **138**: 305.

40 Light, R.W., Muro, J.R., Sato, R.I., *et al.* Effects of oral morphine on breathlessness and exercise tolerance in patients with chronic obstructive pulmonary disease. *Am Rev Respir Dis* 1989; **139**: 126–33.

41 Eiser, N., Denman, W.T., West, C., and Luce, P. Oral diamorphine: lack of effect on dyspnea and exercise tolerance in the 'pink puffer' syndrome. *Eur Respir J* 1991; **4**: 926–31.

42 Poole, P.J., Veale, A.G., and Black, P.N. The effect of sustained-release morphine on breathlessness and quality of life in severe chronic obstructive pulmonary disease. *Am J Respir Crit Care Med* 1998; **157**(6): 1877–80.

43 Cohen, M.H., Johnston Anderson, A., Krasnow, S.H., *et al.* Continuous intravenous infusion of morphine for severe dyspnea. *South Med J* 1991; **84**(2): 229–34.

44 Bruera, E., Macmillan, K., Pither, J., and MacDonald, R.N. Effects of morphine on the dyspnea in terminal cancer patients. *J Pain Symptom Manage* 1990; **5**: 341–4.

45 Bruera, E., MacEachern, T., Ripamonti, C., and Hanson, J. Subcutaneous morphine for dyspnea in cancer patients. *Ann Intern Med* 1993; **119**(9): 906–7.

46 Allard, P., Lamontagne, C., Bernard, P., and Tremblay, C. How effective are supplementary doses of opiates on dyspnoea in terminally ill cancer patients? A randomized sequential clinical trial. *J Pain Symptom Manage* 1999; **17**(4): 256–65.

47 Boyd, K.J., and Kelly, M. Oral morphine as symptomatic treatment of dyspnoea in patients with advanced cancer. *Palliative Med* 1997; **11**: 277–81.

48 Young, I.H., Daviskas, E., and Veena, K.A. Effect of low dose nebulised morphine on exercise endurance in patients with chronic lung disease. *Thorax* 1989; **44**: 387–90.

49 Beauford, W., Saylor, T.T., Stansbury, D.W., Avolos, K., and Light, R.W. Effects of nebulised morphine sulphate on the exercise tolerance of the ventilatory limited COPD patient. *Chest* 1993; **104**: 175–8.

50 Davis, C.L., Hodder, C.A., Love, S., *et al.* Effect of nebulised morphine and morphine 6-glucuronide on exercise endurance in patients with chronic obstructive airways disease. *Thorax* 1994; **49**(4): 393.

51 Masood, A.R., Reed, J.W., and Thomas, S.H.L. Lack of effect of inhaled morphine on exercise-induced breathlessness in chronic obstructive pulmonary disease. *Thorax* 1995; **50**: 629–34.

52 Harris-Eze, A.O., Sridhar, G., Clemens, E., *et al.* Low-dose nebulized morphine does not improve exercise in interstitial lung disease. *Am J Respir Crit Care Med* 1995; **152**: 1940–5.

53 Leung, R., Hill, P., and Burdon, J. Effect of inhaled morphine on the development of breathlessness during exercise in patients with chronic lung disease. *Thorax* 1996; **51**: 596–600.

54 Davis, C.L., Penn, K., A'Hern, R., *et al.* Single-dose randomized controlled trial of nebulised morphine in patients with cancer related breathlessness. *Palliative Med* 1996; **10**: 64–5.

55 Noseda, A., Carpiaux, J.P., Markstein, C., *et al.* Disabling dyspnoea in patients with advanced disease: lack of effect of nebulised morphine. *Eur Respir J* 1997; **10**: 1079–83.

56 Jankelson, D., Hosseini, K., Mather, L.E., Seale, J.P., and Young, I.H. Lack of effect of high doses of inhaled morphine on exercise endurance in chronic obstructive pulmonary disease. *Eur Respir J* 1997; **10**(10): 2270–4.

57 Davis, C.L., Lam, W., Roberts, M., *et al.* The pharmacokinetics of nebulised morphine. Abstract 995. In: *Proceedings of International Association for the Study of Pain* Seattle: IASP Publications, 1993; 379.

58 Wilcock, A., Corcoran, R., and Tattersfield, A.E. Safety and efficacy of nebulised lignocaine in patients with cancer and breathlessness. *Palliative Med* 1994; **8**: 35–8.

59 Rice, K.L., Kronenburg, R.S., Hedemark, L.L., and Niewoehner, D.E. Effects of chronic administration of codeine and promethazine on breathlessness and exercise tolerance in patients with chronic airflow obstruction. *Br J Dis Chest* 1987; **81**: 287–92.

60 O'Neill, P.A., Morton, P.B., and Stark, R.D. Chlorpromazine – a specific effect on breathlessness? *Br J Clin Pharmacol* 1985; **19**: 793–7.

61 Ventafridda, V., Spoldi, E., and De Conno, F. Control of dyspnoea in advanced cancer patients. *Chest* 1990; **6**: 1544–5.

62 Herxheimer, H., and Streseman, E. Ethanol and lung function in bronchial asthma. *Arch Int Pharm Ther* 1963; **144**: 310–14.

63 Reuben, D.B., and Mor, V.M. Dyspnoea in terminally ill cancer patients. *Chest* 1986; **89**(2): 234–6.

64 Heyse-Moore, L., *et al.* How much of a problem is dyspnoea in advanced cancer? *Palliative Med* 1991; **5**: 20–6.

65 Hanks, G.W., *et al.* Morphine in cancer pain: modes of administration. *BMJ* 1996; **312**: 823–6.

66 Back, I.N., *et al.* A study comparing hyoscine hydrobromide and glycopyrrolate in the treatment of death rattle. *Palliative Med* 2001; **15**(4): 329–36.

67 Hughes, A., *et al.* Audit of three antimuscarinic drugs for managing retained secretions. *Palliative Med* 2000; **14**: 221–2.

68 Latimer, E. Ethical challenges in cancer care. *J Palliative Care* 1992; **8**(1): 65–70

69 Twycross, R. Ethics. In: *Pain relief in advanced cancer.* Edinburgh: Churchill Livingstone, 1994; 559.

70 Fainsinger, R., *et al.* Symptom control during the last week of life on a palliative care unit. *J Palliative Care* 1991; **7**(1): 5–11.

71 Cherny, N.I., and Portenoy, R.K. Sedation in the management of refractory symptoms: guidelines for evaluation and treatment. *J Palliative Care* 1994; **10**(2): 31–8.

72 Beauchamp, T., and Childress, J.F. *Principles of biomedical ethics* New York: Oxford University Press, 1994. Quoted in Thorns, A. A review of the doctrine of double effect. *Eur J Palliative Care* 1998; 5(4): 117–20.

73 Quoted in Twycross, R. Ethics. In: *Pain relief in advanced cancer.* Edinburgh: Churchill Livingstone, 1994; 561.

Chapter 10

Oxygen and airflow

Sara Booth

This chapter considers the use of oxygen in the relief of breathlessness. Recommendations are based on the available literature, but there is a paucity of trial data for many of the problems faced daily in clinical practice in palliative medicine.[1] Current thinking, based on the available scientific evidence and 'best practice', is outlined and discussed. Guidelines are suggested for the use of oxygen in the palliation of breathlessness, taking into account the advice for prescribers set out in the UK Royal College of Physicians' (RCP) report *Domiciliary oxygen therapy services*,[2] which is summarized later in the chapter (Box 10.2).

Definitions

Long-term oxygen therapy (LTOT): Provision of oxygen therapy at home on a continuous and long-term basis, ideally for at least 15 h daily, including time spent asleep.
Short-burst oxygen therapy (intermittent oxygen therapy): Intermittent use of oxygen for relief of breathlessness, before exercise or for recovery after exercise.
Ambulatory oxygen therapy: Provision of oxygen therapy during exercise and activities of daily living.
Ambulatory oxygen equipment: Any oxygen equipment that can be carried by most patients 'on their person' during activities of daily living (usually weighing less than 4.5 kg (10 lb)).

Role of oxygen therapy

In UK practice LTOT is used in patients with chronic obstructive pulmonary disease (COPD) and chronic hypoxaemia (PaO_2 < 7.3 kPa, FEV_1 < 1.5 L, FVC < 2.0 L and cor pulmonale with or without hypercapnia). LTOT will not be considered further in this volume as it is not given primarily to palliate breathlessness, but rather to increase survival.[3]

The role of oxygen in the management of the acutely ill medical patient will also not be reviewed. The use of bronchodilators and other inhaled drugs in breathlessness are discussed in Chapters 9 and 17. This chapter concentrates on the use of oxygen therapy not only at home but also anywhere else that a patient might be living or receiving treatment (general practice or community hospital, nursing home, general or teaching hospital, specialist palliative care unit).

The RCP report[2] is of interest to all clinicians who prescribe, administer, or advise on oxygen therapy in the home. It is necessary and informative reading for cardiologists, respiratory, palliative medicine, and general physicians as well as general practitioners. This chapter gives a general review of the place of oxygen specifically in the palliation of respiratory symptoms. Although the recommendations of the RCP report have been followed, there is also discussion of the difficulties of making therapeutic decisions in the absence of hard evidence.

It is widely recognized that more research evidence is needed to give clearer guidance on the role of oxygen therapy in the palliation of breathlessness, which is a complex and distressing experience of the body and the mind for patients with both malignant and non-malignant disease. The recommendations about oxygen therapy given in this chapter assume that it will be part of comprehensive supportive care, never the complete treatment. All patients require a broad range of treatment techniques, at present sometimes described by the unsatisfactory term 'non-pharmacological measures.' These are increasingly recognized to be central to the management of all patients suffering from breathlessness, whatever its aetiology and for patients at every stage in their illness;[4] for discussion of psychosocial therapies, see Chapter 13. Treatments need to be tailored to individuals and their concerns and priorities. Cancer is a multisystem disorder and breathlessness may be one of a cluster of symptoms, sometimes the most troublesome, but for others overshadowed by another such as pain or immobility. Those who are breathless from COPD will often have had a long history of contact with doctors and other medical professionals and a slow descent into breathlessness. They may be accustomed to using oxygen during acute exacerbations of their illness. Lung cancer often occurs in patients who have COPD and who may have been using oxygen therapy for some time. In other patients with cancer and breathlessness the symptom may develop very rapidly. The patient often undergoes a rapid transition from feeling fit and healthy to being disabled by breathlessness. Oxygen is unlikely to be newly prescribed for a patient within hours of death (where pharmacological control of breathlessness is most appropriate), but it would also be unusual to remove it at this stage from a patient. Oxygen therapy in palliative care is more complex than the treatment of hypoxaemia itself.

Evidence for the use of oxygen to help breathlessness

Much of the work carried out on this subject has concerned patients with COPD. In many of the studies reported, the effect of oxygen on breathlessness or the patient's quality of life has not been considered. Usually the outcome measures have included more directly measurable parameters such as work capacity, exercise endurance, pulmonary function tests, and arterial blood gases. Nonetheless, these studies may still give some useful indicators for caring for the breathless patient with cancer.

It should be remembered that breathlessness is a symptom and the population of people who describe themselves as breathless is very heterogeneous, ranging from those who are breathless at rest to those who are troubled more intermittently and inconstantly. The evidence for the use of oxygen in those breathless at rest and on exertion will thus be considered separately.

Breathlessness at rest

Patients who are breathless at rest are very ill. In one study of 38 cancer patients who were breathless at rest rather than on minimal exertion, the median survival was only 19 days.[5] Only six of these patients were initially hypoxaemic. A number of studies have demonstrated that oxygen supplementation can relieve breathlessness at rest in some patients, whether or not they are hypoxic.[5–9] In these studies oxygen was used for a relatively short time (if specified, 10–15 min maximum). The mix of patients with and without hypoxaemia differed, which may have affected the findings and therefore the conclusions of the authors. These papers are summarized in Table 10.1.

Table 10.1 The effects of oxygen on patients who are breathless at rest

Author (year)	Reference	Disease (initially hypoxaemic?)	Number of patients	Setting	Intervention	Results	Conclusion
Liss (1988)	6	COPD (most hypoxaemic)	8	General hospital	Pts received five flows through nasal prongs, zero flow, air then oxygen at 2 and 4 L/min then repeated after nasal mucosa anaesthetized	SOB rated with VAS, no change until mucosa anaesthetized, then SOB increased	Any reduction in SOB after nasal oxygen is a placebo effect or results from flow of gas over nasal receptors altering respiratory pattern
Swinburn (1991)	7	ILD = 10 COPD = 12 (all hypoxaemic)	22	General hospital inpatient	28% oxygen and air by mask, double-blind	Severity of SOB (VAS) reduced: oxygen > air	Oxygen helps SOB more than air in this group
Bruera (1992)	8	Cancer (all hypoxaemic)	14	Hospital palliative care unit	4 L/min oxygen and air by mask, double-blind	Severity of SOB (VAS) reduced by oxygen	Oxygen reduces SOB in this group
Booth (1996)	5	Cancer (6/38 initially hypoxaemic)	38	Hospice	4 L/min oxygen and air by nasal prongs	Severity of SOB (VAS/ Borg) reduced by oxygen and air	Oxygen and air can reduce SOB in this group

COPD, chronic obstructive pulmonary disease; ILD, interstitial lung disease; SOB, short(ness) of breath; VAS, visual analogue scale

The important findings from these studies were:

- Oxygen was not consistently beneficial for all subjects, even those initially hypoxaemic on air and those who had previously reported benefit from oxygen.
- The use of air from a cylinder also reduced breathlessness in some patients.

The proportions falling into the groups helped most by air, most by oxygen, and not helped by either have varied. In a study of cancer patients who were breathless at rest,[5] the authors concluded that the 'administration of either oxygen or air to patients with cancer who are dyspnoeic at rest significantly reduces the severity of the symptom' but also noted that 'individual patients differed markedly in their responses to either oxygen or air.'

In two studies[5,7] the authors noted that:

- The facial cooling produced by the stream of oxygen or air could explain the relief of the symptom in some patients. This provides further confirmation that a fan should be tried in all breathless patients[10] (see Chapter 6).
- Movement of the gases across nasal receptors could also account for the reduction in breathlessness experienced by others.[6]
- Relief of breathlessness was not necessarily related to reversal of hypoxaemia.

In the study by Booth et al.,[5] these points were exemplified in the data shown in Figure 10.1.

Leach and Bateman recommended that oxygen should only be given to those who are breathless at rest if they are hypoxaemic,[11] but other studies have found that some patients who are quite hypoxic are not breathless and other patients who are normoxic benefit from oxygen. All would agree that there must be clear evidence of benefit on some sort of simple, but formal testing, e.g. use of a visual analogue scale (VAS) before and after a test dose, or a more formal blinded 'n of 1' study,[8] before oxygen therapy is prescribed.

In the 1999 RCP report[2] it is recommended that:

> Domiciliary oxygen therapy can be prescribed for palliation of dyspnoea in pulmonary malignancy and other causes of disabling dyspnoea due to terminal disease.

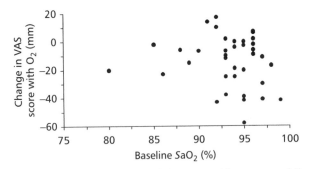

Fig. 10.1 The relationship between improvement of dyspnoea with oxygen and the degree of arterial hypoxaemia in cancer patients. For each of 38 patients the change in visual analogue scale ratings of dyspnoea during oxygen breathing (Change in VAS score with O_2) is plotted against the level of arterial oxygen saturation measured during air breathing (baseline SaO_2). There is no significant correlation ($r = 0.13$) between the effect of oxygen on dyspnoea and the arterial oxygen saturation during air breathing. Oxygen administration always corrected hypoxaemia where this was present. Data from Booth et al.[5]

This is placed alongside indications for LTOT, and later the recommendation is made that all patients who are to be prescribed LTOT should have arterial blood gas tensions measured on 'two occasions not less than 3 weeks apart to ensure clinical stability.'

However, in contrast to patients with COPD having LTOT, who have a prognosis of months to years, palliative care patients disabled by dyspnoea may have an expected survival of days to weeks. For these patients documentation of clear evidence of benefit after oxygen using a simple measuring tool as well as the patient's history would suffice for many clinicians. (For details of suitable assessment methods see Chapters 7 and 8.) Evidence of hypoxaemia by pulse oximetry can give weight to the argument for the use of oxygen although, as stated above, dyspnoea may be present and alleviated by oxygen therapy even when the patient is only mildly hypoxaemic. Because of the known effects of facial cooling, it is important also to explain the use of a fan to patients and to give them an opportunity to try this approach.

Breathlessness on exertion

There is still much to be clarified about the role of oxygen in reducing exercise-induced breathlessness (see Table 10.2 and Box 10.1). Standardized walking tests (see below) with air and oxygen are beginning to be used routinely to establish the efficacy of oxygen for individual patients. It is established that some patients do find relief from breathing oxygen and that in some their exercise capacity is increased.[3,12–25] Supplemental oxygen therapy does not seem to shorten recovery time after exercise in patients with COPD.[26] It is clear that the benefits are not universal, that oxygen therapy may have adverse effects and that we do not have clear-cut indicators to identify those patients who will gain most from oxygen therapy.

The contribution of hypoxaemia

It has been postulated that hypoxaemia is a stimulus for dyspnoea in its own right,[17] though how it promotes breathlessness is unclear. One theory is that because hypoxaemia acts as a respiratory stimulant the work of breathing is increased and this contributes to breathlessness. It is certain that not all hypoxaemic patients are breathless and of those that are, not all obtain benefit from oxygen therapy (see Chapter 6 for full discussion on this topic).

Present evidence suggests that although oxygen supplementation prevents desaturation during exercise, it does not always relieve breathlessness. Exercise tolerance in the short term is enhanced for some people by short-burst oxygen therapy, but this may not translate into an improved quality of life at home.[21,23] It may be that breathlessness during exercise in patients with COPD is related more to airflow limitation than falling arterial oxygen saturation. There is no evidence that giving normoxaemic patients short bursts of oxygen before exertion reduces breathlessness, though some hypoxic patients may be able to exercise for longer, at submaximal levels of effort. This may indeed represent a useful improvement in everyday life.

Careful patient selection is necessary to identify those people who will benefit from oxygen therapy. It is clear that a proportion of people get very useful palliation from both short-burst and ambulatory oxygen but a larger number do not. It is important that those who do benefit can obtain it, and that those for whom it is ineffective are not burdened with its disadvantages. The use of formal exercise testing in COPD patients is recommended by the RCP. This should preferably be a double-blind procedure using both air and oxygen. In cancer patients it may be better to give a trial of oxygen in the home for a predetermined period, assessing its usefulness with diaries or simple quality of life instruments. There is a need for more research on the use of oxygen in patients with advanced cancer and cardiac failure.

Table 10.2 The effect of oxygen on patients who are breathless on exertion

Author (year)	Reference	Disease (initial hypoxaemia?)	No. of patients	Hypoxaemic on exertion?	Intervention	Results	Conclusions
Cotes and Gildon (1956)	12	Pnc and COPD (variable)	29	Variable recorded	Treadmill, walking time measured with air or oxygen	Walking time increased with oxygen in 22 patients	Breathing of 30% oxygen significantly ↑ exercise ability in most such pts. Portable oxygen should be supplied if individual responds to oxygen on exercise
Bradley et al. (1978)	13	COPD (variable)	26	Yes	Treadmill, room air, comp air and 5 l/min oxygen by nasal prongs	Exercise endurance significantly increased with oxygen	Exercise endurance increased by oxygen, change in SaO$_2$ did not predict improvement.
Woodcock et al. (1981)	14	COPD (no)	10	No/slight	Treadmill + 6MWT, 8 of each over 3 days. Compressed oxygen and air, pt/asst carrying cylinder + some tests of preoxygenation	Use of oxygen improved both SOB and exercise endurance	Recommended portable oxygen if shown to be beneficial in individual patient after standardized exercise test
Waterhouse and Howard (1983)	15	COPD, SOB at rest (no)	20	Variable	5MWT;room air, oxygen 2 and 4 L/min and air 3 L/min through prongs.	Substantial decrease in SOB with oxygen. Placebo effect? 2 L/min = 4 L/min	Oxygen clearly beneficial for SOB (VAS) and exercise in some patients.

Study	N	Diagnosis	Desaturation	Method	Results	Comments
Swinburn et al. (1984)	15	COPD (no)	Yes	Two cycle ergometer tests: pts. Received, in random order, 60% oxygen or room air and then the other for 2nd test	Exercise duration increased on oxygen, SOB (VAS).	Hypoxaemia does not contribute to SOB by different mechanism to effect as ventilatory stimulant. Relieving hypoxaemia will not necessarily relieve SOB
Lane et al. (1987)	17	COPD (no)	Yes	Three successive treadmill tests. Room air for tests 1 and 3, oxygen for 2	Oxygen reduced SOB (VAS). Severity of hypoxia not related to scale of ↓ SOB	Some patients may benefit from low flow rate of oxygen during exercise
Davidson et al. (1988)	18	COPD (some)	yes	Cycle ergometer at constant workload. Compressed air and oxygen at 4 L/min +6MWT	Oxygen ↓ SOB (VAS) and ↑endurance. Degree of relief of SOB not related to degree ↑ SaO_2	Trial of oxygen with endurance walk indicated for every severely breathless patient
Dean et al. (1992)	18	COPD (mild)	Not all	Cycle ergometer endurance test, random order of compressed air or 40% oxygen	Increase in exercise duration and ↓ SOB score (VAS) with oxygen	Oxygen supplements may help pts to ↑ exercise and ↓ SOB even if not desaturating on exercise and only mild initial hypoxaemia
Leach et al. (1992)	3	20 COPD, 10 ILD. (variable)	marked in 3 pts, small or none in others.	Endurance and 6MWT breathing air and (2, 4, 6 L/min). oxygen Randomized and double-blind	Exercise ability and SOB (VAS) improved with oxygen but considerable interindividual variation. Best for short bursts of intense exercise than self-paced. Higher flow rates of oxygen more beneficial	Oxygen recommended for pts showing >50% ↑ in exercise tolerance in endurance or 6MWT. Pts who desaturate on exercise most likely to benefit but also others who get relief SOB

Table 10.2 (continued) The effect of oxygen on patients who are breathless on exertion

Author (year)	Reference	Disease (initial hypoxaemia?)	No. of patients	Hypoxaemic on exertion?	Intervention	Results	Conclusions
Mak et al. (1993)	20	42 COPD, 28 asthma	70	Variable	6MWT to assess submaximal exercise capacity	Changes in SaO_2 did not correlate with exercise endurance nor with perceived SOB: VAS/Borg	Pts who rate themselves very SOB (MRC) do shortest 6MWT but do not always desaturate the most
McDonald et al. (1995)c	21	COPD (variable)	26	Yes	Intranasal air and oxygen at 4 L/min during 6MW and step exercise. Used oxygen/air at home, randomized, from cylinder, for two periods of 6 weeks. Daily diary cards used to record respiratory symptoms	General findings that small acute benefits in exercise ability with oxygen but negligible long-term benefit. Similar oxygen and air usage at home. Small improvements in lab exercise do not correlate with ↑QOL	Recommend oxygen given only to pts with COPD and mild hypoxaemia if exercise endurance ↑ exercise by >50% with oxygen
Marques-Magallanes et al. (1998)	26	COPD (yes)	18	Yes	Treadmill exercise test, followed by compressed oxygen or air, or room air random assignment. Time to recovery recorded	No effect of oxygen on post-exercise recovery time	Oxygen not recommended for helping shorten recovery from SOB after exercise
Revill et al. (2000)	22	COPD (variable)	10	Yes	Performed ESWT under five test conditions: baseline walk, inspiratory pressure support (IPS, HIPP) sham IPS, ambulatory oxygen at 2 L/min and sham oxygen	Significant improvements in duration and distance walked with ambulatory oxygen	Confirmed that oxygen does help increase exercise endurance, present portable ventilators unhelpful

	Author (year)	Disease (oxygen dependent)	n		Method	Results	Conclusions
23	Killen, Corris (2000)	COPD (No)	18	Yes	Pulse, SaO$_2$, time of ascent, dyspnoea recorded before during and after climbing stairs on air or oxygen, 2 L/min via facemask, gases at top and bottom of stairs. (i.e. 'air/air', 'air/oxygen' 'oxygen/air') Order ascents randomly assigned	Peak dyspnoea occurred at top of stairs in n = 10, up to 3 min after completion of ascent in 8. Nadir of SaO$_2$ mostly reached within 1 min of stopping. Pts receiving oxygen shown to be significantly less dyspnoeic when groups combined and significantly less arterial oxygen desaturation.	Oxygen treatment reduces dyspnoea associated with short bursts of exertion if this is associated with hypoxia but is unimportant whether oxygen given before or after exertion
24	Knebel et al. (2000)	Alpha-1 antitrypsin deficiency and COPD (no)	31		Double-blind cross-over study. 3 × 6 MWT (practice) and then two walks with ambulatory compressed air and oxygen in random order via nasal cannulae	No reduction in dyspnoea with oxygen compared to air	No reduction of dyspnoea with oxygen
25	Jolly et al. 2001	COPD (variable)	20	Variable	Performed 3 × 6MWT, one with oxygen, one with compressed air and one basal test without either	Most of the COPD pts desaturated during basal WT. Oxygen administration avoided this and could increase walking distance and reduce dyspnoea but this could not be predicted from baseline WT desaturation results	Efficacy of oxygen needs to be individually assessed.

Table 10.2 (continued) The effect of oxygen on patients who are breathless on exertion

Author (year)	Reference	Disease (initial hypox-aemia?)	No. of patients	Hypoxaemic on exertion?	Intervention	Results	Conclusions
O'Donnell, et al. (2001)	41	COPD (variable)	11	Yes	Compared effects of room air and 60% oxygen on dyspnoea (and other parameters) during exercise on a bicycle ergometer	Improvement in dyspnoea did not correlate with baseline pulmonary function, gas exchange, PaO_2, $PaCO_2$, or ventilatory mechanics. The greater the severity of dyspnoea on RA, the greater the relief with oxygen	Oxygen increases ability to exercise in this group of patients with severe stable COPD. Modest changes in submaximal ventilation and dynamic ventilatory mechanics resulted in large changes in exercise capacity and reduction in dyspnoea

5 or 6MWT, 5 or 6 minute walking test; COPD, chronic obstructive pulmonary disease; ESWT, endurance shuttle walking test; ILD, interstitial lung disease; Pnc, pneumoconiosis; QOL, quality of life; RA, room air; SOB, short(ness) of breath

Box 10.1 Conducting an exercise test with oxygen

1 Choose a validated exercise test such as the shuttle walking test.[27,28]

2 The patient should have at least one formal practice test as there is a learning effect.

3 Just before starting the exercise test measure the patient's SaO_2 whilst breathing room air and ask the patient to assess the current level of breathlessness using a VAS.

4 Carry out the test with blinded oxygen or air (i.e. the patient should not know which they are receiving) ideally using a portable cylinder. Measure saturation and breathlessness on a VAS as soon as possible after the patient stops. Some oximeters measure saturation and pulse rate continuously.

5 Repeat the test after a rest period (2 h) or on another day, using the alternate gas from the first test. The oxygen and air administration should be carried out as a double-blind procedure[11] and the patient should not be told their saturation results until both have been completed.

6 For whom should oxygen be prescribed? There is no firm guidance on this for cancer patients as exercise testing before oxygen is prescribed is not routinely carried out at present. Wedzicha[29] recommends oxygen therapy for patients with COPD who in the following circumstances:

   ◆ Desaturated by 4% or more below 90% on formal exercise testing.

   ◆ Able to walk 10% further when they are receiving oxygen supplementation[21] (would only recommend it for those whose exercise tolerance increases by 50%).

   ◆ Experience a significant subjective improvement in their breathlessness when using oxygen.

Assessment of the patient

Before prescribing oxygen ensure that:

◆ The patient has been given a fan, advised how to use it and tried it.

◆ All other suitable palliative techniques are being applied to relieve breathlessness (including for some patients: breathing exercises, relaxation training, education, and family support).

◆ All reversible causes of breathlessness have been treated appropriately, taking into account the patient's general condition and overall prognosis.

The importance of a detailed assessment

◆ The assessment should cover all the information needed to make a firm diagnosis of the causes of the patient's breathlessness. In a patient with advanced cancer breathlessness is usually multifactorial – some of the causes will be reversible and some not. Effective palliation is more likely to follow precise diagnosis.

◆ The pattern of breathlessness – is the patient breathless at rest? on exertion? when anxious? The answers to these questions may help to decide the order in which different therapies for breathlessness are tried.

- The patient who is **breathless at rest** is probably very ill. After ensuring that all disease-modifying therapy has been tried, pharmacological palliation of breathlessness is most likely to be helpful. The management may also include oxygen depending on oximetry and/or a carefully documented clinical trial. It should always include the use of a fan.

- The patient who is **breathless on exertion** may need oxygen but usually only after documented evidence of 4% desaturation below baseline values during exercise on air or a significant improvement of exercise tolerance, using a standardized test, compared with breathing air from a cylinder (see Box 10.1).

- The patient who is most breathless when anxious may respond best to an exploration of their fears, followed by explanation and being shown how to use controlled breathing exercises and relaxation techniques whenever the anxiety/fear attack begins.

- Has the patient had oxygen before? In what circumstances did they use it? Was it useful? If patients have had previous oxygen therapy, this may inform the clinician about the severity of the patient's previous illnesses, how effective they found oxygen therapy, and their familiarity with oxygen therapy equipment.

- What is the patient's prognosis? If it is estimated to be very short, i.e. hours or days, it may be inappropriate to institute oxygen.

Guidelines for the use of oxygen to palliate breathlessness

The patient who is breathless on exertion

- Take an accurate history of precipitating events and find out if modifying these could help (e.g. by assessment and advice from an occupational therapist or physiotherapist).

- Make sure all other non-pharmacological strategies are being used to the fullest extent.

- Consider a formal test of oxygen therapy with an exercise test (see Box 10.1)

The patient who is breathless at rest

- Assess whether the patient is hypoxaemic (resting saturation breathing air below 90% with a pulse oximeter).

- Ensure that the patient has tried all appropriate pharmacological and non-pharmacological treatments.

- If the patient is already using oxygen therapy, find out how useful it is; if it is not helping, discuss withdrawing it gradually.

- Give a controlled trial of oxygen therapy with an easily administered measurement tool (e.g. VAS) and prescribe oxygen as continuing therapy only if there is clear evidence of benefit, confirmed both by the use of the VAS and the patient's assessment (VAS scores are consistent for each individual and 2 mm change may be significant for one person, whereas 8 mm change may be significant for another. VAS scores should not be used to compare between individuals.)

- An 'n of 1' trial[8] can also be used to assess the benefit of oxygen formally – see Box 10.1 and details below.

- If the test dose oxygen does not help, do not prescribe it for continued use. It may be helpful to measure both the VAS and saturation simultaneously to show whether the breathlessness is related to hypoxaemia.

- If the test dose oxygen does help, find out if the patient prefers a mask or nasal prongs and ensure these are available.

- Explain that the oxygen is only part of therapy and that at some stage may no longer be helpful.

In the dying patient

- Use primarily pharmacological methods to control breathlessness and avoid oxygen if it has not been started.

- If oxygen is being used, try to withdraw it gradually with the patient's agreement as soon as other therapies begin to help.

- If the patient is definitely finding oxygen helpful or comforting, do not persist in removing it.

For all patients

- Remember to reassess treatments regularly, as patients with cancer and breathlessness often deteriorate rapidly, and treatment strategies will need to be modified as their condition changes.

- Formal exercise tests are very rarely done in cancer patients – possibly from concern that to make the patient breathless is unkind. In fact, exercise testing may actually be helpful by increasing a patient's confidence as well as having other benefits.[28]

- In a test, the patient becomes breathless and recovers from this in a controlled, safe environment. A patient will either feel better and walk further with oxygen or not, and is therefore convinced about using it or abandoning it for the time being. They also realize just how far they can walk and 'push themselves.'

- Compared to the situation with cancer, exercise testing with oxygen or compressed air is becoming standard practice for COPD or interstitial lung disease patients.[2,3,29] In the latter conditions it is likely that oxygen will be needed for a much greater period of time and its prescription therefore will have a proportionately greater impact on patients and their family life.

Box 10.2 summarizes the RCP recommendations on the use of oxygen in palliative care.

The visual analogue scale

The VAS is described in detail in Chapter 8. For patients who are very unwell, or those completing it in the difficult period after an exercise test, it is recommended that the vertical VAS is used. It has been demonstrated that it is easier to fill in than the horizontally aligned scale for this group of patients.[30]

The 'n of 1' trial

This is a therapeutic trial involving one patient only. A properly conducted 'n of 1' trial is randomized and double-blind and therefore reduces bias in the selection of treatment for an individual patient. Sometimes the results of several 'n of 1' trials may be combined, enabling a conclusion to be reached which may have wider application. An 'n of 1' trial involves crossover of treatments (variable numbers of crossover have been recommended, from one to eight). It should also have agreed outcome measures which the patient finds valid, and should be properly blinded and randomized.

An 'n of 1' trial is a formal trial for which full ethical approval may be required, and certainly discussion with the local ethical committee chairman.[31] Such trials are potentially useful in palliative care because of the difficulty in carrying out randomized controlled trials (RCTs) which has led to a recognized deficit of good evidence in this area of medicine. However, 'n of 1' trials

Box 10.2 Summary of the RCP recommendations on using different patterns of domiciliary oxygen therapy for palliative care

For all these indications it is noted that 'optimum medical management' is required prior to the assessment for oxygen therapy.

Long-term oxygen therapy (LTOT)

- LTOT can be prescribed in patients with interstitial lung disease when the PaO_2 is less than 8 kPa.
- LTOT should be considered in patients with neuromuscular or skeletal disorders, either in combination with ventilatory support or alone. Assessment for LTOT in this situation requires referral to a physician with a specialist interest in these disorders.
- LTOT can be prescribed in patients with cystic fibrosis either when the PaO_2 is less than 7.3 kPa or when it is between 7.3 and 8 kPa in the presence of nocturnal hypoxaemia, secondary polycythaemia, pulmonary hypertension, or peripheral oedema.
- In view of deteriorating pulmonary hypertension once hypoxia develops, LTOT can be prescribed in patients with pulmonary hypertension, without parenchymal lung involvement, when the PaO_2 is less than 8 kPa.
- Domiciliary oxygen therapy can be prescribed for palliation of dyspnoea in pulmonary malignancy and other causes of disabling dyspnoea due to terminal disease.
- Patients with heart failure can be prescribed LTOT if they have daytime hypoxaemia with a PaO_2 on air of less than 7.3 kPa or nocturnal hypoxaemia (with SaO_2 below 90% for at least 30% of the night).

Indications for ambulatory oxygen therapy

- Ambulatory oxygen therapy can be prescribed in patients with interstitial lung disease who show exercise desaturation.
- Ambulatory oxygen therapy can be prescribed in patients with cystic fibrosis who have chronic hypoxaemia requiring LTOT and when ambulation is required. Ambulatory oxygen therapy may also be prescribed to this group if they show evidence of exercise desaturation without chronic hypoxaemia. ($PaO_2 < 7.3$ kPa).
- Ambulatory oxygen therapy should be considered in patients with chest wall and neuromuscular disorders who have exercise desaturation and are limited by dyspnoea.
- Ambulatory oxygen therapy is not recommended in heart failure.
- Patients who are continuing to smoke cigarettes should not be prescribed ambulatory oxygen as the benefits are debatable in this situation and risk from burns is considerable.

Box 10.2 Summary of the RCP recommendations *(continued)*

Indications for ambulatory oxygen therapy

- Despite extensive prescription of short-burst therapy, there is no adequate evidence available for firm recommendations; further research is required.
- Short-burst oxygen should be considered for episodic breathlessness not relieved by other treatments in patients with severe COPD, interstitial lung disease, heart failure, and those in palliative care.
- Short-burst oxygen should be only be prescribed if an improvement in breathlessness and/or exercise tolerance can be documented.

Extracts from RCP report.[2]

---

cannot supplant RCTs. To be properly conducted an 'n of 1' trial needs the input of statistician and a pharmacist.

It is especially important in palliative care that the treatment under investigation has a rapid onset and offset of action, because, if a long washout period is needed between treatments, the result of the trial may be confounded by a clinical change in the patient's condition.

The key advantage of 'n of 1' trials is that they remove the bias that may confound the results of a simple therapeutic trial. They are of most use in long-term chronic illness where a particular treatment will be needed for some time and where there is insufficient evidence from RCTs to guide treatment, or where there may be doubt that the treatment is right for that person. An example of their use in palliative care is quoted by Bruera.[8] Trials of oxygen or air in the palliation of breathlessness are particularly suited to this sort of investigation for an individual because there is a rapid onset and offset of treatment effect, the most important result is subjective, and embarking on oxygen treatment has significant effects on the patient's way of life. (See Box 10.1 for details of oxygen test.)

Adverse effects of oxygen

Oxygen is often prescribed as 'an expensive placebo',[32] but it is not without problems for the patient. These are summarized in Box 10.3.

Box 10.3 Adverse effects of oxygen

- Restriction of day-to-day activities to stay in continuous contact with oxygen.
- Impaired communication between family, caregivers, and patient.
- Anxiety and fear provoked in some patients when oxygen is unavailable, even momentarily.
- Fire hazard for patients who smoke; it should not be prescribed for those who cannot or prefer not to stop smoking.
- It may be very difficult to withdraw oxygen once it has been started, which may be distressing in the patent's last hours.

Restriction of activities

Oxygen apparatus is cumbersome, and for an already disabled patient may act as a disincentive to going out and living as normally as possible. In recent years small, lightweight cylinders have been more readily available and this has lessened the impact of the weight of the cylinder on the patient's mobility.

Impaired communication between patient and family

If patients become psychologically dependent on oxygen they may attend too much on the mechanics of having their oxygen delivered. Some will not remove their mask for even a minute, and conversation with family and friends is impeded. They may also become extremely frightened when there is any interruption in the oxygen supply and refuse to go outside without a continuous supply from a cylinder. This so-called 'oxygen addiction' has been recognized for many years,[12] and it is not necessarily related to the severity of the breathlessness. It can lead to the maintenance of oxygen therapy taking undue precedence and when it is given as a palliative treatment to improve the quality of a short life this is a great disadvantage. The drying of the upper airways (see below) can also make conversation difficult. The impact of LTOT has been described very well by patients in Williams's study of chronic respiratory illness.[33]

Fire hazard

Oxygen promotes combustion. Patients who smoke while receiving oxygen therapy are in great danger of facial burns and some have even been killed. It is pointless and unkind to try to stop a patient who has enjoyed smoking from doing so in order to institute oxygen therapy in the last stages of illness, when the damage caused by tobacco is irretrievable and the benefits of oxygen therapy may be arguable.

Hypercapnic respiratory failure

The dangers of oxygen therapy in those patients with type II (hypercapnic) respiratory failure are well-known. However, an overemphasis on this hazard has led to other patients, who are not at risk of hypercapnia, being given too low an inspired concentration of oxygen when acutely ill. Morning headaches are an important symptom of hypercapnia and an enquiry about this symptom is important to screen for this condition, especially in neurological illnesses such as motor neurone disease, for example. It is possible to identify those at risk by measuring the arterial blood gases. Non-invasive measurement of arterial carbon dioxide tension is now also possible by monitoring end tidal PCO_2 or transcutaneous PCO_2.

Withdrawing oxygen

Once oxygen has been given to a patient it is often difficult to stop its use, even when it is no longer relieving breathlessness or being used appropriately. It is not uncommon to see patients in hospitals or hospices with oxygen masks and nasal prongs anywhere but in the right place,[34] and yet they are still reluctant to discontinue the treatment.

Cost of oxygen

Oxygen is not a cheap remedy (see Table 10.3). Other and possibly more effective methods of palliating breathlessness by pharmacological and non-pharmacological means also carry costs,

Table 10.3 Total cost of usage of oxygen concentrators in the UK

Year	Total annual cost (£)
December 1995–November 1996	10 860 029
December 1999–November 2000	13 962 631

Source: UK Prescription Pricing Authority.

which are difficult to estimate. However, they may overall be more cost-effective in improving the quality of care for patients than oxygen incorrectly employed.

Humidification

It is unnecessary to humidify oxygen in LTOT as this is done adequately by the patient's own upper respiratory tract. Humidifiers tend to be noisy, bulky, and often ineffective. For a few patients it may be necessary for a specific problem such as viscid sputum.[2]

Oxygen production and storage devices

This has been well reviewed by Leach and Bateman[32] and in the RCP report,[2] and only those systems used in the palliation of breathlessness are considered here. The various devices used to produce, store, and deliver oxygen to the patient are summarized in Box 10.4.

In most general hospitals bed-bound patients will receive their supply from large tanks of liquid oxygen held centrally in the hospital and then piped to the bedside. Many hospice units and nursing homes will use the delivery systems described below, which are also suitable for home use.

Box 10.4 Oxygen storage and delivery systems

Production and storage devices

- Oxygen concentration
- Cylinders for static use
- Ambulatory oxygen cylinders
- Liquid oxygen

Oxygen-conserving techniques

- Reservoir cannulae
- Demand pulsing delivery devices
- Transtracheal oxygen

Inhalation devices

- Low-flow/high-concentration oxygen masks
- Low-flow/low-concentration oxygen masks
- Nasal cannulae
- High-flow systems

Oxygen concentrators

These are small machines that can concentrate oxygen from the atmosphere, powered by an electric mains supply: they do not provide a portable supply of oxygen. In LTOT a concentrator is preferred to cylinders because oxygen can be continuously supplied (unlike cylinders, which have to be changed), and because in the long run they are more economical.[35]

Atmospheric air is filtered and passed under pressure through a bed of zeolite which removes the nitrogen and therefore concentrates oxygen from the atmosphere. To maintain a continuous supply of oxygen a concentrator must have two 'beds' of zeolite: while one is active and adsorbing nitrogen the other will be recharging itself by discharging nitrogen back into the air.

♦ The usual/maximum flow rate and FiO_2 delivered by concentrators is 2–4 L/min.

The oxygen supply from a concentrator is suitable for the palliative care of cancer patients because high flow rates are not required and perfect accuracy of inspired oxygen (FiO_2) is not critical.

Oxygen cylinders for static use

Oxygen cylinders come in various sizes (300–6800 L). The smaller sizes can be fixed to a wheelchair, for example, to allow some mobility for patients. To provide long-term oxygen from a cylinder is both inconvenient and expensive. Oxygen cylinders contain compressed oxygen, and the gas is delivered via a regulator valve. Different valves are available to allow either fixed or variable rate delivery. In the UK only a dual flow-rate regulator is available (2–4 L/min) from size F or AF cylinders (both 1360 L capacity).

These cylinders can be wheeled round on a trolley to get them from place to place within the home, but they are too big to provide portable oxygen.

Ambulatory oxygen cylinders

Portable oxygen cylinders and other devices for the provision of ambulatory oxygen, which can be carried by patients, will soon be prescribed on the NHS in the UK. Until recently the patient or hospital unit must incur a direct charge. They are already widely used in the USA and continental Europe. There are small oxygen cylinders weighing 2.3 kg and about the size of a thermos flask (capacity 230 L) which are easy to carry around but the oxygen will last only about 2 h at 2 L/min. They are refillable from an A or AF oxygen cylinders in the patient's home by means of a special adapter. A full-sized AF cylinder is necessary to achieve complete filling and if this is not done the delivery time of oxygen to the patient will be reduced. As portable oxygen cylinders will be used during exercise to keep oxygen saturation above 90%, many COPD patients, and possibly those with advanced cancer, will need a flow rate greater than 4 L/min to maintain oxygen saturation above 90%. Consequently, these lightweight cylinders will last for only a very short time. All other portable oxygen is transported by patients using a small lightweight trolley.

Liquid oxygen

This is widely available in continental Europe and the USA for ambulatory therapy, but it is not widely used in the UK at the moment. It is much more expensive than compressed oxygen but weighs half as much. Liquid oxygen cylinders can provide up to 8 h of oxygen at 2 L/min. The small cylinders are replenished from a compact tank in the patient's home. The oxygen in the store evaporates continuously, so it needs monitoring and refilling frequently.

Oxygen-conserving techniques

Techniques have been developed in order to reduce oxygen usage and therefore the cost of the treatment. There are three main ways in which oxygen usage can be reduced – reservoir cannulae, demand pulsing delivery devices, and using the transtracheal route. Tiep has written a useful review on this subject.[36]

Reservoir cannulae

These conserve oxygen by storing it in a reservoir as it is exhaled so that it can be used in the next breath. There are two main models: the Oxymizer and the Pendant. In the Oxymizer the reservoir is situated under the nose, in the Pendant it consists of a small chamber on the anterior chest wall together with the tubing leading to it. Both work on the principle that as the patient exhales a membrane in the reservoir will move forward so that a chamber is formed to receive the exhaled gas. As the patient inhales again they will receive the continuous flowing oxygen and the oxygen-rich gas in the reservoir. These devices are very efficient (conferring a two- to fourfold benefit) but they are much larger than ordinary cannulae and therefore more cumbersome.

Demand pulsing delivery devices

These devices allow oxygen to be delivered to the patient during inhalation only. They can significantly reduce oxygen usage but some of them make a noise that can be irritating to patients, especially at night. They are structurally quite complex consisting of a transducer, logic circuitry, and a solenoid valve. The pulsing device is interposed in the circuit between nasal cannulae and the oxygen source. As the patient inhales, this is detected by the sensing device through the nasal cannulae. The valve opens and shuts rapidly and a burst of oxygen flows to the patient. The pulse is short so that the oxygen is targeted to the inspiratory phase of the respiratory cycle, avoiding both delivery during exhalation and into the inspiratory deadspace.

Various models are available depending on the setting for giving oxygen, e.g. hospital piped supply or free-standing cylinders.[36] They are not in general use and their performance with an individual patient must be monitored to ensure accuracy and adequacy for that person.

Transtracheal oxygen

This is the delivery of oxygen directly into the trachea by means of a surgically introduced fine-bore catheter. The catheter is inserted, under local anaesthesia, percutaneously between the second and third tracheal cartilages. This technique is currently little used in cancer patients but more commonly in patients with COPD. Its use was first described by Heimlich and Carr in 1982.[37] Its advantages and disadvantages are set out in Box 10.5.

Aspects of transtracheal oxygen therapy

Transtracheal oxygen may be indicated for more patients than currently receive it, and its use has been more widely studied in the USA. There are no trials to indicate its place in the palliative care of patients with advanced cancer. It is probably most useful in those patients who need LTOT for many hours per day, and who wish to go outdoors, as it seems to be well tolerated and is less obtrusive than nasal prongs.[38,39] Its prescription and provision should be from specialized centres which have sufficient numbers of patients to become familiar and practised with the techniques, not only of insertion but also maintenance of the catheter.

Box 10.5 Transtrachael oxygen therapy

Advantages

- Upper airways deadspace is bypassed, so less oxygen is used
- Upper airways filled with oxygen during expiration, which therefore act as a reservoir
- Oxygen delivery device can be hidden easily by clothing, e.g. shirt or scarf
- More comfortable – fewer problems with soreness, e.g. to ears and nasal passages
- More efficient delivery of oxygen leading to higher FiO_2
- Fewer days in hospital needed by patients using oxygen by this route

Disadvantages

- Meticulous care of catheter needed e.g. irrigation with saline about three times daily or removal of catheter for cleaning
- Expense related to insertion of catheter and other procedures associated with its maintenance
- Possible haemoptysis, usually minor, self-limiting, and occurring early after insertion
- Formation of subcutaneous emphysema or pneumomediastinum
- Cellulitis – catheter may have to be removed
- Catheter can blocked by secretions
- Catheter can be dislodged accidentally
- Effective patient education and motivation vital for success of technique

Oxygen inhalation devices

Oxygen can be delivered to patients by means of high- or low-flow systems. The important difference between the two delivery methods is that only high-flow systems can reliably deliver a predetermined oxygen fraction in the inspired gas, no matter what the patient's respiratory pattern. The inspired oxygen fraction is less reliably estimated when a low-flow system is used.

Low-flow systems

These include nasal cannulae, Mary Caterall (MC) masks, and tracheostomy collars. In a low-flow system the patient receives both oxygen and air, the proportions of each depending on the patient's rate of ventilation and the inspiratory flow rate. It is possible to deliver an FiO_2 of between 24% and 90%. For a given flow rate of oxygen the greater the patient's ventilation the lower the FiO_2, as the patient will inspire more room air.

Low-flow/high-concentration oxygen masks

An example of this device is the MC mask. The inspired oxygen concentration can be raised to about 60% by using a flow rate of oxygen of 6 L/minute and above. Rebreathing of carbon dioxide can take place because the mask has a reservoir of about 100 mL and expired air may not be displaced from the gas reservoir. If high flow rates are used to overcome this, the FiO_2 will then be 0.3 or more.

Low-flow/low-concentration of oxygen masks

These are generally inaccurate and are unsuitable if controlled oxygen therapy is needed as the FiO_2 delivered to the patient is very dependent on the tidal volume and breathing pattern.

Nasal cannulae

These are commonly preferred by patients in cancer units and other palliative care settings. These are very convenient for patients and acceptable to those who find a mask frightening and claustrophobic. Patients can eat and drink and talk readily with the cannulae in place. Occasionally irritation of the nostrils and the backs of the ears develops with prolonged use. This can be prevented and relieved by simple application of Vaseline.

There is no possibility of rebreathing, and the FiO_2 delivered can vary between 0.25–0.50 with flow rates of oxygen between 1 and 6 L/min. Nasal cannulae are recommended for palliative care because the inspired oxygen concentration is rarely critical. On the other hand, those with severe COPD will usually require a more accurate delivery of controlled oxygen therapy or frequent monitoring of their arterial oxygen and/or carbon dioxide by oximetry, blood gas measurement, or transcutaneous or end-tidal carbon dioxide.

High-flow systems

In these systems higher flow rates of oxygen, in combination with reservoir systems, are sufficient to meet the patient's inspiratory demand so the FiO_2 becomes independent of the patient's respiratory pattern. The total gas flow (i.e. oxygen and room air combined) has to be 40 L/min or more to meet the peak inspiratory flow rate. As oxygen flows through a narrow hole it causes a velocity stream that entrains a corresponding proportion of room air through side portholes at the base of the mask (the Bernoulli effect). The amount of air entrained depends on the velocity of the stream of oxygen and the size of the side ports. Such masks (e.g. the Venturi mask) can accurately deliver 24–50% inspired oxygen when the appropriate valve is fitted. Rebreathing of inspired air is minimized and there is a low risk of hypercapnia. High-flow systems tend to be bulky, uncontrollable, and expensive.

Occasionally in palliative care it is essential to deliver a known inspired oxygen fraction, for example in the critically ill patient (where the respiratory pattern is often very abnormal) or for those with a hypoxic respiratory drive. In this situation, a low-flow system can be used but blood gas values of oxygen and carbon dioxide must be monitored by direct or indirect methods; alternatively, an accurate high flow system can be employed to deliver oxygen to the patient.

On balance, a low-flow system e.g. nasal cannulae is appropriate for most palliative care patients.

Safety in the home

The fire hazards associated with oxygen use have been mentioned above. It must also be remembered that when oxygen is used in the home, other members of the family and visitors will also be restricted. There are other safety measures which need to be observed when oxygen therapy is given at home (e.g. positioning and maintenance of the necessary equipment). A full list is given in the RCP report.[2]

Using a fan

Schwartzstein *et al.* demonstrated that in normal volunteers, cooling the central part of the face (innervated by the second and third sensory branches of the fifth cranial nerve) could reduce breathlessness.[10] This finding has been reproduced by cooling the face with water. Some breathless patients obtain benefit by using a combination of a handheld fan and larger fixed one beside a bed or chair. Other patients prefer the draught from an open window; conversely, many report that they feel more breathless when in a confined space without air flowing, e.g. behind hospital bed curtains or in a small room. It is therefore useful and relatively cheap to advise patients to increase facial airflow and thus defer or remove the need for oxygen therapy.

Helium and oxygen

Helium is much less dense than oxygen. Sometimes helium/oxygen ('heliox') mixtures are used to palliate large airways obstruction, for example, from primary tracheal tumours or if there is a critical external tracheal narrowing. The lower density of the helium means that there is less turbulence and hence smoother gas flow through narrow orifices. This principle follows from the Reynolds number ($Re = (2 \times$ radius of tube $\times$ gas density $\times$ gas velocity)/ viscosity of gas). When $Re > 2000$, flow is more likely to be turbulent. When there is turbulence, gas flow will vary with the square root of driving pressure and it will be more difficult to propel the gas. Flow laws were worked out for cylindrical tubes rather than the branching irregularities of the respiratory system and flow is more likely to be turbulent *in vivo*, but the use of helium may make a marginal difference to flow, which could have an important effect in a critically narrowed airway. Heliox mixtures are presently regarded as a short-term measure while other definitive treatment, such as surgery or stenting, is being instituted.

More recently it has been used in a prospective RCT in acute severe asthma.[40] Patients received either 30% oxygen or 70%/30% heliox and the authors found that in the group receiving heliox there was more rapid initial improvement (within 20 min) in airflow obstruction and the sensation of dyspnoea. This rate of improvement was, however, not sustained. Patients receiving oxygen alone had a slower resolution of their airflow obstruction and dyspnoea. The authors suggest that heliox may be useful in acute severe asthma until the effects of other treatment (e.g. corticosteroids) start to work.

A small randomized study in lung cancer patients has been reported as showing improved oxygenation and exercise ability with a helium/oxygen mixture compared to 28% oxygen or air.[42]

Key points

- Where oxygen therapy is indicated, it should be seen as one part of supportive care, never the complete treatment.
- Oxygen therapy in palliative care is more complex than the simple reversal of hypoxaemia.
- The automatic prescription of oxygen to a breathless patient is to be avoided in palliative care.
- Nasal cannulae are the most useful device for delivering oxygen to palliative care patients as they do not interfere with speech and the inspired FiO_2 is rarely critical.
- The treatment strategy, including the use of oxygen, may change quite rapidly in advanced cancer and needs frequent reassessment and adjustment as necessary.

References

1 Higginson, I.J. Evidence based palliative care. *BMJ* 1999; **319**: 462–3.

2 Report of the Royal College of Physicians. *Domiciliary oxygen therapy services.* London: Royal College of Physicians, 1999.

3 Leach, R.M., Davidson, A.C., Chinn, S., *et al.* Portable liquid oxygen and exercise ability in severe respiratory disability. *Thorax* 1992; 47: 781–9. [published erratum appears in *Thorax* 1993; **48**(2): 192.

4 Bredin, M., Corner, J., Krishnasamy, M., *et al.* Multicentre randomised controlled trial of nursing intervention for breathlessness in patients with lung cancer. *BMJ* 1999; **318**: 901–4.

5 Booth, S., Kelly, M.J., Cox, N.P., Adams, L., and Guz, A. Does oxygen help dyspnea in patients with cancer? *Am J Respir Crit Care Med* 1996; **153**: 1515–18.

6 Liss, H.W., and Grant, B.J.B. The effect of nasal flow on breathlessness in patients with chronic obstructive pulmonary disease. *Am Rev Respir Dis* 1988; **137**: 1285–8.

7 Swinburn, C.R., Mould, H., Stone, T.M., Corris, P.A., and Gibson, G.J. Symptomatic Benefit of supplemental oxygen in hypoxaemic patients with chronic lung disease. *Am Rev Respir Dis* 1991; **143**: 913–15.

8 Bruera, E., Schoeller, T., and MacEachern, T. Symptomatic benefit of supplemental oxygen in hypoxaemic patients with terminal cancer: the use of the N of 1 randomized controlled trial. *J Pain Symptom Manage* 1992; **7**: 365–8.

9 Bruera, E., de Stoutz, N., Velasco-Leiva, A., Schoeller, T., and Hanson, J. Effects of oxygen on dyspnoea in hypoxaemic terminal-cancer patients. *Lancet* 1993; **342**, 13–14.

10 Schwartzstein, R., Lahive, K., Pope, A., Weinberger, S.E., and Woodrow Weiss, J. Cold facial stimulation reduces breathlessness induced in normal subjects. *Am Rev Respir Dis* 1987; **136**: 58–61.

11 Leach, R.M., and Bateman, N.T. Domiciliary oxygen therapy. *Br J Hosp Med* 1994; **51**: 47–54.

12 Cotes, J.E., and Gilson, J.C. Effect of oxygen on exercise ability in chronic respiratory insufficiency: use of portable apparatus. *Lancet* 1956; **ii**: 872–6.

13 Bradley, B.L., Garner, A.E., Billiu, D., and Mestas, J.M. Oxygen-assisted exercise in chronic obstructive lung disease. *Am Rev Respir Dis* 1978; **118**: 239–42.

14 Woodcock, A.A., Gross, E.R., and Geddes, D.M. Oxygen relieves breathlessness in 'pink puffers'. *Lancet* 1981; **i**: 681–5.

15 Waterhouse, J.C., and Howard, P. Breathlessness and portable oxygen in chronic obstructive airways disease. *Thorax* 1983; **38**: 302–6.

16 Swinburn, C.R., Wakefield, J.M., and Jones, P.W. Relationship between ventilation and breathlessness during exercise in chronic obstructive airways disease is not altered by prevention of hypoxaemia. *Clin Sci* 1984; **67**: 515–19.

17 Lane, R., Cockcroft, A., Adams, L., and Guz, A. Arterial oxygen saturation and breathlessness in patients with chronic obstructive airways disease. *Clin Sci* 1987; **72**: 693–8.

18 Davidson, A.C., Leach, R., George, R.J.D., and Geddes, D.M. Supplemental oxygen and exercise ability in chronic obstructive airways disease. *Thorax* 1988; **43**: 965–71.

19 Dean, N.C., Brown, J.K., Himelman, R.B., *et al.* Oxygen may improve dyspnea and endurance in patients with chronic obstructive pulmonary disease and only mild hypoxaemia. *Am Rev Respir Dis* 1992; **146**: 941–5.

20 Mak, V.H.F., Bugler, J.R., and Roberts, C.M., Spiro, S.G. Effect of arterial oxygen desaturation on six minute walk distance, perceived effort, and perceived breathlessness in patients with airflow limitation. *Thorax* 1993; **48**: 33–8.

21 McDonald, C.F., Blyth, C.M., Lazarus, M.D., Marschner, I., and Barter, C.E. Exertional oxygen of limited benefit in patients with chronic obstructive pulmonary disease and mild hypoxaemia. *Am J Respir Crit Care Med* 1995; **152**: 1616–19.

22 Revill, S.M., Singh, S.J., and Morgan, M.D.L. Randomised controlled trial of ambulatory oxygen and an ambulatory ventilator on endurance exercise in COPD. *Respir Med* 2000; **94**: 778–83.

23 Killen, J.W., and Corris, P.A. A pragmatic assessment of the placement of oxygen when given for exercise induced dyspnoea. *Thorax* 2000; **55**(7): 544–6.

24 Knebel, A., Bentz, E., and Barnes, P. Dyspnoea management in alpha-1 antitrypsin deficiency: effect of oxygen administration. *Nurs Res* 2000; **49**(6): 333–8.

25 Jolly, E.C., Di Boscio, V., Aguirre, L., *et al.* Effects of supplemental oxygen during activity in patients with advanced COPD without severe resting hypoxaemia. *Chest* 2001; **120**(2): 437–43.

26 Marques-Magallanes, J.A., Storer, T.W., and Cooper, C.B. Treadmill exercise duration and dyspnea recovery time in chronic obstructive pulmonary disease: effects of oxygen breathing and repeated testing. *Respir Med* 1998; **92**: 735–8.

27 Singh, S.J., Morgan, M.D.L., Scott, S., Walters, D., and Hardman, A.E. Development of a shuttle walking test of disability in patients with chronic airways obstruction. *Thorax* 1992; **47**: 1019–24.

28 Booth, S., and Adams, L. The shuttle walking test: a reproducible method for evaluating the impact of shortness of breath on functional capacity in patients with advanced cancer. *Thorax* 2001; **56**(2): 146–50.

29 Wedzicha, J.A. Ambulatory oxygen in chronic obstructive pulmonary disease. *Monaldi Arch Chest Dis* 1996; **51**: 243–5.

30 Gift, A.G. Validation of a vertical visual analogue scale as a measure of clinical dyspnoea. *Rehabil Nurs* 1989; **14**: 323–5.

31 Miller, M.G., and Corner, J. The 'n = 1' randomised controlled trial. *Palliative Med* 1999; **13**: 255–9.

32 Leach, R.M., and Bateman, N.T. Acute oxygen therapy. *Br J Hosp Med* 1993; **49**: 637–44.

33 Williams, S. *Chronic respiratory illness.* The Experience of Illness Series. London: Routledge, 1993.

34 Fitzgerald, J.M., Baynham, R., and Powles, A.C.P. Use of oxygen therapy for adult patients outside the critical care areas of a university hospital. *Lancet* 1988; **i**: 981–3.

35 Heaney, L.G., McAllister, D., and MacMahon, J. Cost minimisation analysis of provision of oxygen at home: are the Drug Tariff guidelines cost effective? *BMJ* 1999; **319**: 19–23.

36 Tiep, B. Portable oxygen therapy with oxygen conserving devices and methodologies. *Monaldi Arch Chest Dis* 1995; **50**(1): 51–7.

37 Heimlich, H.J., and Carr, G.C. The Micro-trach: a 7 year experience with transtracheal oxygen therapy. *Chest* 1989; **95**: 1008–12.

38 Hoffman, L.A., Wesmiller, S.W., Sciurba, F.C., *et al.* Nasal cannula and transtracheal oxygen delivery. A comparison of patient response after 6 months of each technique. *Am Rev Respir Dis* 1992; **6**: 827–31.

39 Kampelmacher, M.J., Deenstra, M., van Kesteren, R.G., Melissant, C.F., Douze, J.M.C., and Lammers, J.W.J. Transtracheal oxygen therapy: an effective safe alternative to nasal oxygen administration. *European Respiratory Journal* 1997; **10**: 828–833.

40 Kass, J.E., and Terregino, C.A. The effect of heliox in acute severe asthma: a randomized controlled trial. *Chest* 1999; **116**: 296–300.

41 O'Donnell, D.E., D'Arsigny, C., and Webb, K.A. Effects of hyperoxia on ventilatory limitation during exercise in advanced chronic obstructive pulmonary disease. *Am J Respir Crit Care Med* 2001; **163**(4): 892–8.

42 Ahmedzai, S.H., Laude, E., Robertson, A., Troy, G., and Vora, V. A double-blind, randomized, controlled Phase II trial of Heliox 28 gas mixture in lung cancer patients with dyspnoea on exertion. *Br J Cancer* 2004; **90**: 366–71.

Chapter 11

Rehabilitation and exercise

Jane Lindsay and Roger Goldstein

Pulmonary rehabilitation is being practised all over the world, and is accepted as a mainstay in the treatment of people with chronic respiratory illness.[1–3] Programmes can be offered in small community clinics or state of the art teaching hospitals, but all pulmonary rehabilitation programmes have several things in common.

The goal of pulmonary rehabilitation is to achieve and maintain an individual's maximum level of independence and functioning in the community.[4] This is best achieved by a multidisciplinary team, through an individualized combination of education, counselling, and exercise, assisting patients to reduce or gain control of their symptoms.[3,5]

The need for individualization of education, counselling, and exercise programmes is obvious, given that the spectrum of those referred for rehabilitation could easily include a 50-year-old, severely underweight idiopathic pulmonary fibrosis patient who is still working at a demanding job, and an overweight 70-year-old, former 20 pack-year smoker with mild emphysema and a sedentary lifestyle. Comparison of the efficacy of the same rehabilitation programme for these two individuals would be impossible, because of the wide variation between them.

Research supports the role of rehabilitation in the control of dyspnoea. Of eight interventions common to pulmonary rehabilitation, four have been shown to decrease dyspnoea: lower extremity training, upper extremity training, ventilatory muscle training (in a subset of patients), and psychosocial/behavioural/educational interventions.[3]

Education and counselling

Education assists patients with lung disease to understand their disease process and the various therapies available, so that they have the tools to become active participants in their own health. Education may be relatively theoretical, such as gaining new insight into the anatomy and physiology of the lungs, to provide a better understanding of the benefits and limitations of various therapeutic interventions. Education also encompasses the learning of new skills, such as the correct technique for inhaled medication devices or energy conservation techniques during activities of daily living. The education sessions of a typical pulmonary rehabilitation program might be expected to cover the topics listed in Table 11.1.

When counselling is considered in a broad sense, it will mean different things in different programmes and to different participants. It can mean any intervention in which the patient receives one-to-one advice and assistance in achieving lifestyle changes. This may mean changes in diet, or learning methods of coping with the stress of a chronic illness. Any of the above education topics, for example, might be covered in a counselling session to provide individuals the opportunity to deal with any unique or particularly troublesome issue.

No matter how information and coping strategies are offered, the goal is well-informed patients who understand how their lungs work, how the lungs interact with the rest of the body

Table 11.1 Topics for education and counselling in pulmonary rehabilitation

Anatomy and physiology	Coping	Therapeutics
Normal and abnormal lungs	Living with chronic illness	Drugs
Principles of exercise	Effects of stress and relaxation	Diet – good nutrition
Breathing mechanics and breath control	Leisure lifestyle and travel Energy conservation and work simplification Community resources sexuality Environmental pollutants including second-hand smoke	Weight gain or loss Oxygen and oxygen delivery systems

Source: Pulmonary Rehabilitation Program, Grand River Hospital, Kitchener, Ontario, Canada.

(physically and psychologically) and who are less fearful and more likely to actively and successfully participate in their own health maintenance.[5,6]

The educational and counselling aspects of a pulmonary rehabilitation programme can have a profound impact on the perception of dyspnoea.[1,7] Because normal human lung capacity is so large, and chronic lung diseases usually progress slowly over many years, most people with chronic lung disease do not identify a problem until their lung disease is quite significant. By the time it is noticeable in their normal day-to-day activities, the respiratory system's ability to adapt to strenuous activity is significantly limited. They experience shortness of breath 'all of a sudden', rather than realizing that they have adapted to it over years of progression of their disease. Their shortness of breath is seen as negative feedback from their lungs: 'If this activity makes me short of breath, it shows me that my lungs can't handle it, so I shouldn't do this any more'. In the same way that a headache may seem more ominous to someone who is worried about a brain tumour, shortness of breath can seem overwhelming when you think that the only reason you have it is because of lung disease.

This reaction has many negative outcomes. The most obvious result is usually the downward vicious circle of decreased activity leading to decreased strength and cardiovascular fitness, leading to shortness of breath with lighter activities and so on.[8] It can also result in many more subtle changes in the way people view themselves.

People like to be in control of their own situations, and particularly of their own bodies. When their lungs won't let them do everything as they have always done, they can feel betrayed and reluctant to participate in activities which make their disability obvious. They may stop being as active in their home or community, fearing to show their limitations in front of their loved ones or in public. Friends and family may not understand why they stop being involved – until someone is using oxygen, lung disease is an invisible disability. If your best friend looks the same as always, it is hard to understand why she won't go walking with you any more. In such situations, avoiding contacts can become the easiest way to cope, and social isolation can result, accompanied by a dramatic decrease in physical activity and often depression.[3,9]

In a pulmonary rehabilitation programme, patients with lung disease may for the first time meet other people who truly understand what they are going through. The psychological support that they gain simply by being able to talk about their problems and fears with others in the same circumstances is tremendous.[3,10,11] In a supportive environment they can put their shortness of breath back into a more normal context and get back into activities that they thought were lost for ever. They learn from their peers who are succeeding in coping with shortness of breath and continuing to be active. They can safely exercise and learn that the shortness of breath they feel is still a normal body response to exercise, even if it occurs with lighter activity than they wish it did. The result is that, even though they are still dyspnoeic, they become desensitized to the sensation.[12] The dyspnoea no longer generates the same fear and the vicious cycle is broken. Instead of dyspnoea leading to fear leading to reflex stress reactions, which trigger more dyspnoea, the dyspnoea can be managed, whether by breathing control activities, relaxation techniques, or appropriate use of rescue medication.

Breathing retraining

Breathing retraining, or breath control (unlike respiratory muscle strengthening, which is covered in Chapter 12) refers to a conscious effort to modify breathing patterns, and teaches effective techniques specifically for the prevention and relief of dyspnoea.

The majority of breathless patients who attend pulmonary rehabilitation have chronic obstructive pulmonary disease (COPD). For these people, one of the main causes of breathlessness is static and dynamic hyperinflation. The air trapping which occurs during exhalation is a decades-long progression in most of these patients, but it also occurs on a minute-to-minute basis as dynamic hyperinflation which is sometimes more functionally limiting.[13] Anything that makes someone with COPD inhale deeply may cause them to trap more air. A few deep breaths without a controlled, adequate exhalation between breaths can cause successively more air trapping, until the chest wall dynamics are significantly impaired, and the ability to inhale is extremely limited, with an unpleasant sensation of dyspnoea as a result.

The altered mechanics of breathing associated with increased flattening of the diaphragm, elevation of the ribs, and increased use of accessory muscles can lead to a sensation of shortness of breath sufficient to require cessation of exercise.[13,14]

Breathing retraining addresses this issue by slowing exhalation and teaching pursed-lip breathing and breath control during activities. Cost-free and with no side effects, these techniques can sometimes be as effective in the short term as rescue medication.

Pursed-lip breathing

Pursed-lip breathing has been shown to increase tidal volume and reduce respiratory rate and minute ventilation. Because air trapping is caused in part by the collapse of inflamed and unsupported small airways in expiration, maintaining a more positive pressure in the airways by pursed-lip breathing will help prevent this collapse, allowing more volume to be exhaled.[15] Emptying the lungs effectively improves the mechanics of breathing, and allows for improved inhalation volume during succeeding breaths.

An effective analogy to use when teaching pursed-lip breathing technique is that of a garden hose with low water pressure. If you want to create more pressure, you reduce the size of the hose aperture by putting your thumb across it. Pursing the lips, like putting your thumb on the garden hose, creates back-pressure to 'splint open the floppy airways' to allow more efficient lung emptying and better exhalation.

Breathing retraining also encompasses the notion of using breath control during activities: matching breathing with the workload cycle of activities and matching breathing with changes in chest shape. Many patients also benefit from learning to match the speed of their activities to their breathing rather than vice versa.

Since one of the common denominators in most chronic lung diseases is a loss of elastic recoil, patients should theoretically be able to empty their lungs better if they exhale as they manoeuvre their chest into a smaller shape. Also, since under normal conditions inhaling uses muscle work and exhaling should be effortless, patients should be able to conserve some energy if they do not combine inhaling with activity. These theories lead to three 'rules of thumb' for patients who have dynamic hyperinflation:

1 If an activity causes your chest to expand (for example, lifting your arms up over your head) and then to reduce its size (when lowering the arms after raising them), inhale while reaching up (as the shoulder girdle muscles are elevating the upper ribs) and exhale while lowering your arms. In some situations, trunk flexion may further assist lung emptying, but the effectiveness would have to be weighed against the effort involved and the effect on posture. Combining lung emptying with movement can assist such activities as putting on socks and shoes: inhale while sitting upright, then exhale as you reach down to your feet.

2 If an activity has short cycles of effort and ease, such as working to push a vacuum cleaner forward, and ease while pulling it back or walking up to it, exhale during the hard part of the cycle and inhale during the easy part of the cycle.

3 Rules are made to be broken. If an activity does not fit either rule 1 or rule 2, respect your own comfortable breathing speed and match the activity to that speed. For example, a shallow knee-bend exercise involves work for both lowering the body and raising it, and there is no effect on chest shape. Patients doing this exercise will become breathless faster if they try to breathe as fast as they can move their legs. If instead they move their legs only as fast as their comfortable breathing speed, taking special care to have enough time to exhale efficiently, the exercise will seem easier.

Rule 1 is best suited to patients with minimal or moderate disease. For these patients, the extra stretch during inhalation is one way of incorporating flexibility exercise into their routine. Rule 2 is best suited to those with more severe dyspnoea, for whom splitting the work of inhaling and of the activity into two separate tasks is often more important than enhancing chest expansion.

Patients who practice these relatively artificial rules of thumb in a supervised setting gradually begin to have conscious control over their breathing in normal activities of daily living. Instead of being at the mercy of their lungs, which can seem to make them short of breath on a whim, they are more in control.

Pacing

Another aspect of breathing retraining is **pacing**. This entails breaking activities into manageable portions, so that breathing control is maintained, and patients are not exhausted by necessary tasks. Doing necessary activities in a more energy-conserving way will allow chronic lung patients to have energy left to do other activities which contribute to their quality of life.

Emergency breathing

In a perfect world, a combination of excellent adherence to properly prescribed medication, pacing and breath control would prevent severe episodes of dyspnoea, as all patients would approach every potentially dyspnoea-causing situation proactively. However, since some episodes of dyspnoea are inevitable, teaching patients to handle these frightening episodes is another vitally important component of breath control. One way to do this is to encourage

Case study 11.1 Sheila

Sheila has become exhausted by her normal morning routine, so that she has to lie down to rest before making her lunch. All her life she has arisen, taken a shower, dressed, made the bed, then had breakfast. Now, however, showering leaves her feeling drained – she is tired from keeping her hands raised to wash her face and hair. Towelling herself dry is another chore. She stays breathless as she gets dressed (gathering her clothes from different drawers and cupboards) and becomes even worse when she bends forward to put on her socks. Reaching up to brush her hair seems like more than she can manage. Making the bed makes her wish that she was getting back into it instead, but she pushes herself to go to the living room to watch TV until her mid-morning nap.

After Sheila has learned pacing, she will have her shower but will rest her arms briefly between washing her face and hair. Instead of using a towel, she will put on an absorbent bathrobe, which will dry most of her body for her. After a brief rest she can dry one leg and foot, exhaling as she reaches down and pausing briefly before drying her second leg. Since she laid out her clothes last night, she doesn't have to gather them together now. She dresses her upper body, pauses, then dresses her lower body. Since her breakfast is a relatively simple affair, she eats before making the bed. This allows her to be rested before tackling this difficult task. When she does make the bed, she makes one side at a time, moving from the head of the bed toward the foot, smoothing the sheets and blankets as she goes. She exhales when she has to bend over. She rests briefly on the foot of the bed before moving along the other side of the bed, from foot to head.

patients to follow a routine to bring their breathing back under control, as shown in Box 11.1. The phrases 'get your head down' and 'get your shoulders down' mean that patients should try to relax their neck and upper body before moving on to actual breath control. The phrase

Box 11.1 Coping with episodes of severe dyspnoea

When on the brink . . . think

1 Stop and rest in a comfortable position
2 Get you head down
3 Get your shoulders down
4 Breathe in through your mouth
5 Blow out through your mouth
6 Breathe in and blow out as fast as necessary
7 Begin to blow out longer, but not forcibly; use pursed lips if you find it effective
8 Begin to slow your breathing
9 Begin to use your nose
10 Begin diaphragmatic breathing
11 Stay in position for 5 minutes longer

Remember: Breathlessness on effort is uncomfortable, but not in itself harmful or dangerous.

Source: Physiotherapy Department, West Park Hospital, Toronto, Ontario, Canada 'begin diaphragmatic breathing' must not be interpreted as 'now breathe with the diaphragm only'. Because of the inefficiency of the diaphragm and intercostal muscles, COPD patients must use their accessory muscles of inhalation when they are in distress. Trying to have a COPD patient breathe only with the diaphragm is an exercise in futility and will only make the dyspnoea worse. Patients should be encouraged to use all of their muscles for inhalation. Therefore, point 10 means that they should begin 'sharing the load' among all muscles groups, rather than emphasizing only accessory muscles, as happens in acute distress.

Exercise

Exercise has always been a primary component of pulmonary rehabilitation programmes. Initially it was thought that exercise must be affecting the physiology of the lungs, since anecdotal reports from patients revealed significant improvements in symptoms. However, the discovery that the benefits of exercise relate more to changes in muscle physiology than to changes in pulmonary function tests has not diminished the importance of exercise in helping chronic respiratory patients achieve their goal of greater functional independence. It is not the intent of this chapter to analyse these physiological changes, but rather to give a practical overview of exercise as it relates to relief of dyspnoea.

What is exercise?

This global term may mean anything from simple repetitions of breathing movements, to whole-body exercise which maximally challenges the cardiorespiratory system. The American National Institutes of Health (NIH) defines exercise as 'planned, structured, and repetitive movement done to improve or maintain one or more components of physical fitness'.[16] For someone who is extremely debilitated by lung disease and subsequent deconditioning, to the extent of not being able to participate in normal activities of daily living, planning and then washing the dishes qualifies as exercise – good news for people with severe chronic lung disease! As with education and counselling, exercise must be individualized if the maximum benefit is to be achieved by each patient. Different types of exercise and different intensities of workload will be appropriate for different people. In pulmonary rehabilitation, exercise is a blend of breathing retraining, flexibility exercise, strengthening, and cardiovascular endurance exercise.

Flexibility exercise

Flexibility exercise encompasses general exercise to maintain or increase the range of motion of the limbs and trunk. Since the goal of pulmonary rehabilitation is maintenance of optimal function, maintenance of joint range is an essential part of assisting patients to maintain the ability to be functionally independent. The downward spiral of inactivity experienced by many people with shortness of breath can be so severe in some cases that joint range of motion is affected, and this can eventually lead to permanent loss of range.[17]

As well as general flexibility, special consideration will need to be given to chest wall flexibility for many chronic lung patients. Soft-tissue stretching techniques and other manual therapies are often helpful.

The Canadian Society for Exercise Physiology recommends gentle reaching, bending and stretching of all muscle groups, 4–7 days per week. After a warm-up of 5 min of light activity, slow smooth stretching motions without bouncing or jerking should be used. Stretches should be gentle continuous movements or stretch and hold (10–30s) as appropriate for the activity. Patients should be encouraged to include flexibility activities in their normal day-to-day activities.[18]

Strengthening exercise

Muscle strengthening falls into two categories: respiratory muscle strength training (Chapter 12), or limb and trunk strengthening. Limb strengthening is usually tailored to meet a specific functional need, but it may serve another important purpose: assistance with weight loss. Chronic lung patients who are overweight often have difficulty performing enough cardiovascular effort to lose weight. Developing a higher proportion of lean body mass may help them in this. More study on this topic is needed.

There are several protocols for limb muscle strengthening and descriptions can be found in many sources, but no single technique has been shown to be the most effective.[17] Before beginning an effective strengthening regime, one must determine how much resistance the patient should use. The notion of a repetition maximum (RM) was developed by Delorme and Watkins and is commonly used to establish a baseline and to measure improvement.[19] The RM is the greatest amount of weight the patient can move through the desired range of motion the desired number of times. The number of repetitions used to establish the baseline varies from author to author, from 1 RM to 15 RM.[17,20] Trial and error is required to find the 'perfect' weight, at which the patient can achieve the desired number of repetitions, but is too tired to lift it on the next try.

One example of an exercise protocol using the RM is the Oxford Technique (Box 11.2), a protocol designed to diminish resistance as muscle fatigue develops. Another protocol, Daily Adjustable Progressive Resistance Exercise (DAPRE), provides a formula for determining progression of the exercise (Box 11.3). As with all exercise, a warm-up component must be included before beginning the resistance training.[17]

For a very debilitated patient with chronic lung disease, even a simple protocol of 2–4 sets of 10–15 repetitions of light weightlifting or even antigravity exercise 2–4 times a week will build strength.[18,20]

Cardiovascular endurance exercise

This is the most common component of pulmonary rehabilitation exercise regimes. From a functional point of view, the ability to 'carry on carrying on' is deemed to be more necessary than strength or power. The downward spiral is characterized by people becoming short of breath with normal functional activities, most of which are of a low-intensity, prolonged nature, such as walking or doing chores around the home.

Box 11.2 The Oxford Technique for resistance exercise

1 Determine a 10 RM

2 The patient then performs

   10 repetitions at the full 10 RM

   10 repetitions at 75% of the 10 RM

   10 repetitions at 50% of the 10 RM

Box 11.3 The DAPRE technique for resistance exercise

1 Determine a 6 RM for the *initial working weight*

2 The patient then performs:

Set 1: 10 repetitions of 50% of the working weight

Set 2: 6 repetitions of 75% of the working weight

Set 3: as many repetitions as possible of the full working weight

Set 4: as many repetitions as possible of the *adjusted working weight.*

The *adjusted working weight* is based on the number of repetitions of the full working weight performed during set 3.

3 The number of repetitions done in set 4 is used to determine the working weight for the next day. The 'ideal' maximum number of repetitions (when the patient is asked to perform as many repetitions as possible) is 5–7.

Guidelines for adjustment of the working weight

Number of repetitions performed during Set 3	Adjustment to working weight for Set 4	Next day
0–2	Decrease 2.3–4.5 kg and repeat set	Decrease 2.3–4.5 kg
3–4	Decrease 0–2.3 kg	Same weight
5–6	Keep weight the same	Increase 2.3–4.5 kg
7–10	Increase 2.3–4.5 kg	Increase 2.3–6.8 kg
11	Increase 4.5–6.6 kg	Increase 4.5–9.0 kg

Endurance training follows the same general guidelines whether it is for healthy people or those with respiratory disease, but as the disease state progresses, more differences in approach are needed. For example, many patients who have become sedentary in response to dyspnoea are more limited by leg fatigue or generalized weakness than by their ventilatory status. Others may desaturate significantly during activity, even though their resting blood gases are at an acceptable level. The use of supplemental oxygen during exercise is controversial: it can allow even non-hypoxemic COPD patients to exercise at higher work rates, but if the training stimulus is tissue hypoxia, then supplemental oxygen might make a training effect unachievable. Both theories need further study.[8]

As our understanding of chronic lung diseases as systemic disorders increases, new exercise guidelines are emerging. At present, only general guidelines exist.

Which chronic lung disease patients can exercise?

Given the lenient definition of exercise above, any except extreme end-stage patients (whose quality-of-life goal would be palliation) can exercise; it is only a matter of choosing the best type and intensity of exercise.[20–22] Patients with chronic lung disease often have co-morbid conditions that require some exercise modifications, but even those with cardiac pacemakers can exercise.[23]

At one end of the spectrum are patients with **severe lung disease**, who have shortness of breath at rest or on minimal exertion. These patients will benefit from breathing retraining and pacing as described above, and very low-intensity exercise.

At the other end of the spectrum are those with **mild to moderate disease** and few symptoms, whose lung disease might only have been discovered in a routine check-up or because of dyspnoea on significant exertion. These patients can usually follow exercise guidelines intended for people with normal cardiovascular and respiratory systems.

In between are the bulk of the patients seen in pulmonary rehabilitation, who have **moderate to severe disease**. Unfortunately there are no strict rules for exercise in these patients, and several controversies exist.

These categories of disease severity are purposely vague. The amount of disability experienced by chronic lung patients is due to such a wide range of variables that, for the purposes of rehabilitation, their functional abilities are a more important gauge than FEV_1 or other measures of lung function.

Cardiovascular exercise testing

Lack of sophisticated exercise testing equipment and specially trained personnel should not be a barrier to providing supervised exercise in this population,[5,22] although all patients should be screened for safety. A resting ECG and a thorough medical examination should be performed on anyone before they are prescribed exercise. This will screen out the most at-risk patients, but there is no clear answer about what further testing is required or useful in this population.

No single testing protocol is clearly established as the most appropriate for all patients and programmes.[20,22] Each pulmonary rehabilitation programme will choose its own exercise test, subject to issues such as availability of equipment and trained personnel, cost, type of patients served, and type of exercise programme used.

The range of exercise testing protocols includes direct measurement of expired gases during a maximal exercise test to calculate true maximal oxygen uptake (VO_{2max}), assessment of blood lactate levels, submaximal graded exercise testing with or without cardiac monitoring, a 6- or 12- min walk test, and a shuttle walk test, step test, or other informal test of physical fitness.[20] Each of these has its strengths and drawbacks.[8,24]

VO_{2max} is the highest achievable extraction of oxygen by the body from the volumes of air breathed into the lungs, and is expressed as L/min or, more accurately, mL kg^{-1} min^{-1}. Although direct measurement of maximal oxygen uptake is the gold standard for the measurement of exercise ability, this type of testing offers limited information in the pulmonary rehabilitation population since the test often needs to be stopped at the symptom-limited maximum rather than the true cardiovascular limit. Also, equipment to measure expired gases, specialized exercise equipment such as a treadmill or stationary bicycle, and trained personnel to perform such tests are not always available.

If exercise equipment is available, tests without measurement of expired gases can estimate the VO_{2max}. Many different protocols exist for these tests. The most widely used in general exercise testing, the Bruce Protocol, is not well suited to COPD patients because of its large and unequal increments, which can overestimate exercise capacity. Protocols with smaller workload increments are better suited to patients with respiratory disease (Figure 11.1).[20,25] Newer 'ramp' protocols, which use a nearly continuous and uniform increase in metabolic demand, may be even better for this population.[25] If the tests are stopped at a submaximal level, VO_{2max} can be estimated by extrapolating from the data obtained (Figure 11.2).

Alternately, if pulmonary function testing and/or expired gas analysis equipment is available, VO_{2max} can be estimated using the Armstrong–Workman nomogram. This estimates VO_{2max} for normal and chronic lung disease patients based on maximal voluntary ventilation (MVV),

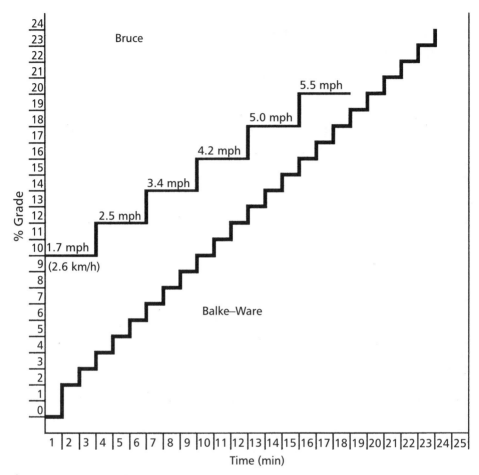

Fig. 11.1 Testing protocols with smaller increments (e.g. Naughton, Balke–Ware, USAFSM) are better suited to people with lung disease. In the Balke–Ware protocol, for example, speed is constant at 5 km/h (3.3 mph) until 25% grade is reached, then increases by 0.3 km/h (0.2 mph) per minute without changing grade. In the Bruce protocol, by contrast, speed and grade change every 3 min.

expired ventilation per minute (V_E) and volume of oxygen consumed per minute (VO_2). This tool provides a method of further estimating the VO_{2max} based only on FEV_1 and an approximate value for V_E/VO_2. Of course, the results become less accurate as more estimates are used.[5]

Timed walk tests, and more recently the shuttle walk test, are used very commonly in pulmonary rehabilitation programmes as approximate measures of fitness. Although they only give limited information, these low-tech tests can still give valuable clues to the patient's exercise capacity for use in the exercise prescription.

The 12-minute walk originally developed by Cooper[26] was later utilized to assess COPD patients.[27] This has evolved into a 6-min test, which is better suited to those with more advanced disease.[24] Both tests are easily administered since they require only a measured hallway, a blood

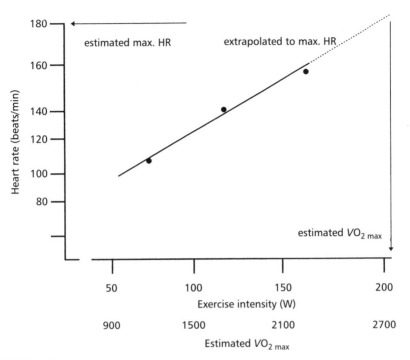

Fig. 11.2 Estimating age-predicted maximal heart rate.

pressure cuff, and an oximeter. Patients are instructed to walk as far/as fast as they reasonably can in the allotted time. Whether a 6-min or a 12-min test is are used, the instructions given to the patient must be standardized, since different instructions can significantly affect the distance walked.[28] The test must also be given more than once (some say more than four times) to decrease the effect of the learning curve.[24,29]

The shuttle walk test introduced by Singh *et al.*[30,31] is gaining popularity. This is an externally paced incremental walk test. Patients walk up and down a 10-m course, matching their pace to the speed of a tape-recorded signal. The speed is increased by a small increment each minute. The test is terminated when the patient is no longer able to maintain the required speed, or when 85% of the predicted maximal heart rate is achieved, using the formula [210 − (0.65 × age)]. The shuttle has a few advantages over the timed walk test. Because of its incremental nature, a higher heart rate is usually achieved before the test is terminated. Also, it is reproducible after only one practice walk.

In the absence of exercise stress-testing facilities, approximate workload can also be measured from a 6-min or 12-min walk test as a metabolic equivalent (MET). An actual MET is calculated by dividing VO_2 during activity by resting VO_2. When estimating VO_{2max} and METs, the constant value for resting VO_2 is 3.5 mL kg^{-1} min^{-1}. MET levels correlate with the patient's level of physical exertion; 1 MET is the amount of energy required while the body is at rest. Activities are expressed as requiring a multiple of this resting requirement. The MET level is therefore helpful in setting up a patient's initial exercise prescription.

Box 11.4 Calculating METs from the 6-min walk test[20,22]

- Calculate walking speed by dividing the number of metres walked in 6 minutes by 6, to give metres per minute:

  MET = (speed in m/min) (0.1 mL^{-1} kg^{-1} min) + (3.5 mL^{-1} kg^{-1} min)/ 3.5 mL^{-1} kg^{-1} min (the basal metabolic rate)

- For example, suppose a person walked 100 m on their 6-min walk test. This would give:

  Speed = 100 m in 6 min = 16.6 m/min

- Therefore MET = (16.6 m/min) × 0.1 mL^{-1} kg^{-1} min) + (3.5 mL^{-1} kg^{-1} min)/3.5 mL^{-1} kg^{-1} min = 1.5

In the absence of exercise stress testing, close supervision during exercise will pick up warning signs. The contraindications to exercise testing suggested by Mahler *et al.*[20] can also be used to help screen patients who should not exercise without further testing (Table 11.2).

Since the risk will increase with the effort level, pulmonary rehabilitation programmes that do not have access to formal testing might not push their patients to their maximum

Table 11.2 Contraindications to exercise testing

Absolute contraindications	Relative contraindications
Recent significant change in the resting ECG suggesting infarction or other acute cardiac event.	Resting diastolic blood pressure >115 mmHg or resting systolic blood pressure >200 mmHg
Recent complicated myocardial infarction (unless patient is stable and pain free)	Moderate valvular heart disease
Unstable angina	Known electrolyte abnormalities (hypokalaemia, hypomagnesaemia)
Uncontrolled ventricular arrhythmia	Fixed-rate pacemaker (rarely used)
Uncontrolled atrial arrhythmia that compromises cardiac function	Frequent or complex ventricular ectopics
Third-degree AV heart block without pacemaker	Ventricular aneurysm
Acute congestive heart failure	Uncontrolled metabolic disease (e.g. diabetes, thyrotoxicosis, or myxoedema)
Severe aortic stenosis	Chronic infectious disease (e.g. mononucleosis, hepatitis, AIDS)
Suspected or known dissecting aneurysm	Neuromuscular musculoskeletal or rheumatoid disorders that are exacerbated by exercise
Active or suspected myocarditis or pericarditis	Advanced or complicated pregnancy
Thrombophlebitis or intracardiac thrombi	
Recent systemic or pulmonary embolus	
Acute infections	
Significant emotional distress (psychosis)	

physiological tolerance. However, as discussed in the intensity section below, even moderately intense exercise is beneficial.

Cardiovascular exercise prescription

Intensity

There is controversy about the appropriate level of intensity of cardiovascular exercise for chronic lung patients. Respiratory patients can often work at or near their maximum aerobic capacity, as established by a maximal exercise stress test, and therefore achieve excellent changes in fitness.[3] However, even exercise of a moderate intensity will make significant changes in muscle physiology over time[8] and may be better tolerated by patients with moderate to severe disease. There are also many different ways to measure workload intensity, and only a few will be discussed here. The choice of intensity, therefore, must be made by the individual pulmonary rehabilitation program

If VO_{2max} test results are available (remembering the limitations), exercise is usually given at about 60–80% of tested maximal workload, but it can be as low as 50% for respiratory patients.[8,20] To put this in context, the normal work capacity for an 8-h occupational work day is between 25–40% of achieved VO_{2max}.[5]

Since there is an almost linear relationship between VO_2 and heart rate, target heart rate (THR) is another measure of workload intensity which is commonly used to establish an exercise prescription in the absence of maximal exercise testing. It is extremely useful for those with only minimal disease, and can be used as an approximate guideline for those with moderate to severe disease.

Exercise THR can be calculated as a straight percentage of maximum heart rate (MHR). If not available from a maximal exercise test, MRH can be estimated by subtracting the patient's age from 220.[5,32] It is assumed that 60–90% of MHR is equivalent to 50–80% of VO_{2max} or heart rate reserve.[20] The heart rate reserve (Karvonen) calculation is very commonly used and is based on age and resting heart rate (RHR).[20,32–34]

Calculating a range of desired exercise heart rate between 60% and 85% of calculated maximum workload gives patients some leeway in their exercise intensity and allows for variation between patients, as well as 'good and bad days' for individual patients. The exercise prescription would include a variety of activities designed to keep the patient's heart rate in the target range.

Box 11.5 Calculating a THR using the Karvonen equation

Maximum heart rate (MHR) = 220 − patient's age

Target heart rate (THR) = [(MHR − RHR) % intensity] + RHR

The % intensity is the percentage intensity that the patient has to achieve during exercise. For example, suppose a patient with chronic lung disease is aged 65 and has an RHR of 85 beats/min.

MHR = 220 − 65 = 155

THR (60% intensity) = 0.6 × (155 − 85) + 85 = 127

THR (80% intensity) = 0.8 × (155 − 85) + 85 = 145

For this patient, THR is between 127 and 145 beats/min.

Intensity can also be extrapolated from a timed walk test. Patients who walk very short distances on a timed test (for example 150–250 m in 6 min) can be considered to be severely debilitated (whether by their lung disease, fitness level, or another co-morbid condition) and may benefit from the use of an ambulation aid such as a wheeled walking aid.[35,36] A very low-intensity exercise prescription is appropriate.

From the walk test, the patient's walking speed can be calculated. A normal adult's brisk walking speed is approximately 5 km/h. A very general guideline would be that a patient who achieves this walking speed during the timed walk test without severe dyspnoea (more than 6 on the modified [10-point] Borg scale), desaturation (below 88%), increased heart rate to near the age-predicted maximum, or a drop in systemic blood pressure (or failure of systemic blood pressure to rise)[20] can probably exercise using guidelines designed for people with normal cardiovascular/respiratory systems.

Walking speed on the test may also be useable as the initial walking speed on a treadmill, if one is to be used in the exercise programme. Some patients unfamiliar with a treadmill may not achieve their normal walking speed until they gain some experience.

Using the calculations discussed in the testing section (above), an exercise prescription can be prepared based on METs. Some very general guidelines exist to estimate a patient's probable performance in METs, which can be compared to activities on a MET table to gain a better understanding of the patient's probable exercise capacity (Table 11.3).[5,17,20] Some exercise equipment is calibrated to show METs, so the exercise intensity can easily be matched with their test results.

With some imagination, the health professional can design exercises that mimic the activities of daily living which patients need or wish to be able to perform. Better yet, since exercising muscles in the way they are used for normal activities will make the most functional gains, exercise sessions should incorporate the functional activities themselves.

Care must be taken not to use the guidelines from MET tables too literally – the activity descriptions given in these tables are not very specific, and the way a person performs an activity can dramatically change the workload. Using MET tables can help health professionals decide which activities of daily living need to be modified. A patient capable of only 2 METs of exercise may still be able to make the bed (2.8) or enjoy a game of 10-pin bowling (3.0) once they are taught energy conservation techniques and pacing.

Another gauge of exercise intensity is perceived exertion or perceived dyspnoea. Numeric or visual analogue scales are excellent tools for measuring these sensations, and for encouraging appropriate exercise intensity. One of the most commonly used, the 10-point Borg scale, has been shown to correlate with VO_2 and heart rate (Figure 11.3). A dyspnoea rating between 3 (moderate) and 6 (between severe and very severe) equates to a peak VO_2 of 50–85%, the desired range for workload intensity.[20,32,37]

The Canadian *Physical Activity Guide* and *Activity Guide for Older Adults*[18] are sets of simple guidelines designed for use by lay people, and may form a suitable starting point for a pulmonary rehabilitation programme. The guidelines for intensity can be graded by the patient's perception of workload (Figure 11.4), and symptoms can be further quantified by using a Borg scale or visual analogue scale.

When you consider that in the absence of a pulmonary rehabilitation programme motivated patients will be active anyway, and that most of their activity can be considered 'exercise', there is no reason for even a minimally equipped programme not to offer supervised exercise. With a small portable oximeter, a blood pressure cuff, and the ability to take a pulse, a healthcare professional can provide sufficient monitoring for low or moderate

Table 11.3 Estimates of MET and VO_{2max} related to symptoms for common activities

Disease severity	Functional capacity	Estimated MET workload achievable	Probable % VO_{2max} achieved (mL kg^{-1} min^{-1})	Equivalent activities	Activity METs
Normal	No limits, no symptoms	≥7 METs	≥21–24	Playing tennis	7.0
				Snow skiing	8.0
				Jogging (8.0 km/h)	7.0–8.0
				Rowing	12.0
				Running (8 km/h)	9.0
Mild	Slight limitations, symptoms with heavy activity	5–6	15–18	Lifting and carrying objects (9–18 kg)	4.5
				Lifting and carrying objects (18–27 kg)	6.4
				Bicycling (15 km/h)	5.0
				Walking upstairs	4.0–8.0
				Playing golf, walking	5.0
Moderate	Marked limitations, symptoms with ordinary activity	3–4	9–12	Scrubbing floors	2.7
				Straightening rooms (for example making beds)	2.8
				Bowling	3.0
				Bicycling	4.0
				Walking (5 km/h)	4.0–5.0
Severe	Discomfort at rest and during all activities	1–2	3–6	Knitting	1.5
				Driving a car, or sweeping floors	2.0
				Hammering nails or playing piano	2.0
				Preparing food while standing	
				Walking (3 km/h)	2.0–3.0

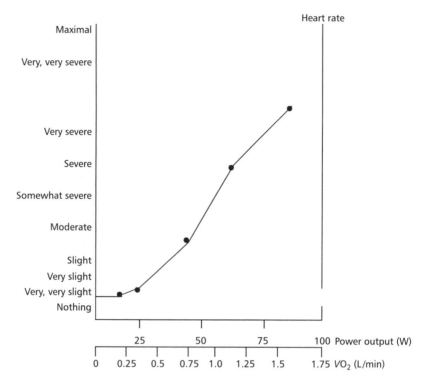

Fig. 11.3 Dyspnoea ratings and heart rate responses during an incremental graded exercise test in a patient with severe COPD. Modifed from Mahler *et al.* (1995).[20]

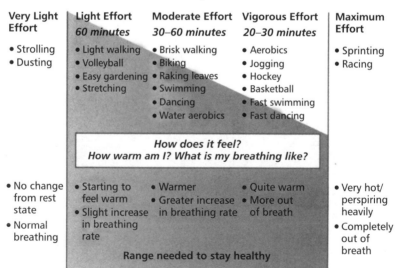

Fig. 11.4 Cardiovascular exercise guidelines for normal adults. Reproduced with permission from *Canada's Physical Activity Guide* (Health Canada and Canadian Society for Exercise Physiology).

workload, at intensities that the patients would do at home. The more experienced and highly trained the staff, and the more sophisticated the monitoring equipment that is available, the higher the intensity of the exercise can be, right up to the patient's symptom limited maximum.

Mode

It is important to remember that there is no perfect exercise or piece of exercise equipment. Patients may stay interested in exercise if a variety of equipment (such as treadmill, cycle ergometer, arm ergometer, and resistance machines) is available. However, a very vigorous and varied workout can be performed with only a staircase or step-stool, some small weights (household objects can suffice), and some therapeutic elastic bands.

Duration

Since many chronic respiratory patients cannot conform to rigid exercise rules as laid out for healthier people, exercise duration may have to be modified to allow realistic participation. General guidelines for duration range from 10-min sessions (repeated 6 times for a total 60 min of exercise daily)[18] to 20–30-min sessions of continuous exercise.[20]

Frequency

Again, a range of recommendations have been made: 4–7 times per week at lower intensity levels or 3–5 days per week at higher intensity levels.[8,18,20] A common guideline is to exercise on alternate days to allow the body to rest and recover between sessions. This is particularly important with resistance training.

Limitations to cardiovascular exercise

The factors that limit exercise in chronic lung patients are many and complex. Wasserman[38] has summarized these, as shown in Table 11.4. The following paragraphs touch on a few important limiting factors seen in the day-to-day operation of a pulmonary rehabilitation program.

Some chronic patients desaturate during exercise, as observed with a portable oximeter. Their working muscles use oxygen faster than their lungs can supply it. Resting blood gases or pulmonary function tests are not sufficient to predict this phenomenon. Although measurement of the lung's diffusing capacity during pulmonary function testing can give some hints that desaturation might occur, we do not yet have a test which accurately predicts which patients will desturate, or how far they will desturate during activity. It is better simply to measure it.

Controversy exists about whether (and how much) oxygen should be used during exercise in this instance. Although many studies show that correcting oxygen desaturation will increase a patient's exercise ability,[24,39,40] there is evidence that this is not true of every patient who desaturates.[41] Tissue hypoxia may be linked to the training stimulus,[8] but maintaining oxygen saturation in the normal or near normal range often means that the patient can achieve a cardiovascular target heart rate, or at least a higher intensity of exercise. If oxygen is supplied for this purpose, it is important to be sure that it actually results in increased exercise tolerance. This can be achieved by a simple test: have the patient perform the same activity on compressed

Table 11.4 Limiting factors for exercise in patients with lung disease

Mechanisms limiting exercise tolerance in obstructive lung diseases	
Increased work of breathing	
Increased ventilatory drive:	decreased PaO_2
	increased VDS/VT
	decreased pH
	increased metabolic requirement
Impaired cardiac output increase:	decreased cardiac filling due to increased intrathoracic pressure during exhalation
	increased pulmonary vascular resistance during exhalation due to increased alveolar pressure and the loss of functional pulmonary vessels because of underlying lung disease
Pathophysiologic responses to exercise in restrictive lung diseases	
Reduced peak VO_2	
Reduced anaerobic threshold	
Reduced ratio of the change in consumption to the change oxygen in work rate ($\Delta VO_2/\Delta WR$)	
Increased VDS/VT	
Increased ventilatory equivalent for O_2 and CO_2	
Hypoxia that is usually progressive	
Ratio of tidal volume to inspiratory capacity (VT/IC) $\sim$ 1 at low levels of work	
Non-cardiopulmonary factors contributing to exercise intolerance in patients with lung disease	
Carboxyhaemoglobinemia	
Anemia	
Obesity	
Chronic metabolic acidosis	

oxygen and on compressed air (using the same delivery method, for example, nasal speculae [cannulae]), blinding them to the choice. This can show you whether the oxygen allows the patient to achieve a desired heart rate, intensity, or duration of exercise if oxygen is used. However, we do not know how much improvement in exercise tolerance, between the oxygen and the air results, is functionally useful.

Another limiting factor in this population can be the mechanics of breathing. A common pitfall when observing someone whose exercise is limited by dyspnoea in spite of normal or near-normal oxygen saturation is to assume that their limitation is general lack of fitness. However, the culprit may be their altered mechanics of breathing.

As mentioned in the section on breath control, hyperinflation interferes with the normal mechanics of breathing. The flattened diaphragm can no longer generate as much change from its resting position to its maximally contracted position. The elevated ribs change the length–tension relationship of the intercostal muscles, making them less efficient. The use of accessory muscles of both inhalation and exhalation may be required in order to augment the primary muscles of respiration.

These altered mechanics may produce a sensation of shortness of breath, sufficient to require cessation of exercise. They have also been shown to contribute to the sensation of leg fatigue. Patients who experience dynamic hyperinflation during exercise will benefit from pursed-lip breathing and breath control techniques including pacing (see above). Also, timing their exercise so that it coincides with their medication dosing may maximize their abilities.

Leg or general body fatigue can also be a profound limiting factor for exercise.[24,42] As discussed above, many chronic lung disease patients have become increasingly less active over time, and their fitness level often outweighs their lung disease as the main cause of symptoms. It is very encouraging for patients to be reminded that shortness of breath is a normal response to effort. If muscle fatigue is found to be the limiting factor for exercise, this is, in many ways, good news. Decreased muscle strength and endurance are relatively easy to change, given the patient's willingness to work at it.

It is important to rule out or to account for other factors which are contributing to dyspnoea and fatigue, whenever possible. The fatigue associated with significantly increased heart rate may only be due to severe deconditioning, or it may represent undiagnosed heart disease. When there is any doubt, the patient must be referred on for further investigation. As we gain more insight into chronic lung disease as a systemic disease, more specific guidelines should emerge.

Putting it all together: interval exercise

The exercise prescriptions for patients with mild, moderate, or severe disease have many similarities. Each contain warm-up, overload, and cool-down sections. During the cardiovascular effort (overload) section, interval exercise (which alternates more challenging exercises with easier exercises or brief pauses) is often preferable in this population to continuous exercise, since it allows patients an opportunity to regain breathing control and helps prevent an excessive rise in heart rate. Mode, duration, and intensity of exercise are individualized to achieve the highest desirable workload and progressed as quickly as the patient tolerates.[21,24] This progression should take into account each individual's main limiting factor to exercise.

Exercise for patients with severe disease

Patients who are dyspnoeic at rest or with minimal exertion will find breathing retraining and pacing most useful. Once they have better control of their breathing, they can usually participate in low-intensity exercises which mimic a normal cardiovascular routine, and train them for specifically problematic activities of daily living. Some of these patients are so severely debilitated that seemingly low-intensity level exercise is actually quite strenuous, and measurable gains from their low starting point can be made.[12,43,44] However, even if the effort level they are capable of sustaining is too low to gain any real cardiovascular training effect, a structured exercise session has several benefits. Participation in any exercise, especially if it is in a supportive setting, provides much-needed psychological benefit. As well as contributing to desensitizing the sensation of dyspnoea, supervised exercise has a beneficial effect on depression.[12] Patients begin to feel more in control of their lungs and less anxious, and are often more willing to become more involved in life. Practicing breath control techniques during repetitive exercises helps patients to learn these new skills, so that they become more natural and are more easily applied to 'real life' situations. In the sample exercise programme in Table 11.5, the patient is following rule of thumb # 2 (see above), even though raising the arms elevates the ribs, so the activity also falls under rule of thumb # 1. For this patient, splitting the work of inhaling and of lifting the arms into two separate tasks is more important than enhancing chest expansion.

Table 11.5 Sample exercise programme for someone who is severely dyspnoeic

	Time (min)	Exercises (done sitting)	
Warm up	2–3	1	Deep breathe, and exhale with pursed lips
		2	Shrug shoulders
		3	Controlled breathing with alternate trunk side bending
Overload ('hard work')	4–6	4	Raise arms to shoulder height (inhale while at rest, exhale while raising and lowering)
		5	Straighten alternate knees
		6	With hands on shoulders, make circles with your elbows
		7	Alternately bring knees toward chest (exhale while raising leg, inhale while lowering foot to floor)
Cool down	2–3	8	Controlled breathing with alternate trunk side bending
		9	With feet on floor, alternately lift toes, then heels
		10	Deep breathe, and exhale with pursed lips

It is surprising how often people who seem very near end-stage can achieve significant increases in their quality of life through low-intensity exercise. People can go from a bed-to-chair existence to being able to participate in self-care and activities of daily life around the home, or can begin to be involved in their communities once more.

Exercise for patients with moderate to severe disease

Patients in this category will follow the general guidelines for cardiovascular exercise, and some will be able to reach a cardiovascular target heart rate. However, many of them will be limited by their ventilatory capacity, severe deconditioning, or another factor. It is important to try to identify their limiting factor for exercise, so that a programme can be individualized for maximum benefit.

An exercise programme for someone with moderate to severe lung disease could follow the warm up (5–10 min) – cardiovascular effort (overload) (20–60 min) – cool down (5–10 min) format, but the overload (whether this includes aerobic endurance exercise alone, or a mix of aerobics and strengthening) might need to be performed for shorter intervals, with more time spent on the easier activities. The need for individualization cannot be stressed enough. Table 11.6 gives one example.

Exercise for patients with mild to moderate disease

Many patients in this category can use standard exercise guidelines safely and effectively. *Canada's Physical Activity Guide*[18] summarizes current thought on endurance, flexibility, and strengthening in easily understood terms. The section on how to judge for yourself whether your exercise routine is sufficiently intense is particularly helpful when educating those with mild lung disease (Table 11.7). Since it uses changes in breathing sensation as one guideline, patients can be reminded that dyspnoea is a normal response to exercise, and dyspnoea of itself is not harmful.

Table 11.6 Sample exercise programme for someone with moderate to severe dyspnoea

	Time (min)	Exercises	
Warm up	5–10	1	Walking at a comfortable pace
		2	Raise arms above your head, deep breathing as you lift
		3	Walk in place and swing your arms
Overload ('hard work')	20–40	4	Punch the ceiling (alternately lift arms above head; hold a small weight if possible)
		5	Standing, shrug shoulders holding a small weight or pulling an elastic exercise band
		6	Shallow knee bending (progress to doing this with your back against the wall)
		7	Sitting, with an elastic exercise band for each hand, tied to something sturdy: do a rowing motion
		8	Treadmill or brisk walking
		9	Standing, heel raises
Cool down	5–10	10	Walk in place and swing your arms
		11	Raise arms above your head, deep breathing as you lift
		12	Walking at a comfortable pace

Table 11.7 Sample exercise programme for someone with mild to moderate dyspnoea

	Time (min)	Exercises	
Warm up	5–10	1	Walking at a comfortable pace
		2	Reaching overhead with deep breathing
		3	Slow marching in place
Overload ('hard work')	20–40[a]	4	Alternately lifting a small weight toward the ceiling
		5	Stepping on and off the bottom step of a staircase, or a sturdy stool
		6	Using an elastic exercise band, pull the band diagonally in both directions
		7	Stationary bicycle
		8	Arm ergometer
		9	Treadmill
Cool down	5–10	10	Slow marching in place
		11	Reaching overhead with deep breathing
		12	Walking at a comfortable pace

a An easy activity between each difficult one will allow better breath control.

Although the Canadian guidelines for people with a normal cardiovascular–respiratory system are designed to be used by lay people, they can also be used by healthcare practitioners who do not have access to sophisticated exercise testing equipment, and whose main exercise goal is functional improvement, rather than maximal physiological change.

People with mild to moderate disease may be able to tolerate continuous exercise, or may require only a few brief intervals of lower intensity exercise during the overload component of their programme. The example in Table 11.7 shows interval exercise using the general guidelines for duration. Appropriate intensity would have to be judged for each patient.

When supervised exercise is not available with the recommended frequency, patients should be provided with a written exercise programme that they can perform on their own between visits.

Follow-up

Maintenance of fitness requires less effort than that required to improve it, and exercise effects are temporary. Obvious loss of work capacity occurs if anyone stops exercising for 2 weeks, and all improvements can be lost in several months.[17] For this reason, follow-up after a structured rehabilitation programme is completed is strongly advised.

Follow-up exercise may take many shapes. First, each patient must be provided with an individualized exercise programme at discharge, with specific instructions on how to proceed on their own. Provision of supervised exercise sessions will encourage some patients to continue to stay active, and provides an opportunity for exercise programmes to be progressed appropriately. A variety of exercise settings or modes will appeal to a broader spectrum of patients. Exercise in the gym with varied equipment, in group walking sessions, or in the pool will appeal to different patients. If the healthcare facility which offered the pulmonary rehabilitation programme cannot offer these services, it may be possible to have exercise sessions provided by private enterprises in the community, such as health and fitness clubs. Continuing contact by the pulmonary rehabilitation programme staff will help to encourage the patients. This contact may be by return visits to the facility, through newsletters or by telephone.[1,3,22]

Ongoing psychosocial support after discharge from a pulmonary rehabilitation programme is another factor which will enhance long-term healthy lifestyles. The new methods which the patients learned for coping with their disease, such as proper medication use, changes in diet, relaxation techniques, or active lifestyle suggestions, can be easily lost once patients return to their former day-to-day routines. Group reunions and other ways of bringing patients together again will provide ongoing opportunities for peer support. Telephone calls or newsletters help patients to feel connected to a community which understands their unique needs. Providing patients with a variety of ways to continue to enjoy life in spite of their disease, and reminding them from time to time of other options available, will help them to maintain a positive outlook on life.

Keypoints

- ◆ The goal of pulmonary rehabilitation is to achieve and maintain an individual's maximum level of independence and functioning in the community
- ◆ This is best achieved by a multidisciplinary team through a combination of education counselling and exercise, assisting patients to reduce or gain control of their symptoms

◆ Important components of a rehabilitation programme are:
 – education and counselling
 – breathing retraining
 – techniques to control abrupt and unexpected breathlessness
 – exercise

◆ Components of an exercise programme are flexibility training, strengthening exercises, and cardiovascular endurance exercise. Patients with almost any level of disability may benefit

◆ Exercise prescription should be preceded by an exercise capacity assessment, for example the 6-min walking distance, a shuttle walk test, or a treadmill test to measure VO_{2max}.

◆ The intensity, mode, duration, and frequency of exercise should be individually prescribed

◆ Exercise programmes require a follow-up policy either in hospital or in the community

References

1 Goldstein, R.S., Gort, E.H., Stubbing, D., Avendano, M.A., and Guyatt, G.H. Randomised controlled trial of respiratory rehabilitation. *Lancet* 1994; **344**: 1394–97.

2 Lacasse, Y., Wong, E., Guyatt, G.H., *et al.* Meta-analysis of respiratory rehabilitation in chronic obstructive pulmonary disease. *Lancet* 1996; **348**: 1115–19.

3 Ries, A.L., Carlin, B.W., Carrieri-Kohlman, V., *et al.* Pulmonary rehabilitation: Joint ACCP/AACVPR evidence-based guidelines. *Chest* 1997; **112**: 1363–96.

4 Fishman, A.P. Pulmonary rehabilitation research. *Am J Respir Crit Care Med* 1994; **149**: 825–33.

5 May, D.F. Exercise and reconditioning in pulmonary patients. In: J.W. Youtsey (ed.) *Rehabilitation and continuity of care in pulmonary disease.* St. Louis, M.O.: Mosby-Year Book, 1991; 72–94.

6 Kaplan, R.M., Eakin, E.G., and Ries, A.L. Psychosocial issues in the rehabilitation of patients with chronic obstructive pulmonary disease. In: R. Casaburi, and T. Petty (eds) *Principles and practice of pulmonary rehabilitation.* Philadelphia: W.B. Saunders, 1993; 351–65.

7 Reardon, J., Awad, E., Normandin, E., *et al.* The effect of comprehensive outpatient rehabilitation on dyspnoea. *Chest* 1994; **105**: 1046–52.

8 Casaburi, R. Exercise training in chronic lung disease. In: R. Casaburi (ed.) *Principles and practice of pulmonary rehabilitation.* Philadelphia: W.B. Saunders, 1993; 204–24.

9 Sotile, W.M. The importance of psychosocial interventions in the treatment of cardiopulmonary patients. In: R.A. Washburn and E. Mustain (eds) *Psychosocial interventions for cardiopulmonary patients.* Champaign, IL: Human Kinetics, 1996; 3–12.

10 Ries, A.L., Kaplan, R.M., Limberg, T.M., *et al.* Effects of pulmonary rehabilitation on physiologic and psychosocial outcomes in patients with chronic obstructive pulmonary disease. *Ann Intern Med* 1995; **122**: 823–32.

11 Emery, C.F., Leatherman, N.E., Burker, E.J., and MacIntyre, N.R., Psychological outcomes of a pulmonary rehabilitation program. *Chest* 1991; **100**: 613–17.

12 Haas, F., Salazar-Schicci, J., and Axen, K. Desensitization to dyspnoea in chronic obstructive pulmonary disease. In: R. Casaburi, and T. Petty (eds) *Principles and practice of pulmonary rehabilitation.* Philadelphia: W.B. Saunders, 1993; 204–24.

13 O'Donnell, D.E., and Webb, K.A. Exertional breathlessness in patients with chronic airflow obstruction. The role of lung hyperinflation. *Am Rev Respir Dis* 1993; **148**: 1351–7.

14 Killion, K.J. Dyspnea: implications for rehabilitation. In: R. Casaburi, and T. Petty (eds) *Principles and practice of pulmonary rehabilitation.* Philadelphia: W.B. Saunders, 1993; 103–14.

15 Faling, L.J. Controlled breathing techniques and chest physical therapy in chronic obstructive pulmonary disease and allied conditions. In: R. Casaburi, and T. Petty (eds) *Principles and practice of pulmonary rehabilitation*. Philadelphia: W.B. Saunders, 1993; 167–82.

16 National Institutes of Health Consensus Development Conference Statement no.101. Physical activity and cardiovascular health. NIH consensus statement, 18–20 December 1995; 1–33. NIH Consensus Program Information Centre, P.O. Box 2577, Kensington, MD 20891.

17 Kisner, C., and Colby, L.A. In: C. McNichol and R. Massey (eds) *Therapeutic exercise foundations and techniques*, 3rd edn. Philadelphia: F.A. Davis, 1996.

18 *Handbook for Canada's physical activity guide to healthy active living*. Ottawa, Ontario: Health Canada and Canadian Society for Exercise Physiology, 1998.

19 Delorme, T.L., and Watkins, A. *Progressive resistance exercise*. New York: Appleton-Century, 1951.

20 Mahler, D.A., Froelicher, V.F., Houston Miller, N., and York, T.D. In: W.L. Kenney, R.E. Humphrey, and C.X. Bryant (eds) *ACSM's guidelines for exercise testing and prescription*, 5th edn. Baltimore, M.d.: American College of Sports Medicine, Williams & Wilkins, 1995.

21 D'Arsigny, C., and O'Donnell, D. Will exercise help my COPD patient?. *Med N America* 1997; (July/August): 40–6.

22 J.A. Marx (ed.) *American Association of Cardiovascular and Pulmonary Rehabilitation Guidelines for pulmonary rehabilitation programs*, 2nd edn. Champaign, IL: Human Kinetics, 1998.

23 Sharp, C.T., Busse, E.F., Burgess, J.J., and Haennel, R.G. Exercise prescription for patients with pacemakers. *J Cardiopulmonary Rehabil* 1998; **18**: 421–31.

24 Patessio, A., Iolo, F., and Donner, C.F. In: R. Casaburi, and T. Petty (eds) *Principles and practice of pulmonary rehabilitation*. Philadelphia: W.B. Saunders, 1993.

25 McKirnan, M.D., and Froelicher, V.F. General principles of exercise testing. In: J.S. Skinner (ed.) *Exercise testing and exercise prescription for special cases, theoretical basis and clinical application*, 2nd edn. Philadelphia, Pa.: Lea & Febiger, 1993; 3–27.

26 Cooper, K.H. A means of assessing maximal oxygen intake. *JAMA* 1968; **203**: 138.

27 McGavin, C.R., Gupta, S.P., and McHardy, G.J. Twelve-minute walking test for assessing disability in chronic bronchitis. *Br Med J* 1976; **3**: 822–3.

28 Guyatt, G.H., Pugsley, S.O., Sullivan, M.J., *et al*. Effect of encouragement on walking test performance. *Thorax* 1984; **39**: 818–22.

29 Swinburn, C.R., Wakefield, J.M., and Jones, P.W. Performance, ventilation, and oxygen consumption in three different types of exercise test in patients with chronic obstructive lung disease. *Thorax* 1985; **40**, 581–6.

30 Singh, S.J., Morgan, M.D., Scott, S., Walters, D., and Hardman, A.E. Development of a shuttle walking test of disability in patients with chronic airways obstruction. *Thorax* 1992; **47**: 1019–24.

31 Singh, S.J., Morgan, M.D., Hardman, A.E., Rowe, C., and Bardsley, P.A. Comparison of oxygen uptake during a conventional treadmill test and the shuttle walking test in chronic airflow limitation. *Eur Respir J* 1994; **7**: 2016–20.

32 Skinner, J.S. General principles of exercise prescription. In: J.S. Skinner (ed.) *Exercise testing and exercise prescription for special cases. Theoretical basis and clinical application*. Philadelphia, Pa.: Lea & Febiger, 1993; 29–40.

33 Karvonen, M., Kentala, K., and Musta, O. The effects of training on heart rate: a longitudinal study. *Ann Med Exp Biol Fenn* 1957; **35**: 307.

34 Hodgkin, J.E., and Litzau, K.L. Exercise training target heart rates in chronic obstructive pulmonary disease. *Chest* 1988; **94**: 305.

35 Wesmiller, S.W., and Hoffman, L.A. Evaluation of an assistive device for ambulation in oxygen dependent patients with COPD. *J Cardiopulmonary Rehabil* 1994; **14**: 122–26.

36 Honeyman, P., Barr, P., and Stubbing, D.G. Effect of a walking aid on disability, oxygenation, and breathlessness in patients with chronic airflow limitation. *J Cardiopulmonary Rehabil* 1996; **16**: 63–7.

37 Borg, G. Psychophysical bases of perceived exertion. *Med Sci Sports Exerc* 1982; **14**: 377–381.

38 Wasserman, K. Exercise tolerance in the pulmonary patient. In: R. Casaburi and T. Petty (eds) *Principles and practice of pulmonary rehabilitation*. Philadelphia: W.B. Saunders, 1993; 115–23.

39 Stein, D.A., Bradley, B.L., and Miller, W.C. Mechanisms of oxygen effects on exercise in patients with chronic obstructive pulmonary disease. *Chest* 1982; **81**: 6–10.

40 Zack, M.B., and Palange, A.V. Oxygen supplemented exercise of ventilatory and nonventilatory muscles in pulmonary rehabilitation. *Chest* 1985; **88**: 669–74.

41 Nixon, P.A., Orenstein, D.M., Curtis, S.E., and Ross, E.A. Oxygen supplementation in cystic fibrosis. *Am Rev Respir Dis* 1990; **142**: 807–11.

42 Killion, K.J., Summers, E., Jones, N.L., and Campbell, E.J. Dyspnea and leg effort during incremental cycle ergometry. *Am Rev Respir Dis* 1992; **145**: 1339–45.

43 Pineda, H., Haas, F., Axen, K., and Haas, A. Ability of standardized pulmonary function tests to predict exercise capability. *Chest* 1984; **86**: 564–7.

44 Celli, B.R. Pulmonary rehabilitation for patients with advanced lung disease. *Clin Chest Med* 1997; **18**: 521–33.

Chapter 12

Dyspnoea and respiratory muscle training

Hans Folgering and Yvonne Heijdra

Dyspnoea in obstructive pulmonary disease

Dyspnoea is a multifactorial condition that can be described by an operational definition: 'the unpleasant awareness of the need to breathe'. It occurs in pulmonary, cardiac, or neurological disease; in anaemia; and also in patients with a hyperventilation problem, or in situations of detraining in normal healthy subjects.[1] This chapter deals mainly with dyspnoea in patients with obstructive pulmonary diseases: asthma and COPD. The underlying mechanisms, respiratory muscle dysfunction, and load on these muscles will be discussed, as well as the effects of general exercise training and of respiratory muscle training on dyspnoea.

The descriptions of dyspnoea, used by patients vary substantially: shortness of breath, 'can't get enough air', suffocation, chest tightness, smothering, fatigue, heaviness of breathing, or plain 'fatigue'.

The underlying mechanisms that contribute to dyspnoea are multiple and complex. There is no single mechanism or receptor stimulus that will fully explain it, nor is there a single therapy that abolishes this unpleasant sensation. Multiple sensory pathways may lead to dyspnoea; when one pathway is alleviated or blocked, another one may take over. (See Chapter 6 for a full discussion of mechanism of dyspnoea.)

A diagram may help the reader to understand some of the underlying mechanisms and their interactions (Figure 12.1). Starting in the upper left corner: isolated increased activity in the 'respiratory centres' of the brain (which do not necessarily result in an actual increase of ventilation) can be perceived as a respiratory sensation, as shown by hypnosis experiments and experiments in patients with spinal cord lesions. When the ventilatory drive produces respiratory muscle activity, the afferent nerve proprioceptor activity in these muscles can be perceived. The magnitude of the perception can be modified by the strength and any possible fatigue of these muscles.[2] This is probably one of the major pathways that mediates dyspnoea in patients with obstructive pulmonary disease. A mismatch between the degree of motor command (effort) and the actual change in length of the respiratory muscles or the actual change in thoracic volume (which means an disproportion between the tension in these muscles and their length) appears to be very dyspnogenic.

Hyperinflation, as occurs in COPD patients, will make the lungs and thoracic wall operate on the flatter upper part of their pressure–volume curves. Hyperinflation means that a relatively large effort has to be made for further small expansions of the lung. Thus hyperinflation itself also contributes to dyspnoea. Reduction of this hyperinflation, as is achieved by lung-volume reduction surgery, will alleviate dyspnoea by improving respiratory muscle function.[3]

An increase in vagal afferent traffic originating from rapidly adapting receptors, from slowly adapting receptors in the airways, or from J-receptors in the lungs, may also lead to dyspnoea.

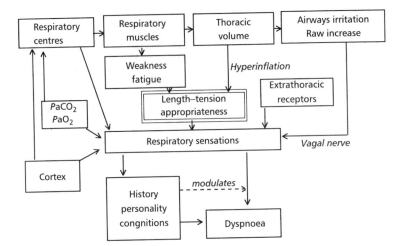

Fig. 12.1 Mechanisms contributing to production of dyspnoea. The following factors contribute to respiratory sensations: increased activity of the 'respiratory centres', increased activity of respiratory muscles modulated by fatigue or weakness; hyperinflation and high thoracic volume; stimulation of airway receptors by an increase in airway resistance (R_{aw}) or irritant receptor stimulation via vagal afferents; chemoreceptor stimulation (by a low arterial PO_2 and/or high PCO_2). The processing of these sensations, influenced by personality factors, personal history, and cognitions, will eventually lead to a more or less intense sensation of dyspnoea.

However, the fact that patients also become dyspnoeic after lung transplantation, in spite of their vagal denervation, suggests that these vagal afferents are not essential for generation of dyspnoea.[4]

Chemoreceptor stimulation from a high arterial PCO_2 and/or a low PO_2 also contributes to dyspnoea. This may work either by direct pathways from chemoreceptors to the cerebral cortex, or via stimulation of respiratory centres, and the perception of the subsequent increased respiratory effort.

The perception of dyspnoea is modulated by a person's history, adaptations to these perceptions, and by his/her personality and cognitions. A patient with unstable asthma, remembering his last severe attack that ended in an acute hospital admission, might feel more dyspnoeic than a stable COPD patient with the same degree of airway obstruction that has gradually developed over a period of years. Cognitive techniques can be useful in the therapy of dyspnoea.[5]

Effects of exercise

During exercise, several stimuli come together to increase the sensation of dyspnoea in patients with obstructive pulmonary disease. Respiratory effort is increased as a result of an increased ventilatory drive.

In these patients, the increased ventilatory drive will cause greater length–tension disparity, more hyperinflation, possible hypoxia and hypercapnia, and more anaerobic metabolism because physical fitness is lower than in healthy subjects. The respiratory load that has to be overcome by these patients is increased because of the increased airways resistance and lung hyperinflation. The 'chemical drive' for breathing may increase due to (relative) hypoventilation and impaired oxygen uptake. Dyspnoea is increased in proportion to the degree of airway obstruction, and in proportion to the peak inspiratory pressures that the patient *has* to generate, relative to the maximal inspiratory pressures that the patient *can* generate (Figure 12.2).[2]

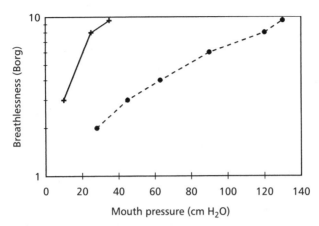

Fig. 12.2 Breathlessness and ventilatory effort. Breathlessness, scored on a modified Borg scale, versus mouth pressure, during a test of loaded breathing, in subjects with two different levels of inspiratory muscle strength ($P_{i\,max}$): 48 cmH$_2$O (4.7 kPa) (solid line) and 180 cmH$_2$O (17.6 kPa) (broken line). Subjects with a low inspiratory muscle strength have high levels of dyspnoea at low inspiratory loads. Reproduced with permission from Kilian and Jones (1988).[2]

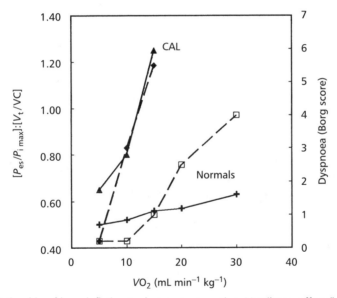

Fig. 12.3 Relationship of hyperinflation to dyspnoea perception. Ventilatory effort (length–tension disparity) on left ordinate, and dyspnoea on right ordinate, in a group of normal subjects and a group of patients with chronic airflow limitation (CAL) during an incremental exercise test, with VO_2 max increasing from left to right (abscissa). The broken lines represent the perceived sensation of dyspnoea at different workloads. $P_{es}/P_{i\,max}$: VT/VC reflects the relationship between effort and ventilatory output. Note that the CAL patients have to generate a high percentage of $P_{i\,max}$ for every percent of their vital capacity (because of their starting hyperinflation). P_{es}, oesophageal pressure generated at each level of exercise; $P_{i\,max}$, maximum static inspiratory pressure; VT, tidal volume; VC, vital capacity; VO_2, oxygen consumption in mL/min per kg body weight. Reproduced with permission from O'Donnell et al. (1997).[6]

The hyperinflation induced by dynamic exercise can be so extreme that the end-inspiratory lung volume approaches the total lung capacity. The oesophageal pressures that are required for maintaining this hyperinflation in exercise approach 50% of the maximal inspiratory intrapleural pressure; the increase in dyspnoea parallels this increase in work by the respiratory muscles (Figure 12.3).[6]

In patients with severe COPD, respiratory pump failure may occur. Thus, in spite of maximal effort of the respiratory muscles, the patient cannot maintain carbon dioxide homeostasis, and arterial PCO_2 rises during exercise. In a study on 50 patients with obstructive pulmonary disease, we found that the work performed by the respiratory muscles during exercise was the main determinant of dyspnoea as long as the patients remained normocapnic. The total work performed by both the inspiratory muscles and expiratory muscles showed the best correlation with dyspnoea. However, as soon as our patients became hypercapnic, the dyspnoea was completely dominated by this chemoreceptor drive.[7]

Dyspnoea often limits exercise capacity in patients with obstructive pulmonary disease. Thus patients tend to avoid exercise and become negatively conditioned to the unpleasant sensations that they experience. This, in turn, leads to a sedentary lifestyle and to further deconditioning, not only of the cardiocirculatory system, but also of peripheral and respiratory muscles, and subsequently aerobic capacity decreases. Any exercise will then lead to early lactate production and more ventilatory drive. This cannot lead to an appropriately increased ventilation, because of the airway obstruction and the hyperinflation. Thus patients are caught in a negative spiral where dyspnoea and deconditioning mutually augment each other.[8]

Respiratory muscle function

Maximal inspiratory pressure ($P_{i\,max}$) is reported to be lower in patients with COPD than in healthy subjects[9,10] (see Table 12.1). The ability of the diaphragm to generate volume is influenced by its length. Hyperinflated patients have a shortened diaphragm, which works at a more unfavourable position on the length–tension curve, and therefore generates lower inspiratory pressures and less volume change.

The effects of hypoxia and hypercapnia on muscle performance have been investigated only in the acute situation. The isolated effects of chronic changes in blood gases, as in patients with COPD, is not known. Administered oxygen seems to delay the onset of diaphragm fatigue in normal subjects.[11]

Corticosteroids may induce myopathy of the respiratory muscles, with reduction in values of $P_{i\,max}$ and $P_{e\,max}$. Malnutrition is important in patients with COPD, since it reduces respiratory muscle strength and maximal voluntary ventilation.[12] Refeeding of malnourished patients can lead to improvement of respiratory muscle strength (see Chapter 14).[13]

Respiratory muscle fatigue was shown to occur in normal subjects when they had to breathe through a resistance and had to use more than 60% of $P_{i\,max}$. The dynamic hyperinflation during exercise in patients with obstructive pulmonary disease often does not allow an increase in respiratory tidal volume. Thus respiratory frequency increases, with a corresponding increase in deadspace ventilation. Tachypnoea is one of the features of respiratory muscle fatigue; another feature is an alternating activity of intercostal respiratory muscles and diaphragm, resulting in paradoxical breathing.[14] Rapid shallow breathing and paradoxical breathing are inefficient ways of breathing, so they lead to further fatigue, with high deadspace ventilation and high levels of dyspnoea.

The lung volume at which the maximal inspiratory and expiratory manoeuvres are performed influences respiratory pressures, since the length of the respiratory muscles and therefore their

Table 12.1 Reference values for maximal inspiratory
and expiratory mouth pressures

Men			Women		
Age (years)	$P_{i\,max}$ (kPa)	$P_{e\,max}$ (kPa)	Height (cm)	$P_{i\,max}$ (kPa)	$P_{e\,max}$ (kPa)
20	12.1	16.2	150	6.4	8.6
25	11.6	15.7	155	6.7	8.9
30	11.1	15.3	160	7.1	9.2
35	10.6	14.8	165	7.4	9.4
40	10.1	14.4	170	7.8	9.7
45	9.6	13.9	175	8.1	10.0
50	9.0	13.5	180	8.5	10.3
55	8.5	13.0	185	8.8	10.5
60	8.0	12.5	190	9.2	10.8
65	7.5	12.1	195	9.6	11.1
70	7.0	11.6			
75	6.5	11.2			

Reference values for $P_{i\,max}$ and $P_{e\,max}$ according to Wilson et al.,[9] measured with a flanged mouthpiece, from residual volume (RV) and from total lung capacity (TLC) respectively.

Equations:

Men: $P_{i\,max} = 14.2 - (0.103 \times \text{age})$, SD = 3.1 kPa; $P_{e\,max} = 10.8 - (0.091 \times \text{age})$, SD = 3.4 kPa.

Women: $P_{i\,max} = -4.3 + (0.071 \times \text{cm})$, SD = 2.2 kPa; $P_{e\,max} = 0.35 + (0.055 \times \text{cm})$, SD = 1.7 kPa.

Figures for men are derived from age alone: reference values for women are derived from these by subtraction from the figure for the appropriate age, with a correction for height.

contractile properties vary with lung volume. The highest static inspiratory pressures ($P_{i\,max}$) are measured at residual volume (RV), while the highest expiratory pressures are measured at total lung capacity (TLC), because at these lung volumes the optimal length of the inspiratory and expiratory muscles respectively is reached. Sniff inspiratory pressures are a more dynamic way of measuring maximal strength, and are measured at functional residual capacity (FRC). The choice of mouthpiece, flanged or tubed, influences the measured respiratory pressures.[15]

Body position can influence pressure measurement. In healthy subjects respiratory pressures are higher in the sitting than in the supine position; in COPD patients it is the other way around.[16] This is caused by the increased phasic and tonic activity of the scalene, sternocleido-mastoid, and parasternal-intercostal muscles and the increased compliance of the ribcage when sitting, as compared to lying supine.

Measurement of respiratory muscle endurance is even more complicated. Respiratory muscle endurance is defined as the capacity of the respiratory muscles to generate and sustain a certain level of inspiratory pressure. Sustained maximal voluntary ventilation and resistive breathing are two types of endurance tests. These methods are highly dependent on flow rates and breathing patterns have to be strictly defined and controlled, otherwise subjects tend to adopt a non-fatiguing breathing pattern with low flow rates. For these reasons, the inspiratory threshold loading test was developed. A weighted plunger is used as inspiratory valve. This ensures that a constant pressure is generated with each breath and it allows subjects to vary tidal volume freely,[17] so the results are independent of flow rates.

Muscle fatigue is defined as a condition in which there is a loss in capacity for developing force or velocity of a contracting muscle, which results from muscle activity under load, and which is reversible by rest. The mechanisms of fatigue are complex and involve changes at various sites within the muscle, the neuromuscular junction, and the central nervous system. Tests have been developed to measure the change from a non-fatigued unloaded condition to a fatigued state. An example of such a test is measurement of oesophageal or transdiaphragmatic pressures generated during tidal breathing at exercise . The pressure time index (PTi) was defined as the product of the mean intrathoracic pressure developed during tidal breathing (P_i) divided by $P_{i\,max}$, multiplied by the duration of contraction (T_i) divided by the total duration of the respiratory cycle (T_{tot}):

$$PTi = [P_i/P_{i\,max}] \times [T_i/T_{tot}]$$

Bellemare and Grassino[18] showed that the critical PTi for fatigue of the diaphragm for normal subjects is 0.15. The PTi of the ribcage muscles was studied by Zocchi et al.[19] They found that the fatigue threshold for these muscles was 0.30. In patients with a similar stage of amyotrophic lateral sclerosis, those with dyspnoea had a lower strength of both inspiratory and expiratory muscles. The authors hypothesized that this was mainly due to a diaphragmatic dysfunction.[20]

Effects of general exercise training

General exercise training has been shown to improve respiratory muscle function in several human and animal studies. Endurance exercise on a treadmill improved oxidative capacity of the costal diaphragm and intercostal muscles in rats. Mitochondrial enzyme activity increased by 20–30%, and antioxidants such as superoxide dismutase were upregulated. Even low intensity endurance training resulted in a 13–20% increase of oxidative fibres in the costal diaphragm in these animals. Also expiratory muscles such as the rectus abdominis and external obliques benefited from general exercise training, in contrast to the internal obliques and transversus abdominis of these rats which did not improve.[21]

O'Donnell et al. trained 20 patients with chronic airflow limitation (mean FEV_1 40 ± 3% predicted) in a 6-week rehabilitation programme.[22] $P_{i\,max}$ increased by 28% and $P_{e\,max}$ by 26%.

Box 12.1 Measures of respiratory muscle strength, endurance, and fatigue

Strength:

Maximum mouth inspiratory pressure (MMIP) and residual volume, and maximum mouth expiratory pressure (as total lung capacity) – voluntary

Twitch stimulation of phrenic nerve – involuntary

Endurance: Inspiratory threshold loading test (weighted plunger)

Fatigue: Oesophageal of transdiagramatic pressures on exercise

Inspiratory muscle endurance increased 2.8-fold. Dyspnoea was reduced significantly: the slope of the Borg score during an incremental exercise test reduced from 0.98 units/min to 0.59 units/min. Endurance exercise (walking, cycling, arm-cranking) increased from 24 to 37 min. The percentage of patients stopping exercise because of dyspnoea was 40% before the training, and 45% after the training (not statistically significant). However, the relief of activity-related breathlessness did not correlate significantly with increased respiratory muscle strength or endurance. The only significant correlation was the inverse relationship between exertional breathlessness and breathing frequency.[22]

Reardon studied 20 patients with COPD (mean FEV_1 33 ± 12% predicted): 10 of them were treated in a 6-week rehabilitation program; 10 were controls who had to wait for admission to the programme. Exercise testing was performed until exhaustion, on a treadmill with increasing speed and grade settings. At the end of the rehabilitation period, the VAS exercise-dyspnoea score in the treatment group decreased from 74.4 to 50.5, whereas in the control group this score did not change significantly (72.0 and 79.4). In the treatment group, the minute ventilation at maximal exercise was 30.5 L/min before rehabilitation, and 32.4 L/min after. Consequently, at the same level of ventilation, the sensation of dyspnoea was substantially reduced (Figure 12.4).[23] This might be interpreted as a consequence of improvement of functioning of the respiratory muscles, learning of different breathing strategies (lower frequencies), or desensitization of the subject to sensations from the respiratory muscles.

Casaburi trained 25 COPD patients (mean FEV_1 36% predicted), and found that minute ventilation was lower after training, at the same level of external workload. A lower respiratory frequency and a higher tidal volume were the characteristics of breathing pattern that made deadspace ventilation decrease, and thus the total ventilation more efficient. He hypothesized that this might be possible, as a result of an increased respiratory muscle endurance.[24] Alternatively, these results could also be explained by an improved cardio-circulatory fitness and lower production of lactate, or by an improved peripheral muscle efficiency. Our current knowledge of effects of general exercise training is summarized in Box 12.2.

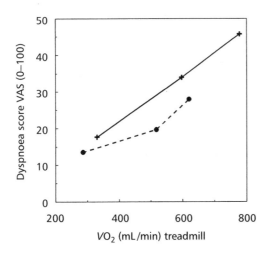

Fig. 12.4 The degree of dyspnoea (FEV_1 33% predicted), during an incremental treadmill test, of 10 patients with COPD after a rehabilitation treatment (circles, broken line), and of 10 matched controls before rehabilitation (crosses, solid line). At the same level of oxygen consumption, the dyspnoea was lower after rehabilitation. (Data from Reardon et al.[23]).

Box 12.2 Effects of general exercise training

♦ General exercise training may improve respiratory muscle function, and does decrease dyspnoea. It is not yet clear what the exact causal relations are: general training reduces dyspnoea possibly through improved strength and endurance of respiratory muscles, probably also through better patient motivation.

♦ The improvement in fitness and in self-efficacy, and the improvement of the efficiency of exercising and the efficiency of breathing, also play a role in diminishing dyspnoea.

♦ The improved ventilation and reduced dyspnoea are a consequence of the change in breathing pattern.

♦ Desensitization to dyspnoea may also occur during a rehabilitation programme.

Inspiratory muscle training

Respiratory muscle strength and endurance can be improved by inspiratory muscle training (IMT). Five methods of training have been described (Table 12.2). Various IMT devices are shown in Figure 12.5.

Voluntary isocapnic hyperpnoea

In this type of training patients perform two or three runs of maximally sustained voluntary ventilation of 15 min under eucapnic conditions each day. This used to be possible only under laboratory conditions. However, Boutellier's group has developed a home-training method for ventilatory muscles which improved endurance performance by 50% in sedentary normal subjects and by 30% in active normal subjects.[25,26] Dyspnoea was significantly reduced in these healthy subjects.

Inspiratory flow resistive training

In this form of training patients breathe through a valve in which the calibre of the inspiratory orifice can be changed (Figure 12.5(a)). When the calibre of the orifice is made smaller the inspiratory effort has to increase. However, the inspiratory pressure depends on the inspiratory flow. The latter needs to be controlled during a training programme, otherwise a non-fatiguing breathing pattern will be adopted. Results from this type of respiratory muscle training are equivocal.

Table 12.2 Inspiratory muscle training (IMT)

Method	Technique
Voluntary hyperventilation with isocapnoea	Constant PCO_2
Inspiratory flow resistive training	Valve with variable opening
Inspiratory threshold loading	Valve loaded with weights or a spring
Targeted flow inspiratory muscle training	Target flow through fixed resistance
Targeted pressure inspiratory muscle training	Target pressure through resistance

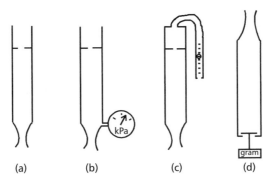

(a)   (b)   (c)   (d)

Fig. 12.5 Four types of inspiratory muscle training devices: (a) Resistive device. Often such devices have variable resistances. Since only a resistance is imposed, the patients have two degrees of freedom in Ohm's law (driving force = resistance × flow) By generating low flows, the patient does not have to generate high mouth pressures, and does not train the respiratory muscles. This type of training device is not recommended. (b) Target-pressure device. This device has a resistance and a manometer. By imposing resistance and target-pressure, the inspiratory muscles can be trained adequately. (c) Target-flow device. A resistor and an incentive flowmeter. When the resistance and flow are imposed, the patient must generate a certain pressure. This device is also adequate for IMT. (d) Threshold-loaded device. At every inspiration through this device, the patient has to generate enough pressure to lift the weighted inspiratory valve. Often the weights on the valve are replaced by an adjustable spring. This is also an adequate IMT device.

Target flow and target pressure inspiratory muscle training

In this method patients are instructed to generate a target inspiratory flow rate through a fixed resistance.[27,28] The flow is measured by an incentive flowmeter with an added resistance (Figure 12.5(c)). In target pressure training (Figure 12.5(b)), the subjects are instructed to inspire through a resistance with a force sufficient to generate a target pressure that can be read from an added manometer.[29] In this way there is a breath-to-breath visual feedback of training intensity, in contrast to training methods with resistive breathing. Both targeted IMT methods have been shown to improve respiratory muscle performance and patient performance, as well as to improve nocturnal saturation in patients with severe COPD.

Inspiratory threshold loading

This uses an inspiratory valve that is loaded with a spring or with weights (Figure 12.5(d)). Thus, a certain level of inspiratory pressure has to be generated with every inspiration, in order to overcome the threshold load and to initiate air flow.

Effects of respiratory muscle training

Accounts of the results of IMT in patients with COPD are conflicting. Some studies show an increase of P_{imax} and/or endurance, whereas other studies are negative.[30,31] The recommendations of the ACCP/AACVPR report on pulmonary rehabilitation[32] are that the evidence for the beneficial effect of respiratory muscle training is 'provided by observational studies or by less consistent results to support the guideline recommendation'. Inspiratory muscle training 'can be considered in selected patients with COPD who have decreased

Box 12.3 Results of inspiratory muscle training

♦ IMT can be considered for patients with obstructive pulmonary disease in whom a low respiratory muscle strength or endurance is established. Respiratory insufficiency, or very high time–pressure product during exercise, can also be a reason for prescribing IMT.

♦ The training device should be a threshold loading device, or a resistance device providing feedback on inspiratory pressure or flow. Mouth pressures of up to 70% of P_{imax} can be imposed during the training sessions.

♦ Two 15-min sessions a day, at least 5 days a week, for 6–10 weeks, are necessary to obtain a training effect. The training should be supervised weekly by a physiotherapist.

♦ Respiratory muscle function will improve, dyspnoea will decrease in most cases, and better exercise performance can be achieved.

respiratory muscle strength and breathlessness'. This working group found 11 randomized trials on respiratory muscle training: 7 showed significant changes in $P_{i\ max}$, but in 4 respiratory muscle function was not improved. Twelve- or six-minute walking distances increased in 5 studies, and respiratory endurance time in 4. Dyspnoea was measured in 2 studies, and improved in both. Improvement was often associated with a decrease in breathing frequency.

Goldstein reviewed a number of studies on respiratory muscle training.[33] He concluded that 'subjects can be trained to improve their performance as measured by a particular test of endurance which is specific to the training modality' Correlations with any improvements in exercise capacity were equivocal. The effects of respiratory muscle training on dyspnoea were not mentioned in this review.

Analysing the studies mentioned above, and others on respiratory muscle training, we found that methodological problems may explain why the results are inconsistent:

♦ In several inspiratory flow-resistive training studies, neither inspiratory flow, nor breathing pattern and inspiratory pressure, was controlled.

♦ Patient compliance was not always assured.

♦ In some studies, no selection criteria were defined: i.e. which patients could possibly benefit from training their inspiratory muscles (those with low P_{imax}, or high PTi and/or hypercapnia at exercise).

♦ Not all studies had a control group.

♦ The duration of the total training period varied from 4 weeks to 6 months.

♦ There were differences in training frequency, duration, intensity, and devices used.

♦ Sometimes the number of patients enrolled was small.

The studies summarized in Table 12.3 seem to fulfil most of the methodological criteria.

Belman and Shadmehr trained respiratory muscles in 17 COPD patients who were randomized into a high- and a low-intensity training group.[34] The training consisted of two 15-minute sessions daily, 6 days a week for 6 weeks, breathing through a resistive device (P-flex) that

Table 12.3 Recent studies on the benefit of inspiratory muscle training in COPD

Authors	Year	Reference	Number of patients	Intervention	Conclusion
Belman and Shadmehr	1988	34	17	Resistive device 6 weeks	$P_{i\,max}$ better
Harver et al.	1989	29	19	Target pressure training	$P_{i\,max}$ better
Dekhuijzen et al.	1991	27	40	Target flow training 6 weeks muscles and a 12-min walk	Better
Lisboa et al.	1994	36	10	Threshold loading	$P_{i\,max}$ and 6-min walk test better
Wanke et al.	1994	35	42	Strength training muscles andexercise performance	Better
Heijdra et al.	1996	28	10	Target flow training diaphragm strength and overnight SaO_2	Better
Larson et al.	1999	37	53	IMT and cycle exercise training	Both improved dyspnoea
Weiner et al.	2000	38	82	IMT	Improved dyspnoea
Weiner et al.	2000	39	30	IMT	No benefit with exercise training, but IMT improved dyspnoea

provided feedback on the negative mouth pressure that had to be generated. The training was supervised in a pulmonary laboratory once a week. The high-intensity training group improved $P_{i\,max}$ from 42 to 50 cmH$_2$O (3.92 to 4.9 kPa) and increased the maximal sustainable ventilatory capacity from 23 L/min to 26 L/min ($p = 0.03$). This study shows that the ventilatory pump can be improved significantly by adequate training methods. No dyspnoea was measured in this study.

Our group studied 40 COPD patients with a ventilatory limited exercise capacity (hypercapnia at maximal work load) during a pulmonary rehabilitation treatment programme. They were randomized either to receiving additional target-flow IMT for 6 weeks, or not. Respiratory muscle function ($P_{i\,max}$, EMG fatiguability of the diaphragm) increased significantly more in the IMT group, as compared to the rehabilitation-only group. The 12-min walking distance increased significantly more in the group with additional IMT (263 versus 194 m improvement, $p < 0.01$). The score for activities of daily life increased more in the group with additional inspiratory muscle training. The changes in scores for anxiety, depression, and for physical complaints were unchanged.[27]

Harver et al. trained 19 COPD patients; 10 with target-pressure IMT and 9 controls.[29] The training group used a resistive device (P-flex) with an added manometer in the mouthpiece, and achieved a significant improvement in $P_{i\,max}$ (measured from FRC) from 47 to 62 cmH$_2$O (4.6 to 6.08 kPa), and a significant decrease in the Transitional Dyspnoea Index subscales on functional impairment, magnitude of task, magnitude of effort, and total score. The training group also seemed to show a lower respiratory frequency, though this was not statistically significant. Significant correlations were found between the changes in inspiratory muscle strength and the Transitional Dyspnoea Index.

Wanke *et al.* applied general exercise training in 42 COPD patients with a mild to moderate obstructive disease (mean FEV_1 46% pred)icted.[35] In this study 21 patients were given additional strength training for their respiratory muscles. The latter group achieved higher levels of exercise performance (99 W versus 80 W), better respiratory muscle strength (8.1 kPa versus 5.8 kPa) and endurance, and higher levels of maximal minute ventilation (55 L/min versus 48 L/min) after the training. The Borg score for dyspnoea at maximal exercise was the same in both groups: 7.2 and 7.0 units. However, since the group that received additional respiratory muscle training reached higher levels of maximal oxygen consumption, and higher levels of minute ventilation, and since neither group reached the maximum Borg score for breathlessness (no 'ceiling-effect'), this must be interpreted as an improvement of the dyspnoea due to the respiratory muscle training.

COPD patients often suffer from nocturnal hypoventilation during REM sleep, because of diaphragmatic weakness. We trained 10 patients (FEV_1 35.5% predicted) with target-flow IMT at a mouth pressure of 60% of $P_{i\,max}$ twice daily for 10 weeks; another 10 patients were given sham training. Mean nocturnal saturation improved from 89% to 91% in the treatment group, whereas it did not change in the control group. The percentage of sleeping time spent at saturations <90% decreased from 55% to 28% in the treatment group, and did not change in the control group. Maximal transdiaphragmatic pressure improved from 6.6 kPa to 10.0 kPa in the treatment group. This shows that the diaphragm can be trained by adequate IMT, and that this leads to better nocturnal oxygenation in severe COPD patients.[28]

In a study by Lisboa *et al.*, isolated IMT was performed with a threshold loading device for 10 weeks, at 30% of $P_{i\,max}$ in a group of patients with chronic airflow limitation (mean FEV_1 36% predicted).[36] A control group 'trained' at 10% of $P_{i\,max}$. In the training group the strength of the inspiratory muscles increased significantly (from 6.8 kPa to 9.12 kPa), the 6-min walking distance increased from 303 to 417 m, and the Borg score decreased from 6.6 to 3.4 units. Thus, even low-level (at 30% of $P_{i\,max}$) IMT was able to improve exercise performance, respiratory muscle function, and dyspnoea.

Larson *et al.* studied 53 COPD patients (FEV_1 50% predicted).[37] They were randomly assigned to one of four categories: (1) home inspiratory muscle training with a threshold loading device at 60% of $P_{i\,max}$ 5 days/week and 30 min/day; (2) cycle ergometer training; (3) inspiratory muscle training and cycle ergometer training; (4) health education. Dyspnoea decreased in groups 2 and 3. There was no difference between the groups in the changes in dyspnoea, suggesting that IMT did not contribute significantly in the reduction of dyspnoea.

Weiner *et al.* supplied long-acting bronchodilators to a group of 82 asthma patients.[38] The perception of dyspnoea during breathing through various resistances did not change from control levels. Next, half of these patients received 3 months (6 days/week and 30 min/day) of IMT with a threshold loading device at 60% of $P_{i\,max}$. The other group received sham training. The perception of dyspnoea decreased significantly in the IMT group. The same research group also performed a study on 30 COPD patients (FEV_1 33% predicted).[39] After a run-in with a long-acting bronchodilator (no effect on dyspnoea), all patients received 6 weeks of exercise training, which also did not improve their dyspnoea as compared with baseline. Next, the patient's inspiratory muscles were trained with a threshold loading device at 60% of $P_{i\,max}$. After this IMT, the sensation of dyspnoea when breathing through various resistances was significantly diminished.

Keypoints

♦ Dysfunction of respiratory muscles occurs in COPD patients, and this contributes to dyspnoea

♦ Respiratory muscles can be trained by general exercise training to improve strength and endurance

♦ IMT in particular may be helpful in reducing dyspnoea

♦ Patients may benefit from education to change breathing patterns

References

1   Manning, H.L., and Schwarzenstein, R.M. Pathophysiology of dyspnoea. *N Engl J Med* 1995; **333**: 1547–53.

2   Kilian, K., and Jones, N. Respiratory muscles and dyspnoea. *Clin Chest Med* 1988; **9**: 237–48.

3   Martinez, F.J., Montes de Oca, M., Whyte, R.I., *et al.* Lung volume reduction improves dyspnoea,dynamic hyperinflation, and respiratory muscle function. *Am J Respir Crit Care Med* 1997; **155**: 1984–90.

4   Kimoff, R.J., Cheong, T.H., Cosio, M.G., and Levy, R.D. Pulmonary denervation in humans:effects on dyspnoea and ventilatory pattern during exercise. *Am Rev Respir Dis* 1990; **142**: 1034–40.

5   Guenard, H., Gallego, J., and Dromer, C. Exercise dyspnoea in patients with respiratory disease. *Eur Respir Rev* 1995; **5**(25): 6–13.

6   O'Donnell, D.E., Bertly, J.C., Chau, L.K.L., and Webb, K.A. Qualitative aspects of exertional breathlessness in chronic airflow limitation. *Am J Respir Crit Care Med* 1997; **155**: 109–15.

7   Cloosterman, S.G.M., Hofland, I.D., van Schayck, C.P., and Folgering, H.T.M. Exertional dyspnoea in patients with airway obstruction, with and without CO2-retention. *Thorax* 1998; **53**: 768–74.

8   Prefaut, C., Varray, A., and Vallet, G. Pathophysiological basis of exercise training in patients with chronic obstructive lung disease. *Eur Respir Rev* 1995; **5**: 27–32.

9   Wilson, S.H., Cooke, N.T., Edwards, R.H.T., and Spiro, S.G. Predictive normal values for maximal respiratory pressures in caucasian adults and children. *Thorax* 1984; **39**: 535–8.

10   Wijkstra, P.J., van der Mark, T.W., Boezen, M., van Altena, R., Postma, D.S., and Koëter, G.H. Peak inspiratory mouth pressure in healthy subjects and in patients with COPD. *Chest* 1995; **107**: 652–6.

11   Pardy, R.L., and Bye, P.T.P. Diaphragmatic fatigue in normoxia and hyperoxia. *J Appl Physiol* 1985; **58**: 738–42.

12   Engelen, M.P.K.J., Schols, A.M.W.J., Baken, W.C., Wesseling, G.J., and Wouters, E.F.M. Nutritional depletion in relation to respiratory and peripheral skeletal muscle function in out-patients with COPD. *Eur Respir J* 1994; **7**: 1793–7.

13   Whittaker, S., Ryan, C.F., Buckley, P.A., and Road, J.D. The effects of refeeding on peripheral and respiratory muscle function in malnourished chronic obstructive pulmonary disease patients. *Am Rev Respir Dis* 1990; **142**: 283–8.

14   Mador, M.J. Respiratory muscle fatigue and breathing pattern. *Chest* 1991; **100**: 1430–5.

15   Koulouris, N., Mulvey, D.A., Laroche, C.M., Green, M., and Moxham, J. Comparison of two different mouthpieces for the measurement of PImax and PEmax in normal and weak subjects. *Eur Respir J* 1988; **1**: 863–7.

16   Heijdra, Y.F., Dekhuijzen, P.N.R., van Herwaarden, C.L.A., and Folgering, H.T.M. Effects of body position, hyperinflation, and blood gas tensions on maximal respiratory pressures in patients with COPD. *Thorax* 1994; **49**: 453–8.

17   Nickerson, B.G., and Keens, T.G. Measuring ventilatory muscle endurance in humans as sustainable inspiratory pressure. *J Appl Physiol* 1982; **52**: 768–72.

18 Bellemare, F., and Grassino, A. Effect of pressure and timing of contraction on human diaphragm fatigue. *J Appl Physiol* 1982; **53**: 1190–5.

19 Zocchi, L., Fitting, J.W., Majani, U., *et al.* Effect of pressure and timing of contraction on human ribcage muscle fatigue. *Am Rev Respir Dis* 1993; **147**: 857–64.

20 Similovski, T., Attali, V., Bensimon, G., *et al.* Diaphragmatic dysfunction and dyspnoea in amyotrophic lateral sclerosis. *Eur Respir J* 2000; **15**: 332–7.

21 Powers, S.K., and Criswell, D. Adaptive strategies of repiratory muscles in response to endurance exercise. *Med Sci Sports Exerc* 1996; **28**: 1115–20.

22 O'Donnell, D.E., McGuire, M., Samis, L., and Webb, K.A. General exercise training improves ventilatory en peripheral muscle strength and endurance in chronic airflow limitation. *Am J Respir Crit Care Med* 1998; **157**: 1489–97.

23 Reardon, J., Awad, E., Normandin, E., *et al.* The effect of comprehensive outpatient pulmonary rehabilitation on dyspnoea. *Chest* 1994; **105**: 1046–52.

24 Casaburi, R., Porszasz, J., Burns, M.R., *et al.* Physiologic benefits of exercise training in rehabilitation of patients with severe obstructive pulmonary disease. *Am J Respir Crit Care Medine* 1997; **155**: 1541–51.

25 Boutellier, U., and Piwko, P. The respiratory system as an exercise limiting factor in normal sedentary subjects. *Eur J Appl Physiol* 1992; **64**: 145–52.

26 Boutellier, U. Respiratory muscle fitness and exercise endurance in healthy humans. *Med Sci Sports Exerc* 1998; **30**: 1169–72.

27 Dekhuijzen, P.N.R., Folgering, H.T.M., and van Herwaarden, C.L.A. Target-flow inspiratory muscle training during pulmonary rehabilitation in patients with COPD. *Chest* 1991; **99**: 128–33.

28 Heijdra, Y.F., Dekhuijzen, P.N.R., van Herwaarden, C.L.A., and Folgering, H.T.M. Nocturnal saturation improves by target-flow inspiratory muscle training in patients with COPD. *Am J Respir Crit Care Med* 1996; **153**: 260–5.

29 Harver, A., Mahler, D.A., and Daubenspeck, A. Targeted inspiratory muscle training improves respiratory muscle function and reduces dyspnoea in patients with chronic obstructive pulmonary disease. *Ann Intern Med* 1989; **111**: 117–24.

30 Guyatt, G., Keller, J., Singer, J., Halcrow, S., and Newhouse, M. Controlled trial of respiratory muscle training in chronic airflow limitation. *Thorax* 1982; **47**: 598–602.

31 Gosselink, R., and Decramer, M. Inspiratory muscle training: where are we? *Eur Respir J* 1994; **7**: 2103–5.

32 Ries, A.L., Carlin, B.W., Casaburi, R., *et al.* Pulmonary rehabilitation. *Chest* 1994; **112**: 1363–96.

33 Goldstein, R.S. Ventilatory muscle training. *Thorax* 1993; **48**: 1025–33.

34 Belman, M., and Shadmehr, R. Targeted resistive ventilatory muscle training in chronic obstructive pulmonary disease. *J Appl Physiol* 1988; **65**: 2726–35.

35 Wanke, T., Formanek, D., Lahrmann, H., *et al.* Effects of combined inspiratory muscle training and cycle ergometer training on exercise performance in patients with COPD. *Eur Respir J* 1994; **7**: 2205–11.

36 Lisboa, C., Munoz, V., Beroiza, T., Leiva, A., and Cruz, E. Inspiratory muscle training in chronic airflow limitation: a comparison of two different trainings loads with a threshold device. *Eur Respir J* 1994; **7**: 1266–74.

37 Larson, J.L., Covey, M.K., Wirtz, S.E., *et al.* Cycle ergometer and inspiratory muscle training in chronic obstructive pulmonary disease. *Am J Respir Crit Care Med* 1999; **160**: 500–7.

38 Weiner, P., Berar-Yanay, N., Davidovich, A., Magadle, R., and Weiner, M. Specific inspiratory muscle training in patients with mild asthma with high consumption of inhaled b2-agonists. *Chest* 2000; **117**: 722–7.

39 Weiner, P., Magadle, R., Berar-Yanay, N., Davidovich, A., and Weiner, M. The cumulative effect of long-acting bronchodilators, exercise, and inspiratory muscle training on the perception of dyspnea in patients with advanced COPD. *Chest* 2000; **118**: 672–8.

Chapter 13

Psychosocial therapies

Rod MacLeod

A broad approach to the management of dyspnoea is essential if the person with dyspnoea is going to maximize their potential. In order to identify the most appropriate components of the therapeutic management of dyspnoea it is vital that an accurate assessment of the perception of dyspnoea is undertaken.

Historically, the assessment of breathlessness has tended to focus on the physical attributes of that symptom and has necessarily focused on the physical or sensory features, without including psychological reactions and subjective observations.

It is often suggested that the most effective treatment for dyspnoea is prevention, so attention to the detail of the non-physical dimensions of this complex symptom are essential. Dyspnoea can be seen as a global symptom, but deconstructing the symptom is often helpful in its management. Adaptive breathing patterns are built up often over months or even years and those patterns become familiar to each individual.

For each individual, however, there can be a disjunction between the rate and depth of breathing, so that the health professional can remain confused by mere observation of dyspnoea. Psychosocial therapies involved in the management of dyspnoea do not only rely on an understanding of an intensity measurement which shows the quantity of breathlessness; attention must be paid to the quality of dyspnoea in order to help to recognize the most appropriate therapeutic intervention. Skevington *et al.* underlined the potential value of the linguistic qualities of dyspnoea, designing a scale of breathlessness that was proposed to help direct the therapy to the most appropriate quality.[1] Those authors reinforced the understanding that breathlessness was not purely a sensation but included significant affective and evaluative features. They also showed that dyspnoea included a distinctive, consistent but relatively small component of low energy (fatigue) which had often been subsumed within physical sensations in other studies (Box 13.1). One outcome was that asking the question, 'How would you describe your breathlessness today?' can prove useful in helping to identify the most helpful therapeutic intervention. For example, if a person describes their dyspnoea by using descriptors such as 'frightening' or 'panicky', then adopting a more psychological approach could be beneficial.

Similar observations had previously been made by Kinsman *et al.* when exploring dyspnoea in people with asthma.[2,3] Their original studies focused on two **mood** symptom categories and two **somatic** categories, and this work was elaborated in later studies identifying categories of dyspnoea and congestion alongside three secondary mood categories: worry, loneliness, and anger.

Non-pharmacological nursing intervention

Non-pharmacological interventions for breathlessness can have a significant impact not only on patients' feeling of well-being but also more generally on their quality of life. In developing a nursing approach to managing dyspnoea in lung cancer patients, Corner *et al.*[4] and Bredin *et al.*[5]

Box 13.1 Structure for a scale of breathlessness

- Physical sensations
- Affective/evaluative
- Low energy
- Hyperventilation
- Speechlessness

Source: Skevington *et al.*[1]

---

adopted the psychosocial model of dyspnoea proposed by Steel and Shaver.[6] In order to help direct their interventions, they developed techniques derived from chronic pulmonary disease rehabilitation. Exercise and physiotherapy, biofeedback techniques and progressive muscle relaxation have all been previously identified as being helpful adjuncts to the management of dyspnoea. It is from this background that Corner *et al* developed their nursing intervention strategies (Box 13.2).[7] Their aim was to increase an individual's response to restricted lung function, to increase fitness and confidence to cope with attacks of breathlessness, and to reduce the disability caused by symptoms. They worked with patients with small-cell and non-small-cell lung cancer randomized to intervention or control group (34 patients in total). The study was not blinded, and randomization was stopped after nursing and medical staff observed a clear benefit from the intervention strategy. The intervention group showed a median improvement in 'breathlessness at worst' of 35%, a median improvement in 'distress' of 53%, a median improvement of 17% in 'functional capacity', and a median reduction in 'difficulty in performing activities of daily living' of 21%. The median scores of the non-intervention group were static or deteriorated over the same period. Patients in the intervention group described how they were able to expand their horizons, acknowledged their physical limitations and, addressed their fears and restrictions caused by their disease in general and their breathlessness in particular.

Box 13.2 Strategies used in sessions with patients

- Detailed assessment of dyspnoea and factors affecting it
- Exploration of meaning of dyspnoea, their disease and feelings about the future
- Advice on methods of managing dyspnoea
- Breathing retraining
- Relaxation and distraction
- Goal setting
- Early recognition of problems warranting pharmacological intervention
- Advice on maintaining health

Source: Corner *et al.*[7]

The model outlined by Corner *et al.*[7] is readily translated into differing settings such as a hospice day unit or the patient's home, and has been adopted for use with people whose breathlessness is derived from diseases other than lung cancer.

The process for identifying an appropriate approach to psychosocial management of dyspnoea should include a number of elements.

Psychological response to dyspnoea

The first is an exploration of the **meaning** of dyspnoea for the patient and family and the **feelings** associated with that meaning. This includes asking how these people respond to dyspnoea psychologically, using the following questions:

- What fears do they have? (One of the most commonly held fears is that the patient will choke to death or suffocate.)

- What has been lost by the development of dyspnoea? (Loss of control, independence, or physical function is often seemingly relentless.)

- What degree of control do those people feel they have? (They may feel that health professionals have control with the use of medications; they may feel that their breathing controls them, rather than the other way round.)

- Do they feel responsible in any way for their dyspnoea? (Exploration of their lifestyle before illness and any 'blame' attached to that for the development of their dyspnoea.)

- How do they respond to feelings of panic, anger, loneliness, or worry? (Most people have learned coping strategies for similar emotions throughout their lives that may not be relevant or effective in this situation.)

- What are their hopes for future management of dyspnoea? (Is their hope realistic, or are they hoping for an impossible cure?)

- What goals do they have for their future? (Again, goals for the future must be set in realistic terms.)

- How can they see themselves developing greater control of their dyspnoea? (This can be a most effective way of rebuilding hope.)

Case studies

Case study 13.1 Pat

Pat was a 28-year-old woman with a neuroendocrine tumour that progressed rapidly. Throughout her involvement with the hospice team her predominant symptom had been severe bone pain in multiple sites. About 3 weeks before her death she developed intermittent but severe dyspnoea with coughing and retching. No physical cause was identified and her distress became intense. She described her breathlessness as 'choking', 'suffocating', 'as if I can't get my breath'. Exploration of her fears revealed that she was indeed fearful of suffocation and ultimately she was able to confide in one of the team that she had previously been in an abusive relationship where her partner had tried to strangle her. Discussion of this with reassurance that there was no reason for her to choke or suffocate led to a dramatic reduction in her perception of breathlessness. Despite the later development of a bronchopneumonia she never expressed feelings of breathlessness in such distressing terms again and remained in control of her breathing until she became unconscious just before her death.

Case study 13.2 James

James was a 72-year-old clergyman with COPD who was dependent on steroids and required continuous oxygen therapy when he was first seen by a hospice team member. He was concerned that he was achieving nothing and had nothing to look forward to. On further inquiry it transpired that he had lost his faith and had serious doubts about his previously strongly held religious convictions. A variety of techniques for relaxation including imagery were discussed, and work with the spiritual care team helped him to make some sense of his doubts and fears. Over a period of 2 weeks he learned the effectiveness of imagery for him and became more relaxed and confident – looking forward to participating in his family life. He was able to discontinue his use of oxygen. He talked of his feelings of guilt for some past events and achieved a sense of resolution and forgiveness for himself.

Educational process

The process of education for both patient and family about the meanings, significance, and process of dyspnoea includes an explanation of how and why dyspnoea has developed, including possible psychosocial and behavioural risk factors (for example, smoking). The anatomy and physiology of dyspnoea can be outlined, if appropriate. A basic understanding of the normal mechanisms for the control of breathing can be a simple and effective way of empowering people with dyspnoea. The efficiency and effectiveness of different breathing techniques should be explained, using examples of positioning, muscle groups involved in breathing, rate and depth of respirations associated with the unlearning of any maladaptive techniques that may have already been utilized (for example, rapid shallow breathing, hyperventilation, or unnecessary reliance on oxygen).

Everyday tasks and activities

It is important for the patient and family to acknowledge that the dyspnoea may be a symptom that will never 'come right' and therefore explore more helpful ways of carrying out everyday tasks and activities.

This aspect of management should include a discussion about the difficulty of maintaining hope while the prospect of 'cure' is no longer possible or likely. It also includes an acknowledgement that the professional carers have a commitment to the patient and family and the confirmation that the carers will not lose interest in them as the illness progresses.

Alternative feedback model

A cyclical feedback model has been proposed (Figure 13.1; J. Corner, personal communication).

When adopting a counselling or psychotherapeutic approach it should be borne in mind that these patients often have little energy and a limited prognosis. The exploration of deep-seated issues should only be undertaken if it is envisaged that the person has the time, the energy, and the inclination to address them. It is possible inadvertently to exacerbate the situation by encouraging a focus on fears or loss of control, or providing too great a concentration on the process of breathing.

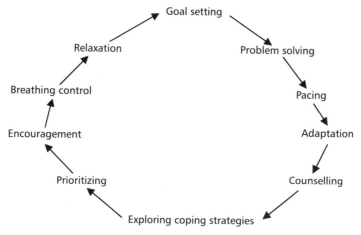

Fig. 13.1 Cyclical feedback model.

Music therapy

Over 20 years ago music therapy was identified as a useful adjunct in aspects of palliative care. The discipline continues to develop, as evidenced by international activity and development of techniques.[8]

Given that dyspnoea has many dimensions, for some patients music therapy could be a useful adjunct in the management of this symptom. In this context, music therapy is the controlled use of music, its elements, and their influences on the human being to aid in the physiological, psychological, and emotional integration of the individual during an illness. It can act as a catalyst in mobilizing deeply held beliefs and feelings, and can assist in communication. From a psychosocial point of view it can help in identifying and reinforcing self-concept and self-worth, it can help to improve the patient's mood, it can help with recall of past significant events, and it can help in exploring fantasy and imagery. From a social point of view it can act as a means of socially acceptable self-expression, recreating a bond and a sense of community with family members, as a link to the patient's life before illness and as entertainment and diversion.

Taylor has described a theory of music therapy that emphasizes the observable effects of music on brain function.[9] His four hypotheses address neurological pathways for the effect of music on pain, neural processing of musical stimuli in the brain for emotion, physiological responses to music associated with communication and movement, and musical influences of stress and anxiety. He ultimately describes music therapy as 'the enhancement of human capabilities through the planned use of music on brain functioning' (ref. 9, p. 121).

It is not within the remit of this chapter to be prescriptive about music therapy, but the options available for the therapist are many. One of the simplest approaches is to prepare an audiotape with a variety of musical selections aimed at inducing relaxation. The therapist can help the patient to choose music that has particular meaning and significance to their life. For example, the use of liturgical music can help a whole family to express religious faith, if that is appropriate. Similarly, the use of ethnic music can help to draw patient and/or family back to their past or their origins.

The therapist can help the patients to play music for themselves. This can be done using percussive instruments or stringed instruments in which the patient may simply have to draw a hand or a bow across the strings of an instrument while the therapist fashions the music.

The therapist may also choose to play music to the patient that may help to elevate mood, encourage relaxation or reflection, or simply as a diversion from the daily routine.

As with all types of therapy, it is essential to stress the need for careful assessment in the introduction and application of music with each person.

Art therapy

Restoring creativity to the dying patient is regarded as an important goal of palliative care teams.[10] As with music therapy, art can be used to help to promote a healthy and safe environment. It can be used as a diversion from pain and breathlessness. It can assist in rehabilitation and can help to build esteem. Where art therapists are not available, this role has sometimes been filled by occupational therapists and physiotherapists. An art therapist has the specific goal of helping patients express themselves, with communication being the prime goal. The artist is concerned with the patient and the artwork is the expression of that patient, nothing more.[11] Patients can be encouraged to become actively involved in creating a picture or painting or they can choose to watch others. Being part of a creative process can provide an escape from everyday life and can help individuals explore their creativity and have fun, which can often be a useful diversion from troublesome or distressing symptoms.

Other strategies that are successfully employed are the creation of collage work, the use of clay for pottery or sculpture and the use of wood or other hard material for creating more permanent art works. Figures 13.2 and 13.3 are examples of works of art created by people with dyspnoea.

Many other media can be used imaginatively in this creative process. As with some of the other strategies outlined, the use of creative art as part of an approach to the management of dyspnoea can help the individual regain some sense of control over aspects of their function that may help in a broader plan for the reduction of dyspnoea.

In this context, 'art' can include all forms of creative and interpretative expression. Other forms of arts, which have been used successfully in the management of symptoms near the end of life include biography work, journalling, reminiscence therapy, and poetry. It has been suggested that we can express in written words things that we find hard to say, and so poetry and prose can have a significant part to play in the discovery of the journey towards the end of life. The arts can also provide a most effective means by which a legacy can be left for the family. During the preparation of such items, a focus on relieving symptoms such as breathlessness can be maintained.

Using some of these approaches as part of a rehabilitative dimension to the management of dyspnoea has been reported by many authors as being useful in complementing a more medical approach by restoring a sense of self-esteem, as a focus for emotional expression, by helping to create goals for the future, and by the creation of a renewed sense of hopefulness.

Staff support

As with all aspects of palliative care, it is essential that there is close and effective communication between team members and the patient and family. A variety of professionals may be involved in this aspect of the management of dyspnoea, and the system adopted by each team

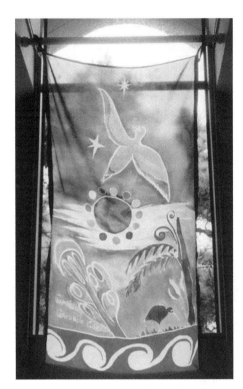

Fig. 13.2 'Bird takes flight'. Silk painting created by a woman with breathlessness from advanced lung cancer.

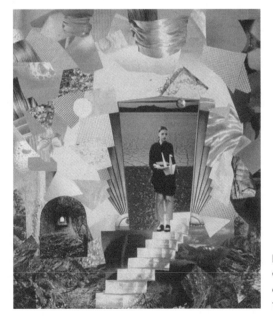

Fig. 13.3 'Focus on release'. Collage created by a man disabled by breathlessness from COPD.

Case study 13.3 Mary

Mary was a 54-year-old woman with widely metastatic breast cancer who became severely breathless towards the end of her life as a result of lymphangitis carcinomatosis. Discussion with her about discharge from the hospice inpatient unit led to a recognition that she was fearful of going home because of the severe limitations she perceived her breathlessness would have on her activity and quality of life. She chose to express this in artwork in which she drew 'her life'. This work indicated to the therapist the areas of her life that she perceived as difficult, and she was able to eliminate some of these through discussion and planning. She later redrew her life with 'boundaries' in place that she felt comfortable with and her discharge was completed successfully. She was confident that she would remain in control of her breathing – this was the case until the end of her life, at home, some weeks later.

must ensure optimal coordination and communication. It is also important to acknowledge that dyspnoea can engender significant distress and anxiety in staff as well as patients and their families and, at times, staff may need opportunities to acknowledge their feelings of frustration, hopelessness, or fear. Personal and professional support for all staff working with people with dyspnoea should be available. Staff need to be responsive and aware of each others' needs to reduce personal distress. This can be facilitated by ensuring staff have professional supervision and an opportunity for debriefing sessions.

Keypoints

- Assessment of dyspnoea should include an understanding of the patient's perception of dyspnoea and a description of the quality of the symptom
- Psychosocial management should include an exploration of the meaning of dyspnoea for patients, helping them to understand that meaning and its significance for them and their families
- It is helpful in some instances to lead patients to an acknowledgement that their dyspnoea may never be completely resolved
- Music therapy can be helpful in facilitating feelings and help in communication
- Art therapies can help restore creativity and can act as a diversion
- All of these interventions should accompany a medical approach and a multidisciplinary team involvement

References

1 Skevington, S.M., Pilaar, M., Routh, D., and MacLeod, R.D. On the language of breathlessness. *Psychol Health* 1997; **12**: 677–89.

2 Kinsman, R.A., *et al.* Observations on patterns of subjective symptomatology of acute asthma. *Psychosom Med* 1974; **36**(2): 129–43.

3 Kinsman, R.A., *et al.* Observations on subjective symptomatology, coping behaviour and medical decisions in asthma. *Psychosom Med* 1977; **39**(2): 102–19.

4 Corner, J., Plant, H., A'Hern, R.A., and Bailey, C. Non-pharmacological intervention for breathlessness in lung cancer. *Palliative Med* 1996; **10**: 299–305.

5 Bredin, M., Corner, J., Krishnasamy, M., *et al.* Multicentre randomised controlled trial of nursing intervention for breathlessness in patients with lung cancer. *BMJ* 1999; **318**(7188): 901–4.

6 Steele, B., and Shaver, J. The dyspnoea experience: nociceptive properties and the model for research practice. *Adv Nurs Sci* 1992; **15**(1): 64–76.

7 Corner, J., Plant, H., and Warner, L. Developing a nursing approach to managing dyspnoea in lung cancer. *Int J Palliative Nurs* 1995; **1**(1): 5–11.

8 Lee, C. Lonely waters. In: C. Lee, (ed.) *Proceedings of the international conference on music therapy in palliative care.* Oxford: Sobell Publications, 1995.

9 Taylor, D.B. *Biomedical foundations of music as therapy.* St Louis: MMB, 1997.

10 Wood, M.J.M. Art therapy in palliative care. Chapter 3 in: M. Pratt, and M.J.M. Wood (eds) *Art therapy in palliative care – the creative response.* London: Routledge, 1998.

11 Eames, P. *The ART and Health Partnership.* Wellington: Arts Access Aotearoa, 1999.

Chapter 14

Nutrition and cachexia

E.F.M. Wouters and A.M.W.J. Schols

The association between weight loss and severe COPD is a phenomenon that has long been recognized. Fowler and Godlee[1] first described the association of weight loss and emphysema in the late 19th century. Attempts to describe different COPD classifications found that body weight might be an important discriminant. This led to the classic description of the **pink puffer** (emphysematous type) and the **blue bloater** (bronchitic type).[2] The pink puffing patient is characteristically thin and breathless with marked hyperinflation of the chest. The blue and bloated patient may not be particularly breathless, at least when at rest, but has severe central cyanosis.

By the 1960s several studies had already reported that a low body weight and weight loss are negatively associated with survival in COPD.[3] However, attention to the therapeutic implications of weight loss and muscle wasting in patients with COPD has gained interest only recently, since it was formerly considered to be a terminal event in the disease progression and therefore inevitable and irreversible. Furthermore, it was suggested that weight loss is an adaptive mechanism to decrease oxygen consumption.

Recent studies have challenged this concept and shown that a low body weight may be a prognostic factor independent of, or at least not closely correlated with, the degree of airflow obstruction.[4] Several studies in the early 1980s established the prevalence of nutritional depletion in selected groups of COPD patients; these ranged from 20% in stable outpatients to 70% in the presence of acute respiratory failure.[5–8] Because of these high prevalences, there has been renewed interest in the nutritional aspects of COPD in recent years.

This renewed interest in nutritional therapy in chronic respiratory disease runs parallel to changing concepts in its management toward an integrated and multidisciplinary approach. Chronic respiratory diseases are progressively disabling disorders causing dyspnoea and impaired exercise performance, reducing quality of life, and consuming healthcare resources. Current pharmacological treatment, consisting of bronchodilation and anti-inflammatory medication, has limited effects on functional performance and quality of life. This is not surprising since, by definition, much of the airflow obstruction is irreversible and only a moderate relationship between airflow obstruction and functional performance has been demonstrated.

Recent studies in patients with COPD have identified both respiratory and peripheral skeletal muscle weakness as important determinants of impaired functional performance.[9,10] Respiratory muscle weakness in patients with chronic respiratory disease is also significantly related to the perceived breathlessness, the degree of carbon dioxide retention,[11] and even to the quality of life.[12] Independent of the underlying lung disease, weight loss and in particular skeletal muscle wasting are accompanied by loss of mass and strength of the respiratory muscles. Muscle wasting is particularly detrimental in those patients whose exercise capacity is already limited by disturbances in ventilation and gas exchange. Therefore, it is not only important to consider changes in body weight but to consider also alterations in body composition: several reports have shown that loss of fat-free mass (FFM) occurs not only in most of the underweight patients, but also in some of the normal-weight patients. The latter group suffers from physical impairment to an even greater degree than underweight patients with a relative preservation of FFM.[7,8]

Pathogenesis of weight loss and muscle wasting

Weight loss is generally seen as a disturbance of the balance between energy expenditure and energy intake. Total energy expenditure can be considered as the sum of resting energy expenditure (REE), diet-induced thermogenesis, and energy spent during daily activities. REE comprises the sleeping metabolic rate and the energy cost of arousal, and amounts to about 70% of total energy expenditure in sedentary individuals. It can now be adequately and easily assessed by indirect calorimetry.

Initially, a lot of attention was focused on assessment of resting or basal energy expenditure in COPD patients, assuming that the contribution of activity-related expenditure would be small in this group of impaired patients. An increased REE in 25–35% of patients with COPD has been reported in different studies.[13,14] In the past this increase in REE was explained by an increase in the work of breathing,[15] but there is increasing evidence that REE reflects not only the work of breathing[16] but also the level of tissue inflammation in COPD patients.[17,18]

Cytokines such as TNFα may increase REE, induce symphatic nervous stimulation, and lead to proteolysis and lipolysis when infused into healthy volunteers. Acute administration of β_2-agonists and theophyllines also induces a transient increase in REE, although the effect of chronic administration of drugs on REE has to be established.[19] The limited role that a raised REE might have on the development of FFM depletion was demonstrated by Creutzberg et al.[14] They showed that a similar distribution of FFM depletion occurs in normometabolic and hypermetabolic COPD patients. This observation was supported by Baarends et al.[21] They showed that there was no significant difference in free living total daily energy expenditure (TDE) between clinically stable COPD patients with an elevated REE and those with a normal REE. Variations in TDE appeared to reflect differences in energy expenditure for activities, but not in REE. Even in COPD patients with severe airflow limitation, TDE was significantly higher than in healthy subjects.[20] These differences were partly attributed to a decreased mechanical efficiency on exercise in COPD patients.

Dietary intake

Systematic analyses of dietary intake in COPD patients are scarce. Schols et al.[22] reported an inadequate dietary intake for energy expenditure especially in more disabled COPD patients. Several factors have been suggested to contribute to this. Chewing and swallowing change breathing patterns and have been shown to decrease arterial oxygen saturation in such patients. Furthermore, gastric filling may reduce the functional residual capacity contributing to an increase in dyspnoea.

Leptin

The role of leptin in energy homeostasis is intriguing. This adipocyte-derived hormone represents the afferent hormonal signal to the brain in a negative feedback mechanism regulating fat mass. This means that leptin levels should be high in patients with an elevated fat mass, and low in patients who are fat-depleted. Leptin also has a regulating role in lipid metabolism and glucose homeostasis, increases thermogenesis, and has effects on T-cell mediated immunity.

There is little data on leptin metabolism in COPD patients. Takabatake *et al.*[23] recently reported that serum leptin levels were significantly lower in COPD patients than in healthy controls. COPD patients in that study had a significantly lower body mass index (BMI) and percentage of body fat than their healthy control group. Circulating leptin correlated well with BMI and % fat, as expected. On the basis of observations that administration of endotoxin or cytokines produces a prompt increase in serum leptin in animals and in humans, the authors have also related circulating leptin to inflammatory markers. However, no relation was found with TNF or with soluble TNF-receptor (sTNF-R) levels.

Schols *et al.*[24] have recently measured leptin levels in both 'emphysema' and 'chronic bronchitis' COPD subtypes. As expected, emphysema patients had a lower BMI and a lower fat mass than patients with chronic bronchitis. Leptin levels were significantly lower in the emphysematous group. Non-detectable levels of leptin were found in 30% of the patients with emphysema, and in 11% of the patients with chronic bronchitis. Leptin was moderately related to fat mass in emphysema and chronic bronchitis. In absolute terms as well as when adjusted for fat mass (FM), leptin was significantly related to sTNF-R55 in emphysema but not in chronic bronchitis. It was also demonstrated that sTNF-R55 and leptin are significantly related to dietary intake in absolute terms as well as when it is adjusted for REE.

These data on the metabolism of leptin in COPD patients are especially intriguing in view of its possible role in ventilatory control. Leptin appears to have a direct effect on respiratory control centres in the brain.[25] In animal studies, it has been shown that the absence of leptin is associated with a reduced hypercapnic ventilatory response. This suggests that in humans, leptin may be an endogenous respiratory stimulant.

The physiology of leptin in COPD patients needs further exploration, but at least is has to be considered to have a central role in energy balance regulation (Figure 14.1).

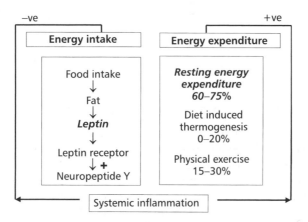

Fig. 14.1 Energy imbalance and inflammation. Inflammation influences energy expenditure by increasing resting energy expenditure. Inflammation negatively influences energy intake by increasing levels of leptin, a fat-derived hormone. Leptin represents the afferent hormonal signal to the brain regulating food intake by the hypothalamic transmitter neuropeptide Y, which suppresses appetite and food intake.

Body composition

As well as a selective loss of fat mass, depletion of FFM is a frequent finding in patients with COPD or other chronic respiratory disorders. At present, only limited information is available to explain this loss of FFM. It can be hypothesized that FFM in patients with advanced lung disease is influenced by metabolic factors as well as by variables such as aging, exercise, inflammation, or pharmacological drug use.

It is well known that during adulthood, body composition changes markedly, with a progressive loss of FFM and an increase in fat mass. The most significant reductions in FFM occur in muscle; non-muscle lean tissue is preserved. These changes in muscle mass explain the reduced basal metabolic rate and exercise capacity in older patients. Physical activity can attenuate this loss of muscle mass and strength.[26,27] However, depletion of FFM is not limited to older patients with advanced lung disease, or to patients with advanced airflow obstruction. Even in patients with moderate airflow obstruction, marked percentages of weight loss[5] as well as depletion of FFM have been reported.[8] Furthermore, the FFM loss is not related to the severity of airflow obstruction. Therefore, it can be concluded that neither age nor severity of airflow obstruction can explain this loss of FFM. Other disease-related factors have to be taken into account.

Accelerated muscle proteolysis is considered as the primary cause of the loss of lean body mass in many chronic conditions. Although many proteolytic systems that serve distinct functions are described in mammalian cells, the ubiquitin–proteasome pathway is the most important in the normal turnover of most cellular proteins and in the accelerated breakdown of muscle proteins in catabolic states. The ubiquitin–proteasome pathway is a multienzymatic process of degradation that requires ATP[28] and consists of two important steps: the ubiquitin conjugation of the proteins, and the process of protein degradation by the proteasomes, leading to release of small peptides.

Activation of the ubiquitin–proteasome pathway has been reported in a variety of models and clinical conditions. The role of inflammatory mediators in activation of this process of protein degradation has been reported.

We have only limited data on the direct effects of inflammatory mediators on differentiated skeletal muscle cells in chronic lung disease. Li et al.[29] recently studied the underlying mechanisms of TNFα-induced effects in differentiated skeletal muscle. They have demonstrated that TNFα stimulates time- and concentration-dependent reductions in total protein content and loss of myosin heavy chain content. These changes were evident at low TNF concentrations that did not alter muscle DNA content and were not associated with a decrease in myosin heavy chain synthesis.

Weight loss and inflammatory mediators in COPD

A relationship between weight loss and TNFα levels has been hypothesized in patients with COPD.[30,31] Increased TNFα serum levels were found in COPD patients who were steadily losing weight, compared to a normal weight group. However, no correlation was found between TNFα levels and recent weight loss.[30] De Godoy et al.[31] reported a significant increase in lipopolysaccharide(LPS)-stimulated TNFα production by monocytes in weight-losing COPD patients compared to weight-stable and control populations. However, TNFα levels have to be interpreted cautiously. Although increased TNFα production by peripheral blood monocytes is reported in healthy subjects during severe deprivation of energy intake,[32] this is suppressed during therapeutic refeeding and suggests that increased levels of TNFα result from, rather than contribute to, the process of muscle wasting.[33] Further studies are needed to unravel the role, if any, of inflammatory mediators in the process of FFM depletion.

Openbrier and co-workers[34] focused attention on the reduction in diffusing capacity for carbon monoxide (DL_{CO}) and malnutrition in COPD patients. This observation was supported by Engelen et al. ,[7] who found a correlation between depletion of FFM and DL_{CO}. Intermittent hypoxaemia during exercise is a possible consequence of this loss of lung parenchyma (low DL_{CO}). Schols et al.[18] also reported that depletion of FFM and muscle mass was most pronounced in patients suffering from chronic hypoxemia. Therefore, the effect of impaired peripheral tissue oxygenation in relation to FFM depletion needs to be investigated.

Medication

It can be hypothesized that medication such as corticosteroids could contribute to muscle wasting by inhibiting protein synthesis and promoting protein catabolism. However, studies of steroid-induced muscle weakness in patients with chronic airflow limitation clearly illustrate that in a considerable number of them, muscle weakness is reduced out of proportion to any reduction in body weight.[35] Other studies have revealed that changes in body composition and especially depletion of FFM are not related to the use of oral corticosteroids.[18]

At present, it can be concluded that the process of muscle wasting is likely to be the resultant of complex metabolic processes in patients with chronic respiratory diseases. Careful analysis of these pathogenic effects is mandatory, especially when strategies for intervention fail.

Nutritional intervention

Despite the general observation that any living organism will die if nutrients are not adequately provided, there has only recently been clinical interest in the therapeutic management of weight loss and muscle wasting in patients with chronic respiratory disorders. Epidemiological insights into the prevalence of depletion and recent concepts of the pathogenesis of depletion have contributed to this.

At present, nutritional intervention based on supplementation has been studied in COPD outpatients and inpatients. Comparison between published nutritional intervention studies is limited owing to the variety of study designs, characteristics of the study populations, nutritional markers, duration of follow-up, and small patient numbers. In only one of them was a substantial weight gain achieved (4.2 kg after 3 months oral support).[36] The average weight gain in the other studies was less than 1.5 kg in 8 weeks. It should be noted, however, that in comparison to other studies, the baseline daily intake in the underweight patients of the successful study was very low. In general, improvements in physiological function were demonstrated only when clear weight gain was obtained. The most consistent changes were improvements in respiratory muscle strength and peripheral skeletal muscle strength.

Unfortunately, it has to be concluded that most trials have shown only limited success with simple, oral nutritional supplementation for outpatients.

Short-term inpatient nutritional intervention strategies are more successful. A significant increase in body weight and respiratory muscle function has been seen after 2–3 weeks of oral or enteral nutritional support.[37] However, it was suggested that the effect of this short period of nutritional repletion might be related more to repletion of muscle water and potassium than to constitution of muscle protein nitrogen.[38] On the other hand, Goldstein et al. demonstrated that 2 weeks of nutritional support increased body weight, nitrogen balance, and improved respiratory and peripheral skeletal muscle function, to a similar degree in malnourished patients with and without lung disease.[39] Possibly supplementation contributes more to improved muscle strength over the short term than to an increase in nitrogen retention.[38] Only one study has examined the immune response to short-term nutritional intervention in patients with advanced COPD. Refeeding and weight gain were associated with a significant increase in absolute lymphocyte count and an increase in reactivity to skin test antigens after 21 days.[40]

Despite the positive outcome of short-term repletion in a trial setting, the progressive weight loss usually seen in COPD demands sustained outpatient nutritional intervention. As an example, the effect of an aggressive nutritional support regimen was studied in 5 patients with severe COPD and weight loss.[41] Over 4 months, nocturnal enteral nutrition was provided via a percutaneous endoscopic gastrostomy. The regimen was effective in producing positive energy balance (0.2 kg/week), but this weight gain was associated with predominant expansion of body fat mass and no significant expansion of the FFM. Therefore, it seems important to incorporate nutritional intervention in a more integrated disease management program for COPD.

In a large clinical trial Schols et al.[42] investigated the effects of a daily nutritional supplement as an integrated part of a pulmonary rehabilitation programme, and found a significant weight gain (0.4 kg/week), despite a daily supplementation of 420 kcal/day (1.76 MJ/day) which was much less than in most previous outpatient studies. The combined treatment of nutritional support and exercise not only increased body weight but also resulted in a significant increase in FFM and respiratory muscle strength.

Schols et al. also investigated the effect of nutritional repletion in combination with supportive treatment with the anabolic steroid nandrolone decanoate[42] (50 mg intramuscularly every 2 weeks for men and 25 mg intramuscularly every 2 weeks for women; total duration 8 weeks) Despite a similar weight gain to the group having nutrition alone, measurements of body composition showed a larger increase of FFM in the group additionally treated with anabolic steroids, as well as a larger improvement in respiratory muscle strength in the absence of side effects.

Preliminary reports have suggested that nitrogen balance in COPD may also be improved by growth hormone therapy.[43,44] This is likely to be due to increased insulin concentrations, since this promotes protein synthesis and inhibits protein degradation and urea synthesis. However, a recent study demonstrated that the daily administration of 0.15 IU/kg recombinant growth hormone for 3 weeks increased lean body mass but did not improve muscle strength or exercise tolerance in underweight patients with COPD.[45]

On the basis of the present findings, it seems important to combine nutritional intervention with an anabolic stimulus as exercise training or anabolic steroids.

As a post hoc analysis of the intervention study by Schols et al.,[46] the effectiveness of nutritional supplementation on mortality was studied. COPD patients able to increase their body weight by nutritional intervention had a significantly better prognosis than non-responders.

A strategy for nutritional supplementation

In routine clinical practice it seems sensible to screen COPD patients on the basis of BMI (body weight corrected for body height) and recent weight loss. Epidemiological data indicate that patients reporting recent weight loss and with a BMI <25 kg/m^2 should be considered for supplementation. When BMI is below 25 kg/m^2 in the presence of stable body weight, further stratification based on FFM assessment has to be advised. If FFM <16 kg/m^2 in men or <15 kg/m^2 in women, nutritional therapy should be considered for a trial period

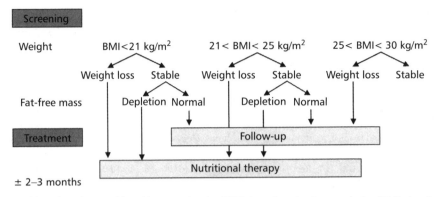

Fig. 14.2 Flowchart for nutritional intervention in COPD based on body mass index (BMI), involuntarily weight, loss and assessment of fat free mass (FFM). Depletion of FFM: FFM index (FFM [kg]/ m²) <16 kg/m² in men and <15 kg/m² in women.

of at least 2 months. Regular follow-up is very important not only during but also after the intervention period. Dietary intake has to amount to 1.9 times calculated basal metabolic rate (based on the Harris and Benedict equations[47]) in many patients with COPD. Therefore, diet supplementation with high-energy, high-protein drinks has to be advised. In general, daily nitrogen intake has to be increased to 1.5 g/kg body weight. A flowchart is shown in Figure 14.2.

Summary

Pulmonary cachexia is a frequently occurring complication in patients with chronic respiratory disorders, and contributes negatively to health status and quality of life. Detection and characterization of these patients, based on measurements of body composition, is a prerequisite of nutritional intervention. Tissue depletion is not only the result of a (temporarily) decreased dietary intake, but often of a complex metabolic process. Important factors contributing to the resulting muscle depletion are systemic inflammation and a decreased mechanical and metabolic efficiency. With respect to the outcomes of nutritional supplementation, we might expect that dyspnoea would be reduced with an improvement in respiratory muscle strength. Whether these interventions improve overall health status is not yet clear, although they have been associated with an improved life expectancy. The possible role of leptin modulation by nutritional intervention strategies in relation to ventilatory control in COPD patients is a fascinating prospect.

Keypoints

♦ Weight loss can occur in any chronic non-malignant respiratory disease if it is severe
♦ Weight loss in chronic respiratory disease is a poor prognostic factor
♦ The physiology of weight loss is complex and has been investigated mainly in COPD
♦ Factors which appear to cause it include an increased work of breathing at rest; an increased energy expenditure during exercise; a poorly understood chronic inflammatory state, which may act via cytokines to influence leptin; and occasionally, prescribed drugs

- Correcting negative energy balance in these patients is difficult
- To increase FFM probably requires a combination of a high energy intake and muscular exercise
- An algorithm for nutritional intervention in chronic respiratory disease is provided.

References

1 Fowler, J., and Godlee, R. Emphysema of the lungs. *Diseases of the lungs.* London: Longmans, Green and Co, 1898; 171.

2 Filley, G.F., Beckwitt, H.J., Reeves, J.T., and Mitchell, R.S. Chronic obstructive bronchopulmonary disease. *Am J Med* 1968; **44**: 26–39.

3 Vandenbergh, E., Van de Woestijne, K.P., and Gyselen, A. Weight changes in the terminal stages of chronic obstructive pulmonary disease. Relation to respiratory function and prognosis. *Am Rev Respir Dis* 1967; **95**: 556–66.

4 Wilson, D.O., Rogers, R.M., Sanders, M.H., Pennock, B.E., and Reilly, J.J. Nutritional intervention in malnourished patients with emphysema. *Am Rev Respir Dis* 1986; 134(4): 672–7.

5 Wilson, D.O., Rogers, R.M., Wright, E.C., and Anthonisen, N.R. Body weight in chronic obstructive pulmonary disease. *Am Rev Respir Dis* 1989; **139**: 1435–8.

6 Braun, S., Keim, N., Dixon, R., *et al.* The prevalence and determinants of nutritional changes in COPD. *Chest* 1984; **86**: 558–63.

7 Engelen, M.P., Schols, A.M., Baken, W.C., Wesseling, G.J., and Wouters, E.F. Nutritional depletion in relation to respiratory and peripheral skeletal muscle function in out-patients with COPD. *Eur Respir J* 1994; **7**: 1793–7.

8 Schols, A.M., Soeters, P.B., Dingemans, A.M., *et al.* Prevalence and characteristics of nutritional depletion in patients with stable COPD eligible for pulmonary rehabilitation. *Am Rev Respir Dis* 1993; **147**: 1151–6.

9 Gosselink, R., Troosters, T., and Decramer, M. Peripheral muscle weakness contributes to exercise limitation in COPD. *Am J Respir Crit Care Med* 1996; **153**: 976–80.

10 Bernard, S., LeBlanc, P., Whittom, F., *et al.* Peripheral muscle weakness in patients with chronic obstructive pulmonary disease. *Am J Respir Crit Care Med* 1998; **158**: 629–34.

11 Begin, P., and Grassino, A. Inspiratory muscle dysfunction and chronic hypercapnia in chronic obstructive pulmonary disease. *Am Rev Respir Dis* 1991; **143**: 905–912.

12 Shoup, R., Dalsky, G., Warner, S., *et al.* Body composition and health-related quality of life in patients with obstructive airways disease. *Eur Respir J* 1997; **10**: 1576–80.

13 Schols, A.M., Fredrix, E.W., Soeters, P.B., Westerterp, K.R., and Wouters, E.F. Resting energy expenditure in patients with chronic obstructive pulmonary disease. *Am J Clin Nutr* 1991; **54**: 983–7.

14 Creutzberg, E.C., Schols, A.M., Bothmer Quaedvlieg, F.C., and Wouters, E.F. Prevalence of an elevated resting energy expenditure in patients with chronic obstructive pulmonary disease in relation to body composition and lung function. *Eur J Clin Nutr* 1998; **52**: 396–401.

15 Donahoe, M., and Rogers, R.M. Nutritional assessment and support in chronic obstructive pulmonary disease. *Clin Chest Med* 1990; **11**: 487–504.

16 Hugli, O., Schutz, Y., and Fitting, J. The cost of breathing in stable chronic obstructive pulmonary disease. *Clin Sci* 1995; **89**: 625–632.

17 Pouw, E.M., Schols, A.M., Deutz, N.E., and Wouters, E.F. Plasma and muscle amino acid levels in relation to resting energy expenditure and inflammation in stable chronic obstructive pulmonary disease. *Am J Respir Crit Care Med* 1998; **158**: 797–801.

18 Schols, A.M., Buurman, W.A., Staal van den Brekel, A.J., Dentener, M.A., and Wouters, E.F. Evidence for a relation between metabolic derangements and increased levels of inflammatory mediators in a subgroup of patients with chronic obstructive pulmonary disease. *Thorax* 1996; **51**: 819–24.

19 Creutzberg, E.C., Schols, A.M., Bothmer Quaedvlieg, F.C., Wesseling, G., and Wouters, E.F. Acute effects of nebulized salbutamol on resting energy expenditure in patients with chronic obstructive pulmonary disease and in healthy subjects. *Respiration* 1998; **65**: 375–80.

20 Baarends, E.M., Schols, A.M., Westerterp, K.R., and Wouters, E.F. Total daily energy expenditure relative to resting energy expenditure in clinically stable patients with COPD. *Thorax* 1997; **52**: 780–5.

21 Baarends, E.M., Schols, A.M., Pannemans, D.L., Westerterp, K.R., and Wouters, E.F. Total free living energy expenditure in patients with severe chronic obstructive pulmonary disease. *Am J Respir Crit Care Med* 1997; **155**: 549–54.

22 Schols, A.M., Soeters, P.B., Mostert, R., Saris, W.H., and Wouters, E.F. Energy balance in chronic obstructive pulmonary disease. *Am Rev Respir Dis* 1991; **143**: 1248–52.

23 Takabatake, N., Nakamura, H., Abe, S., *et al.* Circulating leptin in patients with chronic obstructive pulmonary disease. *Am J Respir Crit Care Med* 1999; **159**(4): 1215–1219.

24 Schols, A.M.W.J., Creutzberg, E.C., Buurman, W.A., *et al.* Plasma leptin is related to pro-inflammatory status and dietary intake in patients with COPD. *Am J Respir Crit Care Med* 1999; **160**(4): 1220–6.

25 O'Donnell, C., Schaub, C., Haines, A., *et al.* Leptin prevents respiratory depression in obesity. *Am J Respir Crit Care Med* 1999; **159**: 1477–1484.

26 Brown, A.B., McCartney, N., and Sale, D.G. Positive adaptations to weight-lifting training in the elderly. *J Appl Physiol* 1990; **69**: 1725–33.

27 Frontera, W.R., Meredith, C.N., O'Reilly, K.P., *et al.* Strength conditioning in older men: skeletal muscle hypertrophy and improved function. *J Appl Physiol* 1988; **64**: 1038–44.

28 Mitch, W.E., and Goldberg, A.L. Mechanisms of muscle wasting. The role of the ubiquitin-proteasome pathway. *N Engl J Med* 1996; **335**: 1897–905.

29 Li, Y., Schwartz, R., Waddell, I., Holloway, B., and Reid, M. Skeletal muscle myocytes undergo protein loss and reactive oxygen-mediated NF-kB activation in response to tumor necrosis factor. *FASEB J* 1998; **12**: 871–80.

30 Francia, M., Barbier, D., Mege, J.L., and Orehek, J. Tumor necrosis factor-alpha levels and weight loss in chronic obstructive pulmonary disease. *Am J Respir Crit Care Med* 1994; **150**: 1453–5.

31 Godoy de, I., Donahoe, M., Calhoun, W.J., Mancino, J., and Rogers, R.M. Elevated TNF-alpha production by peripheral blood monocytes of weight-losing COPD patients. *Am J Respir Crit Care Med* 1996; **153**: 633–7.

32 Vaisman, N., Schattner, A., and Hahn, T. Tumor necrosis factor production during starvation. *Am J Med* 1989; **87**: 115.

33 Vaisman, N., and Hahn, T. Tumor necrosis factor-alpha and anorexia – cause or effect? *Metabolism* 1991; **40**: 720–3.

34 Openbrier, D.R., Irwin, M.M., Rogers, R.M., *et al.* Nutritional status and lung function in patients with emphysema and chronic bronchitis. *Chest* 1983; **83**: 17–22.

35 Decramer, M., Lacquet, L.M., Fagard, R., and Rogiers, P. Corticosteroids contribute to muscle weakness in chronic airflow obstruction. *Am J Respir Crit Care Med* 1994; **150**: 11–16.

36 Efthimiou, J., Fleming, J., Gomes, C., and Spiro, S.G. The effect of supplementary oral nutrition in poorly nourished patients with chronic obstructive pulmonary disease. *Am Rev Respir Dis* 1988; **137**: 1075–82.

37 Whittaker, J.S., Ryan, C.F., Buckley, P.A., and Road, J.D. The effects of refeeding on peripheral and respiratory muscle function in malnourished chronic pulmonary disease patients. *Am Rev Respir Dis* 1990; **142**: 283–8.

38 Russell, D., Prendergast, P.J., Darby, P.L., *et al.* A comparison between muscle function and body composition in anorexia nervosa: the effect of refeeding. *Am J Clin Nutr* 1983; **38**: 229–37.

39 Goldstein, S.A., Thomashow, B.M., Kvetan, V., *et al.* Nitrogen and energy relationships in malnourished patients with emphysema. *Am Rev Respir Dis* 1988; **138**: 636–44.

40 Fuenzalida, C.E., Petty, T.L., Jones, M.L., *et al.* The immune response to short-term nutritional intervention in advanced chronic obstructive pulmonary disease. *Am Rev Respir Dis* 1990; **142**: 49–56.

41 Donahoe, M., Mancino, J., Costatino, J., Lebow, H., and Rogers, R. The effect of an aggressive support regimen on body composition in patients with severe COPD and weight loss. *Am J Respir Crit Care Med* 1994; **149**: A313.

42 Schols, A.M.W.J., Soeters, P.B., Mostert, R., Pluymers, R.J., and Wouters, E.F.M. Physiological effects of nutritional support and anabolic steroids in COPD patients. *Am J Respir Crit Care Med* 1995; **152**: 1268–74.

43 Suchner, U., Rothkopf, M.M., Stanislaus, G., *et al.* Growth hormone and pulmonary disease. Metabolic effects in patients receiving parenteral nutrition. *Arch Intern Med* 1990; **150**: 1225–30.

44 Pape, G.S., Friedman, M., Underwood, L.E., and Clemmons, D.R. The effect of growth hormone on weight gain and pulmonary function in patients with chronic obstructive lung disease. *Chest* 1991; **99**: 1495–500.

45 Burdet, L., de Muralt, B., Schutz, Y., Pichard, C., and Fitting, J.W. Administration of growth hormone to underweight patients with chronic obstructive pulmonary disease. A prospective, randomized, controlled study. *Am J Respir Crit Care Med* 1997; **156**: 1800–6.

46 Schols, A.M., Slangen, J., Volovics, L., and Wouters, E.F. Weight loss is a reversible factor in the prognosis of chronic obstructive pulmonary disease. *Am J Respir Crit Care Med* 1998; **157**: 1791–7.

47 Harris, J.A., and Benedict, F.G. *A biometric study of basal metabolism in man.* Washington: Carnegie Institute of Washington, 1919.

Chapter 15

Occupational therapy and environmental modifications

Louise Sewell and Sally Singh

Occupations fill our daily lives, and each individual task fulfils a specific purpose. The profession of occupational therapy concerns itself with an individual's ability to perform these occupations or activities. It endeavours to promote optimal independence in all areas of daily living and occupational therapists work with clients who have psychiatric or physical problems, or both.

The philosophy of occupational therapy is based on two theoretical assumptions:

- Occupation is fundamental to the basic well-being of a person. Thus, enabling a person to regain their ability to complete daily activities or occupations following some kind of disruption can improve their general health status.

- Occupational therapists base their practice on the belief that each individual is different, has differing roles, and so needs to be independent in a variety of activities. It is therefore essential that the occupational therapist completes an holistic assessment prior to commencing any treatment programme.

Knowledge of people, how they normally function; how to discover what is important to them and how to help them address their difficulties is fundamental to the work of an occupational therapist.[1]

Occupational therapy focuses on the consequences of the disease rather than the diagnosis itself. Diagnosis alone is not a good indicator of outcomes such as an individual's particular service and care needs. Patients will inevitably differ in their perceptions of their abilities. The World Health Organization has developed a scientific model (ICIDH-2) for the study of functioning and disablement which highlights the importance of seeing past the disease process.[2] Examination of this model will illustrate where an occupational therapist's input fits into the breathless patient's care.

The ICIDH-2 is a multipurpose classification consisting of three dimensions:

- **Impairment** is a loss or abnormality of body structure or of a physiological or psychological function.

- **Activity** is the nature and extent of functioning relevant to the requirement of the person. Activities may be limited in nature, duration, and quality. They may be physical or mental and could include personal care tasks, household tasks, or completing paid employment.

- **Participation** refers to the ability to be involved in life situations within all environments, such as participating in work and community activities, family and social relationships, etc.

It is accepted by the model that participation may be restricted or facilitated by social and physical factors (collectively known as **contextual factors**). These include the physical environment, the level of person and social support available, and the availability of economic resources.

The varying difficulties experienced by the breathless patient are accommodated within the context of this conceptual framework. Impairment for breathless patients refers to the level of dysfunction or disease process occurring within their lungs. It is no surprise then that there is no evidence to suggest that the occupational therapist's intervention affects this impairment. However, the ICIDH-2 states that the 'activities' dimension refers to functions such as moving around, daily life, learning, applying knowledge, and performing tasks. The 'participation' dimension then goes on to include specific tasks such as personal maintenance, mobility, and involvement in areas such as education, work, leisure, and social relationships. The breathless patient is clearly restricted in some or all of these areas to a greater or lesser degree. It is within the role of the occupational therapist to assess these needs and enable the individual to problem-solve in order to attain their own optimal level of independence.

The occupational therapist and the breathless patient

Occupational therapists are involved with the breathless patient in a variety of settings, usually within acute hospitals or in community based social services. Typical examples of referrals to an occupational therapist may include:

◆ A 73-year-old man, living alone, who has been admitted to a medical ward following an acute exacerbation of chronic obstructive pulmonary disease (COPD), and now feels that he will be unable to manage personal care tasks upon discharge from hospital.

◆ A 63-year-old woman who has emphysema and severely reduced exercise tolerance, and can no longer use the stairs at home.

◆ A 55-year-old woman with chronic bronchitis, living with her husband, who is anxious to maintain her ability to cope with household tasks.

Regardless of the setting, the occupational therapy process is broadly similar and is summarized in Box 15.1. Specifically the stages of assessment, intervention and evaluation will be examined.

Box 15.1 Steps in the occupational therapy process

◆ Accept the referral and collect relevant information
◆ Complete an initial assessment to identify presenting problems
◆ Negotiate a treatment plan in conjunction with the patient
◆ Initiate and complete intervention
◆ Evaluate intervention
◆ Discharge

Assessment

The location of contact, e.g. hospital or community, will determine the exact nature of the occupational therapist's assessment. However, regardless of the point of contact, the occupational therapist will want to gather information about the breathless patient's home environment and their current level of functioning so that a specific problem list can be formulated with the patient. Assessment methods will vary from therapist to therapist, but generally information is gathered by means of examination of any medical records, observation, and interviews. Increasingly standardized assessments are being employed by therapists in order to evaluate both their input and the patient's progress through the intervention period. These will be discussed later.

An efficient and effective way to gather assessment information is to observe and interview the breathless patient in his or her own home. This allows the therapist to examine any physical, social, and environmental barriers that are preventing the patient from achieving optimal functional independence. Assessment in the home is clearly the norm for occupational therapists based in the community. For occupational therapists working in a hospital setting, home visits can be arranged, if needed, before the patient's discharge. This allows the therapist to assess the patient's needs thoroughly before discharge.

Standardized assessments

In order for the therapist to be able to evaluate the clinical effectiveness of any type of intervention both a baseline measure and a outcome measure needs to be established. Increasingly, therapists are developing and employing standardized assessments to achieve this. Measures are commonly divided into two categories: generic measures and disease-specific measures. (See Chapters 7 and 8 for further discussion of these measures.)

Disease-specific measures

The Chronic Respiratory Disease Questionnaire[3] and the St George's Respiratory Questionnaire[4] have been validated and are used extensively in respiratory practice and research. The Pulmonary Functional Status Scale[5] and the Pulmonary Functional Status and Dyspnea Questionnaire[6] are both self-completed measures designed to establish functional status in areas such as self-care, home management, and mobility. The European Organization for Research and Treatment of Cancer (EORTC) has developed a questionnaire, the EORTC QLQ-C30 LC-13,[7] which specifically examines the health-related quality of life in lung cancer patients.

Generic measures

There is now an increasing number of generic measures that can be used along side disease-specific questionnaires. These range from 'functional checklist' type scores to measures that are based on a semi-structured interview.

Barthel Index[8]

This is an established scale, completed by the clinician. Patients are rated on 10 items including mobility, bladder/bowel management, transfers, and dressing. It takes only a few minutes to complete and has been used in many areas of disability. It is not, however formally validated for patients with respiratory disease. Domestic and leisure activities are not rated.

Canadian Occupational Performance Measure[9]

The COPM takes the form of a semi-structured interview and takes approximately 30 min to complete (Figure 15.1). During the interview patients are asked to identify specific tasks that they are either unable to do or would like to do better. These problems will fall into the areas of self-care, productivity, and leisure. Patients then rate their performance and satisfaction in up to five of the most important of these problem areas. These scores are then reassessed after an agreed period of intervention. This is an individualized measure and so it is the change in each patient's scores that is important. The test–retest reproducibility has now been established in patients with chronic obstructive airways disease.[10] Patients need to have adequate cognitive skills to cope with the interview process. Alternatively, the authors have suggested that carers may be interviewed.

Short Form 36 Health Survey (SF-36)[11]

The SF-36 is a generic measure of health-related quality of life and is a self-completed questionnaire. Developed by the Medical Outcomes Study, the SF-36 measures eight multi-item dimensions: physical functioning, role limitations due to physical problems, role limitations due to emotional problems, social functioning, mental health, energy/vitality, pain, and general health perceptions. Extensive international testing to establish reliability and validity has been carried out and authors suggest that that the SF-36 can be used in a wide range of patient populations including elderly people, smokers and patients with asthma.

Nottingham Extended Activities of Daily Living scale (NEADL)[12]

The NEADL, a self-completed measure, was validated as an overall assessment of functional independence in stroke patients discharged from hospital. The measure consists of 22 items grouped into four categories: mobility, kitchen, domestic, and leisure. This is an easy and inexpensive scale to use but has yet to be validated for use with respiratory patients.

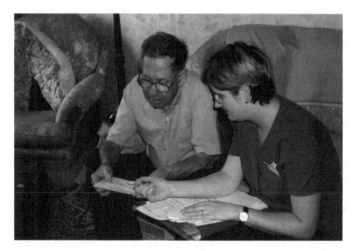

Fig. 15.1 A patient with COPD completes the Canadian Occupational Performance Measure with one of the authors.

London Chest Activity of Daily Living scale (LCADL)[13]

The LCADL is a recent addition to existing measures of functional status and unlike the previous measures reviewed, was developed in the UK. It is a fifteen item self-completed scale. The LCADL is specific in its approach in that it asks only about dyspnoea levels in respect to the fifteen daily activities. The LCADL is a relativly new measure and so further work is needed to establish its clinical utility in patients with COPD.

The Manchester Respiratory Activities of Daily Living scale (MRADL)[14]

The MRADL was developed in the UK, specifically for use in older patients and has been shown to be responsive to change following pulmonary rehabilitation. This is a twenty one item scale and is a combination of items from the NEADL and Breathing Problems Questionnaire that were shown to have good discriminatory properties in COPD patients.

Common problems

Functional difficulties caused by dyspnoea will vary from individual to individual. Some common problems addressed by the occupational therapist are the following.

♦ **Poor exercise tolerance**: Exercise is commonly limited by increasing levels of breathlessness on exertion. This sensation is clearly uncomfortable and frightening, and so typically patients begin to reduce their overall level of activity.[15] Common functional restrictions include decreased ability to climb stairs, walk outside, attend to personal care, or complete domestic tasks.

♦ **Fatigue**: Breathless patients often report high levels of fatigue at differing times during the day which limit their ability to plan their day effectively. Lareau et al.[16] suggest that this is often an important problem that may limit function as much as dyspnoea.

♦ **Muscle impairment**: Once a breathless patient has begun to be limited in terms of activity and exercise by dyspnoea, the downward spiral of deconditioning follows with many patients losing muscle function relatively quickly. Coupled with the effects of dyspnoea and fatigue, muscle impairment compounds the functional limitations already discussed.

♦ **Loss of self-esteem and motivation**: The respiratory disease process will often mean that individuals are forced to withdraw from their established roles. This could mean retirement from paid employment, curtailment of voluntary work, withdrawal from family roles, and decreased participation in sports and hobbies. This can often be measured in terms of self-reported symptoms of depression and self-efficacy.[17]

Intervention

Energy conservation

The cumulative effect of limited exercise tolerance and increasing levels of fatigue mean that the breathless patient has only a reduced amount of energy to take them through their day. The occupational therapist is well placed to assist patients to examine their current daily routine and then to offer advice about how they can gain the optimal level of productivity from the minimal amount of energy expenditure. A useful analogy for the therapist to employ is to liken their energy levels to a daily monetary budget and to explain that some tasks are more 'expensive' than others. Tasks can increase or decrease in 'value' throughout the day. For instance, for some patients taking a bath in the evening may expend more energy than if they were to bath in the morning. The therapist should encourage the patient to examine their own daily routine and begin to identify any patterns of fatigue during their day. Their objective is to budget their energy levels throughout the day.

It has already been stated that individuals often begin to reduce or even curtail activities as their level of breathlessness increases. An understanding of energy conservation techniques can allow patients to increase their overall level of independence and could lead to an improvement in levels of self-esteem and anxiety as patients regain their level of autonomy.

The plan of modifying activities is summarized in Box 15.2.

Anxiety management

The prevalence of anxiety within the breathless patient population is difficult to ascertain. Some studies report levels as low as 2%[18] and other studies state levels of 93%.[19] The measurement of anxiety relies on the accuracy and honesty of self-reported symptoms, and

---

Box 15.2 Modifying activities

Pace activity

- Break activities down into small, manageable parts.
- When beginning new tasks, set small, achievable goals, rather than attempting to complete or master the whole task all at once.
- Pace overall levels of daily activity by alternating heavy tasks with light tasks.

Plan activity

- Allow ample time to complete tasks – do not squeeze too much into one day.
- Consider the times at which medication is taken – often more can be achieved after these times.
- Avoid too many trips up and down stairs – use written prompts to remember what needs to be done/brought down from upstairs.
- Organize the environment to cut down on wasting energy. Consider the layout of kitchens and any storage space.

Be energy efficient

- If objects need to be moved, push them rather than pull them.
- Use correct lifting techniques, keeping objects close to the body in order to use the larger muscle groups.
- Exhale during the most strenuous part of the activity, e.g. pulling the vacuum cleaner towards the body.
- Sit down to complete activities wherever possible.

Delegate

- Consider who really needs to complete each task. Delegating one task could mean more energy to complete two other more enjoyable or essential tasks.

also upon the level of sensitivity of the measure used e.g. the Hospital Anxiety and Depression Scale.[20] However, there can be no doubt that dyspnoea leads to raised anxiety levels in some patients. This anxiety, if unaddressed, will often go on to affect the patients' own management of their respiratory symptoms – they become anxious and so become more breathless.

Management of anxiety is usually based on the cognitive-behavioural approach and often takes place in a group setting. The occupational therapist takes on the role of educator, using a structured course aiming to provide patients with the practical skills and knowledge to enable them to deal with episodes of anxiety or stress.

The content of an anxiety management programme often includes:

- explanation of the physical and psychological processes that occur when a person experiences anxiety
- assertiveness skills
- discussions on how to recognize common, everyday stresses
- relaxation training

Depending on the particular needs of the patient, it is sometimes more appropriate for the occupational therapist to address these issues on a one-to-one basis.

Relaxation training

Relaxation training has its origins rooted in the behavioural approach to treating anxiety. Relaxation techniques are taught on either an individual setting or, more commonly, in a group setting.

Three main techniques are employed by occupational therapists to treat both physical and psychological symptoms of anxiety. There is no evidence currently to suggest that one technique is more effective than another. Therapists rely on subjective feedback from their patients as specific preference of a relaxation technique appears to vary from individual to individual.

Methods of relaxation

- **Progressive muscle relaxation**: This approach teaches the patient to become aware of any tension in different muscle groups and then how to release this tension, working down through the body.
- **Autogenic training**: This involves concentrating on each area of the body in turn and imagining this area becoming warm, heavy, and relaxed. The patient completes this process throughout the whole of the body continually concentrating upon cue words such as 'warm', 'heavy', 'calm', and 'peaceful'.
- **Visual imagery**: This technique involves the patient being talked through a story, e.g. walking along a warm, sunny beach. Patients are encouraged to pay attention to what they may be able to hear, feel, or smell. The aim is to divert any anxious thoughts and replace them with calm, peaceful ones.

Whichever technique is used, the therapist should always emphasize that relaxation is a skill that needs to be first learnt and then practised on a daily basis in order to obtain maximum benefit. See Chapter 13 for further discussion of these approaches.

Case history 15.1 Mrs S

Mrs S is 68 years old and has been an outpatient of the local hospital for 3 years. She retired 18 months ago because of her respiratory problems but has since been able to complete some voluntary work in a local charity shop. Mrs S was widowed 4 years ago and lives alone. She was recently admitted to hospital with a chest infection. Since then she has made good medical progress, but reported to her respiratory physician during a follow-up appointment that she was finding it increasingly difficult to cope with the everyday household tasks and sometimes felt that she might not be able to cope alone any longer. With her permission, her doctor arranged for a referral to the hospital's occupational therapy department.

The occupational therapist was able to complete a comprehensive assessment of Mrs S's recent difficulties with activities of daily living and was able to recommend some items of equipment, including a perching stool and shower seat that Mrs S felt would be of assistance to her. The occupational therapist was then able to discuss some other areas of her daily life that Mrs S may have also been finding difficult. Mrs S reported that since her recent chest infection, she has felt very anxious about being in social situations in case her breathlessness suddenly worsened. She also stated that she felt unable to carry on with her voluntary work and has not been out to visit any family or friends for some months. The occupational therapist was able, over the next four sessions, to discuss some anxiety management techniques with Mrs S and also taught her some relaxation skills. By the end of the course of intervention, Mrs S had planned to return to her work in the charity shop on one day a week and had made good progress in being able to visit her grandchildren. The occupational therapist invited Mrs S back for a follow up appointment in 3 months to discuss her progress.

Environmental modifications

In the UK, The Chronically Sick and Disabled Persons Act (1970) has given local authorities the responsibility to assess the needs of any person who has a chronic disease, including respiratory diseases. Occupational therapists who are employed by social services are often involved in assessment for any major adaptations to the breathless patient's home environment.

Perhaps the largest problem to be addressed by the occupational therapist is that of access, e.g access into the property, the first floor of the house, or bathroom and toilet facilities. Adaptations commonly needed by patients with respiratory problems include:

◆ stair lifts
◆ through-floor lifts
◆ ground floor extensions to incorporate bathroom/bedroom and toilet facilities
◆ installations of walk-in or level access showers with seats.

Procedures for the provision of major adaptations will often vary, depending on the procedures and particular demands of a community's resources. In the UK, the disabled facilities grant procedure is often used to fund these adaptations. This is a means-tested grant and the occupational therapist can be involved throughout the whole process.

Equipment provision

A common part of the occupational therapist's role is to assess for and arrange provision of equipment that may increase the patient's ability to complete activities of daily living independently. During the assessment, the occupational therapist will be able to identify any specific problems that the patient may be experiencing and then decide whether there is a particular piece of equipment that may help.

Equipment commonly found to be helpful by respiratory patients includes:

- chair/bed raisers
- toilet seat raisers/toilet frame
- bath board (Figure 15.2a) and bath seat
- perching stool (for use in kitchen and/or bathroom)
- dressing aids e.g. sock/tights gutter (Figure 15.2b), dressing stick
- helping hand or 'reacher' (Figure 15.2c)

The provision of such equipment will clearly vary from country to country depending on the degree of socialization of the healthcare and social care services. There is now potentially a wide range of equipment available from a variety of sources, and patients may be able to purchase equipment from an increasing number of retail outlets. Larger items of equipment are often available on loan from social services departments and local hospitals. However, loans of smaller pieces of equipment may be subject to a nominal charge.

It is important to remember that although a piece of equipment may appear to improve function there are occasional difficulties in fitting or using it. Patients should seek the advice of a occupational therapist before purchasing equipment themselves.

Other issues

Sexual dysfunction

Problems with sexual intercourse and intimacy are often difficult for both the patient and the therapist to discuss. However, in light of the fact that many relationships could already be under strain due to the pressures of respiratory disease, this may become an important area. Limitations of physical function often lead to the erosion of roles within a relationship and loss of intimacy can only compound this process.

Cole and Hossler[21] suggest that the most important point when discussing sexuality with a patient is to desensationalize sexuality and intimacy. Educational information should be presented just like any other information regarding activities of daily living. It is often helpful to link any advice regarding sexual positions and intimacy to other recommendations in relation to energy conservation and anxiety management.

The role of the carer

The UK government's national strategy for carers[22] states that there are currently a total of 5.7 million carers in the UK with 1.7 million devoting at least 20 h/week. Of these, a substantial proportion may be caring for a relative or friend with a chronic respiratory disease. The pressures placed on the carer can be immense. National statistics state that of the total number of carers in the UK, 49% are still in work. These carers face problems of exhaustion and increased levels of stress due to overwork. However, 25% of all carers are unable to work. This may be due to an established commitment to be the primarly carer for someone. The resulting loss of income will bring with it problems and stresses of its own, and services for carers will vary widely from area to area.[22,23]

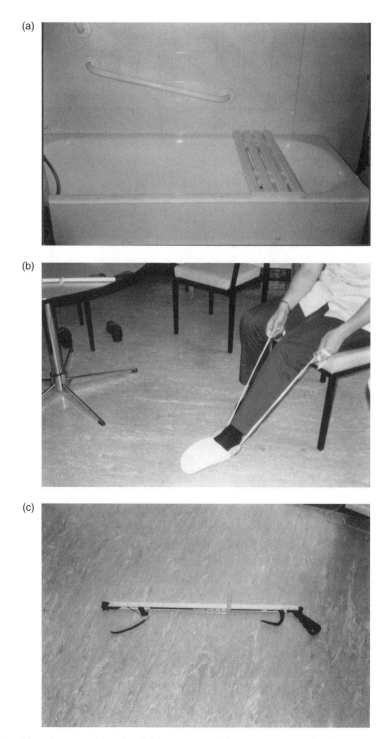

Fig. 15.2 (a) Bath seat and hand rail. (b) Dressing aid for putting on socks. (c) 'Helping hand' or reacher for grabbing articles without bending.

Case history 15.2 Mr J

Mr J is a 72-year-old retired miner who lives with his wife in a two-storey house. He has been on long-term oxygen therapy for 2 years and has regular outpatient reviews at the local hospital's respiratory clinic. For the last 6 months Mr J has been too breathless to leave the house and has, on occasion had to sleep in a chair downstairs as he has not been able to climb the stairs. During the daytime, Mr J sometimes has to use a urinal bottle as he is too breathless to access the toilet which is also situated upstairs. Mr J's wife now has to help him to have a wash at the bathroom sink as he does not feel able to stand to shower and is unable to get in and out of the bath. After washing, Mr J is often too breathless to dress without some help from his wife. Mrs J also has to complete all the other household tasks and is becoming increasingly tired herself.

Mr and Mrs J explained their difficulties to their GP during a routine appointment. The GP was able to refer them to the local social services department who consequently arranged for a visit from a community occupational therapist. After an initial assessment, the occupational therapist was able to recommend that Mr J should be provided with a stair lift. He was considered to be a high priority for provision of a stair lift as he was unable to access toilet facilities. The occupational therapist was also able to arrange provision of a shower seat so that Mr J would be able to take a shower in his own time, safely and independently. Finally, the occupational therapist took time to discuss Mr J's daily routine with him and was able to suggest some basic energy conservation strategies to him. Mr J reported that he was particularly breathless in a morning and so the occupational therapist suggested that he might consider taking a shower in the middle of the day, after his nebulized medication.

After some months' wait, Mr J's stair lift was fitted. He is now able to access his bathroom and bedroom independently.

The role of the occupational therapist has expanded to reflect these changes, and therapists will now fully assess the needs of the carer as well as the patient. Implications of any intervention for the carer must be considered before deciding upon any treatment plan. It may be the occupational therapist who can put the carer in touch with a patient support group. For example, in the UK, Breathe Easy (www.lunguk.org/breathe) is a support group run by the British Lung Foundation which is able to offer help and support to carers, who may also attend locally run clubs that offer information and advice. Respite care may be appropriate in some cases and the occupational therapist is well placed to liaise with the social workers to arrange this.

Conclusion

Occupational therapy aims first to establish what changes in functional performance would improve the breathless patient's quality of life and to then set about formulating an effective treatment plan. The occupational therapist will consider both the physical and psychological needs of the breathless patient during a thorough assessment. It is important to recognize that the work may be usefully done in conjunction with a physiotherapist (see Chapter 11). For cancer patients, nurses also contribute significantly in this area (see Chapter 13).

Interventions may help the many practical problems caused by dyspnoea, fatigue, and limited muscle function, and the related problems of anxiety, depression, and demotivation. Standardized measures are available which can document clinically significant changes in the patient's functional performance.

A referral to an occupational therapist will provide the breathless patient with an opportunity to discuss their functional difficulties in detail. This is can often be the first step to improvements in quality of life. The role of the occupational therapist will be increasingly recognized in the supportive management in the chronically breathless patient, particularly if the revised WHO classifications of disease are adopted.

Keypoints

♦ Occupational therapy aims to enable the breathless patient to attain optimal independence in activities of daily living

♦ Standardized measures of function are now available which enable the occupational therapist to measure the clinical effectiveness of their intervention

♦ Energy conservation techniques allow the breathless patient to make the most efficient use of their reduced level of exercise tolerance

♦ Specific interventions such as anxiety management and relaxation training may be essential in helping the breathless patient to maintain some control over their condition

♦ Occupational therapists are able to arrange provision of equipment that often enables the breathless patient to maintain their independence in activities of daily living as their respiratory condition deteriorates

Useful addresses

College of Occupational Therapists, 106–114 Borough High Street, Southwark, London SE1 1LB, UK (www.cot.co.uk)
British Lung Foundation, 73–75 Goswell Rd, London EC1V 7ER, UK.

References

1 Turner, A. Foundations for practice. In: A. Turner, M. Foster, and S.E. Johnson (eds) *Occupational therapy and physical dysfunction*, 4th edn. Edinburgh: Churchill Livingstone, 1997; 1.

2 World Health Organization. *International classification of impairments, disabilities and handicap – 2*. Geneva, Switzerland: WHO, 1999.

3 Williams, J.E., Singh, S.J., Sewell, L. *et al.* Development of a self-reported Chronic Respiratory Questionnaire (CRQ-SR). *Thorax* 2001; **56**: 954–9.

4 Jones, P.W., Quirk, F.H., Baveystock, C.M., and Littlejohns, P. A. self complete measure for chronic airflow limitation – the St George's Respiratory Questionnaire. *Am Rev Respir Dis* 1992; **145**: 1321–7.

5 Weaver, T.E., Narsavage, G.L., and Guilfoyle, M.J. The development and psychometric evaluation of the Pulmonary Functional Status Scale: an instrument to assess functional status in pulmonary disease. *J Cardiopulmonary Rehabil* 1998; **18**: 105–11.

6 Lareau, S.C., Meek, P.M., Anholm, J.D., and Roos, P.J. How are activities of daily living affected over time in patients with COPD? *Am J Respir Crit Care Med* 1999; **159**: A458.

7 Aaronson, N.K., Ahmedzai, S., Bergman, B., *et al.* The European Organization for Research and Treatment of Cancer QLQ-C30: a quality-of-life instrument for use in international clinical trials in oncology. *J Natl Cancer Inst* 1993; **85**: 365–76.

8 Mahoney, F.I., and Barthel, D.W. Functional evaluation: the Barthel Index. *Maryl State Med J* 1965; **14**: 61–5.

9 Law, M., Baptiste, S., McColl, M.A., *et al. The Canadian Occupational Performance Measure*, 3rd edn. Toronto: CAOT Publications, 1998.

10 Sewell, L., and Singh, S.J. The reproducibility of the Canadian Occupational Performance Measure. *Br J Occup Ther* 2001; **64**(6): 305–10.

11 Ware, J.E., and Sherbourne, C.D. The MOS 36-item short form health survey (SF-36). *Med Care* 1992; **30**: 473–83.

12 Lincoln, N.B., and Gladman, J.R.F. The Extended Activities of Daily Living scale: a further validation. *Disability Rehabil* 1992; **14**: 41–3.

13 Garrod, R., Paul, E.A., Wedzicha, J.A. An evaluation of the reliability and sensitivity of the London Chest Activity of Daily Living Scale (LCADL). *Respiratory Medicine* 2002; **96**(9): 725–30.

14 Yohannes, A.M., Roomi, J., Winn, S., and Connolly, M.J. The Manchester Respiratory Activities of Daily Living questionnaire: development, reliability, validity and responsiveness to pulmonary rehabilitation. *J Am Geriatr Soc* 2000; **48**(11): 1496–500.

15 Griffiths, T.L., Burr, M.L., Cambell, I.A., *et al.* Results at 1 year of outpatient multidisciplinary pulmonary rehabilitation: a randomised controlled trial. *Lancet* 2000; **355**: 362–8.

16 Lareau, S.C., Meek, P.M., and Roos, P.J. Development and testing of the modified version of the Pulmonary Functional Status and Dyspnea Questionnaire (PFSDQ-M). *Heart Lung* 1998; **27**: 159–68.

17 Skilbeck, J., Mott, L., Page, H., *et al.* Palliative care in chronic obstructive airways disease: a needs assessment. *Palliative Med* 1998; **12**: 245–54.

18 Casaburi, R., and Petty, T. *Principles and practice of pulmonary rehabilitation*. Philadelphia: WB Saunders, 1993.

19 Hodgkin, J., Conners, G., and Bell, W. *Pulmonary rehabilitation – guidelines to success*. Philadelphia, Pa.: Lippincott, 1993.

20 Zigmond, A., and Snaith, R.P. The Hospital Anxiety and Depression Scale. *Acta Psychiatr Scand* 1983; **67**: 361–70.

21 Cole, S.S., and Hossler, C.J. Intimacy and chronic lung disease. In: A.P. Fishman (ed.) *Pulmonary rehabilitation*, Lung Biology in Health and Disease, vol. 91. New York: Marcel Dekker, 1996; 251–87.

22 Department of Health. *Caring about carers: a national strategy for carers*. London: HMSO, 1999.

23 Fruin, D. *A matter of chance for carers? Inspection of local authority support for carers*. London: Department of Health, 1998.

Part IV

Dyspnoea in special situations

Chapter 16

Upper airflow obstruction

Martin R. Hetzel

Upper airflow obstruction causes severe distress. The principal symptom in most patients is stridor, and they may feel that they are literally choking to death. Haemoptysis is less common but also frightening, and even modest bleeding from a tumour causing critical airway obstruction can lead to asphyxia. Sedative drugs are appropriate only in terminally ill patients. In fitter patients there is a risk of ventilatory arrest and symptoms will not be well controlled by sedation. Use of a mixture of oxygen and helium may help some patients as a 'first aid' measure while definitive treatment is being arranged (because the lower density of helium versus nitrogen reduces resistance to airflow). This is not practicable for prolonged use, however, as large quantities of this expensive gas are needed.

In many patients surgical resection is impossible, and external beam radiotherapy has significant limitations. Minimally invasive techniques can restore the upper airway in such patients. The relief that they can achieve is often as dramatic as the dyspnoea with which patients present. This chapter is therefore principally devoted to a description of the principles of these techniques.

Causes of upper airflow obstruction

Upper airflow obstruction is principally caused by tumours (benign or malignant), strictures, or inhaled foreign body. The latter should be treated by removal at bronchoscopy and will not be discussed further since this should be a curative treatment (although occasionally foreign body can go undiagnosed for long periods and cause more chronic symptoms). More rarely tracheomalacia and bronchomalacia with destruction or weakening of the airway cartilages result in floppy airways which collapse on inspiration. This is sometimes also seen as a complication of previous radiotherapy.

Upper airways obstruction by laryngeal or oropharyngeal tumours can be palliated with tracheostomy, either short- or long-term depending on whether the causative lesion can be directly treated, for example with radiotherapy. The benefits of tracheostomy are, however, limited to high obstructions where it is possible to place the tracheostomy distal to the inferior margin of the tumour.

External beam radiotherapy has a major role to play in malignant upper airway obstruction. However, it is limited by its slow effect and cumulative toxicity to surrounding structures (oesophagus and spinal cord). Minimally invasive techniques are therefore often needed, either to preserve a viable airway while waiting for a response to radiotherapy or as the only treatment option for recurrence after previous radiotherapy. A large UK study of primary tracheal tumours suggests,[1] however, that external beam radiotherapy may achieve as good results as surgery, even when

Table 16.1 Causes of chronic upper airways obstruction

Tumours	Primary tumours of larynx/trachea. Metastases/direct spread to trachea (usually from primary bronchial carcinomas) Tracheal compression by mediastinal nodes from primary bronchial carcinoma lymphomas/thymomas rarer tumours Severe superior vena caval obstruction with extensive oedema in neck. Compression/invasion by carcinoma of thyroid carcinoma of oesophagus
Benign strictures	Post endotracheal tube/tracheostomy tube Anastamotic stricture after previous resection (for tumours or severe trauma) Anastamotic stricture after lung transplantation Blunt trauma to trachea, e.g. road traffic accidents Inhalation of caustic agents/severe burns affecting upper airway
Rarer causes	Tracheomalacia/bronchomalacia Relapsing polychondritis Tracheobronchomegally (Mounier–Kuhn anomaly) Amyloidosis Sarcoidosis Tracheopathia osteoplastica Bilateral vocal cord palsy (e.g. iatrogenic post-thyroidectomy)

surgery is possible. Once a safe airway has been achieved, therefore, radiotherapy merits serious consideration in all patients with malignant obstruction who have not been given it previously.

A fuller list of chronic causes of upper airways obstruction is given in Table 16.1.

Techniques for relief of upper airways obstruction

Minimally invasive techniques

These are listed, together with their strengths and weaknesses in Table 16.2. They can all be used in patients who have already had maximum safe doses of external beam radiotherapy.

Alternatively, tumour resection or stenting can be used before external beam radiotherapy to relieve symptoms and give a safe airway which is then maintained by the radiotherapy.

Resection techniques

Resection can be undertaken using a fibreoptic bronchoscope, but rigid bronchoscopy under general anaesthesia is safer because there is better control of the airway in the event of severe intraoperative bleeding. General anaesthesia is pleasanter for patients who are unlikely to tolerate a full disobliteration at a single session. Repeated sessions reduce palliative benefit and are potentially dangerous because exudation or bleeding from a partially treated tumour can increase airways obstruction. Rigid bronchoscopy with general anaesthesia has thus been shown to have a better efficacy and safety record than fibreoptic bronchscopy.[2]

Table 16.2 Minimally invasive techniques for palliation of upper airway obstruction

Technique	Examples	Advantages	Disadvantages
Resection techniques		Immediate	Limited to intraluminal lesions
	Biopsy forceps	Cheap	Risk of haemorrhage
	Laser	Relatively safe	Expensive equipment
	Diathermy	Cheaper than laser	Insulated bronchoscope needed
	Radiofrequency resection		
	Cryotherapy	Cheaper than laser	Needs two treatment sessions
Brachytherapy		Treats some surrounding tumour	Delayed effect, expensive, radiation hazard
Photodynamic therapy		Treats some surrounding tumour	Delayed effect, skin photosensitisation, repeat bronchoscopy to clear exudate
Stents		Immediate effect	Displacement, obstruction, difficult to remove, perforation into major vessels, placement sometimes difficult
	Expanding wire, e.g. Gianturco, Ultraflex Silastic, e.g. Dumon Dynamic, e.g. Freitag Wire/silastic, e.g. Orlowski T & TY tube (Montgomery)		Needs tracheostomy for placement and regular suction

These endoscopic techniques are suitable for cases in which there is a significant intraluminal lesion. Because the resistance to airflow varies with the fourth power of the radius, even a modest improvement in airway calibre can produce substantial symptomatic improvement. Their limitation is that obstruction can recur within a few weeks or months; either because of the rate of growth of intraluminal tumour or from the unchecked progression of untreated extraluminal tumour. Nevertheless, in some cases of more benign tumours, e.g. carcinoid tumours of typical histology, prolonged remissions of 6 months or more can be seen and treatment can be repeated as often as required.

There have been descriptions of tumour resection using biopsy forceps alone.[3,4] Serious postoperative bleeding is uncommon. Laser,[5-8] diathermy,[9,10] radiofrequency ablation, and cryotherapy[11-13] have all been used to resect obstructing tumours. There are no good studies of the comparative efficacy of these techniques, but review of the literature suggests that in experienced hands results are comparable.

The carbon dioxide laser is used principally in ENT surgery. It can deal with tracheal and main bronchial lesions.[14,15] It cuts cleanly because of its superficial absorption into tissue (hence its popularity in ENT) but its coagulating effect is relatively weak, making it less reliable than the YAG laser for resecting tracheal tumours.[16] It has limited manoeuvrability, because it can only be transmitted through rigid optical systems. Only a few lasers are capable of transmission through optical fibres for use through rigid or fibreoptic bronchoscopes. The Nd YAG laser has been the most extensively used and has been shown to be particularly effective in treating tracheal tumours.[17] However, it may soon be superseded by the newer gallium arsenide diode lasers (Figures 16.1–16.2). These have similar power (60 W) and slightly better tissue absorption. They are smaller, require no cooling system and run off conventional power supplies. For these reasons, the author's unit has been using this laser for the last 7 years. Lasers are probably the most

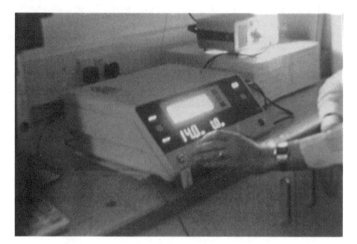

Fig. 16.1 A gallium arsenide diode laser. This newer compact semiconductor laser has a performance comparable to the well-established YAG laser in laser bronchoscopy. Its small size and ability to operate on a conventional power supply make it very versatile for multidisciplinary use on different sites (e.g. urological and gastroenterological tumours). This helps to make the laser more cost effective. These lasers may supersede the YAG in the next few years and their semiconductor design with more robust components may ultimately bring down the equipment costs of laser bronchoscopy.

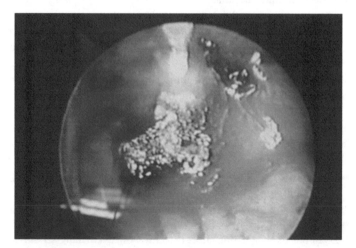

Fig. 16.2 Endoscopic view of laser resection of a lower tracheal tumour. The laser fibre is seen at 12 o'clock. The tumour is situated on the right lateral wall. The view is partly obscured by smoke from the tumour as it is vaporized and coagulated.

popular endobronchial instruments because the optical fibre is very manoeuvrable. They are expensive, but costs are slowly coming down. Diode laser technology, in particular, may lead to cheaper lasers in the future.

Diathermy can be performed with a rigid loop attached to a telescope in a rigid broncho-scope. Some newer fibreoptic bronchoscopes are insulated so that they can be used with flexi-ble diathermy probes. Cryotherapy is also available with both rigid and flexible probes.

Laser bronchoscopy has an excellent safety record, with large series reporting mortality rates of 2% or lower.[5,7,8,18,19] Fewer data are available for the other techniques. Advocates for cryotherapy claim that it is safer than the laser,[11,12] but elect to treat patients in two sessions. This detracts somewhat from the quality of life achieved. The quality of follow-up in papers on laser and other resection techniques is variable. However, the better papers in the literature indicate a symptomatic response and improvement in pulmonary function of 60–95% of cases with an average response rate of around 75%. There are no reliable controlled studies to show any improvement in survival. Two studies have attempted comparison with retrospective controls and suggests a survival advantage.[20,21]

Lasers are rarely suitable for treating benign strictures because they tend to cause further scarring and worse stenosis in the longer term (Figure 16.3). However, they can occasionally be effective in thin diaphragm strictures of the mucosa which do not involve the whole airway wall.[5,22,23] The commoner type of 'bottleneck' stricture should be definitively resected with end-to-end anastamosis if possible, or otherwise treated with a stent. Some strictures will respond reasonably well to dilatation with bougies or balloons at rigid bronchoscopy, or a series of rigid bronchoscopes of increasing diameter can be passed through the stricture to stretch it. However, this technique is limited by the frequency of further dilatations that is likely to be needed and a stent may otherwise be indicated.

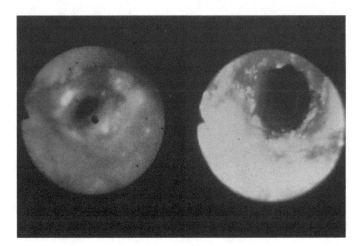

Fig. 16.3 Tracheal stenosis treated with laser resection. The endoscopic view at left shows a pinhole airway through the stricture. This was partly caused by a 'diaphragm' of fibrotic mucosa which has been resected with the laser in the right-hand view. However, there is some involvement of the deeper parts of the tracheal wall so that some airway narro-wing remains. Although laser resection gave good short-term relief, stenting was eventually necessary.

Brachytherapy

This technique is only appropriate for malignant airway obstruction. It employs a high-energy source of gamma radiation which is limited to a radius of a centimetre or two so that the obstructing component of the tumour is treated while surrounding normal tissues are spared. Thus it can be used in patients who have already had external beam therapy where maximum safe cumulative doses have already been given.

Early treatments involved insertion of radioactive gold grains into the tumour using a gun and long needle through the rigid bronchoscope.[24] This was effective, but the patient became a biohazard for several days. Moreover, some needles could detach from necrosing tumour and be coughed up, which further increased the hazard. The high dose rate afterloading machine (e.g. Microselectron) however, uses a pellet of iridium-192 on the end of a flexible drive cable. This is passed through a catheter which is positioned at bronchoscopy within the obstructed airway. Because of the high energy of the radiation, an exposure time of only about 10–15 min is necessary, after which the radioactive source is withdrawn back into the machine. (Figures 16.4–16.5)

Brachytherapy has the advantage over the laser that it can treat tumour outside the airway wall, but its effect is delayed, like that of external beam radiotherapy. Moreover, since the inverse square law applies, more radiation is given to the airway mucosa than to deeper tumour. Although brachytherapy can be repeated this is therefore only possible once or twice because airway strictures will then develop from mucosal fibrosis.[25] There is also a risk of potentially fatal post-treatment haemorrhage which averages about 8% in a number of large series.[25–27]

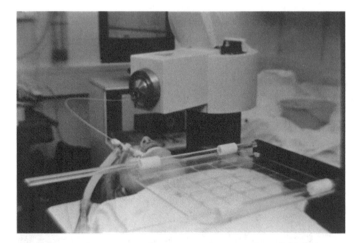

Fig. 16.4 Brachytherapy with the Microselectron high dose rate afterloading machine. The treatment catheter can be seen attached to the head of the Microselectron and passed through an endotracheal tube in an anaesthetized patient. (Most cases can be treated under local anaesthesia alone but occasionally mechanical ventilation is safer.) Under computer control a pellet of iridium-192 on the end of a flexible drive cable is propelled out of a safe in the Microselectron and down the catheter. Once within the lumen of a tracheal or bronchial tumour it progresses in a stepwise fashion, 1 cm at a time. This dwell time is determined by the activity of the radioactive source so that the required dose is given. A grid over the patient's chest (see Figure 16.5) has been used for treatment planning.

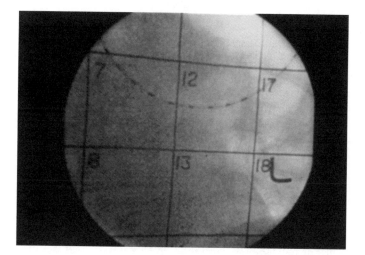

Fig. 16.5 The planning grid as seen on the image intensifier. The grid is marked in 5-cm numbered squares. A guide wire marked at 1-cm intervals has been passed through the treatment catheter. This is used to measure the length of tumour to be treated. The computer in the Microselectron recognizes each interval and can be told at what distance from the catheter tip to start and stop the exposure.

The risk of haemorrhage may, however, relate to the fact that this technique is often used in very advanced tumours where the risk of erosion into a major airway by the tumour itself is also significant. This consideration needs to be born in mind with other minimally invasive techniques as well, but appears to be particularly relevant to brachytherapy. Some workers consider the risk to be increased by combined use of laser and brachytherapy but this has not been the experience of the author's group.[28]

Symptomatic response rates in different large studies range from 70 to 100%, with bronchoscopic evidence of improved airway calibre in 60–90%.

Photodynamic therapy

Photodynamic therapy (PDT) is a form of chemotherapy where laser light is used to activate drugs given systemically to achieve a localized cytotoxic effect. Most work has been done with haemtoporphyrin derivative (HpD), but other drugs including aluminium sulfonated phthallocyanine, aminolaevulinic acid (ALA), and *meso*-tetrahydroxyphenylchlorin (mTHPC) have also been used. These compounds all have an absorption peak in the red. Red light is used because this wavelength has the deepest tissue penetration. When activated the drugs exert a cytotoxic effect with formation of singlet oxygen. PDT has shown most promise in the treatment of small bronchial carcinomas in patients who are unfit for conventional surgery.[29–31] Response is delayed, and there is a risk of airway obstruction by necrotic exudate from the treated tumour which often necessitates a follow-up bronchoscopy after a few days to remove debris. In more critical airway obstruction laser or other resection techniques are therefore clearly safer because they immediately improve the airway. HpD causes skin photosensitization for several weeks, although this is not a problem with ALA which is more rapidly eliminated.

Stents

Many different stents have been developed; their variety results from the lack of an entirely satisfactory design. The two main types are silastic and expanding wire. Both rely on the principle that a structure with a circular cross-section will resist a compressing force, even if it is made of a relatively soft material. Most wire stents also utilize the additional strength of a geodetic mesh in the arrangement of the wire strands in the stent.

Probably the earliest airway stent was that developed by Montgomery[32] for benign subglottic strictures. This involved a 'T' tube with a limb coming out through a tracheostomy. This was necessary for a suction catheter to clear out secretions because a long stent blocks the mucocilliary escalator. Shorter stents such as the Dumon stent[33] can, however, be used without the need for tracheostomy.[33,34]

Thick-walled Silastic stents reduce the airway lumen somewhat. They are inserted at rigid bronchoscopy. Wire stents (e.g. Palmaz, Wallstent, Gianturco, Ultraflex) do not impede mucocilliary clearance and can be positioned at either rigid or fibreoptic bronchoscopy under direct vision[35] or radiographic screening.[36–38] However, tumour can invade through the wire mesh and some earlier types like the Gianturco have occasionally been reported to erode into other structures.[39,40] Covered varieties of wire stent have partly overcome these problems.[41,42] Most published series are small, and often use more than one type of stent. The study by Wilson et al.,[35] however, involved 56 patients treated with a consistent technique using the fibrescope and direct vision. In this study 77% of patients showed symptomatic improvement, two thirds had improved pulmonary function tests, and mean survival was 77 days.

The Ultraflex stent (Figures 16.6–16.12) is a successful modern design which is also available in a covered variety. The Polyflex stent is designed to combine a mesh with a covering but is all made of a plastic material. Unfortunately its wide-bore introducer system requires blind insertion

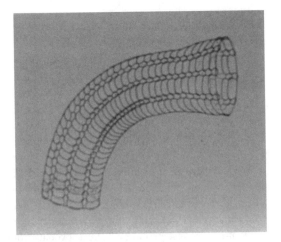

Fig. 16.6 The wire Ultraflex stent has a complex 'knitted' mesh which helps maintain a circular cross-section even when bent as shown in this diagram. It is made of nitenol 'memory metal'. This allows it to be inserted in a relatively soft form but it becomes more rigid once released, when warmed to body temperature.

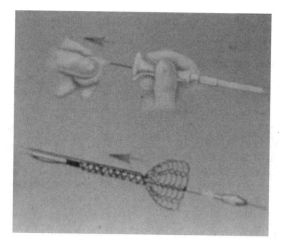

Fig. 16.7 Diagrammatic illustration of stent mechanism. The stent is introduced bound down onto an introducer by a continuous thread. The thread runs back through a central channel in the introducer. When the thread is pulled the stent is progressively freed from the introducer until completely released. The introducer can be placed under direct vision with a rigid bronchoscope and telescope under general anaesthesia (author's preferred method) or passed over a guide wire placed under local anaesthesia with a fibreoptic bronchoscope. It can be released under direct vision or radiographic screening using chest wall markers for guidance.

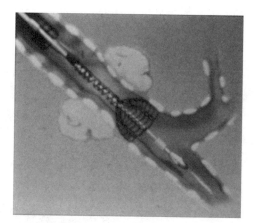

Fig. 16.8 Diagrammatic representation of stent insertion. Under bronchoscopic or radiographic control, the introducer is placed so that the stent straddles the obstructing tumour or stricture. It is then slowly released. It can still be moved proximally or distally in the early stages of release to fine adjust its eventual position. This takes experience to judge, however, because, as with all stents of this type, a stent is longer when compressed than when it has been fully released.

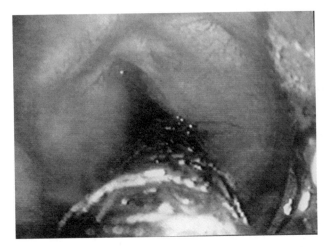

Fig. 16.9 Endoscopic view of stent insertion using the rigid bronchoscope. Using a telescope alongside the introducer, the closed stent on its introducer has been positioned through a tracheal stricture.

without a bronchoscope, which is more hazardous since the airway is completely blocked during insertion. This is also true of the Freitag[43] dynamic stent (Figure 16.13). This complex stent mimics the natural airway, with a soft plastic tube incorporating metal tracheal hoops. On coughing, the soft posterior wall of the stent collapses inwards, like the normal posterior tracheal wall. Thus, as in a normal subject, tracheal cross-sectional area reduces on coughing, increasing the pressure drop across the length of the trachea and facilitating clearance of secretions.

Silicone stents can be removed relatively easily and should be used if there is some prospect for longer-term improvement. Some benign strictures eventually resolve with prolonged stenting over several years. Wire stents should be regarded as permanent implants which become

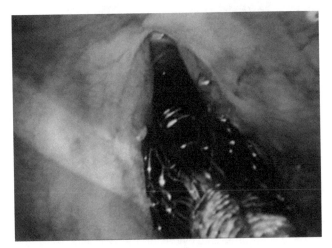

Fig. 16.10 The introducer having been positioned, the stent is now being released. The distal opened portion is now visible beyond and within the lumen of the stricture.

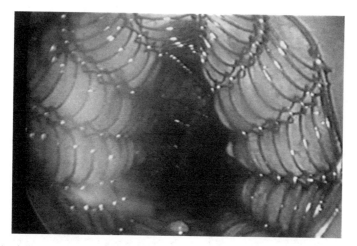

Fig. 16.11 The fully released stent. The empty introducer has been withdrawn. The stent will expand further within the first few hours.

buried in the airway mucosa. There are few long-term data on their safety and efficacy in benign strictures, but they are increasingly being used in this situation.

Conclusions

A wide range of interventions are now possible to palliate upper airway obstruction. If this is severe and acute the most valuable are a resection technique and/or a stent, depending on whether the obstruction is predominantly intra- or extraluminal. Many combinations of these

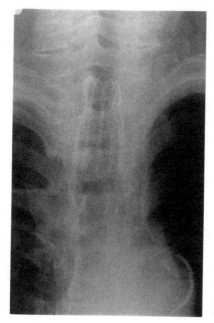

Fig. 16.12 Subsequent chest radiograph confirms that the stent remains stable in the correct position. An indentation is still visible on it at the site of the stricture.

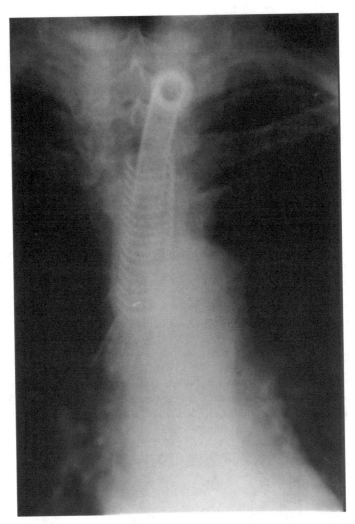

Fig. 16.13 Radiographic view of a Freitag dynamic stent combined with tracheostomy. This patient had prolonged upper airway obstruction from extensive tracheo-bronchomalacia. An earlier permanent tracheostomy had given good palliation initially but stridor had recurred as the lower trachea and main bronchi had become involved. The dynamic stent mimics normal tracheal architecture with metal hoops like cartilages. These can be clearly seen. The device also supports the carina and proximal main bronchi. (The patient felt safer keeping her tracheostomy tube which was re-inserted into the proximal end of the Freitag stent. The tracheostomy tube was successfully removed at a later date.

techniques are possible (with or without subsequent external beam radiotherapy). A discussion of combnation treatment, together with more detailed technical accounts, can be found in other review articles and textbooks.[44,45] These techniques still need to be properly evaluated in controlled trials. Treatments are expensive, require skill and experience, and are best provided in specialist centres. Problems for patients travelling to an appropriate centre and the high cost of treatment are issues which have not yet been properly resolved in the UK or elsewhere. In the authors' opinion these treatments are cost effective when the true cost and quality of life with more conservative management (e.g. hospice care versus continued independent life at home) are taken into consideration.

Patients must, however, be very carefully selected. Some do not want these interventions, and treatment options must be carefully discussed with each individual. It is absolutely crucial to ensure that airways obstruction is the patient's main symptom. The presence of metastatic disease elsewhere is not a barrier to treatment. However, if other symptoms predominate, the risks may then outweigh the benefits. For example, a patient with malignant airway obstruction who is not unduly breathless at rest and has limited mobility through pain or weakness would not normally be a suitable candidate.

Keypoints

- Obstruction of the major airways (trachea and main bronchi) causes severe distress
- In most cases it is better to attempt active palliation rather than employ sedation and conservative measures as a routine
- A number of minimally invasive endobronchial techniques are available – stents, laser therapy, cryotherapy, diathermy, photodynamic therapy, and intraluminal brachytherapy (radiotherapy)
- These techniques are effective in different ways and are complementary
- Prompt referral to a treatment centre is important
- Such centres should offer a range of treatments to cater for different clinical scenarios

Acknowledgements

I am grateful to Boston Scientific/Microinvasive for courteously allowing me to reproduce Figures 16.6–16.8.

References

1 Gelder, C., and Hetzel, M.R. Primary tracheal tumours: a national survey. *Thorax* 1993; **48**: 688–92.

2 George, P.J.M., Garrett, C.P.O., and Hetzel, M.R. Role of neodymium YAG laser in management of tracheal tumours. *Thorax* 1987; **42**: 440–4.

3 Mehta, A.C., and Livingstone, D.R. Biopsy excision through a fibreoptic bronchoscope in the palliative management of airway obstruction. *Chest* 1987; **91**: 774–5.

4 Mathiesen, D.J., and Grillo, H.C. Endoscopic relief of malignant airway obstruction. *Ann Thorac Surg*; 1989; **48**: 469–73.

5 Toty, L., Personne, C., Colchen, A., and Vourc'h, G. Bronchoscopic management of tracheal lesions using the neodymium YAG laser. *Thorax* 1981; **36**: 175–8.

6 Hetzel, M.R., Millard, F.J.C., Ayesh, R., *et al.* Laser treatment for carcinoma of the bronchus. *BMJ* 1983; **286**: 12–16.

7 Hetzel, M.R., Nixon, C., Edmonstone, W., *et al.* Laser therapy in 100 tracheobronchial tumours. *Thorax* 1985; **40**: 341–5.

8 Cavaliere, S., Foccoli, P., and Farina, P.L. NdYAG laser bronchoscopy. *Chest* 1988; **94**: 15–21.

9 Gerasin, V.A., and Shavirovsky, B.B. Endobronchial electrosurgery. *Chest* 1988; **93**: 270–4.

10 Ledingham, S.J.M., and Goldstraw, P. Diathermy resection and radioactive gold grains for palliation of obstruction due to recurrence of bronchial carcinoma after external irradiation. *Thorax* 1989; **44**: 48–51.

11 Maiwand, M.O. Cryotherapy for advanced carcinoma of the trachea and bronchi. *BMJ* 1986; **293**: 181–2.

12 Walsh, D.A., Maiwand, M.O., Nath, A.R., et al. Bronchoscopic cryotherapy for advanced bronchial carcinoma. *Thorax* 1990; **45**: 509–13.

13 Homasson, J.P., Angelbaut, M., and Bonniot, J.P. Cryotherapy of benign and malignant tracheobronchial tumours. Report of 250 cases. *Chest* 1991; **98**(suppl): 1315.

14 Andrews, A Jr., and Horowitz, S. Bronchoscopic CO_2 laser surgery. *Lasers Surg Med* 1980; **1**: 35–45.

15 Goldberg, M., Ginsberg, R., and Basiuk, J. Endobronchial carbon dioxide laser therapy. *Can J Surg* 1986; **29**(3): 180–3.

16 Shapsay, S., Dumon, J., and Beamis, J. Endoscopic treatment of tracheobronchial malignancy. *Otolaryngol Head Neck Surg* 1985; **93**: 205–10.

17 George, P.J.M., Garrett, C.P.O., Nixon, C., *et al.* Laser treatment for tracheobronchial tumours; local or general anaesthesia?. *Thorax* 1987; **42**: 656–60.`

18 Dumon, J.F., Reboud, E., Gerbe, L., *et al.* Treatment of tracheobronchial lesions by laser photoresection. *Chest* 1982; **81**: 278–84.

19 Personne, C., Colchen, A., and Leroy, M. Indications and technique for endoscopic laser resections in bronchology. *J Thorac Cardiovasc Surg* 1986; **91**: 710–15.

20 Brutinel, W.M., Cortese, D.A., McDougall, J.C., *et al.* A two year experience with the Nd YAG laser in endobronchial obstruction. *Chest* 1987; **91**: 159–65.

21 Desai, S.J., Mehta, A.C., Vander Brug Medendrop, S., *et al.* Survival experience following Nd YAG laser photoresection for primary bronchogenic carcinoma. *Chest* 1988; **94**: 939–44.

22 Shapsay, S. Laser applications in the trachea and bronchi: a comparative study of the soft tissue effects using contact and non contact delivery systems. *Laryngoscope* 1987; **97**(suppl 41): 1–26.

23 Ossoff, R., Duncavage, J., Toothill, R., and Tucker, G. Limitations of bronchoscopic carbon dioxide laser surgery. *Ann Otol Rhinol Laryngol* 1985; **94**: 498–501.

24 Law, M.R., Henk, J.H., Goldstraw, P., and Hodson, M.E. Bronchoscopic implantation of radioactive gold grains into endobronchial carcinomas. *Br J Dis Chest* 1985; **29**: 147–52.

25 Speiser, B.L., and Spratling, L. Radiation bronchitis and stenosis secondary to high dose rate endobronchial irradiation. *Int J Radiat Oncol Phys Biol* 1993; **25**: 589–97.

26 Macha, H.N., Koch, K., Stadler, M., *et al.* New technique for treating occlusive and stenosing tumours of the trachea and main bronchi; endobronchial irradiation by high dose iridium-192 combined with laser canalisation. *Thorax* 1987; **42**: 511–15.

27 Stout, R., Burt, P.A., O'Driscoll, B.R., *et al.* HDR brachytherapy for palliation and cure in bronchial carcinoma; the Manchester experience using a single dose technique. *Selectron Brachytherapy J* 1990; **S1**: 48–50.

28 Ornadel, D., Duchesne, G., Wall, P., Ng, A., and Hetzel, M.R. Defining the roles of high dose rate endobronchial brachytherapy and laser resection for recurrent bronchial malignancy. *Lung Cancer* 1997; **16**: 203–13.

29 Cortese, D.A., and Kinsey, J.H. Haematoporphyrin derivative phototherapy in the treatment of bronchial carcinoma. *Chest* 1984; **86**: 8–13.

30 Edell, E.S., and Cortese, D.A. Photodynamic therapy; treatment of early stage lung cancer results and follow up. In: T. Inouye (ed.) *Recent advances in bronchoesophagology: Proceedings of the 6th World Congress on Bronchoesophagology* Amsterdam: Elsevier Science, 1990; 205–10.

31 Kato, H., Kawate, N., and Kinoshita, K. Photodynamic therapy of early stage lung cancer. In: G. Bock, S. Harnett (eds) *Photosensitising compounds: their chemistry, biology and clinical use.* Chichester: John Wiley & Sons, 1990; 531–35.

32 Montgomery, W.W. Reconstruction of the cervical trachea. *Ann Otol* 1964; **73**: 5–9.

33 Dumon, J.F. A dedicated tracheobronchial stent. *Chest* 1990; **97**: 328–32.

34 Tsang, V., and Goldstraw, P. Endobronchial stenting for anastamotic stenosis after sleeve resection. *Ann Thorac Surg* 1989; **48**: 568–71.

35 Wilson, G.E., Walshaw, M.J., and Hind, C.R. Treatment of large airway obstruction in lung cancer using expandable metal stents inserted under direct vision via the fibreoptic bronchoscope. *Thorax* 1996; **51**: 248–52.

36 Simmonds, A.K., Irving, J.D., Clarke, S.W., and Dick, R. Use of expandable metal stents in the treatment of bronchial obstruction. *Thorax* 1989; **44**: 680–1.

37 Varela, A., Maynar, M., Irving, J.D., *et al.* Use of Gianturco self-expandable stents in the tracheobronchial tree. *Ann Thorac Surg* 1990; **49**: 806–9.

38 Spatenka, J., Khaghani, A., Irving, J.D., *et al.* Gianturco self-expanding metallic stents in treatment of tracheo bronchial stenosis after single lung and heart transplantation. *Eur J Cardiothorac Surg* 1991; **5**: 648–52.

39 Hind, C.R.K., and Donnelley, R.J. Expandable metal stents for tracheal obstruction: permanent or temporary? A cautionary tale. *Thorax* 1992; **47**: 757–8.

40 Alfaro, J., Varela, G., De-Miguel, E. *et al.* Successful management of a tracheo-innominate artery fistula following placement of a wire self-expandable tracheal Gianturco stent. *Eur J Cardiothorac Surg* 1993; **7**: 615–16.

41 George, P.J., Irving, J.D., Mantell, B.S., and Rudd, R.M. Covered expandable metal stent for recurrent tracheal obstruction. *Lancet* 1990; **335**: 582–4.

42 Bolliger, C.T., Heitz, M., Hauser, R., Probst, R., and Perruchoud, A.P. An airway wallstent for the treatment of tracheobronchial malignancies. *Thorax* 1996; **51**: 1127–9.

43 Freitag, L., Mohnke, M., Eiker, R., *et al.* Implantation of 156 airway stents of seven types in 94 patients and development of a new dynamic stent. *Am Rev Respir Dis* 1992; **145**: 4.

44 Hetzel, M.R., and Smith, S.G.T. Endoscopic palliation of tracheobronchial malignancies. *Thorax* 1991; **46**: 325–33.

45 Hetzel, M.R., *et al. Minimally invasive techniques in thoracic medicine and surgery.* London: Chapman & Hall, 1995.

Chapter 17

Diffuse airflow obstruction and 'restrictive' lung disease

Martin F. Muers

In this chapter we consider how supportive care can relieve symptoms due to first, chronic diffuse airflow obstruction, and second, pulmonary or pleural disease that causes lung restriction. Together, these conditions provide overwhelmingly the largest number of patients with respiratory problems who may need supportive care.

The first part of the chapter considers the diseases causing chronic diffuse airflow obstruction (otherwise known as chronic airflow limitation, CAL), and briefly discusses their pathophysiology and disease trajectory. Then follows a discussion of the position of supportive measures in a patient's care plan, and a list of the measures available. We also consider the timing of and indications for supportive care and discuss the different modalities of supportive care. Finally, we consider problem areas where physicians and their colleagues seem to have most difficulty.

There is far less evidence for the efficacy of supportive care for restrictive lung disease, but we consider this evidence in the same sequence as for CAL. The chapter closes with a brief summary of some of the key reviews in the field, to assist readers with detailed planning of their own service.

Chronic diffuse airflow obstruction: diseases and their trajectories

By far the commonest disease causing CAL is chronic obstructive pulmonary disease (COPD). This affects now approximately 14 million Americans, outnumbering all adult asthma (10 million). In the UK, about 30 000 adults die from COPD each year. It is defined as 'chronic obstructive pulmonary disease (COPD) is characterised by airflow obstruction. The airflow obstruction is usually progressive, not fully reversible and does not change markedly over several months. The disease is predominantly caused by smoking'. Airflow obstruction is an FEV_1 less than 80%, FEV_1/FVC less than 0.7.[1]

Synonyms are chronic bronchitis and emphysema or chronic obstructive airway disease (COAD). Most cases are caused by tobacco smoking, with smaller contributions from dusty occupations, e.g. long-time coal-mining or welding, and genetic factors, e.g. α_1-antitrypsin deficiency. Pathophysiologically, it is characterized by (1) simple bronchitis, due to large airway mucous gland hypertrophy; (2) bronchiolitis – inflammation of bronchi <2 mm in diameter and with no cartilage, which causes progressive fibrosis and narrowing of these airways; (3) emphysema – destruction of alveolar walls, causing a reduction of gas-exchanging tissue and a loss of elastic tension on the adjacent bronchioles, allowing them to passively narrow and collapse in expiration. In addition, these changes cause the lungs to become hyperinflated (very

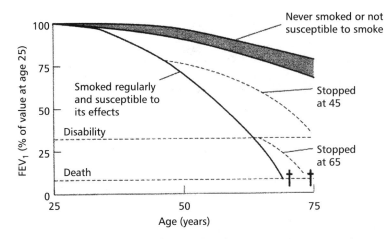

Fig. 17.1 The relationship between lung function (FEV$_1$) and ageing in patients who never smoke or who are not susceptible to it (hatched area) and patients who smoke regularly and who are susceptible. It can be seen that there is an inexorable acceleration of the natural loss of lung function with age in susceptible smokers. The decline resumes the natural track if smoking cessation occurs at any stage. Disability is usual when the FEV$_1$ falls to about 30% of young adult value. Modified from Jones.[51]

large even at rest) because of the concomitant loss of lung elastic recoil which normally tends to balance the outward tension of the chest wall.

The hallmark of COPD is airways obstruction best seen as a low FEV$_1$ (Chapter 1). With normal ageing, the FEV$_1$ progressively but slowly falls during adult life due to an attrition of elastic tissue in the lung (Figure 17.1). In susceptible individuals smoking causes COPD, and there is an acceleration of this loss. This, if unchecked, causes impairment and disability, usually in late middle age. Premature death due to respiratory failure follows in severe cases. Severe disease may be associated with a number of complications such as abnormal blood gases, cor pulmonale (fluid retention, and pulmonary hypertension with right ventricular hypertrophy), and others (Table 17.1). The impact of COPD is

Table 17.1 Possible complications of COPD

Direct	Respiratory failure: chronically abnormal blood gases
	Acute exacerbations: often due to infection
	Cor pulmonale: fluid retention, raised pulmonary artery pressure, and right heart hypertrophy
	Secondary polycythaemia
	Susceptibility to pneumothorax and lung cancer
	Skeletal muscle deconditioning
	Malnutrition, loss of weight
Indirect	Loss of work capacity
	Loss of independence
	Depression and anxiety
	Panic attacks
	Increased impact of co-morbidity

principally to cause exertional dyspnoea, which may progress to dyspnoea at rest in some cases (see below).

Other diseases in which CAL may supervene include asthma, bronchiectasis, some cases of upper lobe tuberculosis or sarcoid, and cystic fibrosis.

Asthma has been described as

> 'a chronic inflammatory disorder of the airways … in susceptible individuals, inflammatory symptoms are usually associated with widespread but variable airflow obstruction and an increased airway response to a variety of stimuli. Obstruction is often reversible, either spontaneously or with treatment'.[2]

It is only in a small minority of patients that irreversible airway narrowing occurs sufficiently severely to cause disability. However, when it does, the clinical features are similar to COPD although respiratory failure and cor pulmonale are less common and the long-term prognosis is much better, with the patients often showing little decline in function over many years.

Bronchiectasis is characterized by abnormally dilated bronchi, which are chronically infected by bacteria, causing the persistent expectoration of mucopurulent or purulent sputum. In most cases the abnormality is confined to one or a few lobes in the lungs, but in others the disease is more diffuse. In these patients airflow obstruction insidiously develops as they age. This may be partially reversible by bronchodilators, but commonly it is not and the condition then resembles COPD in its symptomatology and complications. **Cystic fibrosis** is similar but this disease does in addition have many complications in other organs (Chapter 25). Occasionally, **tuberculosis** and **sarcoidosis** may heal and cause bilateral upper lobe fibrosis and contraction. This leads to distortion and traction of the bronchi of the lower lobes, which may themselves be scarred. The result is obstructive lung disease, which is often severe and fixed. Complications are rare unless secondary pathology occurs, for example a mycetoma. Diffuse airflow obstruction may occasionally be a component of other chronic lung diseases such as extrinsic allergic alveolitis, lymphangioleiomyomatosis (LAM), Langerhans cell histiocytosis (LCH), or post-transplant bronchiolitis obliterans. Such cases are rare, but their problems and need for supportive care are similar to tobacco-related COPD.

Disease-modifying treatment and the place of supportive care

In a sense, all treatments for COPD except long-term oxygen therapy, which improves prognosis but does not affect lung function or quality of life, could be considered 'supportive'. This is because they all have as their goal the relief of symptoms and improvement in patients' functional capacity. However, this chapter focuses on what would generally be described as non-pharmacological treatments, plus the use of drugs which are specifically introduced to treat symptoms (for example opiates for terminal dyspnoea) rather than the underlying disease.

It is crucially important, however, for the disease-modifying treatments (Table 17.2) to be carefully considered in each case. This is best done in parallel with an appropriate assessment of any supportive care needs.

The indicative list of possible supportive care modalities for patients with chronic airflow obstruction is given in Table 17.3. Which modalities should be used for an individual

Table 17.2 Disease-modifying treatments for COPD: outwith the scope of supportive care

Treatment of acute exacerbations

Inhaled and oral bronchodilators

Inhaled and oral corticosteroids

Antibiotics

Treatment of cor pulmonale

Treatment of secondary polycythaemia

Mechanical ventilation

Surgery

Long-term oxygen therapy

patient will depend upon that person's point on their disease trajectory (e.g. mild, moderate, or severe), their disability, and their psychosocial circumstances. In Table 17.3 the most commonly needed modalities are listed first, and modalities required only for the more severely affected patient follow. Other therapies not listed may occasionally be useful, for example complementary medicine (see Chapter 4). Table 17.3 also indicates the chapters where details of these

Table 17.3 Possible supportive care measures in COPD

	Chapter
Smoking cessation assistance	
Exercise rehabilitation	11
Disease education	
Social work advice (patient and family)	
Energy conservation and physical aids advice	15
Posture and breathing technique training	11
Respiratory muscle training	12
Cognitive-behavioural therapy	13
Stress and panic management	13
Drug treatment of depression and anxiety	
Nutrition advice and prescription	14
'Burst' oxygen to relieve dyspnoea	10
Facial airflow to relieve dyspnoea	10
Self-help groups	
Mucolytics	
Drugs for severe dyspnoea and terminal anxiety	9
End of life planning	

treatments can be found in this book. A brief summary of the evidence for the efficacy of these treatments and the others follows later in this chapter.

Assessment of disease severity

The full assessment of a patient with COPD and requiring supportive care needs a multidisciplinary approach including attention to psychosocial as well as physical problems. However, because in general disability follows impairment, and this in turn is easily measured, it has become customary to try to 'hang' ideas of likely disability on measures of airflow obstruction (Figures 17.2 and 17.3). Physical and psychological disability, as measured by questionnaires, are not linearly related to impairment (Figure 17.2). Nevertheless, the concept that patients can be allocated to categories of mild, moderate, or severe disease and treatment adjusted accordingly, has the attraction of simplicity. It is useful in clinical practice, providing it is remembered that (1) the categories are approximate only; (2) some people may be much more or less disabled than others for a given level of FEV_1; and (3) in general, disability accelerates as FEV_1 is lost. The classification in Figure 17.3 is taken from the British Thoracic Society COPD Guideline.[1] This classification is very similar to the US and European statements.[3,4]

◆ Patients with an FEV_1 >80% predicted (for their age, sex, and height) are not regarded as having COPD. An FEV_1 of 50–80% predicted indicates **mild** disease. Such patients are likely to have slight or no breathlessness, and will require only occasional bronchodilators as treatment. Disability is minor.

◆ When the FEV_1 is 30–50% predicted, COPD is likely to be **moderately severe**. Regular dyspnoea on exertion is common, but patients are independent and self-caring, and some can work. At this level, consideration needs to be given both to regular bronchodilator treatment and to some aspects of supportive care.

◆ When the FEV_1 is <30% predicted, COPD is **severe**. There are usually clinically obvious signs of lung hyperinflation, there is dyspnoea on mild exertion, or even at rest in some cases, blood gas abnormalities are usual, and complications common. These patients are nearly always disabled by breathlessness. Supportive care is necessary in addition to conventional medical management.

At all levels of COPD, advice on smoking cessation is required, because of the adverse effect of continued smoking on prognosis (Figure 17.1). At the most extreme level of disability, breathlessness may force patients to a wheelchair-bound existence, confined to home, punctuated by frequent hospital admissions, oxygen dependence, and systemic effects such as cor pulmonale and weight loss. Their prognosis and quality of life is very poor.

Fitting assessments of supportive care needs to conventional management

The physician's first task in managing COPD is to confirm the diagnosis and measure the lung function impairment by a clinical history, examination, and spirometry, and usually a chest radiograph. Other tests, for example full lung function, a CT scan, ECG, reversibility testing, allergy testing, steroid trials, or histamine challenge tests, may be needed in some

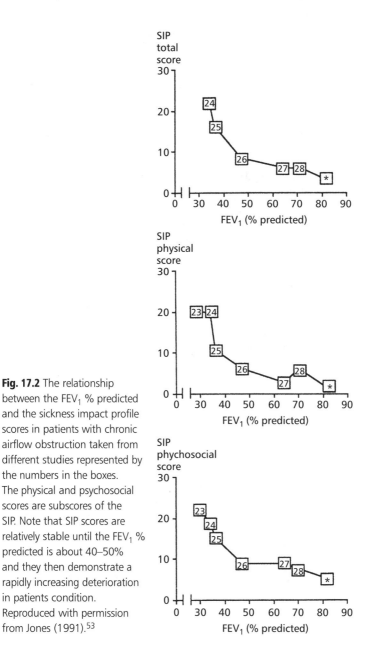

Fig. 17.2 The relationship between the FEV$_1$ % predicted and the sickness impact profile scores in patients with chronic airflow obstruction taken from different studies represented by the numbers in the boxes. The physical and psychosocial scores are subscores of the SIP. Note that SIP scores are relatively stable until the FEV$_1$ % predicted is about 40–50% and they then demonstrate a rapidly increasing deterioration in patients condition. Reproduced with permission from Jones (1991).[53]

cases. At the same time, disability is assessed on history – how much is the disease affecting this person's day-to-day activities at home, work, and leisure? Any obvious psychosocial consequences are noted.

The physician's tasks then are (1) to offer advice on smoking cessation; (2) to explain the diagnosis; (3) to optimize bronchodilator and other disease-modifying treatments such as long-term oxygen therapy; (4) to identify and treat any significant co-morbidity (e.g. heart

The COPD Escalator

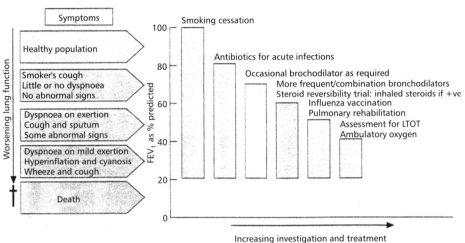

Fig. 17.3 A scheme for a suggested pattern of management for different degrees of severity of patients with COPD. The severity is graded with respect to the post-bronchodilator FEV$_1$ as % of predicted for a patient's age, sex, and height. The gradings are as follows: 80–100% no COPD; 60–80% mild COPD; 40–60% moderate COPD; <40% severe COPD (see text). Reproduced with permission from the BTS guidelines for the management of chronic obstructive pulmonary disease (1997).[1]

failure, arthritis, peripheral vascular disease); and (5) to identify and treat any complications of COPD (e.g. peripheral oedema).

◆ Patients with **mild disease** are not in general likely to have anything other mild impairment, and their COPD is unlikely to interfere with activities of daily living to a significant extent. Their requirements for supportive care are small, confined to simple education and prevention measures as above, together with advice about vaccination against influenza and *Pneumococcus*.

◆ Patients with **moderately severe disease** have usually had to adapt their lifestyles and activities to breathlessness. This means that formal assessment of supportive care needs is usually required. These patients are very suitable for pulmonary rehabilitation programmes with an emphasis on exercise rehabilitation, respiratory muscle training, posture, and breath control techniques, together with perhaps energy conservation, physical aids advice, and social work advice about jobs, benefits, and housing. In practice too few patients are offered these services. Assessments are probably best done by an appropriately trained respiratory nurse specialist or equivalent professional, in parallel with but after separate referral from the managing physician. Primary care physicians need to refer to hospital or ensure that their staff are adequately trained.

◆ Patients with **severe disease** all require assessment for supportive care needs. All the modalities listed in Table 17.3 down to the last two should be considered. These patients usually require an extended one-to-one interview, often at home, with family carers present, and often sessions in addition with a physiotherapist or occupational therapist or equivalent. Other therapists, for example a dietitian or a medical social worker, are brought in as required.

At the **most severe** end of the spectrum, patients may be virtually chair- or bed-bound with very restricted and confined lifestyles and dependent on help for simple activities of daily living. These patients always need assessment as above, but in addition, because prognosis is so poor, end-of-life planning advice is needed usually led by the physician, and a consideration also needs to be given then to direct drug treatment of dyspnoea if distress is evident.

Assessing supportive care needs

Physical needs

Dyspnoea is the principal symptom of and problem with COPD, and a formal assessment of this complements spirometry and direct therapy. Dyspnoea is a complex symptom to evaluate (Chapter 8). For COPD there are in practice several possible levels of assessment, and these instruments are usually usefully added to a formal assessment of **disability** by an exercise test. Levels of assessment may be summarized as:

- Usual clinical history and examination – all patients.
- A simple questionnaire assessing exercise capacity, e.g. the MRC scale.[5]
- A questionnaire incorporating a patient's perception of effort doing various things, e.g. the Baseline Dyspnoea Index (BDI).[6]
- A questionnaire which evaluates the impact of dyspnoea on a patient's quality of life, e.g. the Chronic Respiratory Disease Questionnaire (CRQ),[7] or the St George's Respiratory Questionnaire (SGRQ).[8]

The use of breathlessness scores during or at the end of exercise, for example the Borg scale,[9] is not widespread outside research. In practice most patients would be assessed adequately by the use of a single questionnaire and an objective measure of respiratory disability such as a 6-min walking distance (MWD) test,[10] or a shuttle walk test (SWT).[11] Predicted normal values for the 6MWD are now available,[12] but normative data for the SWT are awaited. For a fuller discussion of dyspnoea assessment the reader is referred to the ATS statement.[13]

Psychosocial needs

It is extremely important not simply to record exercise capacity but to relate this to a person's wishes and situation. Patients with severe COPD have a very poor quality of life, with poor scores on both generic and health-specific measures of quality of life.[15] In my practice, the usual aspects of life which seem moderately frequently to need particular attention in severe COPD are:

- disease education
- advice about mobility outside the home
- benefits advice
- social isolation.

These aspects usually need the input of a trained medical social worker or respiratory nurse specialist.

Psychological needs

Psychological symptoms are probably underrecognized. They consist of depression, anxiety, and panic attacks.

Because the physical impact of COPD or its treatment can cause symptoms akin to endogenous depression, such as weight loss, lack of energy, or anxiety (e.g. palpitations or tremor), most authorities recommend the use of a formal simple screening test. The simplest is probably the HAD score.[16] Abnormal scores need to be followed by a further measure and appropriate referral. It used to be thought that patients with COPD had an unusually high level of psychiatric morbidity, but a recent meta-analysis has highlighted the paucity of reliable evidence.[17]

Organization of supportive care for COPD patients

It is not possible to be prescriptive about this because of the different healthcare systems throughout the world, and the way professions supplementary to medicine have developed in parallel. For example, in the UK most respiratory units have respiratory nurse specialists – senior nurses with particular training in respiratory disease – looking after asthma, COPD, long-term oxygen therapy, etc. In the US, by contrast, a similar role is taken by respiratory therapists who commonly have a physiotherapy background.

Essentially, however, supportive care must be seen as a cooperative effort between patients and their carers on the one hand and health professionals on the other, and also as a multiprofessional service provision. It is necessary for the physician to have access to a colleague who can coordinate this help. Many units subsume this into a formal pulmonary rehabilitation programme (see Chapter 11). This has many benefits, provided that (1) it is seen as not only giving exercise training, and (2) patients who are very disabled are not neglected because they are thought not to be fit enough to benefit. These in fact are the patients who are likely to have the most need of psychosocial support. Whether palliative care services have a role to play in coordinating supportive, holistic care for patients with severe but not terminal COPD is uncertain. It is increasingly being realized that patients with severe non-malignant disease have quality of life and healthcare needs which are as great as those of patients with cancer.[18,19] However, in the absence of research evidence, formal links and referral from respiratory medical units to palliative care remains the exception rather than usual practice, though this may change in the future.

One area where a lesson from palliative care needs to be absorbed into general respiratory practice is the question of follow-up and continuing responsibility. Traditional medical consultations in outpatient clinics or in primary care are poor at considering psychosocial demands since they tend to focus on conventional treatment. The effectiveness of pulmonary rehabilitation is proven in the short term, but fades without reinforcement.[20] The palliative care service model provides parallel and ongoing nurse support for cancer patients at the same time. Regular specialist nurse input is needed for disabled COPD patients. Formal testing of this service model has not so far been encouraging,[21] but more randomized trials are needed.

Summary

For moderate COPD, a formal assessment of supportive care needs is required. This should be coordinated by a nurse specialist, with other professionals being brought in when necessary. After any programme of treatment patients need to be followed up regularly, ideally by a parallel care pathway to their usual medical reviews. Validated instruments for dyspnoea and disability should be used whenever possible. This encourages precision and allows measurement of efficacy and some estimate of cost effectiveness.

Effectiveness in COPD of the components of supportive care

Much of the data on supportive care treatments in other chapters of this book is taken from work with COPD patients, since they are by far the largest group. What follows is a brief review of the conclusions from research on these different modalities, where it is known, together with some comment about the practicalities of applying them.

Advice on smoking cessation

Most patients with COPD are aware that their disease has been caused by tobacco smoking, and wish to quit. Most will have tried, perhaps more than once.[22] Historically, formal quit programmes have been seen as relatively ineffective, with low (<5%) success rates. Now, however, the best techniques are well known and validated, the benefit of nicotine replacement treatment has been shown, and selected antidepressants may in the future raise quit rates from the present 10% to 20% or even more.[23]

Evidence-based summaries of the research are now available.[24,25] The essential components are listed in Box 17.1. Smoking cessation advice and treatment should be a component of all programmes of COPD supportive care, and apply to patients of all disease severity. There is no scientific or moral reason to deliberately and routinely withhold supportive care from patients who continue to smoke, except that ambulatory oxygen does not appear to benefit smokers.

Pulmonary rehabilitation

The present position has been excellently summarized by an ATS Working Party.[26] Meta-analyses have shown that rehabilitation based on exercise improves exercise tolerance probably at any level of disease, although benefit in the severely disabled may be less (Figure 17.4).[27,28] Most studies also show improvement in health-related quality of life (HRQL) although less clearly. It is very difficult to disentangle the benefit of exercise *per se* on HRQL from the benefit of other components or other programmes, e.g. education or medical social work. However,

Box 17.1 The best way of stopping smoking

International medical studies now show that the best way of stopping smoking is as follows:

1 To make a firm decision that **you** want to stop smoking.

2 To discuss with your doctor or specialist nurse a **quit date**, which is best within 2 weeks of meeting that person.

3 To request a supply of **nicotine replacement** for regular use once you have stopped smoking.

4 To tell as many people as you can that you will be stopping smoking on that particular day.

5 To stop smoking **completely and absolutely on that day**.

6 To ensure that you see your doctor or specialist nurse **within a week** of stopping.

7 To ensure that you see your doctor or specialist nurse for further advice **4 weeks** later.

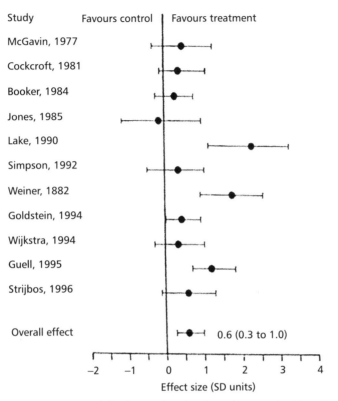

Fig. 17.4 Effects of respiratory rehabilitation on functional exercise capacity. The effect size is given as SD units for different studies with their confidence intervals, and the overall treatment effect is significant at 0.6. Reproduced with permission from the American Thoracic Society official statement on pulmonary rehabilitation (1999).[26]

at present, it is reasonable to infer that programmes should consist of a multidisciplinary approach, and the following sections will assume that.

Referral criteria

These have been listed in the ATS review (Table 17.4).[26] Details of exercise prescription are given in Chapter 11. Rehabilitation seems to be equally effective in the hospital outpatient or home setting, provided that it is adequately supervised. The choice of setting will depend upon local factors, costs, and availability. The need for follow-up has been emphasized above.

Disease and treatment education

An informed patient should be a more self-confident and content patient. Education about the lungs, their disease, its impact, and the treatments available is a usual component of rehabilitation programmes for COPD. There is some formal evidence of benefit.[29] On present evidence there seems no reason to omit education from rehabilitation programmes.

Table 17.4 Common indications for referral for pulmonary rehabilitation

Respiratory disease resulting in:	
Anxiety engaging in activities	
Breathlessness with activities	
Limitations with:	social activities
	leisure activities
	indoor and/or outdoor chores
	basic or instrumental activities of daily living
Loss of independence	

Source: American Thoracic Society official statement on pulmonary rehabilitation.[26] Reproduced with permission.

Social work advice

Most patients with moderate or severe COPD either struggle to work, cannot work, are unemployed, or are retired. Many are elderly and live alone. Their accommodation may not be appropriate and they may be socially isolated with scattered families and little community contact. Formal reviews of rehabilitation do not mention these problems specifically,[26] but personal accounts emphasize them.[30] The author believes, from personal experience, that many people resent their poverty and isolation. Advice about housing, state and other benefits, mobility, and community support seem sensible, and is routine in the palliative care plan of cancer patients.

Energy conservation and physical aids advice

This treatment aims to optimize a patient's exercise capacity by giving them techniques to accomplish activities of daily living more easily and by providing aids for activities such as walking, bathing, ascending stairs, and mobility. These should enable patients to do more, and more comfortably. Domestic assessment is needed, by an occupational therapist or a nurse specialist in the UK or by a respiratory healthcare worker in the US. Benefits are obvious.

Posture, breathing technique training, and respiratory muscle training

The treatments of dyspnoea *per se,* after treatment of the underlying condition, can be listed as (1) those reducing ventilatory drive, e.g. oxygen or opiates; (2) those improving respiratory muscle function; (3) those reducing perception of dyspnoea, e.g. psychotherapy or anxiolytics. This section considers treatments in the second group. Further details can be found in Chapters 11 and 12.

Most patients spontaneously adopt pursed-lip breathing and a forward-leaning posture with shoulder girdle support. This has been shown to reduce dyspnoea in COPD.[31] There is doubt, however, whether voluntary 'diaphragmatic' breathing and abdominal muscle manoeuvres are helpful.[32] The key adaptations seem to be to restore patients' breathing patterns to a slower respiratory rate with more complete emptying of the lungs between each breath. This makes physiological sense as it allows a reduction in dynamic hyperinflation, which is one of the main reasons for their increased sensation of dyspnoea.

Whether respiratory muscle training, used routinely and not in studies, can relieve dyspnoea remains controversial, as shown by a recent meta-analysis of 17 trials.[34] In the author's opinion it is better on present evidence to focus on peripheral muscle training both upper and lower limbs, for which the evidence of efficacy is better.

Cognitive-behavioural therapy

Many patients with severe COPD have severe disabling emotional associations with their breathlessness. These may comprise feelings of worthlessness, a fear of being alone or in a large company of people, a fear of being unable to keep control of their breathing, or anxiety that acute dyspnoea may develop unexpectedly or suddenly. Cognitive therapy is essentially a guided programme of correction of inappropriate thoughts about dyspnoea, desensitization to circumstances thought by the patient to provoke it, and increasing a sense of self-control. Behavioural techniques principally comprise a number different approaches usually subsumed under the title **relaxation therapy**.[35] Patients are encouraged to make use of relaxation tapes, progressive muscle relaxation, and abdominal breathing to slow down the respiratory rate, and treatment may also include visualization and music therapy. There is evidence that these approaches have short-term effects, but my own experience is that longer-term domiciliary benefit is hard to identify and often patients themselves find it hard to apply these techniques when they are really frightened. The topic of respiratory panic has been well reviewed by Somoller et al.[36]

Drugs for depression and anxiety

Although there may be uncertainty about whether depression and anxiety are more prevalent in COPD patients than in a controlled population, the background frequency of depression is so high in elderly people that these conditions need to be sought and diagnosed in any patient housebound or severely disabled by COPD. The treatment of identified depression is straightforward. Tri- or quadricyclic antidepressants can be used in standard doses, but it must be noted that in elderly people it may take far longer than the anticipated 2 weeks for benefits to emerge.

The use of anxiolytics, such as benzodiazepines or haloperidol, is far more difficult. There are legitimate worries about respiratory depression and habituation. They should be avoided if the blood gases are not known, especially if cor pulmonale is present. Nevertheless, personal observation suggests that even a small dose of benzodiazepine, e.g. diazepam 2 mg three times daily or lorazepam 1mg three times daily, may produce a gratifying subjective response on occasions. For patients with severe disease they probably should only be introduced under the direct supervision of a respiratory physician. There is no reason to withhold these drugs in terminally ill patients.

Nutrition advice and prescription

Loss of weight, particularly of fat-free mass, is increasingly common as COPD becomes more severe, and it is a prognostic factor independent of lung function (Chapter 14). The causes are multifactorial and not yet fully understood. The problem with this weight loss is that it is in practice very difficult to reverse. Oral supplements to raise energy intake by more than 30% over baseline have been shown in some trials to increase respiratory muscle strength and improve 6 MWD,[36] but reproducing these results in routine clinical practice is hard. Oral corticosteroids, progesterone, and growth hormone are not effective at substantially increasing fat-free mass. Percutaneous enterogastric feeding (PEG) works, but is invasive and again weight gain is predominantly fat. These results are disappointing. Until research produces novel drugs (such as leptin antagonists), simple dietary advice and frequent high-energy, easy-to-eat meals, which require little chewing, seems to be the optimal strategy for most patients. Expensive proprietary supplements are probably overprescribed and have not been shown to be cost-effective in any randomized trial in COPD.[37]

'Burst' oxygen and facial airflow

A rationale for the assessment and prescription of long-term oxygen therapy (LTOT) is beyond the scope of this chapter. Ambulatory oxygen, on the other hand, may provide relief of exercise-induced dyspnoea in patients who desaturate by at least 4% to <90% on exercise.[38] These recent guidelines suggest that it should only be prescribed if, when used during an exercise test, oxygen provides a 10% benefit over baseline (air) in distance walked or in subjective breathlessness. Patients who are hypoxic (PaO_2 <8 kPa at rest) can be considered for assessment. Review of the provision is important, because many patients will use it little. Housebound patients may benefit from an oxygen supply that allows them to become mobile out of doors. Formal exercise tests may be difficult in these patients, and an assessment of subjective benefit is all that can be done. Patients who continue to smoke should probably not have ambulatory oxygen, because of the risk of burns.

Short-burst oxygen is extensively prescribed for dyspnoea relief in COPD. Unfortunately there is a totally inadequate research base for which to proceed to firm recommendations about prescriptions. There is no physiological rationale for prescription in patients whose SaO_2 is >92% at rest on air and during and after exercise. If these patients report relief, this is a placebo effect due to facial cooling or relief of anxiety. Escalation of treatment from occasional to near-continuous use in very breathless but not hypoxaemic patients is commonly seen in late stage COPD. These patients ideally need a comprehensive assessment of their dyspnoea and use of other strategies such as facial cooling, posture, or anxiolytics.

It is likely that much of the reported benefit of oxygen treatment by mask in this situation is due to a facial cooling effect. Facial cooling appears to reduce the perception of dyspnoea without altering physiological measurements, i.e. tidal volume or respiratory rate.[39,40] Options include oxygen (because air is not usually available in cylinders), fans, open windows, hand-held 'windmills', or facial sponging. Experimentation is needed in every case.

Self-help groups

These groups are popular with some patients and can ameliorate social isolation, provide a focus for charitable work, and reinforce previous educational and rehabilitation programmes. They work best for people who have adapted to their disabilities and are relatively mobile. They need motivated and enthusiastic lay organizers and the regular support of health workers, usually nurses or physiotherapists. An example in the UK is the Breathe-Easy organization (www.lunguk.org/breathe).

Mucolytics

These are discussed in Chapter 26. In studies statistically significant benefits are small, even for rhDNase in cystic fibrosis. Just occasionally mucus impaction may respond to nebulized acetyl-cysteine, but otherwise it is the author's view that these drugs should not be used widely before better research evidence is available. The uncertainty about what to measure in sputum – volume, 'consistency', or 'pourability'– has impeded the assessment of clinical value of these drugs.

Drugs for severe dyspnoea and terminal anxiety

The model for the direct treatment of dyspnoea due to COPD parallels the model for cancer. This suggests that when dyspnoea is present on effort alone, non-pharmacological measures should predominate. When dyspnoea worsens, until breathlessness occurs not quite at rest but on minimal exertion, this still probably holds true, but some use can be made of desensitization using drugs such as weak opioids or antihistamines. When dyspnoea occurs at rest and is distressing, strong opiates or anxiolytics are needed as non-drug methods to control dyspnoea are usually ineffective particularly in frail patients near to death. In the 1980s and early 1990s, nine studies were published examining the effect of promethazine, dihydrocodeine, morphine, and diamorphine on dyspnoea in ambulatory COPD patients. These gave variable results, which have been well summarized by Stulbarg et al.[41] More recently, a well-controlled randomized prospective double-blind placebo-controlled trial examining the effects of slow release morphine in doses up to 20 mg twice daily in severe COPD, showed no benefit from this treatment on either dyspnoea, exercise tolerance, or HRQL.[42] This study suggests strongly that these drugs cannot be recommended for routine use; they can of course be tried on an individual patient basis but should first have their effectiveness formally assessed by a visual analogue scale (VAS) assessment (or a 6MWD, if the patient can walk) and they should be promptly withdrawn if not effective.

For the terminally ill patient with cancer there is good evidence from randomly controlled trials (RCTs) that opiates relieve dyspnoea (see Chapter 6). There have been no RCTs in COPD patients. However, there is no reason to withhold these drugs providing that: (1) their prescription follows discussion of the patient about the prognosis and the possible effects on respiratory control and life shortening has been explained; (2) they are then given a short-acting preparation with frequent (<24 h) dose adjustments. In practice I find that patients with end-stage disease which is predominantly emphysema without carbon dioxide retention tolerate opiates very well. However, drowsiness is almost always an accompaniment of an adequate dose and relatives need to be warned of this. Nebulized opioids are of unproven benefit in the majority of RCTs (see Chapter 6).

There is also no RCT data to support the use of anxiolytics in these patients. Nevertheless, again as in cancer, where anxiety and fear of death or intolerable dyspnoea are obvious there is no reason to withhold these drugs in informed patients whose carers are aware of the balance between the likely benefits and side effects. Oral diazepam, e.g. 5 mg three times daily, lorazepam 1–2 mg three times daily, or later midazolam 10 mg/24 h by syringe driver are needed, as in cancer patients.

Problem areas

Home ventilation

This is appropriate supportive care for patients with respiratory failure due to neuromuscular disease or thoracic cage deformity (Chapter 18). There are some patients with type II respiratory failure in whom nocturnal non-invasive ventilation (NIPPV) maintains a lower overall PCO_2, prevents episodes of hypercapnoeic ventilatory failure and improves quality of life by reducing unpleasant effects of a chronically raised PCO_2, e.g. headache and peripheral oedema

However, there is as yet no RCT evidence to justify regular introduction of NIPPV as an adjunct to LTOT or other treatment for patients with severe and disabling COPD and respiratory failure. Trials are awaited.

Prognosis and end-of-life planning

It is very difficult and often misleading to apply population data without hesitation to an individual patient, because of the wide variation in outcome of patients with a similar % predicted FEV_1. Nevertheless the % predicted FEV_1 is easily the strongest predictor of overall mortality and Figure 17.5 shows that the average median survival of patients with an FEV_1 of <40% predicted (severe disease) over 60 years is about 3 years.[43]

There is research evidence to suggest that additional features worsening the prognosis for such patients are:

- severe hypoxaemia (PaO_2 air <7 kPa)[43]
- weight loss, e.g. 10% ideal body weight[44]
- significant co-morbidity, especially left ventricular failure.[45]

There is surprisingly no evidence (1) that physicians can predict the outcome of an isolated episode of acute respiratory failure needing intubation, or (2) that the occurrence of such an episode has an influence on prognosis over and above that of the underlying lung function and functional state. An exception to the last point is that the prognosis appears to be poor if the pH is very low (e.g. <7.22–7.26) during such an episode.[46]

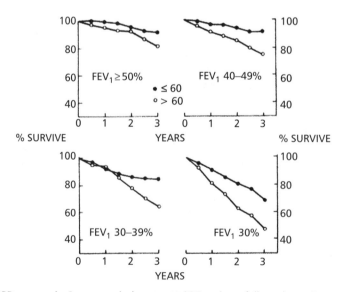

Fig. 17.5 COPD prognosis. 3-year survival amongst 985 patients followed over 3 years in the US intermittent positive pressure breathing trial. The patients were segregated with respect to their ages and enrolment, less or greater than 60 years. It can be seen how the prognosis is inversely related to the FEV_1, and that the most severely affected patients have a 3-year survival of <50%. Reproduced with permission from Poole et al. (1998)[42]

Informally, personal observation suggests that the following may be adverse prognostic factors to consider in addition:

- increasingly frequent admissions with exacerbations of COPD without obvious infection as a cause
- reducing performance status, for example housebound but mobile, progressing to chairbound, progressing to bedbound
- persistent infection developing otherwise uncomplicated severe COPD
- increasingly frequent use (dependence) on nebulizer therapy and 'burst' oxygen for dyspnoea relief.

Unfortunately there is no published data to help the physician synthesize these factors and experience, careful measurement and assessment are the best guides. Prognosis is important in two situations (Figure 17.6):

- in a deteriorating patient, to advise him or her about the (relative) imminence of death
- to determine the patient's wishes regarding invasive ventilatory support for a future exacerbation
- to help families decide whether intensive care should be continued if it is manifestly failing to aid recovery from acute episodes.

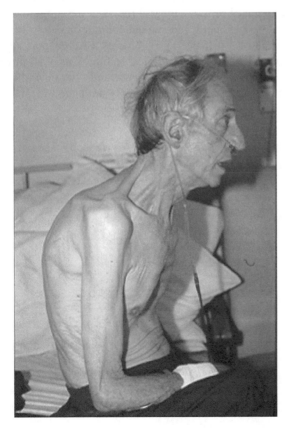

Fig. 17.6 A 70-year old patient with severe COPD in whom end-of-life planning would be appropriate. He is dyspnoeic at rest, hypoxic despite LTOT, has lost weight rapidly, and is chairbound. FEV_1 0.6 L (28% predicted).

Such discussions are necessary, but difficult. Staff need to have formal training in communication skills as they would for cancer work – the problems are the same. Particularly where there is advice to be given about withholding or withdrawing life-sustaining therapy, doctors need to behave in a manner consistent with nationally agreed ethical guidelines, for example those in the US.[47] In such cases second opinions from other physicians are often necessary, valuable and reassuring for patients and their families.

Non-obstructive ('restrictive') lung disease

This section will consider the evidence for the use of supportive care for diseases of the lungs and pleura, which cause disability in the absence of airflow obstruction (Table 17.5). Diseases causing chest-wall deformity and respiratory failure due to neuromuscular conditions are considered in Chapter 16. Non-obstructive lung diseases are often severe, but even collectively they are much less common than obstructive lung disease. In the UK at present, compared with the 30 000 patients dying of COPD, the annual mortality rate from cryptogenic fibrosing alveolitis (CFA) is about 1500. Probably for this reason, supportive care needs of patients like this have not been much studied.

Diffuse parenchymal lung diseases (DPLD) comprise a large number of disparate and relatively rare disorders, which affect the interstitium. Essentially they cause inflammation and subsequent destruction and scarring of the alveolar capillary units of the lung acini (Chapter 2). Gas exchange is impeded by inflammation, scarring and distortion, but airway function is normal. With the onset of fibrosis, the lungs shrink, and the end result is lungs which are retracted, stiff with a low compliance and marked diminution in tests of gas diffusion in the laboratory (DL_{CO} and K_{CO}) (Table 17.5). Patients usually report a gradual onset of exertional dyspnoea, which is the cardinal clinical feature. This often progresses inexorably to dyspnoea at rest with a fast resting respiratory rate and a low tidal volume and persisting and severe hypoxaemia but a well preserved PCO_2 until the terminal stages.

Table 17.5 Examples of non-obstructive lung disease which may require supportive care

Diffuse parenchymal lung disease (DPLD)	Fibrosing alveolitis	Cryptogenic Occupational (asbestosis) Drug-induced (antineoplastics) Radiation (therapeutic RT) Systemic vasculitis (systemic sclerosis)
	Pneumoconiosis	Coalworker's pneumoconiosis Silicosis
	Postinflammatory	ARDS Tuberculosis, sarcoidosis
Post-pneumonectomy		
Diffuse pleural thickening		Asbestos-induced (benign) Drug-induced (bromocriptine) Mesothelioma
Pulmonary vascular disease		Primary pulmonary hypertension Recurrent pulmonary emboli

Complications include persistent cough, secondary infection and cor pulmonale. The commonest disease in this category worldwide is probably CFA. Its prognosis is surprisingly poor; the median survival of a group of 1000 patients presenting to UK physicians in a recent study was only 2 years.[48] Most patients die of respiratory failure or from lung cancer to which they are very susceptible.

Essentially, the lung fibrosis of pneumoconiosis due to coal dust or silica, although quite different in aetiology and pathological appearances, produces a similar pattern of respiratory disability. These conditions may progress long after dust exposure ceases, and there is no effective anti-inflammatory treatment for them, or for fibrosing alveolitis, except for the occasional patient with CFA who may respond to oral steroids and anti-inflammatory drugs. Nevertheless, these are often used, often in high doses with subsequent side effects.

Patients surviving acute respiratory distress syndrome (ARDS) may have persistent lung fibrosis, although often an initially appalling chest radiograph will slowly clear over succeeding months. For cancer, surgeons try to avoid operating on patients with poor preoperative lung function who they think may become disabled by a pneumonectomy. However, occasionally, patients do become unexpectedly breathless postoperatively. Their dyspnoea often seems out of proportion to their residual lung function. This may be because of the activation of chest-wall mechanoreceptors on the operated side causing a marked disparity between respiratory effort and achieved ventilation. The same phenomenon is seen in mesothelioma and unilateral diffuse pleural thickening due to asbestos.

Patients with chronic pulmonary vascular disease have normal lung architecture and mechanics but are breathless because of a very abnormal gas exchange. Active treatment is sometimes possible – e.g. embolectomy, prostacycline, and vasdilators – but if these patients are not transplanted they usually progress to disabling breathlessness comparatively rapidly.

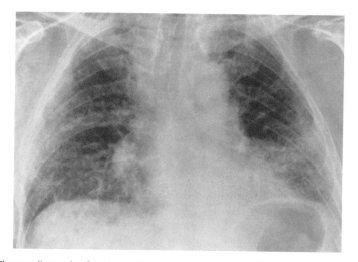

Fig. 17.7 Chest radiograph of patient with advanced cyptogenic fibrosing alveolitis (CFA or UIP). FVC_1 30% predicted; transfer factor (DLCO) 22%. He requires high-flow nasal oxygen to maitain an SaO_2 of >92%. He has a wheelchair and a stair lift at home. His perceived quality of life and psychological state improved rapidly after two home assessments by a respiratory nurse specialist and a social worker

Assessment and treatment

The usual mistake that clinicians make with these patients is to concentrate too much on manipulating usually largely ineffective treatments directed at the primary pathology. The reason is probably that there is not a general appreciation of the potential role for supportive care – again because of the paucity of the literature and the relative rarity of these patients in most physicians' practices. The approach to the symptomatic patient with non-obstructive lung disease should in my view be the same as for COPD:

- The physician should ensure an accurate diagnosis, treat the underlying disease whenever possible, recognize and treat any complications, and assess and treat any co-morbidity.
- The physician should also ensure that the supportive care needs of these patients are assessed and met by a multiprofessional approach considering the modalities listed in Figure 17.4.

There are no published guidelines to help with the timing of referral or selection of these patients for a comprehensive supportive care assessment. However, by analogy with COPD, it would seem sensible to consider patients for this when they have troublesome limitation and/or dyspnoea with activities of work, pleasure, and daily living, or they suffer anxiety about these or are losing previous independence.

Again, the usual deficiency of care, I suggest, is that these patients are assessed far too late in their disease trajectories. For example, in a review of the only 32 of 350 patients referred to their lung rehabilitation centre with non-obstructive lung disease, Foster and Thomas[49] found a mean 6MWD of only 276 feet (84 m) on admission, which is likely to have been only about 15% of predicted. Given the poor prognosis of many of these patients, a much earlier referral for assessment by a nurse-led team seems sensible.

Components of supportive care likely to be helpful for non-obstructive lung disease patients

Table 17.3 indicates the chapters in which more detailed descriptions of some of these topics are to be found.

Smoking cessation advice

These patients have major problems with tissue oxygen delivery. Heavy smoking can cause a carboxyhaemoglobin level of >10%. Although no change in prognosis is to be expected, advice on smoking cessation seems rational and can be guided by measures of carboxyhaemoglobin now possible with hand-held meters.

Exercise rehabilitation

The one study known to me[49] demonstrated a highly significant increase in 6MWD after a 4-week inpatient rehabilitation course in 32 patients with a mixture of lung fibrosis, fibrothorax, and other conditions. However, there were no measures of HRQL, and only 3 patients had alveolitis. More data is required, and possibly a multicentre study is needed.

General measures

Logically, it would seem to be worthwhile assessing and providing disease education, social work advice, energy conservation, cognitive-behavioural therapy, stress management, and drug treatment for depression and anxiety, as for disabled COPD patients. It seems unlikely, however, that respiratory muscle training or breathing control would be beneficial. There is no evidence that such patients become nutritionally depleted before they become very ill, although this would not be unexpected since the metabolic costs of a very considerably increased respiratory workload would require a correspondingly increased energy input. Weight loss therefore should be assessed as in COPD. Many of these patients are treated with relatively high doses of oral corticosteroids. Steroid-induced myopathy can affect both peripheral and respiratory muscles, as demonstrated by biopsy.[50]

Oxygen therapy

Patients with alveolitis, but not necessarily those with coarse fibrosis or pleural disease, have very abnormal gas exchange and readily become hypoxic on exertion with desaturation at rest following. Oxygen therapy, often at high flow rates, can correct hypoxaemia. However, the cause of their breathlessness is not solely hypoxaemia but is almost certainly due, too, to abnormal afferent nerve traffic from receptors in their shrunken and inflamed lungs and from chest-wall mechanoreceptors. Thus, the impact of oxygen therapy on dyspnoea is likely to be variable. As for COPD patients, it seems sensible to limit this treatment to patients who have been formally assessed for either 'burst' or ambulatory oxygen and who have been shown to benefit form this in a laboratory or inpatient setting. The use of continuous oxygen, again often at high flow rates, may be needed to correct resting hypoxaemia in the more severely disabled patients and requires measurement. Again, physiological correction may not be accompanied by any symptom relief. The facial cooling effect of oxygen by mask may be beneficial, as in COPD.

Self-help groups

There is a gradual move towards national registries of patients with some of these rare and disabling diseases. Systemic sclerosis and LAM have support groups in the UK. Others may be formed in future. The internet provides a possible source of information, but patients and their carers should be aware that some of the material may not necessarily have been medically approved.

Drug treatment of severe rest dyspnoea

As for COPD, opiates should be tried. There is much less risk of carbon dioxide retention and loss of ventilatory drive. High doses of drugs may be needed to desensitize patients to their difficult combination of hypoxaemia and high ventilatory drive. A reduction in respiratory rate is likely to worsen hypoxaemia and should be particularly allowed for.

Transplantation

This is more often considered for these patients than for people with COPD, because they are often younger and usually do not have other smoking-related disorders. Difficulties than then arise are

- There may be a long delay (perhaps up to 2 years in the UK) between acceptance on a programme and any surgery. There is a tendency to overlook any deterioration in the meantime and not refer for supportive care assessment because the definitive treatment is being contemplated and may occur at any time.

- Many patients are turned down for transplantation. This naturally leads to increased distress, and sometimes bitterness that needs to be recognized and assuaged.

Transplanted patients usually have comprehensive support from their transplant unit. It is notable that exercise rehabilitation may not return patients to a level of exercise capacity predicted by their (new) lung and cardiorespiratory function. This seems to be because of persistent peripheral skeletal muscle abnormalities which are due principally to the previous underlying disease and perhaps previous immobility and anti-inflammatory treatment. For reasons which are not clear, these abnormalities do not reverse after transplantation, and there is also a concern that post-transplant drugs may have a deleterious affect on skeletal muscle function. This particular problem emphasizes the importance of pulmonary rehabilitation and exercise in patients with DPLD in particular who may be awaiting transplantation.[51]

Medicolegal issues

Some DPLDs and pleural diseases are occupationally induced. It is part of supportive care, and usually the physician's responsibility, to ensure that patients receive timely advice about their statutory rights to compensation and whether they should seek redress at common law.

Prognosis and end-of-life planning

Patients with advanced non-obstructive lung disease who gradually slip into severe respiratory failure with marked breathlessness should not normally be mechanically ventilated. This is because there is virtually no possibility of improvement. Therefore, it is an advantage if this problem is discussed with the patient and their carers in good time. Intercurrent episodes, for example pneumonia, may be appropriately managed by mechanical ventilation, but in these cases a return to an acceptable quality of life should be anticipated.

Keypoints

- COPD is the commonest respiratory disease requiring supportive care
- Supportive care needs should be assessed and supplied in parallel with conventional medical management
- The severity of a chronic airflow limitation (CAL) (especially in COPD) is best measured by the post bronchodilator FEV_1, expressed as % predicted and graded as mild, moderate, or severe
- Patients with restrictive lung disease have similar problems to those with CAL
- Assessment of supportive care needs has physical and psychosocial dimensions
- Supportive care provision for patients with COPD should be multidisciplinary
- A suitable framework for supportive care in these diseases is a formal pulmonary rehabilitation programme based around, but not confined to, an exercise prescription. Additional modalities should be provided on an individual basis
- Sedatives and opioids should not be withheld from patients with a very poor prognosis
- End-of-life planning is important in patients with severe disease
- Referrals for supportive care in patients with restrictive lung disease are usually made too late in the disease trajectory
- The evidence base for efficacy of supportive care in restrictive lung disease is small and more data are badly needed

References

1 National Collaborating Centre for Chronic Conditions. Chronic obstructive pulmonary disease: National clinical guideline on the management of chronic obstructive pulmonary disease in primary and secondary care. 2004; *Thorax* **59** S1, 1–232. (NICE guideline–www.nice.org.uk/CG012niceguideline).

2 British Thoracic Society and Intercollegiate Guidelines Network: British guideline on the management of asthma: A national clinical guideline. 2003; *Thorax* **58** S1, 1–94.

3 American Thoracic Society. Standards for the diagnosis and care of patients with chronic obstructive pulmonary disease. *Am J Respir Crit Care Med* 1995; **152**: S77–120.

4 Celli, B.R., MacNee, W., and Committee Members. Standards for the diagnosis and treatment of patients with COPD: A summary of the ATS/ERS position paper. *Eur Respir J*; **2004**: 932–46.

5 Fletcher, C.M., Elms, P.C., and Wood, C.H. The significance of respiratory symptoms and the diagnosis of chronic bronchitis in the working population. *BMJ* 1995; **1**: 257–66.

6 Mahler, D., Weinberg, D., Wells, C., and Fienstine, A. The measurement of dyspnea: Inter-observer agreement and physiologic correlates of two new clinical indexes. *Chest* 1984; **85**: 751–8.

7 Guyatt, G.H., Berman, L.B., Townsend, M., Pugsley, S.O., and Chambers, L.W. A measure of quality of life for clinical trials in chronic lung disease. *Thorax* 1987; **42**: 733–78.

8 Jones, P.W., Quirk, F.H., Baveystock, C.M., and Littlejohn, T. A self-complete measure of health status for chronic airflow limitation. *Am Rev Respir Dis* 1992; **145**: 1321–7.

9 Borg, G. Psychophysical bases of perceived exertion. *Med Sci Sports Exerc* 1982; **14**: 377–81.

10 Butland, R.J.A., Pang, A., Gross, E.R., Woocock, A.A., and Geddes, D.M. 2, 6 and 12 minute walking tests in respiratory disease. *BMJ* 1982; **284**: 1607–8.

11 Singh, S.J., Morgan, M.D.L., Scott, S., Walters, D., and Hardman, A.E. Development of a shuttle walking test of disability in patients with chronic airways obstruction. *Thorax* 1992; **47**: 1019–24.

12 Enright, P.L., and Sherrill, D.L. Reference equations for 6-minute walk in healthy adults. *Am J Respir Crit Care Med* 1998; **158**: 1384–7.

13 American Thoracic Society. Dypnea: Mechanisms, assessment, and mangement: A consensus statement. *Am J Respir Crit Care Med* 1999; **159**: 321–40.

14 Gore, J.M., Brophy, C.J., and Greenstone, M.A. How well do we care for patients with end stage chronic obstructive pulmonary disease (COPD)? A comparison of palliative care and quality of life in COPD and lung cancer. *Thorax* 2000; **55**: 1000–6.

15 Curtis, J.R., Dayo, R.A., and Hudson, L.D. Health-related quality of life among patients with chronic obstructive pulmonary disease. *Thorax* 1994; **49**: 162–70.

16 Zigmond, A.S., and Snaith, R.P. Hospital anxiety and depression scale. *Acta Psychiatr Scand* 1983; **67**: 361–70.

17 van Ede, L., Yzermans, C.J., and Brouwer, H.J. Prevalence of depression in patients with chronic obstructive pulmonary disease: A systematic review. *Thorax* 1999; **54**: 688–92.

18 Addington-Hall, J. Reaching out: *Specialist palliative care for adults with non-malignant diseases.* London: National Council for Hospice and Specialist Palliative Care Services, 1998.

19 Skillbeck, J., Mott, L., Page, H., *et al.* Palliative care in chronic obstructive airways disease: a needs assessment. *Palliative Med* 1998; **12**: 245–54.

20 Reis, A.L., Kaplan, R.M., Limberg, T.M., and Prewitt, L.M. Effects of pulmonary rehabilitation on physiologic and psychosocial outcomes in patients with chronic obstructive pulmonary disease. *Ann Intern Med* 1995; **122**: 823–32.

21 Cockroft, A., Bagnall, P., Heslop, A., *et al.* Controlled trial of respiratory health worker visiting patients with chronic respiratory disability. *BMJ* 1987; **294**: 225–8.

22 Muers, M.F. Quitting smoking and the lungs. *Lancet* 1999; **354**: 177–8.

23 Jorenby, D.E., Leischow, S.J., Nides, F.A., *et al.* A controlled trial of sustained-release Bupropion, a nicotine patch, or both for smoking cessation. *N Engl J Med* 1999; **340**: 685–91.

24 Fiore, M.C., Bailey, W.C., Cohen, G., *et al. Smoking cessation.* Clinical practice guideline no 18. Rockville, M.D: Agency for Healthcare Policy and Research, US Department of Health and Human Services, Publication No. 96-0692; 1996.

25 Raw, M., McNeill, A., and West, R. Smoking cessation guidelines for health professionals. *Thorax* 1998; **53**: s5 part 1.

26 American Thoracic Society: Pulmonary rehabilitation – 1999. Official statement of the American Thoracic Society. *Am J Respir Crit Care Med* 1999; **159**: 1666–82.

27 Lacasse, Y., Wong, E., Guyatt, G.H., *et al.* Meta-analysis of respiratory rehabilitation in chronic obstructive pulmonary disease. *Lancet* 1996; **348**: 1115–19.

28 Wedzicha, J.A., Bestall, J.C., Garrard, R., *et al.* Randomised controlled trial of pulmonary rehabilitation in severe chronic obstructive pulmonary disease patients stratified with the MRC dyspnoea scale. *Eur Respir J* 1998; **12**: 363–9.

29 Neish, C.m., and Hopp, J.W. The role of education in pulmonary rehabilitation. *J Cardiopulm Rehabil* 1998; **11**: 439–41.

30 Williams, S.J. *Chronic respiratory illness.* The experience of illness series, eds. R. Fitzpatrick, and S. Newman, London: Routledge, 1993.

31 Sharp, J.T., Drutz, W.S., Mosin, T., and Machnach, W. Postural relief of dyspnea in severe chronic obstructive pulmonary disease. *Am Rev Respir Dis* 1980; **122**: 201–11.

32 Gosselink, R.A.A.M., Wagenaar, R.C., Rijswijk, H., Sargeant, A.J., and Decramer, M. Diaphragmatic breathing reduces efficiency of breathing in chronic obstructive pulmonary disease. *Am J Respir Crit Care Med* 1995; **151**: 1136–42.

33 Belman, M.J., Botnik, W.C., and Shin, J.W. Inhaled bronchodilators reduce hyperinflation during exercise in patients with chronic obstructive pulmonary disease. *Am J Respir Crit Care Med* 1996; **153**: 967–75.

34 Smith, L., Cooke, D., Guyatt, G., Madhaven, J., and Oxman, A. Respiratory muscle training in chronic airflow limitation; a meta-analysis. *Am Rev Respir Dis* 1992; **145**: 533–9.

35 Jurman, A., and Campbell-Haggerty, M. Relaxation and bio-feedback: coping skills training. In: R. Casaburi, and T.L. Petty (eds) *Principles and practices of pulmonary rehabilitation.* Philadelphia: W.B. Saunders, 1993; 366–81.

36 Smoller, J.W., Pollock, M.H., Otto, M.W., Rosenbaum, J.F., and Cradin, R.L. State of the art: panic, anxiety, dyspnea and respiratory disease. *Am J Respir Crit Care Med* 1996; **154**; 6–17.

37 Efthimiou, J., Flemming, J., Gomes, C., and Spiro, S.G. The effect of supplementary oral nutrition in poorly nourished patients with chronic obstructive pulmonary disease. *Am Rev Respir Dis* 1998; **137**: 1075–82.

38 Royal College of Physicians of London. *Domiciliary oxygen therapy services: Clinical guidelines and advice for prescribers.* London: RCP, 1999; 1–49.

39 Schwartztein, R.M., Lahive, K., Pope, A., Weinberger, S.E., and Weiss, J.W. Cold facial stimulation reduces breathlessness induced in normal subjects. *Am Rev Respir Dis* 1987; **136**: 58–61.

40 Simon, P.M., Basner, R.C., Weinberger, S.E., *et al.* Oral mucosal stimulation modulates intensity of breathlessness induced in normal subjects. *Am Rev Respir Dis* 1991; **144**: 419–22.

41 Stulbarg, M.S., Belman, M.J., and Reis, A.L. Treatment of dyspnea: physical modalities, oxygen and pharmacology. In: D.A. Mahler (ed.) *Dyspnea.* Lung biology in health and disease series, vol. 3. New York: Marcel Dekker, 1998; 321–61.

42 Poole, P.J., Veale, A.G., and Black, P.M. The effect of sustained-release morphine on breathlessness and quality of life in severe chronic obstructive pulmonary disease. *Am J Respir Crit Care Med* 1998; **157**: 1877–80.

43 Anthonisen, N.R. Prognosis in chronic obstructive pulmonary disease: Results from multi-centre clinical trials. *Am Rev Respir Dis* 1989; **140**: s95–9.

44 Wilson, D.O., Rogers, R.M., Wright, E.C., and Anthonisen, M.R. Bodyweight in chronic obstructive pulmonary disease. *Am Rev Respir Dis* 1989; **139**: 1435–8.

45 Burrows, B. The course and prognosis of different types of chronic airflow limitation in a general population sample from Arizona: Comparison with the Chicago 'COPD' series. *Am Rev Respir Dis* 1989; **140**: s92–4.

46 Mador, M.J., and Tobin, M.J. Acute respiratory failure. In: P.M.A. Calverley, and N.B. Pride (eds) *Chronic obstructive pulmomary disease.* London: Chapman & Hall, 1995; 461–94.

47 President's Commission for the study of ethical problems in medicine and biomedical and behavioral research. *Making healthcare decisions: The ethical and legal implications of informed consent in a patient-practitioner relationship.* Vol. 1. Washington, DC: US Government Printing Office, 1982.

48 Hubbard, R., Johnston, I., and Britton, J. Survival in patients with cryptogenic fibrosing alveolitis. *Chest* 1998; **113**: 396–400.

49 Foster, S., and Thomas, H.M. Pulmonary rehabilitation in lung disease other than chronic obstructive pulmonary disease. *Am Rev Respir Dis* 1990; **141**: 601–4.

50 Decramer, M., de Bock, V., and Dom, R. Functional and histological picture of steroid-induced myopathy in chronic obstructive pulmonary disease. *Am J Respir Crit Care Med* 1996; **153**: 1958–964.

51 American Thoracic Society/European Respiratory Society statement: Skeletal muscle dysfunction in chronic obstructive pulmonary disease. *Am J Respir Crit Care Med* 1999; **159**(4s2): 1–40.

52 Fletcher, C., and Peto, R. The natural history of chronic airflow obstruction. *BMJ* 1977; **1**: 1645–8.

53 Jones, P.W. Quality of life measurement for patients with diseases of the airways. *Thorax* 1991; **46**: 676–82.

Further reading

American Thoracic Society statement on dyspnoea; mechanisms, assessment and management: A consensus statement. *Am J Respir Crit Care Med* 1999; **159**: 321–40. (An authoritative review of the mechanisms, assessment and treatment of dyspnoea.)

American Thoracic Society statement on pulmonary rehabilitation. *Am J Respir Crit Care Med* 1999; **159**: 1666–82. (An authoritative review of the evidence for and limitations of pulmonary rehabilitation.)

Breathe Easy Club, British Lung Foundation: http:/ /www.lunguk.org/breathe.asp

P.M.A. Calverley, W. Mac Nee, N.B. Pride, and S. Rennard (eds) *Chronic obstructive pulmonary disease.* London: Arnold, 2003. (A multiauthor textbook describing all aspects of COPD including pulmonary rehabilitation and oxygen therapy.)

R. Casaburi, and T.L. Petty (eds) *Principles and practices of pulmonary rehabilitation.* Philadelphia: W.B. Saunders, 1993. (A multiauthor textbook on pulmonary rehabilitation.)

Johnston, I.D.A. Diffuse parenchymal lung disease (DPLD). *Nurs Times* 2001 March 22–28; 92(12) II–IV.

MacNee, W., and Calverley, P.M.A. Chronic obstructive pulmonary disease 7: Management of COPD. *Thorax* 2003; **58**: 261–5.

Muers, M.F., and Congleton, J. Energy and intermediate metabolism in chronic lung disease. *Monaldi Arch Chest Dis* 1998; **53**(5): 564–73. (A review of the metabolic abnormalities of lung disease with respect to weight loss and its treatment.)

M.F. Muers, and M. Polkey (eds) *Medicine,* vol. 31(11–2), vol. 32(1–2), *Respiratory disorders.* Abingdon, Oxon: Medicine, 2003–4 (a concise summary of the topic.)

Reis, A.L. (Chair) and the ACCP/AACVPR Pulmonary Rehabilitation Guidelines Panel. Pulmonary rehabilitation; Joint ACCP/AACVPR evidence based guidelines. *J Cardiopulmon Rehabil* 1997; **17**: 371–405.

Royal College Physicians of London. *Domiciliary oxygen therapy services: clinical guidelines and advice for prescribers.* London: RCP, 1999; 1–45. (An evidence-based review of the indications for and application of oxygen therapy for use at home.)

Chapter 18

Neuromuscular and skeletal diseases

John Shneerson

Neuromuscular and skeletal disorders affecting respiratory function may cause a variety of symptoms, of which breathlessness is the most prominent. Respiratory insufficiency usually occurs during sleep before it is apparent in wakefulness and can lead to episodes of breathlessness during sleep, early morning headaches due to carbon dioxide retention, and excessive daytime sleepiness due to fragmentation of sleep. This chapter focuses on the symptom of breathlessness, emphasizes the importance of the analysis of the factors contributing to this symptom, and describes the modern methods of supportive care. The following chapter by Oliver describes in detail one of the commonest clinical conditions causing neuromuscular respiratory insufficiency, motor neurone disease (MND/ALS)

Clinical features

Mild shortness of breath on exertion is common in many chronic neuromuscular and skeletal disorders. Patients usually adapt their activities to cope with this and rarely complain specifically about breathlessness unless it changes. This may be the result of an intercurrent illness such as a chest infection or the development of related disorders such as left ventricular failure. This may be due to a cardiomyopathy associated with the skeletal muscle disorder as in Friedreich's ataxia and dystrophia myotonica. Cardiac dysrhythmias may also cause temporary breathlessness and are a feature of dystrophia myotonica and Duchenne muscular dystrophy.

Worsening of breathlessness over weeks or months in an otherwise stable disorder such as a thoracic scoliosis or following a thoracoplasty should raise the suspicion that respiratory failure is developing. This may arise after many years of clinical stability and is often associated with other symptoms such as ankle swelling.

Breathlessness may also appear at night rather than during the day. The sensation of waking with shortness of breath is usually related to arousal at the end of a central sleep apnoea (i.e. a temporary cessation of central drive to breathing), or hypopnoea, or linked to Cheyne–Stokes respiration. Repeated arousals from sleep cause sleep fragmentation which leads to the sensation of waking unrefreshed in the mornings and increasing daytime sleepiness. Occasionally neuromuscular disorders cause weakness of the upper airway dilator muscles and predispose to obstructive sleep apnoeas. These cause snoring or snoring-like noises. Arousal at the end of the apnoea may simply lead to the awareness of waking suddenly, to awareness of a snoring noise, or to an inability to breathe if the airway remains closed at the moment of arousal. This combination of nocturnal breathlessness and choking should be distinguished clinically from gastrooesophageal reflux, asthma, and left ventricular failure. Vocal cord adduction during sleep is a feature of motor neurone disease and multisystem atrophy, and presents with stridorous noises associated with breathlessness which may occur either at night or during the day.

The pattern of respiratory muscle weakness also influences the clinical presentation. Diaphragm paralysis out of proportion to weakness of the other respiratory muscles causes breathlessness on exertion and when swimming or wading in water up to the level of the lower ribcage. It also causes **orthopnoea**, i.e. breathlessness on lying supine. When weakness is severe it is apparent within the first few breaths on assuming the supine position, but if it is milder breathlessness may take a few minutes to develop. Patients with this condition rarely sleep lying flat, but may adopt either an unusual sleeping position or prefer to sleep sitting up in a chair. Sleep fragmentation is common and thus daytime sleepiness is a feature. Conversely, weakness of the abdominal muscles with preservation of diaphragmatic function causes **platypnoea**, in which breathlessness is worse when sitting up. This arises, for instance, in low cervical spinal cord injuries (where diaphragm function is preserved).

Physical examination will confirm the nature of any skeletal abnormality and reveal specific features of neuromuscular disorders (Figure 18.1). The pattern of respiratory muscle weakness should be identified. For example, weakness and atrophy of the sternomastoid muscles is an early sign of dystrophia myotonica, whereas in Duchenne muscular dystrophy respiratory muscle weakness is global. Respiration should be observed in both the sitting and the supine position. The presence of diaphragm weakness is confirmed by observing paradoxical inward inspiratory abdominal movement in the supine position. Unilateral diaphragm weakness is hard to diagnose with certainty, but similar findings may be found unilaterally.

Hypoxia may be revealed by the finding of central cyanosis. This clinical sign is only reliable when the oxygen saturation falls below around 80%, which is equivalent to a PO_2 of less than around 6.7 kPa. Hypercapnia causes a variety of cardiovascular and central nervous system physical signs. These include tachycardia with large-volume pulse, peripheral venous dilatation, papilloedema, flapping tremor (asterixis), loss of tendon reflexes, small pupils, and, with severe hypercapnia, confusion, or coma (carbon dioxide 'narcosis').

It should be remembered that breathlessness in these patients may also be due to unrelated additional causes such as asthma, or to cardiac diseases.

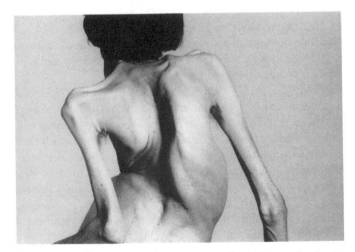

Fig. 18.1 Severe thoracic scoliosis associated with intercostal muscle atrophy due to previous poliomyelitis.

Pathophysiology

Breathlessness in neuromuscular and skeletal disorders may have a variety of causes.

Weakness of chest wall muscles

Each of the chronic neurological disorders has its own characteristic pattern of muscle weakness. It is also important to be aware of whether the disorder is stable, slowly progressive, or rapidly progressive. In some conditions the sequence of respiratory muscle involvement is unpredictable. This is particularly the case with motor neurone disease, and careful analysis of the pattern of weakness at each stage of the illness is essential in planning treatment.

The relationship of breathlessness to the severity of the chest wall muscle weakness is variable because of individual differences in awareness of the symptom of breathlessness and of complaining about it.[1] Breathlessness is in general related to the percentage of the maximal force that can be generated by the chest wall muscles which is actually developed in these patients. The implication of this is that if the muscles are weak, the maximal force is reduced and a level of work of breathing that would not in normal circumstances cause breathlessness, will now do so. As the muscles become weaker or the thorax becomes more deformed, the threshold for becoming breathless gradually falls. The moment at which breathlessness is complained of also depends on the level of physical activity. Breathlessness is much less likely to be a problem if the patient is confined to a wheelchair or bed because of other aspects of the neuromuscular disorder, than if the limb muscles are relatively spared.

The most important chest wall muscle is the diaphragm.[2] Unilateral weakness reduces the tidal volume and the mechanical efficiency of breathing since the affected hemidiaphragm moves upwards (paradoxically) into the thorax during inspiration, instead of descending. This is worse in the supine position when the weight of the abdominal contents pushes the paralysed hemidiaphragm even further into the thorax. In effect, the diaphragm is fixed ('splinted') in an expiratory position. When the whole diaphragm is paralysed bilaterally, it moves paradoxically during both inspiration and expiration and the intrapleural pressure changes are transmitted across it so that the abdominal pressure falls during inspiration and the anterior abdominal wall moves inwards.

Symptoms usually appear when the maximum transdiaphragmatic pressure falls to around 25 cm H_2O (2.45 kPa) compared to a normal value of 70 cm H_2O (6.86 kPa). When the diaphragm is completely paralysed, the vital capacity falls by 50% in moving from the sitting to the supine position. Ventilation is reduced, particularly at the bases of the lungs when supine, with shunting of blood past the alveoli, so that the arterial PO_2 falls.

Breathlessness in skeletal disorders without any involvement of the muscles also has a variety of causes. In scoliosis, for instance, the compliance of the ribcage is reduced, as is also the compliance of the lungs, primarily because of their small volume. The ribcage distortion puts the inspiratory muscles at a mechanical disadvantage on the convexity of the scoliosis. They become shortened and on the concavity they are lengthened. Diaphragmatic function is impaired, as shown by low transdiaphragmatic pressures and a fall in the vital capacity when changing from the sitting to the supine position. Exercise ability and breathlessness on exertion are linked to the reduction of vital capacity. The tidal volume increases initially, then remains constant and the respiratory frequency rises as exercise becomes more intense. The rise in pulmonary artery pressure on exertion, which is related to the severity of the restrictive defect, may also limit the cardiac output and contribute to breathlessness.

Upper airway muscles

Weakness of the upper airway muscles may cause obstructive sleep apnoeas and stridor as described above. Bulbar impairment may also cause dysarthria, dysphagia, and impaired coughing and swallowing, and can lead to aspiration of material into the tracheobronchial tree. This may cause sudden severe major airway obstruction, an intermittent cough which is worse during meals, or recurrent episodes of pneumonia. Weakness of the chest wall muscles, particularly the expiratory muscles, may significantly impair the ability to clear tracheobronchial secretions, and can thus lead to pneumonia.

Sleep

Normal sleep is associated with loss of the voluntary respiratory drive and a reduction in the reflex drive in response to hypoxia, hypercapnia, and other stimuli.[3] Muscle activity is reduced and whereas in non-rapid eye movement sleep (NREM) this affects all the respiratory muscles to an equal extent, in rapid eye movement sleep (REM) diaphragmatic activity is selectively retained. Relaxation of the other respiratory muscles is more intense than during NREM sleep and loss of activity in the upper airway dilator muscles increases the upper airway resistance and the work of the chest wall muscles. These changes during sleep are particularly important in scoliosis where the diaphragm is attached to an asymmetrical ribcage and where the respiratory pump often has little reserve.[4] The effects of sleep are accentuated in neuromuscular disorders causing scoliosis because of the presence of muscle weakness in addition to the skeletal deformities. A reduction in tidal volume and increase in respiratory frequency may result in alveolar hypoventilation and an increase in the deadspace ventilation. Arousals from sleep occur initially in REM, which becomes fragmented, and at a later stage in NREM sleep, particularly with loss of stages 3 and 4. Sleep fragmentation itself further reduces the respiratory drive and impairs the strength and probably the endurance of the respiratory muscles, promoting a vicious circle in which there are progressively more respiratory-induced arousals and a deterioration in respiratory drive and muscle function. Central apnoeas and hypopnoeas are seen and hypercapnia then develops during the day as well as at night.

Abnormalities of respiratory drive

The respiratory centre in the medulla functions normally in most neuromuscular and skeletal disorders, with the exception of central alveolar hypoventilation in which it is reduced or absent. Breathlessness is correspondingly diminished and these subjects may for instance be able to swim for prolonged episodes under water, and take physical exercise without being aware of any breathlessness, despite becoming intensely centrally cyanosed. Reversible impairment of the respiratory centres may arise because of chronic hypercapnia, sleep deprivation, or a metabolic alkalosis and these situations may be associated with less breathlessness, despite the severity of the underlying respiratory failure and muscle weakness.

Treatment

Most of the chronic neuromuscular and skeletal disorders are not amenable to curative treatment, but there is a wide range of supportive measures which can reduce breathlessness and other symptoms and improve the quality of life. Most of these have been inadequately evaluated. It is important to assess each individual's needs carefully before planning any type of rehabilitation or palliative treatment.[5]

Physiotherapy

The physiotherapist should recognize inefficient patterns of movement and teach the patient how to correct them. Coordination of limb and other muscles can be improved by exercise training so that, for instance, walking can be performed with a lower oxygen consumption and less breathlessness. Coordination of the respiratory movements with those of the arms and legs may be helpful. The muscles of the upper arm may be used both as accessory muscles of respiration and in arm functioning, and coordination of these two activities can easily be disrupted. Synchronization of respiratory and leg movements during walking is often helpful.

It is important that the speed of movement, particularly walking, is adjusted to the patient's respiratory capacity. It is common for patients to walk too fast, and the increased oxygen consumption exacerbates their breathlessness. Breathlessness may be less severe while, for instance, standing leaning forward, or resting the arms on a surface so that the accessory muscles of respiration can be used. Energy can be conserved by the use of physical aids such as a walking stick or handrail.

The physiotherapist should also try to improve the patient's confidence and aid relaxation, which reduces oxygen uptake by the skeletal muscles. Advice about taking periods of rest between exercise, and stopping exercise before becoming breathless, may help.

Breathing techniques

A range of breathing exercises has been developed to try to reduce breathlessness and to improve the respiratory pattern both at rest and during physical exertion. **Pursed-lip breathing** is useful in emphysema, but not in neuromuscular and skeletal disorders. **'Diaphragmatic' breathing** and **deep breathing exercises** may, however, be of help. The diaphragm cannot be selectively activated, but this type of breathing encourages abdominal expansion during inspiration. Deep breathing manoeuvres, such as sighing, open distal airways and prevent subsegmental lung collapse and thereby increase lung compliance, and reduce the work of breathing and the degree of breathlessness. This technique, and diaphragmatic breathing, also reduce the respiratory rate, which can help to reduce breathlessness.

Frog breathing is a technique which utilizes the upper airway muscles.[6] Air is pushed through the open larynx into the trachea under pressure generated by the oral muscles. This requires coordination of the upper airway muscles so that the soft palate seals off the nasopharynx while the glottis remains open at the time that air is gulped from the mouth downwards into the pharynx. The glottis then closes to trap air in the lungs until the next frog breath, which further inflates the lungs. Frog breaths of around 50–80 mL are common, and 10–20 gulps can be taken before expiration occurs. This type of breathing is completely independent of chest wall and abdominal muscles and is of particular value in those with tetraplegia, poliomyelitis, Duchenne muscular dystrophy, and similar disorders.[7]

Exercise training

This has been widely used in COPD, but there is little evidence about its effectiveness in neuromuscular and skeletal disorders (see Chapter 17). Programmes involving leg exercises, combined with educational programmes, have been used and may be of benefit, but in muscular dystrophies and myopathies the diseased muscles have a limited capacity to be improved by training.

Specific respiratory muscle training programmes have been attempted. These have been most effective in cervical spinal cord lesions where it is the spared normal muscles that are capable of being trained.[8,9] They may increase the vital capacity and the effectiveness of coughing. However, in muscular dystrophies such as Duchenne muscular dystrophy the results have been disappointing and improvements have been noticed only in mildly affected subjects who have least to gain from the training programme.

A separate type of training in neuromuscular disorders is aimed at improving upper airway function during and after intubation for episodes of respiratory failure. Coordination between the respiratory and swallowing related function of the larynx may be lost, with an increased risk of aspiration and of breathlessness during weaning.[10] Deflation of the cuff on the tracheostomy or endotracheal tube so that air passes through the upper airway and enables speech to resume helps to coordinate the muscles and improve the likelihood of successful weaning.

Cough assistance

Weakness of the cough mechanism may lead to aspiration of material from the pharynx into the tracheobronchial tree or failure to expectorate tracheobronchial secretions. These problems may lead to worsening breathlessness because the material retained within the airways partially obstructs them and increases the work of breathing.

A normal cough requires a deep inspiration, closure of the glottis and then a rapid forceful expiration as the glottis opens (see Chapter 21). Each of these functions may be impaired in people with neuromuscular disorders. In Duchenne muscular dystrophy, the inspiratory muscle weakness is a major factor. In motor neurone disease glottic function is often impaired and spinal cord lesions often reduce expiratory muscle strength.[11]

The depth of inspiration can be increased by frog breathing and by specially designed cough assistance machines, such as the insufflator–exsufflator (J Emerson Co, Cambridge, Massachusetts, USA). This provides an approximately square wave of positive pressure which inflates the lungs. It can then be switched, either automatically or manually, to generate a sudden negative pressure. This assists exhalation of air with sputum and other material which is in the airways.

Assistance to expiration can also be provided either manually through thoracic or abdominal compression, or by functional electrical stimulation of the abdominal muscles.[12] This technique increases intra-abdominal pressure by producing a coordinated activation of the abdominal muscles by multiple cutaneous electrodes.

Psychotherapy

Anxiety and depression are common in those with neuromuscular and skeletal disorders, especially in people who live alone or who have developed poor coping strategies.[13] Antidepressants may be of value, but encouragement to develop new behaviours may help, including a positive approach to problems and the ability to feel in control of situations rather than attributing events to external forces or feeling a victim of these. Self-confidence can be increased; education, motivation, and encouragement to retain or develop social contacts, can all improve the quality of life and reduce awareness of breathlessness.[14] Reassurance and encouragement from healthcare professionals is important, and support from family, carers, and friends is often a vital factor.

Oxygen

Oxygen is frequently prescribed for breathlessness in neuromuscular and skeletal disorders. In general it is contra-indicated for use at rest because of the risk that it will worsen hypercapnia by abolishing any residual hypoxic drive. Oxygen should only be prescribed after careful estimation of blood gases during the day and also sleep studies, including transcutaneous PCO_2 recordings at night.

Oxygen may, however, be of value in relieving breathlessness on exertion, during which oxygen desaturation is common. Exertion itself increases the respiratory drive and reduces the risk of hypercapnia during oxygen treatment.

Walking tests, with or without oxygen, should be used to determine the optimal flow rate, and a small lightweight portable oxygen cylinder may be of help. Liquid oxygen is preferable, but may have limited availability. Oxygen can also be used briefly after exertion in order to speed recovery and reduce the time for which breathlessness is present.

Ventilatory support

Ventilatory support provides a back-up for patients with neuromuscular and skeletal disorders who have developed respiratory failure, and it may also improve respiratory function. It probably resets the respiratory drive, partly through relieving sleep deprivation and partly through reducing the cerebrospinal fluid bicarbonate concentration and thereby increasing the ventilatory response to hypercapnia. It probably improves respiratory muscle function and so increases the vital capacity and raises the threshold at which breathlessness is likely to develop. Respiratory muscle rest may also diminish respiratory muscle fatigue, but there is doubt about the clinical significance of this.

Non-invasive ventilation is usually required. The most commonly used system is a nasal mask (Figure 18.2), although occasionally a face mask which includes the mouth is required, particularly if there are mouth leaks. An alternative is a negative pressure system, such as a cuirass or jacket (Figure 18.3). With these systems the ribcage and abdomen are covered by an airtight and rigid enclosure from which air is evacuated by a negative pressure ventilator. This expands the ribcage and abdomen and air is drawn in through the mouth and nose. No appliance is required around the airway.

Both these non-invasive techniques can adequately ventilate most patients with respiratory failure due to neuromuscular and skeletal disorders. They are usually only required at night while the patient is asleep, but occasionally an extra 1–2 h during the day is of benefit.

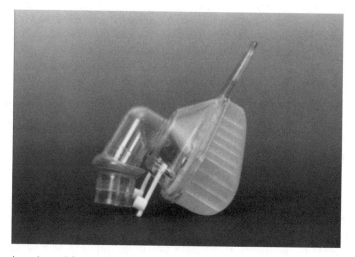

Fig. 18.2 Nasal mask used for non-invasive ventilation.

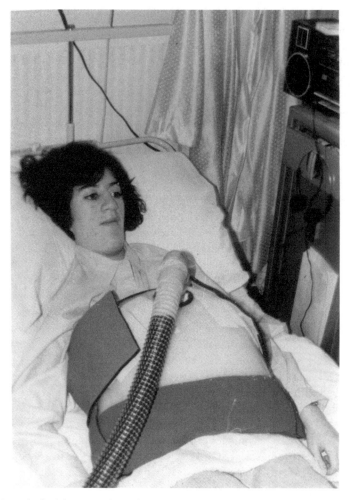

Fig. 18.3 Cuirass shell with connecting tubing which leads to the negative pressure ventilator. Reproduced with permission from Shneerson JM, *Handbook of sleep medicine*, Oxford: Blackwell Science, 2000.

As respiratory muscle weakness worsens, the duration of the ventilation gradually increases. This is seen particularly with Duchenne muscular dystrophy and motor neurone disease, where in the later stages the ventilator may be used almost continuously to minimize breathlessness. Tracheostomy ventilation may be preferred to a non-invasive system if respiratory support is required for more than around 16 h/day, or if there is a weak cough or the airway needs to be protected.[15]

The non-invasive systems can considerably improve the quality of life and reduce breathlessness at rest.[16] Small portable ventilators have been developed, but they do not have the capacity to provide the ventilatory requirements of most patients during exercise. As many of these patients find it difficult to communicate it is important to note that quality of life with respiratory failure treated by non-invasive ventilation to relieve symptoms such as breathlessness is usually underestimated by the carer, relative to the patient's own assessment.[17,18] Relief of breathlessness at night enables a better quality of sleep to be obtained with less subsequent tiredness during the day.

Sedative drugs

Opioids and other centrally sedating drugs may be of value in the preterminal phase and when patients are approaching death, to relieve intense breathlessness, but should not be initiated at an earlier stage in the natural history. Diazepam has been recommended to relieve breathlessness due to vocal cord adduction in motor neurone disease and may work either by relaxing the adductor muscles of the larynx or by reducing anxiety about the airway obstruction (see Chapter 19 for discussion of sedatives).

Keypoints

◆ Breathlessness in neuromuscular and skeletal disorders may be due to global respiratory muscle weakness or selective weakness (e.g. the diaphragm) and it is important to carefully assess the pattern of respiratory muscle weakness in order to plan appropriate treatment

◆ Respiratory muscle weakness causes respiratory failure during sleep before this is apparent in wakefulness

◆ Physiotherapy techniques such as relaxation, improvement of coordination, and education in specific types of respiratory breathing patterns may be of value

◆ Cough assistance and prevention of tracheobronchial aspiration is often important, particularly in the presence of bulbar muscle weakness

◆ Oxygen may induce carbon dioxide retention and non-invasive ventilatory techniques are usually preferable in respiratory failure

◆ Central sedatives should be reserved for the advanced stages of disease

References

1 Laroche, C.M., Moxham, J., and Green, M. Respiratory muscle weakness and fatigue. *Q J Med, NS* 1989; **71**(265): 373–97.

2 Gibson, G.J. Diaphragmatic paresis: pathophysiology, clinical features, and investigations. *Thorax* 1989; **44**: 960–70.

3 McNicholas, W.T. Impact of sleep in respiratory failure. *Eur Respir J* 1997; **10**: 920–33.

4 Midgren, B., Petersson, K., Hansson, L., *et al.* Nocturnal hypoxaemia in severe scoliosis. *Br J Dis Chest* 1988; **82**: 226–36.

5 Shneerson, J.M. Rehabilitation in neuromuscular disorders and thoracic wall deformities. *Monaldi Arch Chest Dis* 1998; **53**: 415–18.

6 Dail, C.W. Glossopharyngeal breathing by paralyzed patients. A preliminary report. *Calif Med* 1951; **75**: 217–18.

7 Montero, J.C., Feldman, D.J., and Montero, D. Effects of glossopharyngeal breathing on respiratory function after cervical cord transection. *Arch Phys Med Rehabil* 1967; **48**: 650–3.

8 Gross, D., Ladd, H.W., Riley, E.J., Macklem, P.T., and Grassino, A. The effect of training on strength and endurance of the diaphragm in quadriplegia. *Am J Med* 1980; **68**: 27–35.

9 Biering-Sorensen, F., Knudsell, J.L., Schmidt, A., Bundgaard, A., and Christensen, I. Effect of respiratory training with a mouth-nose mask in tetraplegics. *Paraplegia* 1991; **29**: 113–19.

10 Shneerson, J.M. Are there new solutions to old problems with weaning? *Br J Anaesth* 1997; **78**: 238–40.

11 Siebens, A.A., Kirby, N.A., and Poulos, D.A. Cough following transection of spinal cord at C-6. *Arch Phys Med Rehabil* 1964; **45**: 1–7.

12 Linder, S.H. Functional electrical stimulation to enhance cough in quadriplegia. *Chest* 1993; **103**: 166–9.

13 Tate, D., Kirsch, N., Maynald, F., *et al.* Coping with the late effects: differences between depressed and nondepressed polio survivors. *Am J Phys Med Rehabil* 1994; **73**: 27–35.

14 Shneerson, J. Quality of life in neuromuscular and skeletal disorders. *Eur Respir Rev* 1997; **7**: 71–3.

15 Bach, J.R. A comparison of long-term ventilatory support alternatives from the perspective of the patient and care giver. *Chest* 1993; **104**: 1702–6.

16 Pehrsson, K., Olofson, J., Larsson, S., and Sullivan, M. Quality of life of patients treated by home mechanical ventilation due to restrictive ventilatory disorders. *Respir Med* 1994; **88**: 21–6.

17 Bach, J.R., Campagnolo, D.I., and Hoeman, S. Life satisfaction of individuals with Duchenne muscular dystrophy using long-term mechanical ventilatory support. *Am J Phys Med Rehabil* 1991; **70**: 129–35.

18 Bach, J.R. Ventilator use by muscular dystrophy association patients. *Arch Phys Med Rehabil* 1992; **73**: 179–83.

Chapter 19

Dyspnoea in motor neurone disease (amyotrophic lateral sclerosis)

David Oliver

Motor neurone disease (MND in the UK, also known as amyotrophic lateral sclerosis or ALS in other countries) is marked by a progressive degeneration of motor neurones leading to progressive muscular weakness. The aetiology is unknown for the majority of patients, although there is a family history in approximately 5% of cases – of these about 20% have been found to have a mutation of the copper/zinc superoxide dismutase (*SOD1*) gene. At present there is no curative treatment, although the glutamate blocker, riluzole, has been shown in trials to slow the progression and reduce the risk of death, probably prolonging life by about 3–6 months, on average, after 18 months treatment.[1]

Dyspnoea is a common symptom, due to degeneration of motor neurones in the cervical region, leading to diaphragmatic and intercostal inspiratory muscle weakness.[2,3] This diaphragmatic weakness, coupled with poor chest expansion, leads to paradoxical indrawing of the abdominal wall in inspiration. As dysphagia is also common (because of bulbar muscle weakness) there is an increased risk of aspiration due to a weak cough reflex and the poor clearance of the airway. Atelectasis may occur as a result of the reduction in chest wall compliance.[3,4]

The prevalence of dyspnoea increases during the progression of the disease and studies have shown that 47–85% of patients in the later stages complain of dyspnoea.[5,6] Occasionally patients may present with acute respiratory failure and may then require resuscitation and ventilation, before the diagnosis is made.[7]

Respiratory failure may be suspected when there is evidence of nocturnal hypoventilation – poor sleep, nightmares, morning headaches, and lethargy in the daytime. Further questioning may elucidate the need for the patient to sleep with the head elevated, and examination may show paradoxical abdominal movement on inspiration when the patient is lying down. Measurement of the FVC when lying and standing is useful and further sleep studies may be necessary.

Dyspnoea can be treated in many different ways. As the patient becomes generally weaker, especially where there is neck muscle weakness, it is important to ensure that positioning allows the free movement of the chest wall, allows the diaphragm to work efficiently, and reduces airway obstruction.[8] The patient should usually be reclined so that the centre of gravity passes through the thorax.[9] Physiotherapy is helpful in maintaining chest expansion and diaphragmatic breathing.[8] Other non-pharmacological measures include ensuring a calm and positive approach, the support of patient and family to reduce anxiety, and the use of a fan to keep the air moving around the patient.[10] Careful assessment of swallowing, usually by a speech and language therapist, will ensure aspiration is minimized and a percutaneous endoscopic gastrostomy may be considered to reduce the problems associated with feeding.[11]

A comprehensive supportive care approach should be used in the treatment of dyspnoea. Thus the management of respiratory symptoms in these patients should be handled within the wider multidisciplinary assessment of the 'whole patient' in the context of their family. There is often associated anxiety, and anxiolytics, such as lorazepam or diazepam, can be helpful. The control of other symptoms is essential, in particular the control of pain, by simple analgesics or opioids, and the reduction of salivation to prevent drooling and the potential aspiration of excess saliva, by anticholinergic medication. (See Chapter 24 for more details on the management of respiratory secretions.)

Patients and families fear dyspnoea and the possibility of 'choking', and many medical books for the general public stress the distress of dying with MND. Although there is much evidence that with good symptom control death is peaceful,[5,12] these fears remain. In the UK in 1997 a patient with MND, Annie Lindsell, went to the High Court to allow her doctor to prescribe and administer medication when her distress was such that she no longer wished to continue. Her arguments were based on the fears of choking and increasing dyspnoea and respiratory distress, and the public discussion which ensued in the media caused distress to many other people with MND. After several court hearings she withdrew her case before any ruling was made, as it was agreed that it was acceptable for her doctor to give medication with the aim of controlling her distressing symptoms.[13]

Opioid medication has been shown to be very helpful in the reduction of dyspnoea in this patient group.[5,6,14] The dose should be titrated carefully to the symptom and, as in terminally ill cancer patients,[15] evidence is accumulating that there is no deterioration in respiratory function if opioids are used carefully. The safety of opioids has been shown in one study with the median oral dose of 60 mg/24 h and a median duration of use of 51 days.[14] If there is a sudden episode of dyspnoea in the terminal stages of the disease an injection of an opioid, together with an anxiolytic such as midazolam and an anticholinergic such as hyoscine to reduce secretions, can reduce distress.

In the UK the MND Association has developed the Breathing Space Kit (Figure 19.1), which is provided to patients if there are concerns about their breathing or swallowing. A box

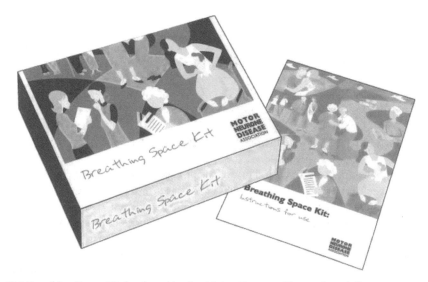

Fig. 19.1 Breathing Space Kit developed by the Motor Neurone Disease Association.

is provided to store medication: diamorphine for analgesia and dyspnoea; midazolam as anxiolytic and sedative; an anticholinergic, such as hyoscine hydrobromide or glycopyrronium bromide, to reduce secretions. There is also a leaflet on the use of the medication and this allows discussion between the doctor and nurse and the patient and their family, so that all are clear as to the action to be taken, including the use of medication, in the event of a crisis or in the terminal stages of the disease.[6,16,17]

As the disease progresses there may be evidence of respiratory failure. The treatment of this will need to be carefully discussed with the patient and family and non-interventional management, as described above using medication such as opioids, can be started. Respiratory support, in the form of non-invasive ventilation, can be used to prevent or delay the onset of respiratory failure. It can also be started once respiratory failure has occurred, to palliate subsequent progression of symptoms. In the past cuirass and negative pressure ventilation have been used,[18] but, increasingly, non-invasive ventilation using positive pressure ventilation by mask is being favoured (Figure 19.2).[16,19] There is evidence that this can extend the length of survival, and the technique may be very effective in the reduction of symptoms arising from nocturnal hypoventilation, such as sleep disturbance, morning headache, anorexia, and breathlessness.[16] However, not all patients can tolerate the tight-fitting mask, especially if there are bulbar symptoms.[16,20] As the disease progresses there may be increasing problems, particularly with pressure on the nose. The patient and family will need support and explanation of the effectiveness and limitations of this form of respiratory support. Because of these potential difficulties, it is essential that a respiratory specialist with experience in this technique is involved in setting up the equipment. Subsequent monitoring can be done by palliative and supportive care professionals, provided that they have had training and have access to respiratory specialists for advice.

Non-invasive ventilatory support may be provided at home, provided that adequate support can be given – the patient may need assistance to secure the mask and start the ventilator.[16] Palliative care providers, including hospices and nursing homes, can support a patient receiving ventilation. A survey in 1998 of the hospices in the UK showed that nine hospices had cared for a person requiring non-invasive ventilation.[21] The survey showed that there was good symptom relief, but it was essential that staff were given training in the use of the ventilator and received adequate support themselves. The majority of patients were able to die peacefully, although on occasions it was felt that the period of dying may have been prolonged. Careful

Case history 19.1 Medical management of progressive distress

Mr JP was a 45-year-old man with primary lateral sclerosis and increasing weakness over a period of 5 years. His speech and swallowing deteriorated and he was only able to move his arms and support himself for short times. He became more breathless and there were episodes of coughing as he found it difficult to swallow his own saliva. The use of sublingual hyoscine reduced his drooling and morphine sulfate controlled-release tablets at a dose of 40 mg/24 h relieved his feelings of dyspnoea.

One day he became more breathless. He had made his views very clear that he wanted to die and did not want any life-prolonging treatment. The dose of morphine was therefore increased in response to his increased distress. Two days later he was unable to take oral medication and a continuous subcutaneous infusion by syringe driver was commenced, which included diamorphine 40 mg/24 h, midazolam 40 mg/24 h, and hyoscine hydrobromide 1.6 mg/24 h. He remained peaceful for the next 2 days and was able to die at home, with his family around him.

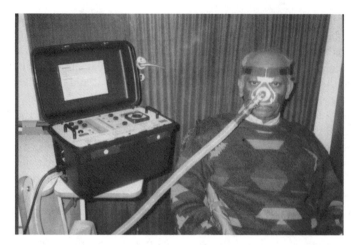

Fig. 19.2 Patient receiving assisted ventilation with nasal mask. This equipment allows a patient with respiratory muscle weakness to have ventilatory support on demand, without restricting eating/drinking or speech. By kind permission of Dr Rebecca Lyall, Department of Respiratory Medicine, Guy's, King's and St Thomas's School of Medicine.

discussion amongst the caring team is important so that all are aware of the need of this intervention for the control of dyspnoea.[16]

The use of tracheostomy and positive pressure ventilation have been suggested as the disease progresses and if non-invasive ventilation is no longer adequate or possible, due to progressive bulbar symptoms.[4,22] Studies have shown that these forms of ventilation can continue at home for long periods of time and patients express the wish to continue, and up to 90% would choose the option again.[23] Although patients may express satisfaction with their quality of life there is, however, a large load on caregivers. In one study caregivers felt that their lives were consumed with the ventilator responsibilities, that the burden was excessive, and their own out-

Case history 19.2 Non-invasive ventilation and MND

Mr GR was a 49-year-old married man with two teenage sons who had developed a foot drop in 1996. He had become weaker and in June 1998 investigations confirmed the diagnosis of MND. At the time of diagnosis it had been noted that the FVC was 103% of the expected value. He became weaker and was restricted to a wheelchair. In April 2000 he was noted to have a raised serum bicarbonate but had no complaints of dyspnoea.

In June 2000 he felt less well and complained of morning headache, a reduced appetite, and feeling sleepy in the day. Investigations showed that the FVC had fallen to 50% of expected and the bicarbonate was 38 mmol/L with a PO_2 of 6 kPa and PCO_2 of 9.2 kPa. He was started on non-invasive ventilation at night and within a month the bicarbonate was 26 mmol/L and the PCO_2 was 5 kPa. His symptoms improved and he felt more alert and was eating more. He developed an ulcer on his nose due to the mask, and many adjustments were necessary.

He continued to use the non-invasive ventilation only at night and in February 2001 he deteriorated over a single night and died peacefully at home.

side activities were severely limited.[24] Moreover, if survival is prolonged, then there is the risk of patients on ventilation eventually losing all means of communication and becoming 'locked in'.[22] The use of advance directives (living wills) may allow patients to retain some control on their care, by advising carers of their wishes if communication becomes impossible.[23,25] This area of care needs very careful discussion and planning, early in the disease process before respiratory support is required. Unfortunately, in most cases the decision is taken as an emergency and without previous discussion.[22]

Keypoints

♦ Dyspnoea is a common symptom in MND/ALS

♦ Non-pharmacological measures can relieve symptoms in many cases

♦ Opioids are effective in reducing the distress of dyspnoea

♦ Non-invasive ventilation may be considered for some patients, but careful discussion with patient and family is essential

References

1 Mitsumoto, H. Riluzole – what is its impact in our treatment and understanding of amyotrophic lateral sclerosis. *Ann Pharmacother* 1997; **31**: 779–81.

2 Polkey, M.I., Lyall, R.A., Green, M., Leigh, N., and Moxham, J. Expiratory muscle funtion in amyotrophic lateral sclerosis. *Am J Crit Care Med* 1998; **158**: 734–41.

3 Tidwell, J. Pulmonary management of the ALS patient. *J Neurosci Nurs* 1993; **25**: 337–42.

4 Oppenheimer, E.A. Decision-making in the respiratory care of amyotrophic lateral sclerosis: should home mechanical ventilation be used? *Palliative Med* 1993; **7** (Suppl 2): 49–64.

5 O'Brien, T., Kelly, M., and Saunders, C. Motor neurone disease: a hospice perspective. *BMJ* 1992; **304**: 471–3.

6 Oliver, D. The quality of care and symptom control – the effects on the terminal phase of ALS/MND. *J Neurol Sci* 1996; **139** (Suppl): 134–6.

7 Chen, R., Grand'Maison, G., Strong, M.J., Ramsay, D.A., and Bolton, B.F. Motor neuron disease presenting as acute respiratory failure: a clinical and pathological study. *J Neurol Neurosurg Psychiatr* 1996; **60**: 455–8.

8 O'Gorman, B., and Oliver, D. Disorders of nerve I: motor neurone disease. In: M. Stokes, (ed.) *Neurological physiotherapy*. London: Mosby, 1998; 171–9.

9 O'Gorman, B. Physiotherapy. In: D. Oliver, G.D. Borasio, and D. Walsh, (eds) *Palliative care in amyotrophic lateral sclerosis*. Oxford: Oxford University Press, 2000; 105–11.

10 Voltz, R., and Borasio, G.D. Palliative therapy in the terminal stage of neurological disease. *J Neurol* 1997; **244** (Suppl 4): S2–10.

11 Wagner-Sonntag, E., Allison, S., Oliver, D., *et al.* Dysphagia. In: D. Oliver, G.D. Borasio, D. Walsh (ed.) *Palliative care in amyotrophic lateral sclerosis*. Oxford: Oxford University Press, 2000.

12 Neudert, C., Oliver, D., Wasner, M., and Borasio, G.D. The course of the terminal phase in patients with amyotrophic lateral sclerosis. *J Neurol* 2001; **248**: 612–16.

13 Corner, J. More openness needed in palliative care. *BMJ* 1997; **315**: 1242.

14 Oliver, D. Opioid medication in the palliative care of motor neurone disease. *Palliative Med* 1998; **12**: 113–15.

15 Bruera, E., Macmillan, K., Pither, J., and MacDonald, R.N. Effects of morphine on the dyspnea of terminal cancer patients. *J Pain Symptom Manage* 1990; **5**: 341–4.

16 Lyall, R., Moxham, J., Leigh, and N. Dyspnoea. In: D. Oliver, G.D. Borasio, and D. Walsh, (eds) *Palliative care in amyotrophic lateral sclerosis*. Oxford: Oxford University Press, 2000; 43–56.

17 Sykes, N. End of life care in ALS. In: D. Oliver, G.D. Borasio, and D. Walsh (eds) *Palliative care in amyotrophic lateral sclerosis*. Oxford: Oxford University Press, 2000; 159–68.

18 Howard, R.S., Wiles, C.M., and Loh, L. Respiratory complications and their management in motor neuron disease. *Brain* 1989; **112**: 1155–70.

19 Meyer, T.J., and Hill, N.S. Noninvasive positive pressure ventilation to treat respiratory failure. *Ann Intern Med* 1994; **120**: 760–70.

20 Aboussouan, M.D., Khan, S.U., Meeker, D.P., Stelmach, R.R.T., and Mitsumoto, H. Effect of non-invasive positive-pressure ventilation on survival in amyotrophic lateral sclerosis. *Ann Intern Med* 1997; **127**: 450–3.

21 Oliver, D., and Webb, S. Ventilation of patients with motor neurone disease – the experience of specialist palliative care. Poster, 10th International Symposium on ALS/MND, Vancouver, 1999.

22 Gelinas, D. Amyotrophic lateral sclerosis and invasive ventilation. In: D., Oliver, G.D., Borasio, and D. Walsh, (eds) *Palliative care in amyotrophic lateral sclerosis*. Oxford: Oxford University Press, 2000; 55–62.

23 Moss, A.H., Oppenheimer, E.A., Casey, P., *et al.* Patients with amyotrophic lateral sclerosis receiving long-term mechanical ventilation. Advance care planning and outcomes. *Chest* 1996; **110**: 249–55.

24 Gelinas, D.F., O'Connor, P., and Miller, R.G. Quality of life for ventilator-dependent ALS patients and their caregivers. *J Neurol Sci* 1998; **160** (Suppl 1): S134–36.

25 Borasio, G.D., and Voltz, R. Advance directives. In: D. Oliver, G.D. Borasio, and D. Walsh (eds) *Palliative care in amyotrophic lateral sclerosis*. Oxford: Oxford University Press, 2000; 36–41.

Chapter 20

Hyperventilation and disproportionate breathlessness

William N. Gardner and Alex Lewis

The physiological definition of hyperventilation is 'alveolar ventilation that is inappropriately high for the metabolic production of carbon dioxide'. This leads to reduction of arterial PCO_2 ($PaCO_2$) below the normal range (hypocapnia) and respiratory alkalosis. The combination can lead to symptoms involving most systems of the body. Dyspnoea, or shortness of breath, is often associated with hyperventilation and vice versa, but the two are not necessarily synonymous.

There is currently little consensus about the clinical definitions, diagnosis, or for that matter, the clinical management of hyperventilation and 'unexplained' disproportionate dyspnoea and this account will inevitably reflect a personal view. Nevertheless, patients with these conditions present to most hospital clinics and accident and emergency departments and are usually inappropriately managed. There are a number of recent reviews,[1–8] all of which also inevitably reflect the personal views of the authors based on the patient population currently available in their departments.

Physiology

Alveolar ventilation (expired minus deadspace ventilation) is inversely related to $PaCO_2$ as long as carbon dioxide production remains constant. Carbon dioxide is released from bicarbonate as described by the Henderson–Hasselbach equation, leading to respiratory alkalosis with rapid rise of blood pH, fall of bicarbonate, and induction of a negative base excess. At the beginning of hyperventilation, carbon dioxide is washed out of extensive stores in bone, skeletal muscle and viscera.[9] Renal compensation is probably unimportant in humans[10] and CSF compensation is also incomplete.[11]

At a clinical level, it is usually not possible to document the increase in alveolar ventilation, and hypocapnia is used as an indirect marker of hyperventilation. However, an obvious increase in either rate or depth of respiratory movement is not necessarily associated with increase in alveolar ventilation and hypocapnia if the other parameter decreases *pari passu* or if tidal volume becomes so low that it encroaches on the deadspace. Details of respiratory control in hypocapnia are uncertain, and whereas chemoreceptors probably prevent $PaCO_2$ from rising much above the resting value, there appear to be few feedback control mechanisms to prevent $PaCO_2$ from falling during hyperventilation.

Symptoms

Hypocapnia is probably of little clinical relevance if it does not produce symptoms, and the way in which patients perceive or interpret these symptoms often influences the subsequent clinical course. Most symptoms of hypocapnia are due either to an increase in neuronal excitability, or

Box 20.1 Hyperventilation

Possible definition

Alveolar ventilation which is inappropriately high for the metabolic production of carbon monoxide.

Causes

- psychogenic (e.g. anxiety)
- organic (e.g. asthma, pulmonary embolism)
- physiological (e.g. progesterone in pregnancy)

vasoconstriction.[5,8] In normal subjects, symptoms occur at a mean end-tidal PCO_2 (see below) of 20 mmHg (2.66 kPa) with an outside range of 14–29 mmHg.[12]

An increase in neuronal excitability causes peripheral paraesthesiae ('pins and needles') which is often mistaken for a neurological disease and may eventually lead to cramps or, rarely, tetany.[13] No change in any aspect of serum calcium has ever been documented in response to hyperventilation,[14] and a fall in serum phosphorus provides a more likely explanation[3] for these effects.

Other symptoms are due to reduction in regional blood flow secondary to the fall of $PaCO_2$. Reduction in cerebral blood flow[15] induces cerebral hypoxia and a range of cerebral symptoms including dizziness, fainting, headaches, derealization, and unilateral somatic symptoms[16] which are often misdiagnosed as neurological disease.[17] Hyperventilation is associated with reduction in peripheral resistance and mean arterial blood pressure, an increase in heart rate and cardiac output, and skin vasoconstriction inducing cold extremities which is a common complaint.[18]

Coronary blood flow is linearly related to $PaCO_2$ in humans in the absence of chest pain[19] and hyperventilation is probably a cause of atypical chest pain,[20,21] but the mechanisms are uncertain. This symptom is particularly important as patients often misattribute such pain to cardiac disease with induction of a vicious cycle of increasing anxiety, panic and further hyperventilation. Hyperventilation may mimic coronary disease by producing S-T segment depression and end-tidal PCO_2 should be routinely measured during treadmill exercise.

Symptoms can arise from most other systems. In the gastrointestinal system, epigastric pain, a bloated feeling and vomiting have been described[22] but it is uncertain whether these symptoms are due to hypocapnia, or to anxiety and misattribution.

Signs

Signs of hyperventilation may be minimal. An increase in chest wall movement and rate may be obvious in acute hyperventilation, but in chronic hyperventilation this may not be so and resting end-tidal PCO_2 can be halved with only a 10% increase in minute ventilation,[23] which is not clinically detectable. Patients with hyperventilation often sigh repeatedly (see below). Even in acute hyperventilation as discussed above, dramatic sighing or panting may not necessarily be associated with reduction of $PaCO_2$.

Diagnosis

The gold standard for diagnosis of hyperventilation and respiratory alkalosis is measurement of arterial PCO_2 and blood gas parameters. However, arterial puncture is invasive and will fail to diagnose patients with variable hyperventilation. Alternative measures are less satisfactory.

End-tidal PCO_2

End-tidal PCO_2 ($P_{ET}CO_2$)[23,24] is equivalent to $PaCO_2$ in subjects at rest and with normal lungs. It can be measured by capnograph or mass spectrometer from a small sample extracted continuously from a manifold through which the subject breathes to and fro, or by taping a fine catheter a few millimetres inside the entrance to a nostril. Care is required to ensure that a valid end-tidal plateau is obtained and that the analyser has a sufficiently fast response time.[25] There is uncertainty about the lower limit of the normal range, and measurements in conscious humans may be confounded by cortical influences and additional respiratory stimulation induced by the measuring apparatus.[26] In our laboratory, we found that the lower limit of the normal range was 32.2 mmHg (4.28 kPa),[23] and we take 30 mmHg (3.99 kPa) as a rough lower limit below which we might expect the patient to report symptoms in clinical practice. We suggest, however, that the normal range should be determined for each laboratory.

Transcutaneous PCO_2

Transcutaneous PCO_2 measured via a skin electrode and recorded on to an ambulatory system has been used to measure PCO_2 changes over a number of hours under home conditions.[27–29] The time constant of response of the electrode to a step change of arterial PCO_2 is a number of minutes, making interpretation of changes difficult; the skin heating necessary to 'arterialize' the skin can only be tolerated for a few hours; and the calibration is subject to drift.[30] Future technical advances may make this technique more useful for routine monitoring

Measurement of PCO_2 with provocations

Hyperventilation can be induced in many patients by stressors that mimic, in the laboratory, factors that may induce hyperventilation in everyday life. The most widely studied stressor is voluntary overbreathing. This can reproduce symptoms which the patient recognizes and can be associated with an abnormally slow recovery of $PaCO_2$ following the cessation of overbreathing.[2] Because voluntary overbreathing may mimic everyday activities such as talking, this can be useful for diagnosis, but recent studies have questioned the technique.[29]

Hyperventilation screen

These studies have provided us with the basis for a test that we perform in selected patients as part of lung function testing. $P_{ET}CO_2$ is measured via a fine nasal catheter for 5–10 min at rest, during and after up to 10 min of exercise at a level appropriate for the patient, and during and after up to 3 min of voluntary overbreathing. We regard $P_{ET}CO_2$ over 30 mmHg (4 kPa) at rest, during and after exercise and at 10 min after overbreathing as normal. This procedure is not diagnostic in isolation but is an aid to clinical assessment. A positive test suggests either that the patient is overbreathing at rest, or responds excessively to provocations and thus may do so at other times. A negative test is a more powerful indication that the patient is unlikely to be precipitated into hyperventilation by relevant triggers but does not exclude hyperventilation at other times.

Breath hold time

Breath hold time is used by many as an indication of a tendency to hyperventilate. However, this is very dependent on the skill of the operator in persuading the patient to continue to the limit, and the normal range of breath hold times is wide.[31]

Aetiology

Hyperventilation is due to increase in respiratory drive and the causes of this should be sought and documented as for any other clinical abnormality. 'Hyperventilation' *per se* is not an adequate diagnosis. The causes of increased drive may be psychogenic, organic, physiological, or unknown, but it is also useful clinically to recognize a range of clinical presentations in which hyperventilation is of predominant clinical importance.

There is a multifactorial aetiology in most cases in which hyperventilation contributes to the presenting symptoms and attempts to attribute hyperventilation to a single cause are probably unrealistic. Many psychiatric, respiratory, and other organic disorders are associated with documented hyperventilation, and these can be classified as psychogenic, organic, and physiological. Most patients have a combination of organic and psychiatric factors, and it should not be forgotten that most organic disease is associated with significant abnormalities of mental health. It is useful to distinguish disorders that can initiate hyperventilation from those that sustain it, and to distinguish acute and chronic time courses. Conditions of relevance to a physician are listed in Table 20.1.

Table 20.1 Disorders that can initiate hyperventilation

Type of disorder	Examples
Respiratory disorders	Asthma
	COPD
	Interstitial fibrosis
	Pneumonia
	Heart failure
	Pulmonary embolism
	Pulmonary hypertension
Other organic disorders	CNS disorders
	Pain
	Aspirin overdose
	System failures
Physiological	Progesterone
	Speech
	Altitude
	Pyrexia
	Control of breathing disorders

Initiating factors

Anxiety

Although anxiety was a key component in the original description of hyperventilation syndrome, the relation of hyperventilation to anxiety is not simple and hyperventilation can occur without anxiety.[23,32,33] Anxiety may be induced by the hyperventilation, rather than itself being a primary initiating factor.[34] Anxiety can be associated with both mild hyperventilation and abnormalities of breathing pattern.[35] Endogenous non-retarded depression can be associated with hyperventilation,[36] and phobic patients have a high prevalence of breathing difficulties.[37,38] The predisposition to overbreathe in response to stress may be dependent on biological vulnerability, personality and cognitive variables[39] as well as individual interpretation of the hyperventilation-induced somatic symptoms,[40] and may become a conditioned response.[41]

Most recent research has focused on the issue of panic disorder, but there is a complex relationship between anxiety, hyperventilation, and panic and the association between the two is controversial.[39,41] The mechanisms of panic are uncertain, but cognitive misinterpretation (or misattribution) of the somatic symptoms of hyperventilation to a life-threatening illness such as a myocardial infarction or a stroke[42] has been suggested as a possible contributing factor.[14]

Factitious hyperventilation leads to bizarre clinical syndromes, which often require considerable time to investigate. Covert observation of the patient can be helpful, as can prolonged and overnight recording of $P_{ET}CO_2$.

Respiratory disorders

The best known example is asthma, in which $PaCO_2$ can fall below 25 mmHg (3.3 kPa) in association with only mild or moderate reduction of FEV_1 during acute attacks.[43] The mechanism is uncertain, but stimulation of airway vagal afferents by mucosal inflammation, stimulation of chest wall receptors by hyperinflation, or stimulation of breathing by hypoxia and psychogenic factors may be involved. In mild chronic asthma, hyperventilation is related to bronchial smooth muscle reactivity and not to inflammation or psychogenic factors.[44]

In practice, asthma, especially if mild, previously undiagnosed and atypical in presentation, can contribute to symptomatic hyperventilation or be the sole aetiological factor in a significant proportion of patients.[45,46] Demeter et al.[45] reported that most of their patients with hyperventilation syndrome had asthma, hypocapnic symptoms being eliminated by treatment with a combination of bronchodilators and explanation. In these patients, standard lung function tests are often normal, or are difficult to interpret due to anxiety, panic, or dyspnoea. Wheeze can also be due to bronchoconstriction induced by hyperventilation.[47] There is documented evidence of hypocapnia in chronic obstructive pulmonary disease (COPD), fibrosing alveolitis, pneumonia, and pulmonary hypertension but it is less likely that hyperventilation will be the primary presenting complaint in these conditions. Pulmonary embolus is a potent cause of hyperventilation and hypocapnia, and is usually associated with hypoxia. Pulmonary hypertension can present with dyspnoea, hyperventilation, depression, and panic disorder.[48]

Other organic disorders

Cheyne–Stokes breathing can be associated with hypocapnia in patients with acute bilateral pontine infarctions, and has been reported in an astrocytoma of the medulla, pons, and midbrain but Plum and Leigh have more recently argued that primary neurogenic hyperventilation is extremely rare, if it exists at all.[49] Hyperventilation is induced by pain[50] and yet patients with chest pain due to coronary artery disease had a surprising absence of hyperventilation when genuine angina was induced by exercise testing.[51] Chest pain is rare in normal subjects during voluntary overbreathing.[12] Hyperventilation is also used in anaesthesia to increase the pain threshold.[52] Hyperventilation can be a predominant symptom in overdose of drugs such as aspirin and in major system failures, and can mimic those of both diabetic ketoacidosis[53] and hypoglycaemia.[54] These conditions have all been missed in emergency departments in patients too readily labelled as having 'hyperventilation syndrome'. It is commonly assumed that thyrotoxicosis is associated with hyperventilation. Although these patients complain of dyspnoea, there is little evidence for hypocapnia in the literature.

Physiological abnormalities

There are a variety of physiological conditions that can induce hyperventilation. Although these alone rarely cause symptomatic hypocapnia, they often combine with other factors to reduce $PaCO_2$ closer to the frontier of hypocapnic symptoms so that any small additional stress, whether psychological or physical, may push a patient over into symptoms, and trigger a vicious circle.[1]

The most important physiological abnormality causing hyperventilation is the effect of progesterone in women which reduces $PaCO_2$ by up to 8 mmHg (1.06 kPa) in the second half of the menstrual cycle and even lower in pregnancy.[55] Hyperventilation is induced by speech and, in our experience, acute attacks are sometimes precipitated following prolonged conversations. Pyrexia can stimulate breathing due to a direct effect on the carotid bodies.

It is often suggested that hyperventilation is the result of imbalance between the action of the diaphragm and chest wall muscles, poor posture, or other abnormalities of respiratory pattern, but the evidence for these mechanisms is poor.[56] Excessive use of the upper chest in relation to the diaphragm has been described in these patients,[1] but it remains to be demonstrated whether this is a cause or an effect of increased ventilation.

Sustaining factors

Sighing and habit

Sighing is a common finding in these patients and may contribute to the continuation of hyperventilation. Sighing may be linked to 'air hunger' (see below) but it is also almost universal for a patient, when faced with unexplained symptoms, to take large breaths in order to 'get more oxygen in' as patients describe it. In normal subjects after 15 min of sustained hyperventilation, hypocapnia can be maintained with only an occasional large breath[57] and this may be one of the causes of continuation of overbreathing in patients with chronic hyperventilation.[23]

Lum believes that anxiety is secondary to hyperventilation and that hyperventilation is triggered by a range of factors and is a normal response to stress or any mood change.[1] With frequent repetition, the response takes on the characteristics of a habit or conditioned reflex. However, it produces 'illness' only when the hyperventilation response is excessive, inappropriate or continues after stress is withdrawn – when the patients' distress may be enhanced by the indifference or incomprehension of doctors and the absence of clear-cut pathology.

Abnormalities of respiratory control

Folgering has reviewed a range of abnormalities of respiratory control that may, under some circumstances, contribute both to the initiation and particularly to the continuation of hyperventilation.[8] The role of these abnormalities in clinical practice remains uncertain. He suggested that stress and anxiety might contribute to increase in muscle tone and upper thoracic breathing by increased gamma-motor input on muscle spindles. Anticipatory or conditioned responses that have been shown to contribute to the initial increase in ventilation at the start of exercise may also contribute to hyperventilation in patients who are anticipating phobic symptoms. The time constant of 'afterdischarge' (a 'flywheel' effect in which ventilation remains raised for some minutes after a range of different respiratory stimuli) is inversely related to $PaCO_2$,[58] and this may contribute to maintaining hyperactivity of the respiratory centres once activated. Both an increase in tidal volume and an increase in respiratory frequency contribute to the increased ventilation in chronic hyperventilation.[23] $P_{ET}CO_2$ has been noted to fall progressively with time during resting breathing in patients with a tendency to hyperventilation.[59] The influence of measuring apparatus in these patients is controversial, and the mouthpiece has been shown to have both a minimal[23] and an excessive influence[60] on breathing. Finally, Folgering has found that, at very low levels of $PaCO_2$, increasing the $PaCO_2$ actually causes a decrease in ventilation which then remains constant as $PaCO_2$ increases until the threshold of the chemoreceptors is reached at about 40 mmHg (5.3 kPa). This could contribute to continuation of hyperventilation at low levels of $PaCO_2$.

Clinical syndromes involving hyperventilation

Hyperventilation syndrome

Problems with definition

Some of the controversies about the use of this term have been reviewed by Folgering[8] and by Gardner and colleagues.[61] Many psychosomatic syndromes have been described in the past in which hyperventilation has a variable and uncertain role, but the term 'hyperventilation syndrome' was first used in 1938 to describe patients with the somatic symptoms of both hypocapnia and anxiety.[62] This theme was extended by subsequent authors[14,63,64] and the definition arrived at by Lewis and Howell in 1986 on the basis of a questionnaire of delegates at a psychophysiology meeting[65] was: 'a syndrome induced by physiologically inappropriate hyperventilation and usually reproduced in whole or in part by voluntary hyperventilation'. However, this definition did not proved entirely satisfactory and the term is now used in so many different contexts that in our personal view it has ceased to have any universal meaning. Some physicians diagnose it in the presence of the somatic symptoms of hypocapnia either at rest or induced by voluntary overbreathing without assumptions about aetiology.[66] Others regard it primarily as an abnormality of respiratory control[67] or as a variant of disproportionate breathlessness.[6,68] Folgering has suggested a new definition as: 'a dysregulation of ventilation, causing hypocapnia, in the absence of organic causes for hyperventilation, with symptoms and complaints not exclusively associated with hypocapnia'. Many authors, however, refuse to recognize it as a separate entity[29] or regard it as secondary to organic disease and especially asthma.[45,69] Many would not use the term in the presence of any organic cause of hyperventilation, and yet organic and psychiatric factors are usually difficult to separate. Lum regarded hyperventilation as a form of conditioned response and he did not use the term 'hyperventilation syndrome',[1] but he has been criticized for underdiagnosing asthma in his patients.[69] These uncertainties reflect the complexity of this subject which falls between psychiatry, clinical medicine, and physiology.

A practical approach

In our view, it is not useful in the clinical context to label a patient with hypocapnia as having 'hyperventilation syndrome'. We believe that in all cases, the initiating and sustaining cause or causes of the increased respiratory drive causing the hyperventilation should be sought. The use of a label such as 'hyperventilation syndrome' tends to preclude further search for underlying aetiological factors and can be dangerous in the emergency room context.

The clinical finding of a low arterial or end-tidal PCO_2 is of little relevance *per se* if there are no associated symptoms of hypocapnia, or if the symptoms are of minor importance compared with the symptoms of the disorder causing the hyperventilation. In other situations, the symptoms of hyperventilation are pivotal to the patients' clinical presentation. One or more of the above aetiological factors can usually be identified as contributing to the presenting symptoms, and organic and psychiatric factors are usually inextricably linked.

We find it clinically useful to distinguish hyperventilation with a short (acute) and long time course (chronic) because of implications for treatment and prognosis. If no cause of causes for the hyperventilation can be found, however, we are happy to leave the question of aetiology open and unexplained.

Acute/subacute hyperventilation

Patients may occasionally present with acute anxiety or depressive states combined with symptomatic hyperventilation in the absence of panic, misattribution, or other organic or physiological factors. Hyperventilation can also occasionally be the main presenting complaint in patients with a single organic disorder such as asthma in the absence of psychogenic or physiological factors.[46] These patients respond to treatment of the underlying condition.

It is more common for patients to present with a multifactorial aetiology and symptoms extending over a time span of up to about 2 years. We described such patients presenting to an emergency department.[70] Due to a combination of factors but often mild asthma combined with anxiety, drug abuse, excessive talking, etc., there is a sudden onset of alarming symptoms of hypocapnia. The patient panics and takes large breaths to relieve symptoms, worsening the hyperventilation and associated symptoms which are misattributed by both patient and attending doctor to serious disease such as a heart attack, epilepsy, or stroke. The patient is often admitted to a coronary care or other acute medical unit but the underlying basis for the attack is not recognized and investigations fail to reveal a diagnosis, leading to heightened anxiety and fear of further attacks, which thus inevitably reoccur. The patient has increasingly unrewarding visits to a variety of medical and psychiatric clinics and rapidly descends into chronic invalidism. This sequence can destroy the life of an otherwise fit young person within months. Rapid recognition of this sequence and positive management is essential, with a rapid return to their normal daily functioning.

These patients can usually be treated by a chest physician. The sequence of events can be reconstructed from a careful history, which is crucial, and the patient's decline can be reversed over weeks or months by explanation, demonstration of the effects of hypocapnia, and continual reassurance, combined with adequate investigations to exclude the feared disorders and treatment of initiating factors such as asthma. Antidepressants such as serotonin-selective reuptake inhibitors (SSRIs) and/or a cognitive-behavioural approach may be required for panic. The presence of depression can be easily elicited by asking the patient, and can be treated with a SSRI antidepressant; these are particularly suitable for pulmonary patients because of a low incidence of side effects.[72] Relaxation and breathing exercises (see below) administered by a physiotherapist help some patients to control breathing during panic but are usually not required.

Chronic hyperventilation

We have described a group of patients who presented with a long history of varied and unimpressive symptoms.[23,29] 'Air hunger' was common, suggesting a psychogenic aetiology, but only 50% had evidence of psychiatric morbidity in the form of a mild phobic state. $P_{ET}CO_2$ was either chronically low at rest and throughout all provocations, or was precipitated into prolonged reduction by either exercise or voluntary overbreathing. Minute ventilation was only increased by about 10%. The initiating and sustaining causes of the hyperventilation were uncertain, but there was no resetting of the carbon dioxide response curve.[72]

These patients can be identified by a hyperventilation screen (see above) and usually have a low resting $P_{ET}CO_2$, but it is often difficult to prove that the vague symptoms are related to the hypocapnia. These patients are resistant to all known treatments. However, by reassurance, and psychiatric support for any associated anxiety or depressive disorder, they can often be kept at work even if there is no improvement in the hypocapnia. It is important that patients continue to be seen in one clinic to prevent multiple referrals and reinvestigation.

There may be an overlap between chronic hyperventilation and other syndromes with a similar chronic presentation. The similarity of chronic fatigue syndrome to the older 'effort syndrome'[73] has been emphasized. However, we found that a group of patients with well-documented chronic fatigue syndrome were mostly not hypocapnic at rest and did not hyperventilate excessively in response to either exercise or voluntary hyperventilation.[74]

Psychogenic, disproportionate, and unexplained breathlessness

There is very little literature about psychogenic breathlessness. It would be reasonable to define **psychogenic breathlessness** as breathlessness assumed to be related to psychogenic factors in the absence of demonstrable organic causes. **Disproportionate breathlessness**, on the other hand, is breathlessness which is out of proportion to the severity of any underlying respiratory disease, again with the assumption that the additional breathlessness is related to either psychiatric abnormalities or an excessive sensitivity to stress. Breathlessness and hyperventilation are not synonymous.

If a patient is breathless, that is the condition for which a cause should be sought; if hyperventilation is also present, it is usually secondary to the breathlessness and of little clinical importance. Patients are often referred because of 'psychogenic dyspnoea' when the degree of

---

Box 20.2 Types of Breathlessness

Psychogenic breathlessness: Breathlessness assumed to be related to psychogenic factors in the absence of demonstrable organic causes.

Disproportionate breathlessness: Breathlessness which is out of proportion to the severity of any underlying respiratory disease.

Clinical syndromes

- during or after exercise
- inability to breathe in fully: "pathological air hunger" (may be asthmatic)

distress seems disproportionate to the clinical findings of lung function or blood gas data, but there is almost no literature.[75,76] Dyspnoea is what the patient reports, and is therefore difficult to dispute. Our clinical experience is that psychogenic factors alone rarely provide a complete explanation for dyspnoea. Studies of breathlessness are impeded by uncertainty about the basic mechanisms,[77] and there are probably many different forms; however, we have found that there are two particular situations in which unexplained and possibly psychogenic factors may be involved in breathlessness:

◆ When disproportionate breathlessness occurs during or immediately after exercise[78] in the absence of any demonstrable causes of dyspnoea. The aetiology of the breathlessness in these patients is obscure, but there is usually little evidence of a psychogenic aetiology. Bronchospasm immediately after exercise has been occasionally documented in the absence of a history of asthma.[79] These patients can be identified during an exercise test by reduction of $P_{ET}CO_2$ with progressive rise of SaO_2 and appropriate increase in heart rate, combined with absence of any other cause for dyspnoea on exertion. A trial of inhaled steroids and bronchodilators is worth trying, but is usually unhelpful.

◆ Patients whose primary report is of inability to 'breathe in', inability to 'take a satisfying breath' or inability to 'fill the lungs'('I can't get enough air in'). These patients usually have no history suggestive of respiratory disease and have near normal lung function. Hyperventilation is often mild or absent. We refer to this presentation as **pathological air hunger**. The mechanism of 'air hunger' is uncertain and there are few descriptions of this symptom in the literature. We suspect that some cases may be initiated by very mild undiagnosed chronic asthma and about half of our cases respond well to inhaled steroids. It can also be a precursor of panic, which in turn can lead to a vicious spiral of hyperventilation, and is probably one of mechanisms of frequent sighing. 'Air hunger' is thus within the province both of the physician and psychiatrist. It is difficult to treat, but may resolve spontaneously. Patients can be taught not to sigh and this reduces the risk of hyperventilation. In some cases, treatment with antidepressants (such as the SSRIs outlined above) provide dramatic relief, but this is not universal.

Howell[6,68] has described a slightly different group of patients who present with attacks of breathlessness at rest for no apparent reason, often associated with sweating and hyperventilation, or breathlessness on exertion poorly related to severity of exertion. 'Air hunger' was not a particular feature of these patients. Anxiety, depression, and hysterical reactions with premorbid hysterical or obsessional personalities were more common than in a control group of patients mostly with severe COPD in whom breathlessness was appropriate to the severity of the disease. A family history of depression, bereavement, and separation; current marital disharmony; gross secondary gain from illness; living alone; and a previous surgical operation were more common than in control groups. A conditioned response ensures that minor stimuli

---

Box 20.3   Empirical treatment of hyperventilation

◆ breathing retraining
◆ ? antidepressants ? beta-blockers

can provoke recurrent attacks of a similar pattern. Howell recognized that either hyperventilation or breathlessness may be absent but he nevertheless referred to this sequence of events as 'hyperventilation syndrome' rather than 'behavioural breathlessness'. It appears to us to be unnecessary to continue to attempt to force breathlessness and hyperventilation into a single straitjacket.

Symptomatic management of hyperventilation

The identification and treatment of the causes of hyperventilation must be a priority, but in some cases the causes cannot be identified and pragmatic treatment is required to control the hyperventilation *per se*. Many regimes have been developed, summarized in a book edited by Timmons and Ley[56] and critically reviewed by Garssen.[80,81]

Management of acute hyperventilation

There are few established regimes for management of severe acute hyperventilation, but rebreathing from a paper bag is widely prescribed. The mode of action and efficacy has not been formally determined and may involve distraction as much as accumulation of CO_2. Its use can be lethal in the presence of preexisting hypoxia due to lung disease.[82]

Breathing retraining

In some patients, and especially those verging on panic, a regime involving breathing exercises and diaphragmatic retraining may be of benefit.[1] Lum's principles of treatment[84] were:

- to cultivate awareness of habits such as sighing and sniffing and to suppress them
- to suppress thoracic movements at rest and minimize them on exercise
- to inculcate slow, regular diaphragmatic breathing
- to teach relaxation.

He first taught his patients to detect upper thoracic and diaphragm movements with the palm of one hand over the manubrium and the other over the umbilicus. The patient is then taught to inhale and exhale with palpable movements of the abdominal wall while attempting to suppress thoracic movements, and this is combined with general relaxation exercises, and desensitization for phobic anxiety disorder.

Some believe that the effect of such training is non-specific, but a recent study showed some long-term benefit.[84] However, other controlled studies suggest that these techniques have only limited effectiveness.[85,86] Our clinical view is that they should *not* be offered routinely to all patients. They can be helpful when no cause for the hyperventilation can be found and in selected patients who require techniques for relaxation and for self-control of breathing in mild panic. In other patients, they can be positively harmful in inducing excessive introspection about the respiratory act.

Drugs

Drugs have only a limited role in symptomatic treatment of hyperventilation,[80] and treatment should be directed to the underlying cause whenever possible. The use of SSRIs for management of co-morbid depression, anxiety, or panic has been discussed above, and these can be combined with a cognitive-behavioural approach. Beta-blockers have been suggested to remove sympathetically mediated symptoms such as palpitations, trembling, and sweating,[87] but must not be used if there is any suspicion of asthma. Benzodiazepines reduce subjective complaints,[88] but a lasting effect has not been demonstrated and their addictive potential limits long-term use.

Treatment – a clinical approach

It would be reasonable to propose the following treatment regime for patients with both hyperventilation and disproportionate dyspnoea.

- Take a careful history of the presenting complaints, associated clinical features, and especially any factors such as chronic wheeze or cough, hay fever, or childhood chestiness that might suggest asthma. Order a chest radiograph, routine blood tests, ventilation–perfusion scan (if available), lung function tests (or twice daily ambulatory peak flow), and hyperventilation screen (if available). If organic disorders are found, treat these. Normal lung function tests do not exclude asthma, but a reduction of morning peak flow by more than say 50 L/min below the evening reading is suggestive.

- If there are any clinical features to suggest asthma, give a low-dose inhaled steroid twice daily as a trial for a month.

- If there is any suggestion of depression, panic, or a phobic state, refer the patient to a psychiatrist, or commence an SSRI on a trial basis. Psychiatric referral is also sometimes required for reassurance even in the absence of a psychiatric disorder if the patient has been previously labelled as a psychiatric case.

- In selected cases with mild panic, breathing and relaxation exercises may help.

- Continue with support and reassurance **in the same clinic**.

Conclusion

In summary, we believe that the management of these difficult patients is firmly within the remit of the chest physician, or a combined clinic with a chest physician and a psychiatrist. Clinical and physiological assessment in combination with psychiatric support can supply a prompt, positive, and informed approach usually leading to a clear treatment strategy which is vital to prevent a rapid descent into iatrogenic chronic invalidism and somatization which is all too commonly the fate of these otherwise fit and often young patients.

Keypoints

- Hyperventilation, psychogenic breathlessness, and disproportionate breathlessness are complex states, difficult to define, but not synonymous

- Patients with these complaints commonly present to a surgery, clinic, or emergency department, and are frequently misdiagnosed

- Hyperventilation because of hypocapnia may cause multiple symptoms in addition to the common ones of parasthesiae, dizziness, weakness, and cold extremities

- Physiological confirmation of hyperventilation requires measurement of $PaCO_2$

- A number of organic disorders can cause hyperventilation; its association with anxiety and asthma are clinically the most important

- Sighing and 'air hunger' are common accompaniments of hyperventilation of any cause
- Causes for apparent hyperventilation should always be sought. A clinical division into acute, subacute, and chronic hyperventilation is useful
- Two particular situations in which unexplained and possibly psychogenic factors may be involved with breathlessness are
  - when it occurs during or immediately after exercise in the absence of any physiological cause
  - where patients complain of an inability to 'breathe in fully' (pathological air hunger).
- The management of hyperventilation should include explanation and reassurance, and a consideration of rebreathing, breathing, and retraining, and in some cases drug treatment

References

1 Lum, L.C. The syndrome of habitual chronic hyperventilation. *Recent Adv Psychosom Med* 1976; **3**: 196–229.

2 Hardonk, H.J., and Beumer, H.M. Hyperventilation syndrome. In: P.J. Vinken, and G.W. Bruyn, (eds) *Handbook of neurology*. Amsterdam: North Holland Biomedical Press, 1979; **38**: 309–60.

3 Magarian, G.J. Hyperventilation syndromes: infrequently recognized common expressions of anxiety and stress. *Medicine* 1982; **61**: 219–36.

4 Brashear, R.E. Hyperventilation syndrome. *Lung*, 1983; **161**: 257–73.

5 Gardner, W.N. Review: The pathophysiology of hyperventilation disorders. *Chest*, 1996; **109**: 516–34.

6 Howell, J.B. The hyperventilation syndrome: a syndrome under threat? *Thorax*, 1997; **52**(Suppl 3): S30–34.

7 Bass, C. Hyperventilation syndrome: a chimera? (editorial). *J Psychosom Res*, 1997; **42**: 421–6.

8 Folgering, H. The hyperventilation syndrome. In: M.D. Altose, and Y. Kawakami, (eds) *Control of breathing in health and disease*. New York: Marcel Dekker, 1999; 633–60

9 Fahri, L.E. Gas stores of the body. In: W.O. Fenn and H. Rahn, (eds) *Handbook of physiology*. Section 3: *Respiration*, vol. 1. Washington, DC: American Physiological Society, 1964; 873–85.

10 Arbus, G.S., Hebert, L.A., Levesque, P.R., Etsten, B.E., and Schwartz, W.B. Potassium depletion and hypercapnia. *N Engl J Med* 1969; **280**: 670.

11 Gledhill, N., Beirne, G.J., and Dempsey, J.A. Renal response to short-term hypocapnia in man. *Kidney Int* 1975; **8**(6):376–84.

12 Rafferty, G.F., Saisch, S.G.N., and Gardner, W.N. Relation of hypocapnic symptoms to rate of fall of end-tidal PCO_2 in normal subjects. *Respir Med* 1992; **86**: 335–40.

13 Macefield, G., and Burke, D. Paraesthesiae and tetany induced by voluntary hyperventilation. Increased excitability of human cutaneous and motor axons. *Brain* 1991; **114**: 527–40.

14 Ames, F. The hyperventilation syndrome. *J Mental Sci* 1955; **101**: 466–525.

15 Kety, S.S., and Schmidt, C.F. The effects of active and passive hyperventilation on cerebral blood flow, cerebral oxygen consumption, cardiac output, and blood pressure of normal young men. *J Clin Invest* 1946; **25**: 107–19.

16 Perkins, G.D., and Joseph, R. Neurological manifestations of the hyperventilation syndrome. *J Roy Soc Med* 1986; **79**: 448–50.

17 Blau, J.N., and Wiles, C.M. Unilateral somatic symptoms due to hyperventilation. *BMJ* 1983; **286**: 1108.

18 Kontos, H.A., Richardson, D.W., Raper, A.J., Zubair-Ulhassan, and Patterson, J.L. Jr. Mechanisms of action of hypocapnic alkalosis on limb blood vessels in man and dog. *Am J Physiol* 1972; **223**(6): 1296–307.

19 Neill, W.A., and Hattenhauer, M. Impairment of myocardial O_2 supply due to hyperventilation. *Circulation* 1975; **52**: 854–6.

20 Evans, D.W., and Lum, L.C. Hyperventilation: an important cause of pseudoangina. *Lancet* 1977; i: 155–7.

21 Bass, C., Wade, C., Hand, D., and Jackson, G. Patients with angina with normal and near normal coronary arteries: clinical and psychosocial state 12 months after angiography. *BMJ* 1983; **287**: 1505–8.

22 McKell, T.E., and Sullivan, A.J. The hyperventilation syndrome in gastroenterology. *Gastroenterology* 1947; **9**: 6–16.

23 Gardner, W.N., Meah, M.S., and Bass, C. Controlled study of respiratory responses during prolonged measurement in patients with chronic hyperventilation. *Lancet* 1986; **ii**: 826–30.

24 DuBois, A.B., Fowler, R.C., Soffer, A., and Fenn, W.O. Alveolar CO_2 measured by expiration into the rapid response infrared gas analyser. *J Appl Physiol* 1952; **4**: 526–34.

25 Saish, S.G. An introduction to capnography *Biofeedback Self Regul* 1994; **19**(2): 115–34.

26 Gilbert, R., Auchincloss, J.H.J., Brodsky, J., and Boden, W. Changes in tidal volume, frequency and ventilation induced by their measurement. *J Appl Physiol* 1972; **33**: 252–4.

27 Pilsbury, D., and Hibbert, G. An ambulatory system for long-term continuous monitoring of transcutaneous PCO_2. *Bull Eur Physiopathol Respir* 1987; **23**(1): 9–13.

28 Pilsbury, D., and Hibbert, G. Time-dependent variations transcutaneous PCO_2 level in normal subjects. *J Appl Physiol* 1988; **64**(5): 1858–63.

29 Hornsveld, H.K., Garssen, B., Dop, M.J., van Spiegel, P.I., and de Haes, J.C. Double-blind placebo-controlled study of the hyperventilation provocation test and the validity of the hyperventilation syndrome. *Lancet* 1996; **348**(9021): 154–8.

30 Pilsbury, D., and Hibbert, G. An ambulatory system for long-term continuous monitoring of transcutaneous PCO_2. *Bull Eur Physiopathol Respir* 1987; **23**: 9–13.

31 Lin, Y.C., Lally, D.A., Moore, T.O., and Hong, S.K. Physiological and conventional breath-hold breaking points. *J Appl Physiol* 1974; **37**(3): 291–6.

32 Lewis, B.I. The hyperventilation syndrome. *Ann Int Med* 1953; **38**: 918–27.

33 Bass, C., and Gardner, W.N. Respiratory and psychiatric abnormalities in chronic symptomatic hyperventilation. *BMJ* 1985; **290**: 1387–90.

34 Lum, L.C. Hyperventilation syndromes in medicine and psychiatry: a review. *J Roy Soc Med* 1987; **80**: 229–31.

35 Tobin, M.J., Chadha, T.S., Jenouri, G., Birch, S.J., Gazerigky, H.B., and Sackner, M.A. Breathing patterns. 2. Diseased subjects. *Chest* 1983; **84**(3): 286–94.

36 Damas Mora, J., Grant, L., Kenyon, P., Patel, M.K., and Jenner, F.A. Respiratory ventilation and carbon dioxide levels in syndromes of depression. *Br J Psychiatr* 1976; **129**: 457–64.

37 Arrindell, W.A. Dimensional structure and psychopathology correlates of the Fear Survey Schedule (FSS-III) in a phobic population: a factorial definition of agoraphobia. *Behav Res Ther* 1980; **18**(4): 229–42.

38 Hallam, R.S., and Hafner, R.J. Fears of phobic patients: factor analyses of self-report data. *Behav Res Ther* 1978; **16**(1):1–6.

39 Bass, C., Kartsounis, L., and Lelliott, P. Hyperventilation and its relationship to anxiety and panic. *Integr Psychiatry* 1987; **5**: 274–91.

40 Clark, D.M., and Hemsley, D.R. The effects of hyperventilation; individual variability and its relation to personality. *J Behav Ther Exp Psychiatry* 1982; **13**: 41–47.

41 Garssen, B., Buikhuisen, M., and van Dyck, R. Hyperventilation and panic attacks. *Am J Psychiatry* 1996; **153**: 513–18.

42 Salkovskis, P.M., and Clark, D.M. Affective responses to hyperventilation: a test of the cognitive model of panic. *Behav Res Ther* 1990; **28**: 51–61.

43 McFadden, E.R., and Lyons, H.A. Arterial blood gas tension in asthma. *N Engl J Med* 1968; **278**(19): 1027–32.

44 Osborne, C.A., Lewis, A.J., Orr, L.M., Kanabar, V., O'Connor, B.J., and Gardner, W.N. Mechanisms of hyperventilation in mild asthmatic subjects. *Eur Respir J* 1999; **14**(suppl 30): 469s.

45 Demeter, S.L., and Cordasco, E.M. Hyperventilation syndrome and asthma. *Am J Med* 1986; **81**: 989–94.

46 Gardner, W.N., Bass, C., and Moxham, J. Recurrent hyperventilation tetany due to mild asthma. *Respir Med* 1992; **86**: 349–51.

47 Deal Jr, E.C., McFadden, E.R., Ingram Jr, R.H., Strauss, R.H., and Jaeger, J.J. Role of respiratory heat exchange in production of exercise-induced asthma. *J Appl Physiol* 1979; **46**: 467–75.

48 Sietsema, K.E., Simon, J.I., and Wasserman, K. Pulmonary hypertension presenting as a panic disorder. *Chest* 1987; **91**: 910–12.

49 Plum, F., and Leigh, R.J. Abnormalities of central mechanisms. In: Hornbein (ed.) *Regulation of breathing. Lung biology in health and disease*, vol. 17. New York: Marcel Dekker, 1981; 989–1067.

50 Glynn, C.J., Lloyd, J.W., and Folkhard, S. Ventilatory response to intractable pain. *Pain* 1981; **11**: 201–11.

51 Chambers, J.B., Kiff, P.J., Gardner, W.N., Jackson, G., and Bass, C. Value of measuring end tidal partial pressure of carbon dioxide as an adjunct to treadmill exercise testing. *BMJ* 1988; **296**: 1281–5.

52 Geddes, I.C., and Gray, T.C. Hyperventilation for the maintenance of anaesthesia. *Lancet*, 1959; **ii**: 4–6.

53 Treasure, R.A.R., Fowler, P.B.S., Millington, H.T., and Wise, P.H. Misdiagnosis of diabetic ketoacidosis as hyperventilation syndrome. *BMJ* 1987; **294**: 630.

54 Steel, J.M., Masterton, G., Patrick, A.W., and McGuire, R. Hyperventilation or hypoglycaemia? *Diabet Med* 1989; **6**: 820–1.

55 Damas-Mora, J., Davies, L., Taylor, W., and Jenner, F.A. Menstrual respiratory changes and symptoms. *Br J Psychiatry* 1980; **136**: 492–7.

56 B.H. Timmons, and R. Ley, (eds) *Behavioral and psychological approaches to breathing disorders*. New York: Plenum Press, 1994.

57 Saltzman, H.A., Heyman, A., and Sieker, H.O. Correlation of clinical and physiologic manifestations of sustained hyperventilation. *N Engl J Med* 1963; **268**: 1431–6.

58 Folgering, H., and Durlinger, M. Time course of posthyperventilation breathing in humans depends on alveolar CO_2 tension. *J Appl Physiol* 1983; **54**: 809–13.

59 Vansteenkiste, J., Rochette, F., and Demedts, M. Diagnostic tests of hyperventilation syndrome. *Eur Respir J* 1991; **4**: 393–9.

60 Han, J.N., Stegen, K., Simkens, K., *et al.* Unsteadiness of breathing in patients with hyperventilation syndrome and anxiety disorders. *Eur Respir J* 1997; **10**: 167–76.

61 Saisch, S.G., Wessely, S., and Gardner, W.N. Patients with acute hyperventilation presenting to an inner-city emergency department. *Chest* 1996; **110**(4): 952–7.

62 Kerr, W.J., Gliebe, P.A., and Dalton, J.W. Physical phenomomena associated with anxiety states: the hyperventilation syndrome. *Calif West Med* 1938; **48**: 12–16.

63 Lewis, B.I. Chronic hyperventilation syndrome. *J Am Med Assoc* 1954; **155**(14): 1204–8.

64 Lewis, B.I. Hyperventilation syndrome: a clinical and physiological evaluation. *Calif Med* 1959; **91**: 121–6.

65 Lewis, R.A., and Howell, J.B.L. Definition of the hyperventilation syndrome. *Bull Eur Physiopath Respir* 1986; **22**: 201–5.

66 Stoop, A., de Boo, T., Lemmens, W., and Folgering, H. Hyperventilation syndrome: measurement of objective symptoms and subjective complaints. *Respiration* 1986; **49**: 37–44.

67 Folgering, H., and Colla, P. Some anomalies in the control of $PaCO_2$ in patients with hyperventilation syndrome. *Bull Eur Physiopathol Respir* 1978; **14**: 503–12.

68   Howell, J.B.L. Behavioural breathlessness. *Thorax* 1990; **45**: 287–92.

69   Dent, R., Yates, D., and Higenbottam, T. Does the hyperventilation syndrome exist? *Thorax* 1983; **38**: 223.

70   Saisch, S.G.N., Wessely, S., and Gardner, W.N. Patients with acute hyperventilation presenting to an inner-city emergency department. *Chest* 1996; **110**(4): 952–7.

71   Smoller, J.W., Pollack, M.H., Otto, M.W., Rosenbaum, J.F., and Kradin, R.L. Panic anxiety, dyspnea, and respiratory disease. Theoretical and clinical considerations. *Am J Respir Crit Care Med* 1996; **154**: 6–17.

72   Gardner, W.N., Bass, C., and Meah, M.S. Response to CO_2 in chronically hyperventilating man. *Am Rev Respir Dis* 1988; **137**(suppl 4): A409.

73   Soley, M.H., and Shock, N.W. The etiology of effort syndrome. *Am J Med Sci* 1938; **196**: 840–51.

74   Saisch, S.G., Deale, A., Gardner, W.N., and Wessely, S. Hyperventilation and chronic fatigue syndrome. *Q J Med* 1994; **87**: 63–7.

75   Mahler, D.A., Harver, A., Lentine, T., Scott, J.A., Beck, K., and Schwartzstein, R.M. Descriptors of breathlessness in cardiorespiratory diseases. *Am J Respir Crit Care Med* 1996; **154**: 1357–63.

76   American Thoracic Society. Dyspnoea. Mechanisms, assessment and management: a consensus statement. *Am J Respir Crit Care Med*, 1999; **159**: 321–40.

77   Tobin, M.J. Dyspnea. Pathophysiologic basis, clinical presentation, and management. *Arch Intern Med* 1990; **150**: 1604–13.

78   Gardner, W.N., Meah, M.S., and Bass, C. Controlled study of respiratory responses during prolonged measurement in patients with chronic hyperventilation. *Lancet* 1986; ii(8511): 826–30.

79   Ferguson, A., Addington, W.W., and Gaensler, E.A. Dyspnea and bronchospasm from inappropriate postexercise hyperventilation. *Ann Int Med* 1969; **71**: 1063–72.

80   Garssen, B., and Rijken, H. Clinical aspects and treatment of the hyperventilation syndrome. *Behav Psychother* 1986; **14**: 46–68.

81   Garssen, B. Hyperventilation and panic attacks. *Am J Psychiatry* 1996; **153**(4): 513–18.

82   Callahan, M. Hypoxic hazards of traditional paper bag rebreathing in hyperventilating patients. *Ann Emerg Med* 1989; **18**: 622–8.

83   Lum, L.C. Physiological considerations in the treatment of hyperventilation syndromes. *J Drug Res* 1983; **8**: 1867–72.

84   De Guire, S., Gevirtz, R., Kawahara, Y., and Maguire, W. Hyperventilation syndrome and the assessment of treatment for functional cardiac symptoms. *Am J Cardiol* 1992; **70**: 673–7.

85   de Ruiter, C., Rijken, H., Garssen, B., and Kraaimaat, F. Breathing retraining, exposure and a combination of both, in the treatment of panic disorder with agoraphobia. *Behav Res Ther* 1989; **27**: 647–55.

86   Salkovskis, P.M., Clark, D.M., and Hackmann, A. Treatment of panic attacks using cognitive therapy without exposure or breathing retraining. *Behav Res Ther* 1991; **29**: 161–6.

87   Folgering, H., and Cox, A. Beta-blocker therapy with metoprolol in the hyperventilation syndrome. *Respiration* 1981; **41**: 33–8.

88   Aronson, P.R. Evaluation of psychotropic drug therapy in chronic hyperventilation syndrome. *J New Drugs* 1966; **6**: 305–7.

Part V

Cough and haemoptysis

Chapter 21

Physiology and pathophysiology of cough

John Myers

Cough is one of a number of protective and defensive reflexes which have evolved to facilitate clearance of foreign material from the airways and limit their exposure to noxious stimuli (Table 21.1). This is vital to the survival of the individual. Absence of these reflexes is virtually incompatible with prolonged life. Troublesome cough is common, with a prevalence of 2–40% in the general population. It may be an indicator of serious underlying disease (e.g. bronchogenic carcinoma, asthma) and may in itself be socially disabling. Cough is associated with a number of physical complications including musculoskeletal injuries such as rib fractures, pneumothorax, cough syncope, and stress incontinence.

Symptomatic treatment of cough remains unsatisfactory. Despite its prevalence, the physiology and pathophysiology of cough is poorly understood. It is hoped that greater understanding of the mechanisms involved in normal and pathological cough will lead to progress in this difficult area of management.

This chapter first outlines the physiology of cough. The first section deals with the afferent limb of the cough reflex covering the laryngeal, tracheobronchial, and other sites from which the reflex may be elicited. Next, the role of neuropeptides as sensory neurotransmitters is discussed. In the following section, the poorly understood area of central processing of the cough reflex is outlined along with a description of the most likely central neurotransmitters involved. The reflex arc is completed with an account of the efferent limb and effector mechanisms that result in an individual or series of coughs. A discussion of pathophysiology follows, with sections on the cough reflex in disease and the involvement of airway inflammation, inflammatory mediators and bronchial hyperresponsiveness. Finally, current methods of quantifying and assessing cough are reviewed.

Cough reflex

Cough may be elicited by a variety of stimuli acting at a number of different anatomical sites (Figure 21.1 and Table 21.2). Such stimuli are sensed by a poorly defined set of nerve termini.[1] Afferent impulses are relayed proximally, via the vagus nerve to a putative medullary cough centre. Central processing occurs predominantly in the dorsal medulla, though voluntary initiation of cough and modulation by the cerebral cortex are also important. Connections to appropriate efferent (motor) nuclei produce the motor manifestation of cough. The efferent outflow of the cough reflexes is mediated via the bulbospinal tracts to motor nuclei of the cranial nerves and to nerves of the anterior horns of the spinal cord and hence to the innervation of the diaphragm and intercostal muscles and accessory muscles of respiration as well as the

Table 21.1 Defensive and protective reflexes in humans

Airway	Cardiovascular	Behavioural
Cough	Bradycardia	Avoidance
Expiration reflex	Hypotension	Flight
Augmented breaths		
Apnoea		
Laryngospasm		
Bronchospasm		
Sneeze		
Nasoconstriction		
Swallow		
Gag		

recurrent laryngeal and lower cranial nerves responsible for the upper airway movements involved. The resulting cough is characterized by an initial brief inspiration, usually to a little above the inspiratory end-tidal volume. A brief compressive phase follows, with expiration against a closed glottis. Glottic opening results in a sudden expiratory flow propelling alveolar gas and material from the bronchial tree out through the mouth at high velocity.[2]

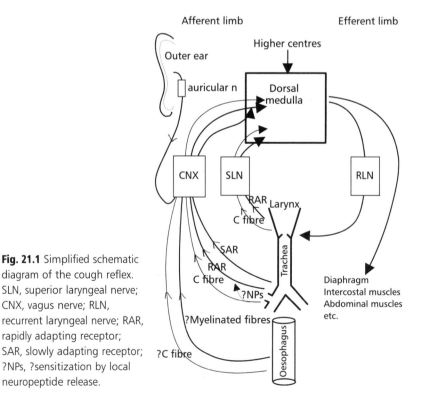

Fig. 21.1 Simplified schematic diagram of the cough reflex. SLN, superior laryngeal nerve; CNX, vagus nerve; RLN, recurrent laryngeal nerve; RAR, rapidly adapting receptor; SAR, slowly adapting receptor; ?NPs, ?sensitization by local neuropeptide release.

Table 21.2 Summary of the cough reflex (see also Figure 21.1)

Afferent limb	
Larynx	
Tracheobronchial tree	Slowly adapting stretch receptors (SARs)
	Rapidly adapting (stretch) (irritant) receptors
	Unmyelinated nerve fibres(C-fibres)
Other sites	Outer ear
	Nasopharynx and sinuses
	Oesophagus
	Heart
Neuropeptides which may have a role in initiating the reflex	Substance P
	Neurokinin A
	CGRP
	Other neuropeptides
Central processing	
Central neurotransmitters	Opioids
	Serotonergic neurones
	γAminobutyric acid
Efferent limb	Inspiratory phase
	Compressive phase
	Expiratory phase
	Cessation

Afferent limb of the cough reflex

A common feature of all anatomical sites that may elicit cough is their sensory innervation by fibres arising from the vagus nerve. This observation led to the development of the anatomic-diagnostic protocol for the investigation of chronic cough[3] (see Chapter 22). The major sites involved are the intrathoracic airways and the larynx, but diseases affecting the upper airways, outer ears, and oesophagus may also give rise to cough.[4]

Larynx

The larynx receives a rich sensory supply of both myelinated and unmyelinated fibres via the superior laryngeal and, to a lesser extent, the recurrent laryngeal nerves. Mechanical stimulation of the vocal cords and infraglottic larynx potently provoke cough and expiration reflex responses. However, the larynx may play a lesser role in chemically (as opposed to mechanically) provoked cough. The cough response to inhaled tussive agents is markedly reduced in heart–lung transplant recipients in whom the innervated larynx is intact,[5] is not attenuated by local anaesthesia of the superior laryngeal nerves,[6] and is preserved in laryngectomees.[7,8] Furthermore, in a study using nebulized capsaicin – a potent cough stimulant – small peripherally deposited droplets were more effective at provoking cough than larger, more centrally deposited ones.[9]

Physiological studies have identified a number of receptors in the larynx (Table 21.3). Little is known about their different roles, but myelinated fibres that respond to irritants such as cigarette smoke, ammonia, and sulfur dioxide have been identified. These also respond to mechanical stimulation. Fibres that respond to low-chloride solutions are thought to be

Table 21.3 Sensory receptors in the airways

Laryngeal		
Mechanoreceptors	Pressure receptors	Respond to change in intraluminal pressure
	Drive receptors	Activation dependent on laryngeal motor drive and related to intrinsic muscle function
	Cold/flow receptors	Respond to cold airflow, hence active in inspiration
Irritant receptors		
Chemoreceptors	Myelinated fibres	
	C fibres	
Proprioceptors		Function related to control of cartilaginous laryngeal
skeleton		
Tracheobronchial		
Slowly adapting stretch receptors (SARs)		
Rapidly adapting (stretch) (irritant) receptors (RARs)		
C-fibres	Bronchial C-fibres	
	Pulmonary C-fibres	

involved in the cough response, as are unmyelinated fibres, though there is no conclusive evidence for this. Anatomically, a rich plexus of nerve fibres – both sub- and intraepithelial – have been described throughout the airways. There is marked species variation in fibre type and distribution, and the proportion of unmyelinated and myelinated fibres may change from neonate to adult. At least some of these fibres are ideally located for a role as irritant receptors, terminating close to the tight junctions between epithelial cells of the respiratory mucosa.

Tracheobronchial tree

Almost any disease of the lungs may cause cough. However, irritation of smaller airways is less likely to provoke cough than stimulation of large or medium-sized ones. This is reflected by the relative prominence of cough in diseases affecting the larger airways such as asthma and chronic bronchitis where cough may be the main or even sole manifestation, compared to small airway and parenchymal lung disease such as emphysema and pulmonary fibrosis where breathlessness predominates.

Airway nerves are clearly important. Those species that lack intraepithelial nerve fibres are unable to cough in response to irritant stimuli. In humans, denervation of the airway after heart–lung transplantation[5] and nebulized local anaesthetic agents[10] inhibit the cough response to irritant stimuli.

Three subtypes of airway nerves may play a role in the cough response in humans (Table 21.3):

♦ **Slowly adapting stretch (irritant) receptors** (SARs) are the classic stretch receptors of the Hering–Breuer reflex. Their activation is not thought to cause cough directly but may augment its force and lower the cough threshold to other stimuli. Patients with persistent non-productive cough often cough on deep inspiration, which may suggest a role of SARs. However, changing baseline SAR activity by continuous positive airway pressure (CPAP) did not affect the cough threshold to intratracheal water instillation in anaesthetized humans.[11]

- **Rapidly adapting receptors** (RARs) are classically described as the 'irritant receptors' of the lung. Anatomically they are ideally located for maximum exposure to inhaled irritants, being concentrated around the carina and main bronchi. They are highly sensitive *in vitro* to numerous chemicals that provoke cough *in vivo*.

- **Unmyelinated nerve fibres** or **C-fibres** within the lungs are divided into pulmonary and bronchial groups according to their blood supply. The bronchial C-fibres are believed to be important in chemically provoked cough in a number of species, including humans. Much of the evidence for this is derived from studies using the alkaloid, capsaicin. This extract of hot peppers of the genus *Capsicum* is a selective but non-specific stimulator of unmyelinated fibres. Thus at threshold doses it acts via C-fibres though at higher concentrations it probably also affects thin myelinated (Aδ) fibres. At still higher concentrations, capsaicin is neurotoxic, causing oedema and cell death of capsaicin-sensitive nerve fibres. Capsaicin at low concentration stimulates cough in many species, including humans. The cough threshold is reduced in diseases associated with persistent dry cough and returns toward normal with successful treatment.[12,13] The sensory neurotransmitters of C-fibres are the neuropeptides which are discussed below.

Other sites

As well as the larynx and lungs, irritation at other sites may cause cough. The posteroinferior external auditory meatus and tympanic membrane are innervated by the auricular branch of the vagus nerve (Arnold's nerve). The ear–cough reflex is a well-described consequence of instrumentation of the outer ear, occurring in 2–16% of the population. Cough may also occur in conditions affecting the outer ear including otitis externa, tumours, hairy ears, and foreign bodies.

Cough may be the presenting symptom of rhinitis with or without sinusitis.[3] It is likely that this is due to postnasal drip irritating the larynx, as instrumentation of the nasopharynx and sinuses does not provoke cough. Furthermore these areas are innervated via the trigeminal nerve, whereas other anatomical sites associated with cough have a vagal innervation.

Gastrooesophageal reflux (GOR) may also manifest as cough.[3] Measurements of intratracheal pH suggest that microaspiration may be important in asthmatics with severe GOR.[14] The presence of posterior laryngitis suggests that aspiration may also be a factor in GOR cough.[15] However, proximal oesophageal reflux is not prominent in patients with GOR cough and their cough may be reproduced in the upright position by distal oesophageal instillation of acid.[16] This cough is blocked by local anaesthesia of the oesophageal mucosa, suggesting a reflex mechanism involving oesophageal afferent nerves.

Whether cardiac afferent nerves can play a role in cough is unknown. Their vagal origin and the association of cough with cardiac conditions, including the pacemaker syndrome,[17] would make this feasible but there is no direct evidence for such an effect.

Role of neuropeptides in cough

The possible role of unmyelinated nerve fibres in cough has been discussed above. The neurotransmitters for these fibres are a group of small peptides known as the neuropeptides. Their exact role is unclear, and some possible mechanisms are illustrated in Figure 21.2.

Conventional, orthodromic transmission in unmyelinated fibres may result in neuropeptide release at their central connections. These may provide a direct afferent signal for the cough reflex or may amplify input from other sources so acting as a central, upregulatory mechanism. Alternatively, stimulation of unmyelinated fibres may lead to local neuropeptide release via an axon reflex with a variety of possible protussive consequences (Figure 21.2).

A number of peptides with neurotransmitter properties have been identified and many of these are thought to be important sensory neurotransmitters in unmyelinated nerves (Table 21.4).[18],[19] Much of the evidence for their role comes from studies using capsaicin (see above).

In animal models, neurotoxic doses of capsaicin abolish the cough response to challenge with capsaicin or citric acid. Simultaneously, substance P (SP) and calcitonin gene related peptide (CGRP) immunoreactivity within the lungs is depleted. The cough response to nicotine and mechanical stimulation are preserved, suggesting a separate neural pathway for different cough stimuli.[20] SP, CGRP, and neurokinin A (NKA) are thought to be important sensory neuropeptides in unmyelinated nerves and have been shown to co-localized within nerve fibres of the respiratory tract. It is for these peptides that the greatest evidence of a role in cough exists.

SP is encoded by the same gene as NKA – the preprotachykinin gene. SP is an agonist at the neurokinin 1 (NK1) receptor. *In vivo* it is rapidly metabolized by a variety of proteolytic enzymes including angiotensin converting enzyme (ACE) and neutral endopeptidase (NEP). It is known to promote neurogenic inflammation in the airways and may play an important pathological role in asthma. In animal studies, SP causes cough and bronchoconstriction which is potentiated by NEP inhibitors and antagonized by nebulized recombinant NEP.[21] The response to SP is enhanced in animals with upper respiratory tract infection in which levels of NEP are reduced.[22] In rabbits SP enhanced activity in single airway RAR nerve fibres, and in guinea-pigs it enhanced responses to capsaicin and citric acid, suggesting a role in sensitization of the cough reflex.[23],[24]

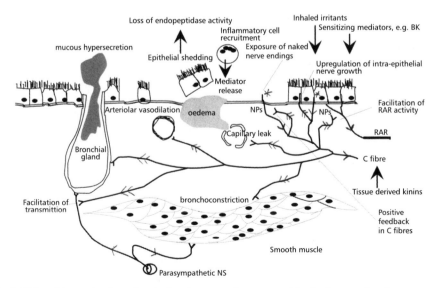

Fig. 21.2 Possible mechanisms for the involvement of neuropeptides in the cough reflex.

Table 21.4 Neuropeptides in the respiratory tract

Afferent	Substance P
	Neurokinin A
	Neuropeptide K
	CGRP
	Gastrin releasing peptide
	Neurokinin B?
Parasympathetic nervous system	VIP
	Protein histidine isoleucine/methionine
	Protein histidine valine-42
	Helodermin
	PACAP-27
	Galanin
Sympathetic nervous system	Neuropeptide Y
Others/uncharacterized	Cholecystokinin
	Somatostatin

Studies of inhaled SP in humans are conflicting. No cough response has been shown in normal subjects, asthmatics,[25] or patients taking ACE inhibitors.[26] A cough response to SP has been demonstrated in human subjects with upper respiratory tract infection[27] and idiopathic persistent non-productive cough.[28]

Studies using NK1 receptor antagonists in animals have shown conflicting results,[23] possibly reflecting differences in receptor subtype affinity of the different agents used as well as methodological differences. There are no published studies of the antitussive actions of NK1 receptor antagonists in humans.

NKA is co-transcribed and co-expressed with SP by neural tissue. It acts via the neurokinin 2 (NK2) receptor provoking airways hyperresponsiveness, bronchoconstriction, and cough in guinea-pigs.[29] Inhaled NKA caused bronchoconstriction but not cough in asthmatics.[25] There are no published NKA cough challenge studies in humans, but NKA is the most abundant neuropeptide recovered from bronchoalveolar lavage in normal subjects and asthmatics and increases after allergen challenge.[30]

Studies with NK2 receptor antagonists in animals have demonstrated consistent though partial antitussive effects against a range of challenges. They may also prevent sensitization of the cough reflex to other stimuli.[23] Studies using NK2 antagonists have not been reported in humans.

CGRP is an alternative post-transcriptional product of the calcitonin gene. It is a potent vasodilator and may play a role in neurogenic inflammation.[31] CGRP immunoreactivity has been shown to be increased in guinea-pigs with increased cough sensitivity induced by cigarette smoke[32] and in humans with increased cough sensitivity associated with idiopathic persistent non-productive cough. Challenge studies have not been reported in humans and suitable receptor antagonists are not available.

Other neuropeptides, including neurokinin B[33] and vasoactive intestinal polypeptide (VIP), may be implicated in the cough reflex though evidence for this is sparse.

The **site of action** of neuropeptides in the cough reflex is debated. Neuropeptides may act peripherally. They are released by unmyelinated nerve endings in the airway mucosa and may thus sensitize both myelinated and unmyelinated afferent fibres directly or via neurogenic inflammation (Figure 21.2). Evidence for this hypothesis comes from positive inhalation studies and studies showing increased neuropeptide immunoreactivity in the airways of patients with cough. An alternative but not exclusive suggestion is that the central connections of these nerves upregulate the cough reflex. Different routes of administration of neurokinin receptor agonists and antagonist or agents with differing ability to penetrate the blood–brain barrier[33,34] have produced conflicting results. As with other biological systems where a large response to a minor stimulus is required, amplification of the signal may occur at many levels.

Central processing of the cough reflex

Neurophysiology

Understanding of the central processing of the cough reflex remains far from complete. Afferent nerves from the vagus and superior laryngeal nerves synapse with second-order neurones in the medullary nucleus tractus solitarius which in turn relay by multiple, as yet uncharacterized, pathways to the motor 'cough centre' comprising two groups of medullary neurones. The rostral ventral respiratory group (VRG) is involved in respiratory rhythmogenesis and has connections with the facial and glossopharyngeal nuclei as well as the bulbospinal neurones of the phrenic, intercostals, and abdominal pools. The dorsal respiratory group (DRG) relays to inspiratory premotor fibres of the intercostal and phrenic nerves.[35]

Cough can be voluntarily initiated or suppressed and is reduced by distraction, so cortical influences are clearly important as is level of consciousness.[11] Psychogenic cough is uncommon in adults, but psychological therapies may be effective in this condition.[36] There are no published data on such methods in the treatment of persistent dry cough not thought to be psychogenic.

Central neurotransmitters

Pharmacological studies suggest that a number of central neurotransmitters are involved in modulating of the cough reflex:

♦ **Opioids** are the best known antitussive agents, though their efficacy is less than generally appreciated. High-dose, systemic treatment can attenuate provoked cough in normal subjects but opioids are completely ineffective when inhaled, confirming their central action. Naloxone has no effect by either route,[37] suggesting that no tonic, baseline suppressive opioid mechanism exists.

♦ **Serotonergic neurones** may be the final pathways of opiate effects upon cough. In animal studies serotonin appears to be antitussive and in humans pizotifen, a serotonin 1/2 receptor antagonist, blocked the antitussive effect of morphine.[38]

♦ **γ-Amino butyric acid (GABA)** has recently been implicated as a neurotransmitter with antitussive actions by studies using the GABA agonist baclofen.[39] This agent may prove to have a therapeutic role.

Efferent limb of the cough reflex

The motor manifestation of cough represents a complex interaction of the muscles of respiration, upper airways and facial muscles, not to mention the maintenance of postural equilibrium, during what may be a violent spasmodic movement. The cough response is divided into four phases (Figure 21.3):[2]

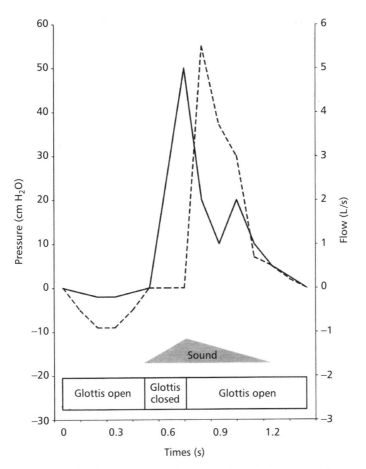

Fig. 21.3 Changes in subglottic pressure (solid line), and airflow (broken line) during a typical cough.

- The **inspiratory phase** lasts for about 0.5 s. The vocal cords are actively abducted and there is a brief inspiration. The degree of inspiration varies between individuals and between coughs. Cough initiated at a greater lung volume is likely to be more effective because of the greater pressure generated and flow rates achieved.

- The **compressive phase** occurs when the cords are actively adducted almost simultaneously with the onset of forced expiration. Subglottic pressure rises abruptly reaching a peak of about 50 cm H_2O (4.9 kPa) after approximately 0.2 s. Compression of alveolar gas results in a reduction in lung volume. As well as activation of the muscles of expiration, antagonist groups such as the diaphragm are also activated.

- The **expiratory phase** follows when the cords are abruptly and actively abducted over a period of 20–40 ms. Subglottic pressure falls rapidly to atmospheric but the intra-alveolar pressure continues to rise for a few seconds as a result of expiratory muscle activity. This allows material to be propelled from the distal airways, proximally. Dynamic compression of the airways dramatically narrows more central airways, proximal to the equal pressure point. This is the point at which intraluminal pressure equals intrapleural pressure. The cartilaginous rings of the airways prevent complete collapse. This abrupt narrowing increases the kinetic energy of airflow producing spikes of 'supramaximal', turbulent flow. The vibration effect of this turbulence and resultant rapid decelerations of the bronchial walls help loosen adherent secretions. Lung volume and flow rate fall approximately exponentially. In some coughs, expiratory muscle activity ceases abruptly after glottic opening. Maximal airflows are maintained by the re-expansion of compressed alveolar gas. These processes result in alveolar air being forced out through the glottis at peak flows of about 10 L/s, typically achieving velocities of 5000 cm/s.

♦ The **cessation phase** occurs with relaxation of the expiratory muscles, sometimes accompanied by activation of antagonist muscle groups. Intrathoracic pressures fall rapidly to atmospheric and flow becomes submaximal. The glottis may close.

The initial cough may be an isolated event or the first of a series, or epoch of coughs. Subsequent coughs may occur without an initial inspiration. Thus a series of coughs starts from progressively lower lung volumes. The equal pressure point moves progressively distally and this ensures the clearance of more peripheral airways.

Cough in disease

Pathological cough is often subdivided into productive and non-productive cough. This classification is clinically useful, as the causes and hence treatments differ, though this distinction has recently been challenged.[40] There is evidence of a difference in mechanism of cough in the two groups. Patients with productive cough do not differ in cough sensitivity from normal subjects. In contrast, non-productive cough is associated with increased sensitivity of the cough reflex. This is well demonstrated in uncomplicated upper respiratory tract infections, where about one third of patients develop a productive cough with normal reflex sensitivity while a further third develop a dry cough with enhanced cough response. Cough sensitivity is enhanced in all groups of patients studied with non-productive cough, and returns toward normal with successful treatment.

Productive cough therefore appears to be due to increased stimulation of the normal cough reflex by intraluminal material. The situation is likely to be more complex in that the range of cough sensitivities seen in productive cough is wide. Furthermore, this may change during the natural history of the disease: cough sensitivity is normal in stable bronchiectasis, but enhanced during exacerbations.[41]

Non-productive cough, on the other hand, is associated with a hypersensitive cough reflex, trivial stimulation leading to an excessive response.[42] The mechanism of this enhanced sensitivity is not fully understood. It is not known whether the site of upregulation is peripherally in the airway nerves, centrally in the central nervous system, or a combination of the two. Possible involvement of neuropeptides and inflammatory mediators in upregulation of the cough reflex is discussed above.

Airways inflammation and the cough reflex

Airway inflammation is a cardinal feature of asthma and chronic bronchitis – conditions in which cough is a major symptom. The role of airways inflammation in other forms of cough is less clear. A group of patients with airway eosinophilia, cough, and a clinical response to inhaled corticosteroids is being increasingly recognized.[43] They do not exhibit bronchial hyperresponsiveness and cannot be classified as asthmatic. The term eosinophilic bronchitis has been coined. The initial description was of 7 patients with productive cough,[44] though a recent report suggests that this entity may account for a substantial proportion of chronic cough patients.[45] Airway inflammation has been suggested by bronchoalveolar lavage fluid (BALF) and bronchial biopsy findings in a mixed group of non-asthmatic cough patients[46] and in steroid-responsive, non-asthmatic cough patients.[47] More recently, increased neutrophilia and expression of neutrophil-associated cytokines was reported in induced sputum from chronic cough patients including a sub-group with idiopathic persistent non-productive cough (IPNPC).[48] However, in other studies, patients with IPNPC did not have airway inflammation on bronchial biopsy or in BALF.[49]

Inflammatory mediators

Studies of inflammatory mediators suggest possible roles for bradykinin and for prostanoids in the sensory upregulation of the cough reflex seen in disease states.

Bradykinin

Bradykinin is a peptide inflammatory mediator. It acts locally via bradykinin receptors before being rapidly degraded by proteolytic enzymes including ACE.[50] In healthy volunteers inhalation of bradykinin resulted in retrosternal discomfort and cough.[51] In dogs bradykinin stimulated bronchial C-fibres but had little effect on pulmonary C-fibres or myelinated afferent fibres.[52] By contrast, in rabbits bradykinin has been shown to stimulate RARs and this effect is enhanced by enalapril.[53] Both bradykinin and ACE inhibition enhanced the cough response to citric acid in guinea-pigs and these effects were attenuated by the bradykinin antagonist HOE140. In vitro bradykinin also sensitized single vagal C-fibres to capsaicin.[54] In another guinea-pig study, HOE 140 and indomethacin both attenuated citric acid cough and it was suggested that prostanoids may be the final mediator of bradykinin-induced cough.[55]

Because ACE inhibitors were originally identified by their ability to impair the degradation of kinins, there has been considerable attention to the hypothesis that ACE inhibitor cough may be mediated by an accumulation of bradykinin. ACE inhibition has been reported to increase the wheal and flare response to intradermal bradykinin in guinea-pigs and humans.[56] The increase in skin blood flow in response to intradermal captopril in rabbits is mediated by a bradykinin-dependent mechanism, being abolished by bradykinin receptor antagonists.[57] The cough response is enhanced in patients with ACE inhibitor cough and returns toward normal on withdrawal of ACE inhibition.[26]

However, bronchial responsiveness to bradykinin was unaffected in asthmatics treated with captopril.[58] Furthermore, bradykinin does not sensitize the response to capsaicin in normal human subjects.[59] Studies of the effect of ACE inhibition on plasma bradykinin levels have produced conflicting results. Tissue bradykinin levels may be of more relevance.[50] It is possible that some of its effects are mediated by neuropeptide release from unmyelinated nerve fibres. There are no published data on the effects of bradykinin receptor antagonists in human cough.

Prostaglandins

Prostaglandins are synthesized from arachidonic acid via the cyclooxygenase pathway. Both prostaglandin F_{2a} (PGF_{2a}) and prostaglandin E_2 (PGE_2) are potent tussive agents in asthmatics and normal subjects.[60] This is independent of effects on airway tone, which vary between agents. They also potentiate the response to other tussive stimuli.[61]

The mechanism of their action is unclear, but an analogy has been drawn with their ability to enhance the pain response to intradermal inflammatory mediators.[61] In animals they enhance activity in both myelinated and unmyelinated vagal afferents.[62–64] A possible role in cough reflex upregulation in humans is supported by studies showing attenuation of capsaicin cough by NSAIDs, which reduce prostaglandin synthesis. Sulindac reduced the capsaicin cough response in ACE-inhibitor cough patients,[65] and indomethacin had similar effects in those with the sinobronchial syndrome or asthma.[66] However, sulindac had no effect on capsaicin sensitivity in IPNPC.[65]

Bronchial hyperresponsiveness and cough

Cough is a cardinal symptom of asthma and occurs during pharmacologically provoked bronchoconstriction. Many agents that provoke cough also produce bronchoconstriction in asthmatic patients, but there is ample evidence that the two processes are separate.

In asthma, bronchial hyperresponsiveness (BHR) is not accompanied by increased cough sensitivity. Futhermore, BHR does not correlate with cough sensitivity in airways disease.[67] Manipulation of airway calibre in normal volunteers does not affect cough sensitivity,[68] and a number of studies have blocked cough[10,69] or bronchoconstriction[69,70] independent of the other.

Quantification and measurement of cough

In clinical practice formal quantification of cough is rarely attempted. Patients are asked directly how severe their cough is or indirectly, in terms of its effect on their quality of life (sleep disturbance, social inconvenience, etc.). Further enquiry is directed at ascertaining the presence of complications such as injuries, cough syncope, and stress incontinence. Where attempts have been made to quantify cough more precisely this has been done in one of three ways: patient- or observer-administered subjective scoring systems; indirect quantification by measurement of the sensitivity of the cough reflex using inhaled agents; and direct, objective measurement of cough.

Subjective methods of cough quantification

A variety of subjective methods of scoring cough have been used. Many studies have described the proportion of patients whose cough has 'disappeared' or 'substantially' or 'markedly' improved. However, such endpoints lack definition. Other workers have attempted to use visual analogue scales (VAS), cough diaries, or specifically designed verbal category descriptive scoring systems (VCD). There is little published data on the correlations between these different subjective scores themselves and between these and other measures of cough. VAS (Figure 21.4) appear to accurately reflect daytime cough but may be less reliable for nocturnal cough.[71] The poor correlation between actual and perceived nocturnal cough may be due to the disproportionate sleep disruption resulting from a few bouts of nocturnal cough. VCDs appear to perform better than VAS when assessed by comparison with objectively recorded cough frequency. VCDs constrain the response by series of graded statements to which specific scores are attached, reducing the subjectivity of patient responses. Cough severity recorded by means of cough diaries (Figure 21.5) appears to relate particularly poorly to recorded cough,[72] though this may reflect the different time periods sampled by the different systems.

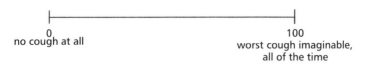

Fig. 21.4 Visual analogue scale. The patient is asked to mark the scale using a single vertical pen mark at the point representing the severity of their cough during the chosen time period (typically the preceding day, night, or 24 h). They are unable to see their own or other patients' previous responses at the time of marking the scale. The score in mm is obtained by measuring from the zero point to the patient's mark.

The author's conclusion is that VCDs best reflect cough frequency of the same time period. They appear to be the best subjective method of cough quantification. However, other factors such as the intensity and timing of cough may be equally important contributors to the patient's interpretation of cough severity and VCDs may be too selective to be the sole measure used. Further studies using validated quality-of-life measures may be revealing.

Quantification of cough reflex sensitivity by inhalation challenge

Cough provocation challenge is an indirect method of assessing cough severity by assessment of the sensitivity of the cough reflex. Cough reflex sensitivity is enhanced in dry cough and returns toward normal with successful treatment of the underlying cause. A variety of tussive agents have been used (Table 21.5) but the most commonly employed are capsaicin, citric acid and iso- or hypo-osmolar solutions low in permeant anion (1.26% sodium bicarbonate solution or ultrasonically nebulized distilled water). The reproducibility of cough challenge varies with different agents. Cough sensitivity to inhaled tussive stimuli is a useful tool and has

DATE							
COUGH							
SPUTUM							
MEDICATION USE?	Y/N	Y/N	Y/N	Y/N	Y/N	Y/N	Y/N

0 = NIL

1 = MILD

2 = MODERATE

3 = SEVERE

Please record the severity of your symptoms by writing a number in the box at the same time each day according to the above scale.

Fig. 21.5 Example of a cough diary card.

Table 21.5 Inhalation challenges used in the investigation of cough

Vanilloids	Capsaicin
	Pseudocapsaicin
Organic acids	Citric acid
	Tartaric acid
Altered electrolyte solutions	Isotonic (1.26%) sodium bicarbonate
	Isotonic (5% dextrose)
	Urea
	Distilled water
	Hypertonic (3–5%) saline
Other	Nicotine
	Cigarette smoke
	Sulfur dioxide
	Bradykinin
	Prostaglandins
	Lactose
	Dust
	Acetylcholine
	Metabisulfite
	Histamine

been successfully used to demonstrate differences between patient groups[41] and treatment effects within individuals as well as pharmacologically induced within-subject changes in reflex sensitivity in normal volunteers.[65] Such studies have provided useful information about the physiology and pathophysiology of the cough reflex, but have a limited role in the assessment of symptoms in patients (because of the wide inter-individual variation in response) and assessment of antitussive agents (because they are only an indirect indicator of symptomatic response).

Methodology of cough challenge

The cough response to a tussive agent is affected by a number of external influences, and careful attention to methodology is essential.

Comparisons between groups must take into account factors likely to influence cough reflex sensitivity including age,[73] gender,[74] and smoking history.[75] Severe diabetic autonomic neuropathy reduces cough sensitivity, whereas it may be enhanced in conditions known to cause dry cough even in the absence of overt cough, e.g. ACE inhibitor therapy and GOR.

The initial exposure to an agent may result in a greater response than subsequently. Where repeated challenges are envisaged, a screening day with a challenge that is not used in the subsequent analysis is desirable. The cough response to citric acid has been shown to be subject to diurnal variation,[76] and so time of challenge should be standardized during a study.

Cough is subject to important cortical influences. Subjects should therefore be encouraged to rest quietly for a period before inhalation challenge. A placebo response to the tussive agent can be minimized either by randomizing the order of administration of concentrations or by introducing inhalations of vehicle at random intervals during the challenge. The former approach has the disadvantages of increasing the effects of tachyphylaxis and potentially exposing subjects to concentrations of tussive agent higher than they may comfortably tolerate.

Within-subject variability in response is a problem with all inhaled agents. Strategies to minimize its effects include the use of dose–response curves rather than individual concentrations of agents, and administration of multiple doses at each concentration. Both these approaches must be tempered against the increased potential for tachyphylaxis.

The dose range selected for a challenge will depend upon the purpose of the study. Where comparisons are to be made between groups that may include both sensitive and resistant individuals, a wide range of concentrations of agent must be used in order to produce dose–response curves across the whole possible range of responses. In within-subject studies of a drug or other intervention, a broad range of concentrations may not be necessary or desirable. At screening, subjects with extremes of responsiveness can be excluded and a truncated challenge administered. This may consist of a number of concentrations tailored to the responsiveness of the study population or even to each individual. This reduces the effect of tachyphylaxis and limiting it to the mid-dose range allows an effect in either direction to be detected in all subjects.

Inhaled agents may be administered either by tidal breathing or by single inhalation of nebulized solution. Single inhalation is suitable for administration of agents that are potent tussogens at low volume such as capsaicin and citric acid. A brief (e.g. 1 s) burst of mist is generated by a jet nebulizer triggered by a breath-actuated dosimeter. The discharge is timed to start shortly after the onset of a full inspiration. This method has the disadvantage that patients with non-productive cough often cough on deep inspiration, making interpretation of the response difficult. An alternative method is that of tidal breathing of tussive mist. This method is more commonly employed for challenge with distilled water or isotonic low chloride solutions. These agents provoke cough by altering the constitution of the airway lining fluid and must thus be administered at high rates of nebulization.[77] The necessary volumes require ultrasonic nebulizers, which have outputs in the range of 1–3 mL/min. Administration of increasingly potent solutions is generally limited to 1 min at each step as marked tachyphylaxis is seen with these agents.

Selection of tussive agent

The agents most used for cough challenge fall into three categories: vanilloids such as capsaicin, organic acids such as citric acid, and iso- or hypotonic solutions of low chloride content. The mechanisms of action of these different agents is incompletely understood and although broad statements are often made about the type of nerve fibre which each affects, there is no consensus on this point.

Capsaicin is thought to act predominantly on unmyelinated bronchial C-fibres. Inhalation of capsaicin in humans causes reproducible, dose-dependent cough and short-lived, mild bronchoconstriction. Capsaicin responsiveness exhibits tachyphylaxis, but to a lesser extent than other commonly used agents. In healthy volunteers the only peripherally acting agents that have been shown to attenuate capsaicin cough are local anaesthetics[10] and menthol (O'Connell, unpublished data). An antitussive linctus effect of orally administered liquid agents has also been demonstrated.[37] Of centrally acting agents, intravenous opiates alone consistently attenuate the cough response, oral opioids producing variable results.[37,78]

Baclofen, a GABA receptor agonist, may also attenuate capsaicin cough in humans, probably via a central mechanism.[79]

Organic acids are potent tussive agents in humans and animals. Their effectiveness appears to depend upon their ability to donate several hydrogen ions per molecule. The nerve population on which they act in humans remains undefined. Citric acid challenge is markedly tachyphylactic and this has been taken as evidence that it acts via RARs in humans. However, it has been suggested that the time-course of the tachyphylaxis precludes this interpretation. Studies in humans[80] and other animals[20] suggest that citric acid and capsaicin act via similar or at least overlapping populations of sensory nerves.

Isotonic low-chloride solutions are effective tussive agents when administered in amounts sufficient to alter the constitution of the airway lining fluid. The tussive effect appears to be related to the absence of a permeant anion and is probably mediated via myelinated nerves arising from rapidly adapting stretch/irritant receptors.[77,61,82] However, reproducibility is poor and less than half of normal subjects cough to this challenge.[83]

Ultrasonically nebulized distilled water (UNDW) is another commonly used cough stimulus. This probably acts predominantly via the same mechanism as low-chloride solutions, though hypo-osmolality also contributes. This latter property also accounts for a bronchoconstrictor effect,[77] which limits its usefulness. Distilled water may be a more potent stimulus than isotonic low-chloride solutions because of its dual mechanism of action. Sensitivity is affected by ACE genotype. It is possible that ACE activity may be impaired in the low-chloride airway lining fluid produced by these challenges, as chloride is necessary for ACE function. Thus neuropeptide accumulation might be the mechanism of action of these challenges.

Cough counting using recording devices

Since the late 1950s there have been a number of attempts to record and measure cough objectively, mostly in terms of cough numbers over a period of observation or recording.[84] Detailed analysis using tussiphonography or spectral analysis can accurately identify cough sounds. However, high sampling rates are required, making this impractical for prolonged ambulatory recording. Another approach has been to record cough sounds both digitally for computer analysis and on audiotape which may be played back to confirm identification of cough events.[85] This method remains very labour intensive, though it provides a great deal of data over a range of cough parameters. The system is well validated but is not suitable in its current form for true ambulatory monitoring.

An alternative approach is to measure audio signal and simultaneously another parameter characteristically affected by cough. Cough is then identified by synchronous changes in the two channels. Such a system is Medtronic's Digitrapper device. In this the audio signal is compared to intrathoracic pressure change recorded from an oesophageal balloon. The system is fully portable and cough should be accurately identifiable. It has the disadvantage of requiring the introduction of the balloon. The Logan–Sinclair system (Figure 21.6) relies on identification of synchronous deflections in the audio channel and in electromyographic signal recorded from surface electrodes on the upper abdominal wall (Figure 21.7). This system has been better validated with accurate distinction of cough from other sounds.[71,86] A similar system has recently been described using an adapted Holter monitor.[72] Further work using these systems is required to assess the repeatability and relationship to other measures of cough severity.

(a)   (b)

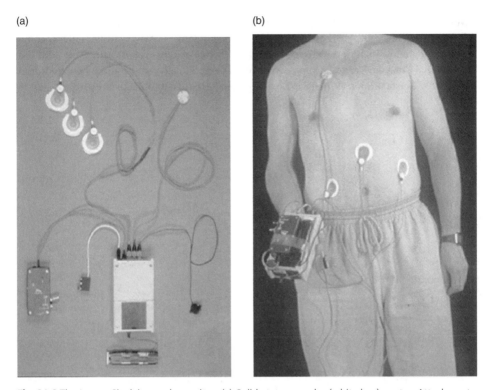

Fig. 21.6 The Logan-Sinclair cough monitor: (a) Solid-state recorder (white box) centre. Attachments clockwise from 1 o'clock: unidirectional microphone; accelerometer (motion detected as surrogate for wake/sleep); auxiliary battery pack; event marker; optional oesophageal pH module (probe not shown); abdominal EMG leads (three surface electrodes). (b) Unidirectional microphone attached to chest wall over right anterior second intercostal space to record audio signal. Three surface electrodes attached over upper abdomen to record electromyogram (EMG). The solid-state recording unit is carried in a shoulder bag.

It is unlikely that these systems will gain widespread use until their cost in terms of both capital expense and investigator time can be substantially reduced. However, they are of great potential value in pharmacological studies of potential antitussives, which until now have lacked reliable and validated objective endpoints.

Relationship between different methods of measuring cough severity

There are few studies comparing symptom severity and cough reflex sensitivity. Those that exist show weak correlations or fail to demonstrate a relationship,[87,88] perhaps reflecting the indirect nature of reflex sensitivity in symptom production. This echoes observations in asthma where bronchial hyperresponsiveness poorly predicts asthma symptoms.

We have found no consistent relationship between reflex sensitivity to inhaled agents and objectively recorded cough frequency using an ambulatory monitor in 21 patients being investigated for persistent non-productive cough.[89] In view of the day-to-day variability of cough frequency and in the absence of a 'gold standard' of cough measurement, cough assessment should include a VCD and cough challenge as outcome measures. In addition, a cough diary may give a closer approximation to overall quality of life and where nocturnal cough is of especial interest, there is no adequate alternative to objective recording.

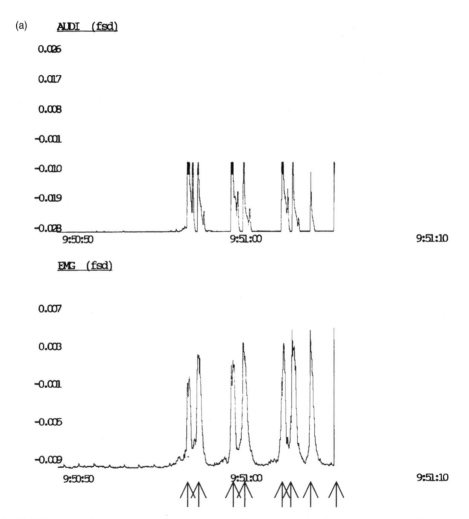

Fig. 21.7 Typical tracings obtained using the Logan–Sinclair recorder. Coughs are indicated by an arrow: (a) Simultaneous audio and EMG deflections during voluntary cough. The trace shows eight coughs recorded as a single epoch, as the internal between coughs does not exceed 2 s. (b) Spontaneous cough can be less distinct than voluntary cough. Two episodes of spontaneous cough are shown, the first consisting of 11 and the second of 5 individual coughs. The characteristics of the groups of deflections between the two cough epochs (black arrow) differ, and it probably represents throat clearing.

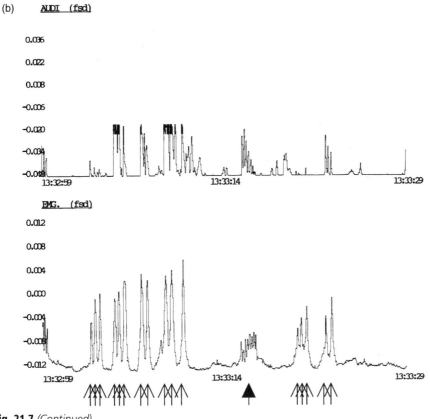

Fig. 21.7 *(Continued)*

Keypoints

- The cough is an essential variable reflex, which protects the respiratory tract. A tiny afferent stimulus is amplified to produce a major expulsive effort, which involves many muscle groups
- The afferent limb comprises laryngeal and pulmonary nerve endings including C-fibres
- Central processing is in the dorsal medulla
- The efferent limb is a coordinated set of muscular actions: inspiration – compression – expiration – cessation
- Axon reflexes in vagal C-fibres may allow a variety of neuropeptides released locally to modulate the cough reflex sensitivity
- The reflex is also modulated by cortical impulses
- Productive cough appears to be due to an increased stimulation of the normal cough reflex by intraluminal material; non-productive cough is usually associated with a hypersensitive cough reflex and trivial stimulation leads to an excessive response

- Airway inflammation releases mediators such as bradykinin and prostaglandins which can upregulate vagal afferents, increasing the cough reflex sensitivity
- Methods for measurement of cough are complex and difficult to apply in clinical practice
- The best combination is probably verbal category descriptive scores, together with a cough challenge, to determine the sensitivity of the reflex
- Ambulatory continuous cough recording devices are under development

References

1 Widdicombe, J.G. Neurophysiology of the cough reflex. Eur Respir J 1995; 8: 1193–202.

2 Leith, D.E., Butler, J.P., Sneddon, S.L., Brain, J.D. and Cough. In: N.S. Cherniack, and J.G. Widdicombe (eds) *Handbook of physiology*. Bethesda, M.D.: American Physiological Society, 1986; 315–36.

3 Irwin, R.S., Corrao, W.M., and Pratter, M.R. Chronic persistent cough in the adult: the spectrum and frequency of causes and successful outcome of specific therapy. *Am Rev Respir Dis* 1981; **123**: 413–17.

4 Widdicombe, J.G. Sensory neurophysiology of the cough reflex. *J Allergy Clin Immunol* 1996; **98**: S84–9.

5 Higenbottam, T., Jackson, M., Woolman, P., Lowry, R., and Wallwork, J. The cough response to ultrasonically nebulized distilled water in heart-lung transplantation patients. *Am Rev Respir Dis* 1989; **140**: 58–61.

6 Stockwell, M., Lang, S., Yip, R., *et al.* Lack of importance of the superior laryngeal nerves in citric acid cough in humans. *J Appl Physiol* 1993; **75**: 613–17.

7 Cross, B.A., Guz, A., Jain, S.K., *et al.* The effect of anaesthesia of the airway in dog and man: a study of respiratory reflexes, sensations and lung mechanics. *Clin Sci Mol Med* 1976; **50**: 439–54.

8 Fontana, G.A., Pantaleo, T., Lavorini, F., *et al.* Coughing in laryngectomized patients. *Am J Respir Crit Care Med* 1999; **160**: 1578–84.

9 Hansson, L., Wollmer, P., Dahlback, M., and Karlsson, J.A. Regional sensitivity of human airways to capsaicin-induced cough. *Am Rev Respir Dis* 1992; **145**: 1191–5.

10 Choudry, N.B., Fuller, R.W., Anderson, N., and Karlsson, J.A. Separation of cough and reflex bronchoconstriction by inhaled local anaesthetics. Eur Respir J 1990; 3: 579–83.

11 Nishino, T., Sugimori, K., Hiraga, K., and Hond, Y. Influence of CPAP on reflex responses to tracheal irritation in anesthetized humans. *J Appl Physiol* 1989; **67**: 954–8.

12 O'Connell, F., Thomas, V.E., Pride, N.B., and Fuller, R.W. Capsaicin cough sensitivity decreases with successful treatment of chronic cough. *Am J Respir Crit Care Med* 1994; **150**: 374–80.

13 O'Connell, F., Thomas, V.E., Studham, J.M., Pride, N.B., and Fuller, R.W. Capsaicin cough sensitivity increases during upper respiratory infection. *Respir Med* 1996; **90**: 279–86.

14 Jack, C.I., Calverley, P.M., Donnelly, R.J., *et al.* Simultaneous tracheal and oesophageal pH measurements in asthmatic patients with gastrooesophageal reflux. *Thorax* 1995; **50**: 201–4.

15 Jacob, P., Kahrilas, P.J., and Herzon, G. Proximal esophageal pH-metry in patients with 'reflux laryngitis'. *Gastroenterology* 1991; **100**: 305–10.

16 Ing, A.J., Ngu, M.C., and Breslin, A.B. Pathogenesis of chronic persistent cough associated with gastroesophageal reflux. *Am J Respir Crit Care Med* 1994; **149**: 160–7.

17 Cohen, S.I., and Frank, H.A. Preservation of active atrial transport; an important clinical consideration in cardiac pacing. *Chest* 1982; **81**: 51–4.

18 Barnes, P.J., Baraniuk, J.N., and Belvisi, M.G. Neuropeptides in the respiratory tract. Part I. *Am Rev Respir Dis* 1991; **144**: 1187–98.

19 Kamei, J. Role of opioidergic and serotonergic mechanisms in cough and antitussives. *Pulm Pharmacol* 1996; **9**: 349–56.

20 Forsberg, K., Karlsson, J.A., Theodorsson, E., Lundberg, J.M., and Persson, C.G. Cough and bronchoconstriction mediated by capsaicin-sensitive sensory neurons in the guinea-pig. *Pulm Pharm* 1988; **1**: 33–9.

21 Kohrogi, H., Nadel, J.A., Malfroy, B., *et al.* Recombinant human enkephalinase (neutral endopeptidase) prevents cough induced by tachykinins in awake guinea pigs. *J Clin Invest* 1989; **84**: 781–6.

22 Borson, D.B., Brokaw, J.J., Sekizawa, K., McDonald, D.M., and Nadel, J.A. Neutral endopeptidase and neurogenic inflammation in rats with respiratory infections. *J Appl Physiol* 1989; **66**: 2653–8.

23 Advenier, C., Lagente, V., and Boichot, E. The role of tachykinin receptor antagonists in the prevention of bronchial hyperresponsiveness, airway inflammation and cough. *Eur Respir J* 1997; **10**: 1892–906.

24 Kohrogi, H., Graf, P.D., Sekizawa, K., Borson, D.B., and Nadel, J.A. (1988) Neutral endopeptidase inhibitors potentiate substance P- and capsaicin-induced cough in awake guinea pigs. *J. Clin. Invest.* **82**, 2063–2068.

25 Joos, G., Pauwels, R., and van der Straeten, M. Effect of inhaled substance P and neurokinin A on the airways of normal and asthmatic subjects. *Thorax* 1987; **42**: 779–83.

26 Katsumata, U., Sekizawa, K., Ujiie, Y., Sasaki, H., and Takishima, T. Bradykinin-induced cough reflex markedly increases in patients with cough associated with captopril and enalapril. *Tohoku J Exp Med* 1991; **164**: 103–9.

27 Katsumata, U., Sekizawa, K., Inoue, H., Sasaki, H., and Takishima, T. Inhibitory actions of procaterol, a beta-2 stimulant, on substance P-induced cough in normal subjects during upper respiratory tract infection. *Tohoku J Exp Med* 1989; **158**: 105–6.

28 Myers, J.D., Shakur, B.H., El-Khushman, H., and Ind, P.W. Sensitivity to prostaglandin F2a, substance P and low chloride in persistent cough (abstract). *Am J Respir Crit Care Med* 1998; **157**: A842.

29 Takahama, K., Fuchikami, J., Isohama, Y., Kai, H., Miyata, T., and Neurokinin, A., but not neurokinin B and substance P, induces codeine-resistant coughs in awake guinea-pigs. *Regul Pept* 1993; **46**: 236–7.

30 Heaney, L.G., Cross, L.J., McGarvey, L.P., *et al.* Neurokinin A is the predominant tachykinin in human bronchoalveolar lavage fluid in normal and asthmatic subjects. *Thorax* 1998; **53**: 357–62.

31 Barnes, P.J., Baraniuk, J.N., and Belvisi, M.G. Neuropeptides in the respiratory tract. Part II. *Am Rev Respir Dis* 1991; **144**: 1391–9.

32 Karlsson, J.A., Zackrisson, C., and Lundberg, J.M. Hyperresponsiveness to tussive stimuli in cigarette smoke-exposed guinea-pigs: a role for capsaicin-sensitive, calcitonin gene-related peptide-containing nerves. *Acta Physiol Scand* 1991; **141**: 445–54.

33 Advenier, C., and Emonds, A.X. Tachykinin receptor antagonists and cough. *Pulm Pharm* 1996; **9**: 329–33.

34 Bolser, D.C., DeGennaro, F.C., O'Reilly, S., McLeod, R.L., and Hey, J.A. Central antitussive activity of the NK1 and NK2 tachykinin receptor antagonists, CP-99,994 and SR 48968, in the guinea-pig and cat. *Br J Pharm* 1997; **121**: 165–70.

35 Shannon, R., Baekey, D.M., Morris, K.F., and Lindsey, B.G. Brainstem respiratory networks and cough. *Pulm Pharm* 1996; **9**: 343–7.

36 Riegel, B., Warmoth, J.E., Middaugh, S.J., *et al.* Psychogenic cough treated with biofeedback and psychotherapy. A review and case report. *Am J Phys Med Rehabil* 1995; **74**: 155–8.

37 Fuller, R.W., Karlsson, J.A., Choudry, N.B., and Pride, N.B. Effect of inhaled and systemic opiates on responses to inhaled capsaicin in humans. *J Appl Physiol* 1988; **65**: 1125–30.

38 O'Connell, F., Thomas, V.E., Fuller, R.W., and Pride, N.B. Effect of pizotifen on the antitussive action of morphine in healthy humans using the capsaicin model. *Eur Respir J* 1995; **8**: 347s (abstract).

39 Dicpinigaitis, P.V., *et al.* Inhibition of capsaicin cough by GABA agonist, baclofen (abstract). *Eur Respir J* 1996; **9**(suppl 23): 30s.

40 Smyrnios, N.A., Irwin, R.S., and Curley, F.J. Chronic cough with a history of excessive sputum production. The spectrum and frequency of causes, key components of the diagnostic evaluation, and outcome of specific therapy. *Chest* 1995; **108**: 991–7.

41 Choudry, N.B., and Fuller, R.W. Sensitivity of the cough reflex in patients with chronic cough. *Eur Respir J* 1992; **5**: 296–300.

42 O'Connell, F., Springall, D.R., Moradoghli, H.A., *et al.* Abnormal intraepithelial airway nerves in persistent unexplained cough? *Am J Respir Crit Care Med* 1995; **152**: 2068–75.

43 Gibson, P.G., Hargreave, F.E., Girgis, G.A., *et al.* Chronic cough with eosinophilic bronchitis: examination for variable airflow obstruction and response to corticosteroid. *Clin Exp Allergy* 1995; **25**: 127–32.

44 Gibson, P.G., Dolovich, J., Denburg, J., Ramsdale, E.H., and Hargreave, F.E. Chronic cough: eosinophilic bronchitis without asthma. *Lancet* 1989; **i**: 1346–8.

45 Brightling, C.E., Ward, R., Goh, K-L., Wardlaw, A.J., and Parvod, I.D. Eosinophilic bronchitis is an important cause of chronic cough. *Am J Respir Crit Care Med* 1999; **160**: 406–10.

46 Boulet, L.P., Milot, J., Boutet, M., St, G.F., and Laviolette, M. Airway inflammation in nonasthmatic subjects with chronic cough. *Am J Respir Crit Care Med* 1994; **149**: 482–9.

47 Gibson, P.G., Zlatic, K., Scott, J., *et al.* Chronic cough resembles asthma with IL-5 and granulocyte-macrophage colony-stimulating factor gene expression in bronchoalveolar cells. *J Allergy Clin Immunol* 1998; **101**: 320–6.

48 Jatakanon, A., Lalloo, U.G., Lim, S., Chung, K.F., and Barnes, P.J. Increased neutrophils and cytokines, TNF-alpha and IL-8, in induced sputum of non-asthmatic patients with chronic dry cough. *Thorax* 1999; **54**: 234–7.

49 McGarvey, L.P., Forsythe, P., Heaney, L.G., MacMahon, J., and Ennis, M. The cellular profile of BAL in non-asthmatics with chronic non-productive cough (abstract). *Eur Respir J* 1996; **9**: 463s.

50 Trifilieff, A., Da, S.A., and Gies, J.P. Kinins and respiratory tract diseases. *Eur Respir J* 1993; **6**: 576–87.

51 Fuller, R.W., Dixon, C.M., Cuss, F.M., and Barnes, P.J. Bradykinin-induced bronchoconstriction in humans. Mode of action. *Am Rev Respir Dis* 1987; **135**: 176–80.

52 Kaufman, M.P., Coleridge, H.M., Coleridge, J.C., and Baker, D.G. Bradykinin stimulates afferent vagal C-fibers in intrapulmonary airways of dogs. *J Appl Physiol* 1980; **48**: 511–17.

53 Hargreaves, M., Ravi, K., Senaratne, M.P., and Kappagoda, C.T. Responses of airway rapidly adapting receptors to bradykinin before and after administration of enalapril in rabbits. *Clin Sci Colch* 1992; **83**: 399–407.

54 Lalloo, U.G., Fox, A.J., Belvisi, M.G., Chung, K.F., and Barnes, P.J. Bradykinin sensitisation of airway nerves: a mechanism for captopril-induced enhancement of the cough reflex (abstract). *Am J Respir Crit Care Med* 1996; **153**: A162.

55 Featherstone, R.L., Parry, J.E., Evans, D.M., *et al.* Mechanism of irritant-induced cough: studies with a kinin antagonist and a kallikrein inhibitor. *Lung* 1996; **174**: 269–75.

56 Lindgren, B.R., Rosenqvist, U., Ekstrom, T., *et al.* Increased bronchial reactivity and potentiated skin responses in hypertensive subjects suffering from coughs during ACE-inhibitor therapy. *Chest* 1989; **95**: 1225–30.

57 Warren, J.B., and Loi, R.K. Captopril increases skin microvascular blood flow secondary to bradykinin, nitric oxide, and prostaglandins. *FASEB J* 1995; **9**: 411–18.

58 Overlack, A., Muller, B., Schmidt, L., *et al.* Airway responsiveness and cough induced by angiotensin converting enzyme inhibition. *J Hum Hypertens* 1992; **6**: 387–92.

59 Choudry, N.B., Fuller, R.W., and Pride, N.B. Sensitivity of the human cough reflex: effect of inflammatory mediators prostaglandin E2, bradykinin, and histamine. *Am Rev Respir Dis* 1989; **140**: 137–41.

60 Costello, J.F., Dunlop, L.S., and Gardiner, P.J. Characteristics of prostaglandin induced cough in man. *Br J Clin Pharm* 1985; **20**: 355–9.

61 Nichol, G., Nix, A., Barnes, P.J., and Chung, K.F. Prostaglandin F2 alpha enhancement of capsaicin induced cough in man: modulation by beta 2 adrenergic and anticholinergic drugs. *Thorax* 1990; **45**: 694–8.

62 Coleridge, H.M., Coleridge, J.C., and Luck, J.C. Pulmonary afferent fibres of small diameter stimulated by capsaicin and by hyperinflation of the lungs. *J Physiol Lond* 1965; **179**: 248–62.

63 Coleridge, H.M., Coleridge, J.C., Baker, D.G., Ginzel, K.H., and Morrison, M.A. Comparison of the effects of histamine and prostaglandin on afferent C-fiber endings and irritant receptors in the intrapulmonary airways. *Adv Exp Med Biol* 1978; **99**: 291–305.

64 Coleridge, J.C., and Coleridge, H.M. Afferent vagal C fibre innervation of the lungs and airways and its functional significance. *Rev Physiol Biochem Pharm* 1984; **99**: 1–10.

65 McEwan, J.R., Choudry, N.B., and Fuller, R.W. The effect of sulindac on the abnormal cough reflex associated with dry cough. *J Pharm Exp Ther* 1990; **255**: 161–4.

66 Fujimura, M., Kamio, Y., Kasahara, K., *et al.* Prostanoids and cough response to capsaicin in asthma and chronic bronchitis. *Eur Respir J* 1995; **8**: 1499–505.

67 Taylor, D.R., Reid, W.D., Pare, P.D., and Fleetham, J.A. Cigarette smoke inhalation patterns and bronchial reactivity. *Thorax* 1988; **43**: 65–70.

68 Smith, C.A., Adamson, D.L., Choudry, N.B., and Fuller, R.W. The effect of altering airway tone on the sensitivity of the cough reflex in normal volunteers. *Eur Respir J* 1991; **4**: 1078–9.

69 Sheppard, D., Rizk, N.W., Boushey, H.A., and Bethel, R.A. Mechanism of cough and bronchoconstriction induced by distilled water aerosol. *Am Rev Respir Dis* 1983; **127**: 691–4.

70 Fuller, R.W., and Collier, J.G. Sodium cromoglycate and atropine block the fall in FEV_1 but not the cough induced by hypotonic mist. *Thorax* 1984; **39**: 766–70.

71 Hsu, J.Y., Stone, R.A., Logan, S.R., *et al.* Coughing frequency in patients with persistent cough: assessment using a 24 hour ambulatory recorder. *Eur Respir J* 1994; **7**: 1246–53.

72 Chang, A.B., Newman, R.G., Carlin, J.B., Phelan, P.D., and Robertson, C.F. Subjective scoring of cough in children: parent-completed vs child-completed diary cards vs an objective method. *Eur Respir J* 1998; **11**: 462–6.

73 Newnham, D.M., and Hamilton, S.J. Sensitivity of the cough reflex in young and elderly subjects. *Age Ageing* 1997; **26**: 185–8.

74 Fujimura, M., Kasahara, K., Kamio, Y., *et al.* Female gender as a determinant of cough threshold to inhaled capsaicin. *Eur Respir J* 1996; **9**: 1624–6.

75 Pounsford, J.C., and Saunders, K.B. Cough response to citric acid aerosol in occasional smokers. *Br Med J Clin Res Ed* 1986; **293**: 1528.

76 Pounsford, J.C., and Saunders, K.B. Diurnal variation and adaptation of the cough response to citric acid in normal subjects. *Thorax* 1985; **40**: 657–61.

77 Eschenbacher, W.L., Boushey, H.A., and Sheppard, D. Alteration in osmolarity of inhaled aerosols cause bronchoconstriction and cough, but absence of a permeant anion causes cough alone. *Am Rev Respir Dis* 1984; **129**: 211–15.

78 Hutchings, H.A., and Eccles, R. The opioid agonist codeine and antagonist naltrexone do not affect voluntary suppression of capsaicin induced cough in healthy subjects. *Eur Respir J* 1994; **7**: 715–19.

79 Dicpinigaitis, P.V., Dobkin, J.B., Rauf, K., and Aldrich, T.K. Inhibition of capsaicin-induced cough by the gamma-aminobutyric acid agonist baclofen. *J Clin Pharm* 1998; **38**: 364–7.

80 Morice, A.H., Higgins, K.S., and Yeo, W.W. Adaptation of cough reflex with different types of stimulation [see comments]. *Eur Respir J* 1992; **5**: 841–7.

81 Boggs, D.F., and Bartlett, D. Chemical specificity of a laryngeal apneic reflex in puppies. *J Appl Physiol* 1982; **53**: 455–62.

82 Godden, D.J., Borland, C., Lowry, R., and Higenbottam, T.W. Chemical specificity of coughing in man. *Clin Sci* 1986; **70**: 301–6.

83 Cavigioli, G., Pelucchi, A., Mastropasqua, B., *et al.* Prevalence and repeatability of the cough response induced by inhalation of low chloride ion solutions in normal subjects. *Monaldi Arch Chest Dis* 1995; **50**: 352–5.

84 Piirila, P., and Sovijarvi, A.R. Objective assessment of cough. *Eur Respir J* 1995; **8**: 1949–56.

85 Subburaj, S., Parvez, L., and Rajagopalan, T.G. Methods of recording and analysing cough sounds. *Pulm Pharm* 1996; **9**: 269–79.

86 Munyard, P., Busst, C., Logan, S.R., and Bush, A. A new device for ambulatory cough recording. *Pediatr Pulmonol* 1994; **18**: 178–86.

87 Riordan, M.F., Beardsmore, C.S., Brooke, A.M., and Simpson, H. Relationship between respiratory symptoms and cough receptor sensitivity. *Arch Dis Child* 1994; **70**: 299–304.

88 Yeo, W.W., Chadwick, I.G., Kraskiewicz, M., Jackson, P.R., and Ramsay, L.E. Resolution of ACE inhibitor cough: changes in subjective cough and responses to inhaled capsaicin, intradermal bradykinin and substance-P. *Br J Clin Pharm* 1995; **40**: 423–9.

89 Myers, J.D., Shakur, B.H., Ind, P.W., and Pride, N.B. Use of ambulatory cough recording to validate other measures of cough. *Eur Respir J* 1997; **10**: 422s.

Chapter 22

Chronic cough with a 'normal' chest radiograph

J. Mark Madison and Richard S. Irwin

Cough is a reflex that serves as a clearance mechanism when normal mucociliary clearance of the tracheobronchial tree is inadequate or overwhelmed. In the absence of excessive secretions or foreign bodies, however, cough can still be stimulated by disease processes, and in this setting, the reflex serves no purpose.

Chronic cough can be physically and psychologically debilitating. Patients with complaints of cough have been shown to account for up to 38% of a pulmonologist's outpatient practice. Non-specific, symptomatic treatment of chronic cough is usually ineffective and should be avoided. Fortunately, careful evaluation of patients with chronic cough usually identifies an underlying diagnosis that leads to specific and effective treatment (Figure 22.1)[1,2].

The approach to cough depends on the duration of symptoms.[3–6] It has been proposed that cough be divided into three categories based on the duration of cough at the time of patient presentation: acute, defined as cough lasting less than three weeks; subacute, lasting three to eight weeks; and chronic, lasting more than eight weeks.[1] This chapter focuses mainly on the diagnosis and management of chronic cough. However, because earlier definitions of chronic cough included cough of three to eight weeks duration, this chapter will discuss cough due to pertussis infection as well.[6]

A chest radiograph is an important step in evaluating chronic cough.[3–6] When present, abnormalities on chest radiograph direct subsequent evaluation. A common clinical problem, however, is chronic cough with a normal chest radiograph.

Evaluation of chronic cough with a normal chest radiograph begins with a history and physical examination (Figure 22.1). For identifying the cause of cough, the character of the cough (barking, honking, dry, etc.), the timing of the cough (nocturnal, with meals, etc.) and the complications of cough (e.g. syncope) have not been predictive. Instead, the main, but not exclusive, emphasis of evaluation should be on the most common causes of chronic cough: angiotensin converting enzyme inhibitor (ACEI) medications, smoking, postnasal drip syndrome (PNDS), asthma, and gastroesophageal reflux disease (GERD).

Because it is highly contagious, the first diagnosis to consider is pertussis infection. Cough due to pertussis can persist at least 6 weeks and, therefore, the differential diagnosis of cough present for longer than 3 weeks must include pertussis infection.[6] Typically, as the upper respiratory tract symptoms of pertussis infection improve, the cough worsens. Adult patients may not have the inspiratory whoop at the end of coughing but they often vomit after coughing.[7] One should consider pertussis in patients with cough–vomit syndrome, characteristic whoop, recent close contacts, or severe cough in a high endemic area. Acute serology for *Bordetella pertussis*-specific IgA is a sensitive test. If taken early, a nasopharyngeal culture, direct

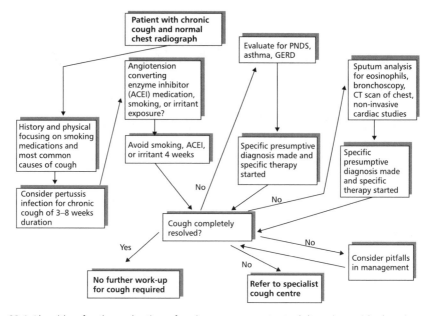

Fig. 22.1 Algorithm for the evaluation of an immunocompetent adult patient with chronic cough and a normal chest radiograph. PNDS, asthma, and GERD contribute to chronic cough in approximately 40%, 25%, and 20% of cases, respectively. Multiple causes of chronic cough may exist simultaneously.

fluorescent antibody (DFA), or polymerase chain reaction for *Bordetella pertussis* will confirm the diagnosis. Erythromycin is used to treat pertussis and as prophylaxis for exposed persons. For persistently troublesome cough during the chronic phase of pertussis infection, it is reasonable to consider treating with corticosteroids also.

The next step in evaluating chronic cough is to determine whether the patient is taking an ACEI and/or is a current smoker.[8] ACEI-induced cough is suggested by medication history. Cough is a class effect of these drugs and not dose related. Cough may begin within a few hours of starting the medication or may not become apparent for months. Chronic bronchitis due to smoking should be considered as a cause of cough in smokers who expectorate phlegm on most days during periods spanning at least 3 consecutive months for more than 2 successive years. It is important to recognize that in the general population, chronic bronchitis is a very common cause of cough, but smokers have not been a group that commonly seeks medical attention for cough. It is in this latter group that cigarette smoking quit rates have been quite high.[9] Physical examination may reveal wheezing or rhonchi due to airway secretions. Additional diagnostic studies for cough should not be done until the response to cessation of smoking or discontinuation of the ACEI for 4 weeks can be assessed.

Although hundreds of diseases and conditions cause cough, further evaluation of cough depends on recognizing that three conditions account for most cases.[3] Among patients that included smokers, PNDS, asthma, and GERD accounted for 41%, 24%, and 21% of cases, respectively.[3,6,10] It is also important to recognize that for 18–62% of patients, in different series, multiple diagnoses may contribute to chronic cough simultaneously.[6] When the chest radiograph is normal, even when there a history of smoking, occult bronchogenic carcinoma as a cause of cough is an unlikely diagnosis and, therefore, bronchoscopy is not a procedure performed early in the evaluation of chronic cough with a normal chest radiograph.[11] Much more likely causes of cough are PNDS, asthma, and GERD, alone or in combination.

PNDS is the most common cause of chronic cough in adults.[10] PNDS refers to cough, dyspnoea, and wheeze due to drainage of secretions into the hypopharynx/larynx. Patients with PNDS have the sensation of postnasal discharge dripping in their throats, nasal discharge, and/or the need to frequently clear their throats. Examination of the nasopharynges and oropharynges may reveal mucoid or mucopurulent secretions and/or a cobblestone appearance of the mucosa. For adults with chronic cough due to PNDS, sinusitis is the cause of the PNDS in 30–60% of cases. The other major cause of PNDS is rhinitis of any cause.

Rhinitis causing PNDS is treated with an antihistamine–decongestant combination, e.g. dexbrompheniramine maleate plus D-isoephedrine, and avoidance of environmental precipitating factors. Note that decongestants should not be used for prolonged periods. All forms of rhinitis generally respond to first-generation antihistamines. For patients with allergic rhinitis who do not tolerate the sedating effects of first-generation antihistamines, the newer, non-sedating H1 antagonists also are effective. However, it should be noted that non-allergic rhinitis – which is not histamine mediated – does not respond to the newer, non-sedating H1 antagonists because these drugs lack significant anticholinergic activity. When theraphy with antihistamine–decongestant therapy is not possible rhinitis may respond to intranasal corticosteroids or intranasal ipratropium bromide. These agents should be used preferentially over antihistamine decongestants whenever there is glaucoma, benign prostatic hypertrophy, or poorly controlled hypertension. Unless there is strong clinical suspicion of sinusitis (e.g. purulent nasal discharge), antibiotics should be withheld initially.

When patients with PNDS fail to respond to treatment for rhinitis, sinus imaging studies should be obtained. Some authorities advocate sinus CT, but, for the evaluation of chronic cough, there are no prospective studies establishing the clinical superiority of sinus CT over four-view sinus radiographs. Based on data from retrospective and prospective descriptive studies, successful initial treatment of cough due to chronic sinusitis has usually consisted of antibiotics and decongestants that facilitate sinus drainage. If this fails, a specialist's opinion should be sought.

Asthma is the second most common cause of chronic cough in non-smoking adults not taking an ACEI.[10,12] Asthmatics usually complain of wheezing and shortness of breath. However, it should be recognized that cough may be the sole presenting manifestation of asthma (i.e. cough-variant asthma).[12] Non-specific, pharmacologic bronchoprovocation challenge testing with methacholine or histamine is helpful in ruling out asthma as a cause of cough. Although it only has a positive predictive value of 60–80%, it has a negative predictive value that approaches 100%. Therefore, when methacholine inhalation challenge (MIC) is negative, asthma is essentially ruled out. However, it should be recognized that MIC can be falsely positive for predicting that asthma causes cough and this has been reported for up to 22% of such patients. Therefore, a positive MIC, by itself, without a subsequent favourable response to asthma therapy, is not diagnostic of asthma as a cause of cough. Uncomplicated cough-variant asthma responds to asthma medications including inhaled or oral β_2-adrenergic agonists, theophylline, inhaled nedocromil, and either inhaled or systemic corticosteroids. In general, cough will begin to improve within 1 week of beginning inhaled β_2-adrenergic agonists and will resolve within 6–8 weeks of beginning inhaled corticosteroids. Therefore, we recommend initial therapy with inhaled β_2-adrenergic agonist plus inhaled corticosteroids. If any of these agents themselves provoke cough, different proprietary formulations and the use of spacer devices is often helpful. Although a trial of systemic corticosteroids may sometimes be necessary for initial control of cough-variant asthma, it is important to recognize that a response to prednisone does not, by itself, make a diagnosis of asthma because other conditions such as non-asthmatic eosinophilic bronchitis, a condition distinct from asthma, may respond as well.[6]

GERD is the third most common cause of chronic cough in adults.[10, 13,14] Failure to obtain a history of nocturnal coughing does not exclude GERD as a cause of cough, because the coughing commonly occurs while the patient is awake and upright and it often is not noted during the night. GERD should be suspected when there is frequent heartburn, regurgitation, or a sour taste. These symptoms allow a diagnosis of GERD without obtaining barium oesophagography and/or 24-h oesophageal pH monitoring. In the evaluation of cough, barium oesophagography and/or 24-h oesophageal pH monitoring are reserved for identifying 'silent' GERD – i.e. GERD producing cough without other symptoms. Prolonged 24-h oesophageal pH monitoring is helpful in linking 'silent' GERD to chronic cough. GERD is linked to chronic cough when reflux events (either acid or alkaline) are temporally correlated before instances of cough and/or any reflux parameter falls out of the normal range (e.g. percentage of time that pH is less than 4.0). Although less sensitive and specific for diagnosing GERD, barium oesophagography can sometimes reveal significant reflux that is not detected by pH probe testing[14] and, therefore, both tests are necessary to rule out 'silent' GERD as a cause of cough.

Less common causes of chronic cough with a normal chest radiograph include bronchiectasis, non-asthmatic eosinophilic bronchitis, left ventricular failure, aspiration syndromes, and, rarely, psychogenic or habit cough.[6] The following additional testing may be useful if cough persists following initial evaluation and treatment:

◆ ear, nose, and throat consultation when sinusitis fails to respond to medical therapy

◆ sputum cytology to detect eosinophilia

◆ bronchoscopy to assess for endobronchial abnormalities not detected on chest radiograph

◆ high-resolution CT scan to assess for parenchymal lung disease and/or bronchiectasis not apparent on chest radiograph; and non-invasive cardiac studies.

A detailed assessment of possible allergies may also be helpful when PNDS fails to respond to therapy but suspicion of an allergic aetiology remains high. In those cases, identification of a specific allergic aetiology by skin or *in vitro* testing may be helpful in devising a strategy to reduce ongoing environmental exposures that are preventing a response to medication.

Habit or psychogenic cough is reported to be common, but in our experience it is a rare diagnosis of exclusion.[6] Some have suggested that patients with psychogenic cough typically do not cough at night and have barking or honking coughs. However, these characteristics of cough are not diagnostically helpful. For instance, cough due to a variety of diseases is unlikely to occur during sleep and can be barking or honking in quality. Consequently, because there are no distinguishing clinical features for psychogenic cough, it should only be a diagnosis of exclusion. A referral to a specialty cough clinic has been shown to be successful in diagnosing and eliminating cough in many patients who had been previously told the cause could not be determined or was psychogenic in origin.[9] In our experience, cough due to PNDS is commonly misdiagnosed as habit cough. In those rare instances where an organic cause of cough can not be identified, we have found treatment by behavioural medicine or psychiatry to be helpful, but this has not been established by clinical studies.

A definitive diagnosis of a cause of cough always depends on observing a favourable response to specific treatment (Figure 22.1). If there is at least partial resolution of cough on specific therapy, then at least one diagnosis is confirmed. After additional evaluation, new potential causes of cough may be identified and specific treatments are added to the regimen.[1–3,6,15] The common pitfalls in management are:

- prescribing non-specific antitussive therapy without attempting to make specific diagnoses
- failure to consider other common causes of cough when one diagnosis is seemingly obvious
- failure to consider the possibility that cough has more than one cause simultaneously
- failure to consider ACEI as a cause of cough
- failure to use the older H1 antagonists when treating non-allergic rhinitis
- failure to recognize that a bronchoprovocation challenge test may be falsely positive in suggesting that cough is due to asthma and that inhaled asthma medications may themselves cause cough
- failure to utilize oesophageal pH monitoring to diagnose 'silent GERD' or to assess response to medical therapy for GERD
- failure to consider that treatment for GERD may require 2–3 months before being even partially effective and that maximal medical treatment for GERD sometimes fails
- failure to make referral to a specialist respiratory physician before resorting to non-specific suppressive therapy.

References

1   Irwin, R.S., and Madison, J.M. Primary care: The diagnosis and treatment of cough. *N Engl J Med* 2000; **343**: 1715–21.

2   Irwin, R.S., and Madison, J.M. The persistently troublesome cough. *Am J Respir Crit Care Med* 2002; **165**: 1469–74.

3   Cough. In: R.S. Irwin, F.J. Curley, and R.F. Grossman (eds) *Diagnosis and treatment of symptoms of the respiratory tract*. Armonk, NY: Futura, 1997; 1–54.

4   Poe, R.H., and Israel, R.H. Chronic cough: A strategy for work-up and therapy. *J Respir Dis* 1997; **18**: 629–41.

5   Yu, M.L., and Ryu, J.H. Assessment of the patient with chronic cough. *Mayo Clin Proc* 1997; **72**: 957–9.

6   Irwin, R.S., Boulet, L-P., Cloutier, M.M., *et al*. Managing cough as a defense mechanism and as a symptom: a consensus panel report of the American College of Chest Physicians. *Chest* 1998; **114**: 133S–81S.

7   Olsen, L.C. Pertussis. *Medicine* 1975; **54**: 427–69.

8   Lacourciere, Y., Brunner, H., Irwin, R.S., *et al*. Effects of modulators of the renin-angiotensin-aldosterone system on cough. *J Hypertension* 1994; **12**: 1387–93.

9   Irwin, R.S., Corrao, W.M., and Pratter, M.R. Chronic persistent cough in the adult: the spectrum and frequency of causes and successful outcome of specific therapy. *Am Rev Respir Dis* 1981; **123**: 413–17.

10 Irwin, R.S., Curley, F.J., and French, C.L. Chronic cough: the spectrum and frequency of causes, key components of the diagnostic evaluation, and outcome of specific therapy. *Am Rev Respir Dis* 1990; **141**: 640–7.

11 Markowitz, D.H., and Irwin, R.S. Is bronchoscopy overused in the evaluation of chronic cough? Bronchoscopy is overused. *J Bronchol* 1997; **4**: 332–6.

12 Irwin, R.S., French, C.T., Smyrnios, N.A., *et al.* Interpretation of positive results of a methacholine challenge and 1 week of inhaled bronchodilator use in diagnosing and treating cough-variant asthma. *Arch Intern Med* 1997; **157**: 1981–7.

13 Harding, S.M., and Richter, J.E. The role of gastroesophageal reflux in chronic cough and asthma. *Chest* 1997; **111**: 1389–402.

14 Irwin, R.S., French, C.L., Curley, F.J., *et al.* Chronic cough due to gastroesophageal reflux: clinical, diagnostic, and pathogenetic aspects. *Chest* 1993; **104**: 1511–17.

15 Poe, R.H., Harder, R.V., Israel, R.H., *et al.* Experience in diagnosis and outcome using an anatomic diagnostic protocol. *Chest* 1989; **95**: 723–8.

Chapter 23

Massive haemoptysis: causes, assessment, and management

Peter R. Mills and Jadwiga A. Wedzicha

The expectoration of sputum streaked with blood is a common occurrence in pneumonic illnesses and infective exacerbations of chronic obstructive pulmonary disease (COPD), bronchiectasis, and cystic fibrosis. The source of the bleeding is usually from areas of mucosal inflammation, and it invariably settles with appropriate antibiotic therapy. Lung neoplasms often present with minor degrees of haemoptysis, again due to mucosal disruption, and hence any report of haemoptysis should be investigated thoroughly, even in the absence of radiographic signs.

Thus, minor haemoptysis is a common manifestation of a wide range of respiratory diseases and is usually self-limiting. **Massive haemoptysis**, however, is a much rarer occurrence and potentially life threatening, with a mortality of 30–40%, even with optimal management.[1,2] Massive haemoptysis has been variously described as the expectoration of 200–1000 mL fresh blood from the lungs in a 24–48-h period.[3,4] In reality, once an individual has been identified as having a significant haemoptysis the exact volume of blood expectorated becomes immaterial as the threat to life is not from volume depletion, as with other forms of organ haemorrhage, but from asphyxiation. An estimation of the rate of bleeding is a more important indicator of severity, and the expectoration of 200 mL or more of fresh blood over a 24-h period should be considered a massive haemoptysis with the subsequent train of investigations and therapeutic interventions rapidly deployed for this medical emergency. This chapter concentrates on the practical aspects of diagnosis and management of patients with haemoptysis, with particular emphasis on massive haemoptysis.

Aetiology

Most patients who present with massive haemoptysis have significant underlying structural lung disease. The bleeding in most cases usually originates from the systemic rather than the pulmonary circulation.[3] There is often enlargement and an increased tortuosity of the bronchial arteries with an increase in bronchial artery blood flow. In addition, the dilated bronchial arteries may be thin walled and more friable, predisposing them to rupture and bleed into the lung.

The incidence of massive haemoptysis in the general population is difficult to quantify, and there are no clear estimates of relative frequency. Mortality statistics do not fully reflect the true life-threatening nature of this condition, with only eight deaths recorded in England and Wales due to haemoptysis in 1997. This is probably an indication of the way death certification occurs; recording the underlying disease takes precedence over describing the actual terminal event. Classically the most common cause for pulmonary haemorrhage was either active or old tuberculous lung disease. The combination of effective chemotherapeutic regimens and a marked decline in the incidence of tuberculosis in most developed countries over the last four decades has resulted in other diseases becoming more common causes of major bleeds. There are, however, still significant numbers of individuals with old tuberculous pulmonary cavities who remain at risk by virtue of chronic lung scarring and altered architecture, as well as the possibility of disease reactivation. A recent study of 208 patients who presented with significant haemoptysis in Israel showed that 20% were due to bronchiectasis, 19% to lung cancer, 18% to pneumonia, and 16% to bronchitis. Active tuberculosis accounted for only 1.4% of cases seen.[2] This contrasts with data from South Africa where 85% of all cases of massive haemoptysis at a single institution were due to tuberculosis.[5] A US study reported tuberculosis as a cause of massive haemoptysis in 16% of cases, which is probably a reflection of the socio-economic status of the centre's surrounding population.[6] Clearly the relative contributions of differing pulmonary disease states to the incidence of massive haemoptysis varies according to the demographics of the region.

Patients with cystic fibrosis are particularly prone to haemoptysis, with minor degrees occurring during infective exacerbations in approximately two thirds of affected individuals.[7] With life expectancy approaching, and in some cases exceeding, 30 years of age there has been an increase in the incidence of severe pulmonary complications. The incidence of massive haemoptysis in cystic fibrosis is 5–10% of all affected individuals, with an immediate mortality of approximately 11%, due in the main to respiratory compromise.[8]

Several studies of massive haemoptysis have shown that primary and secondary pulmonary malignancy was the cause in 6–19% of cases.[1,2,6,9] This is more frequent than is generally thought (see Figure 23.1). In the absence of a suspicious chest radiograph, however, lung cancer is the cause of a major haemoptysis in only 5–6% of cases of bleeding. Age >50 years and a significant smoking history make this diagnosis more likely.[10,11]

Pulmonary mycetomas (e.g. aspergillomas) are an important cause of massive haemoptysis. Bleeding occurs from aberrant vessels surrounding and traversing the cavity that contains the fungal ball. Previous tuberculosis and chronic sarcoidosis are the most common diseases

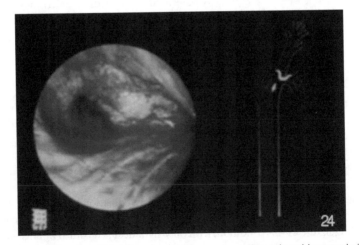

Fig. 23.1 Bronchoscopic view of bleeding necrotic lung cancer. Reproduced by permission of Boehringer Ingelheim Ltd.

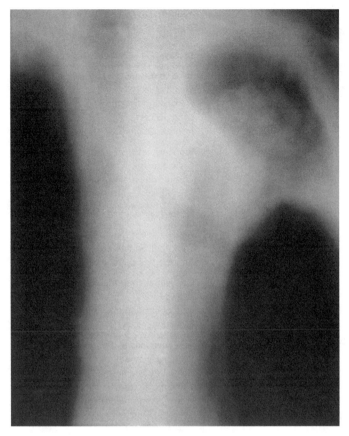

Fig. 23.2 CT scan of apical cavity containing aspergilloma. Mycetomas are frequently a source of severe haemoptysis.

predisposing to development of a mycetoma (Figure 23.2). HIV-positive patients with *Pneumocystis carinii* infection have also recently been described as being at increased risk.[12] Systemic vasculitides can frequently present with haemoptysis, the severity of which may initially be underestimated due in the main to alveolar haemorrhage being retained in the lung and not expectorated. Other notable but rarer causes of haemoptysis include lung abscess, pulmonary embolism, and arteriovenous anomalies and malformations (Table 23.1).

Diagnosis and treatment

Massive haemoptysis must be considered a medical emergency, because of its morbidity and high mortality.[2] Patients need to be nursed in a high dependency or intensive care unit where they can be constantly monitored. This should preferably be in a centre with specialist radiological and thoracic surgical facilities. Initial management should concentrate on securing the airway and maintaining adequate circulatory volume. Fluid resuscitation and oxygen therapy should be administered to all patients, depending on their physiological parameters. Oxygen therapy should be administered by face mask in order to maintain oxygen saturations above 92%. Central venous access should be established at the outset, with colloid and blood

Table 23.1 Some reported causes of haemoptysis. Those marked with an asterisk are the most common aetiologies

Category	Disease
Infective	Tuberculosis (active and old)*
	Pneumonia*
	Pulmonary mycetoma*
	Lung abscess
	Invasive aspergillosis
Structural lung disease	Bronchiectasis*
	Cystic fibrosis*
	Chronic obstructive pulmonary disease (COPD)*
	Sarcoidosis
Neoplastic	Primary and secondary lung neoplasms*
Drugs	Anticoagulant therapy*
	Thrombolytic therapy
	Amiodorone pulmonary toxicity
Congenital	Congenital abnormalities of cardiopulmonary vasculature
	Intralobar pulmonary sequestration
	Bronchogenic cysts
Vascular disease	Anteriovenous malformations
	Pulmonary emboli
	Hereditary haemorrhagic telangiectasia
	Vasculitic disease
	Wegener's granulomatosis
	Behçet's disease
	Takayasu's arteritis
Connective tissue disease	Systemic sclerosis
	Ehlers–Danlos syndrome
Iatrogenic	Pulmonary artery catheter induced pseudoaneurysms
	Post bronchoscopy or transcutaneous needle biopsy*
Miscellaneous	Bronchiolitis obliterans organizing pneumonia (BOOP)
	Thoracic endometriosis

administered in order to maintain haematocrit and circulating volume. Overt hypertension should be corrected, as this can worsen the haemorrhage. Likewise, any bleeding diathesis should be reversed with fresh frozen plasma and cryoprecipitate as necessary and all drugs with detrimental effects on bleeding time or platelet activity should be stopped for as long as possible, dependent upon other co-morbid conditions, and certainly for at least 48 h. All patients should receive intravenous broad-spectrum antibiotics for at least 24–48 h, because of the likelihood of an infective exacerbation of an underlying lung disease contributing to the bleeding episode. Patients with proven or suspected tuberculosis should be started on standard quadruple antituberculous chemotherapy (see Chapter 32).[5] Additionally, nebulized bronchodilators may provide symptomatic relief of dyspnoea in patients with obstructive lung disease. Nursing care should concentrate on airway maintenance with regular oropharygeal suction and appropriate positioning of the patient to aid the expectoration of blood and secretions.

Light sedation is often necessary during active bleeding, as haemoptysis can be extremely distressing. As with sedation in other pulmonary disease states, it should be titrated to ventilatory function and symptom relief. Benzodiazepines such as midazolam or lorazepam are commonly used as they can be administered intravenously in small easily titratable dosages (e.g. midazolam 2–5 mg), and their effects are readily reversed if necessary with the specific antidote flumazanil. Antifibronolytic agents such as tranexamic acid and haemostatic agents such as ethamsylate are often used in an attempt to slow bleeding, although there is very little evidence for a beneficial effect and no controlled trial data available to recommend their routine use.

The major objective in all cases of massive haemoptysis is to identify the site of bleeding as precisely as possible. A standard chest radiograph is mandatory, although, if significant pulmonary haemorrhage has occurred, blood within the lungs may mask any localizing underlying pulmonary or bronchial pathology. CT scanning has been shown to be a useful diagnostic investigation in identifying the site and cause of the bleeding, being particularly useful in diagnosing central lung neoplasms and bronchiectasis (Figure 23.3).[6,13] In cases of bronchiectasis CT is also useful in guiding the physiotherapist in subsequent postural drainage manoeuvres, although these should not be attempted until bleeding has completely ceased for at least 48 h.

If the patient is haemodynamically stable, with adequate gas exchange, fibreoptic bronchoscopy should be performed immediately in order to ascertain firstly which lung the bleeding is coming from, and secondly to try to identify the precise lobe. In addition, samples can be taken for microbiological and cytological examination. The patient can be nursed lying on one side, with the non-bleeding lung uppermost once this information is available. All patients should have a laryngoscope and double-lumen endotracheal tube ready at the side of the bed in case bleeding becomes uncontrolled and there is impairment of ventilatory function. In such cases the patient should be anaesthetized and the endotracheal tube inserted and the cuff to the non-bleeding lung inflated to prevent the aspiration of blood from the affected to the non-affected side, thereby preserving gas exchange. If ventilatory function is insufficient to allow fibreoptic bronchoscopy, or bleeding is greater than can be suctioned effectively with a flexible bronchoscope, the patient should be immediately anaesthetized and ventilated. Rigid bronchoscopy can then be performed to localize the bleeding site. This is better at clearing the bronchial tree of clot and should be performed if there is any concern about the patency of the main brochi.

If bleeding continues, the treatments to consider are immediate surgery or bronchial arteriography and embolization. Lobectomy has been shown to reduce mortality by over a half as compared to conservative management alone, with some reporting an improvement in mortality from 75% to 23% with surgery.[1,14] Furthermore, early and late recurrence of haemoptysis is significantly reduced in patients who undergo surgery, as opposed to other treatment modalities.[5] The risks associated with such a procedure are those that are commonly encountered postoperatively, namely infection and postoperative bleeding, as well as longer-term problems that can occur with the reduction of pulmonary reserve capacity in individuals with preexistent pulmonary compromise.

Certain patients are not suitable for surgical intervention because of poor pulmonary function or non-resectable malignancy. Bronchial arterial angiography and embolization has been shown to be a safe and effective means of identifying the site and controlling the bleeding (Figure 23.4). Bronchoscopic localization of the site of bleeding is helpful before bronchial artery angiography, although not mandatory. A prerequisite to localizing the bleeding site by this method is that active bleeding needs to be occurring at the time of the angiogram in order

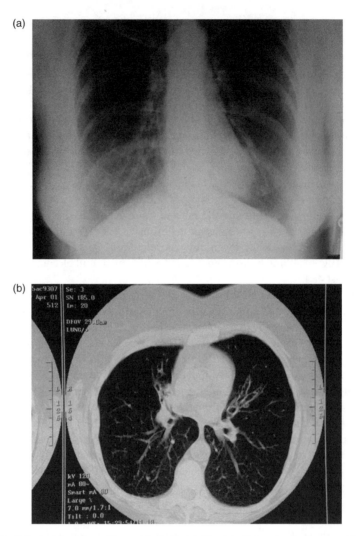

Fig. 23.3 Radiological imaging of bronchiectasis: (a) Chest radiograph of woman with bilateral basal bronchiectasis who presented with major haemoptysis. (b) CT scan showing bilateral basal bronchiectasis in the same patient.

for the leaking vessel to be identified. A catheter is inserted via the femoral artery and passed retrogradely up the aorta to the origin of the four bronchial arteries, which are located in the area where the left main bronchus crosses in front of the descending thoracic aorta. Once the site of bleeding has been localized, the supplying circulation can be embolized with foam-based material or coils. Recent studies have reported success rates of 75–85% in massive haemoptysis, although recurrence of bleeding requiring further embolization occurred in up to 50% of cases.[15–17] Note should be made of aberrant arterial anatomy, particularly spinal arteries arising from the intercostal or bronchial vessels, as a possible major side effect of this procedure is infarction of the spinal cord. Although this is rare (in the region of 1%), the risk should be

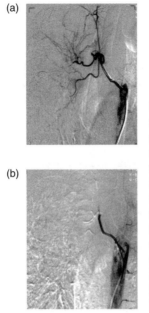

Figure 23.4 (a) Bronchial arterial angiography in female patient with bronchiectasis showing a leash of abnormal vessels responsible for recurrent massive haemoptysis. (b) Postembolization image showing complete occlusion of supplying vessel resulting in complete cessation of haemoptysis. (Pictures courtesy of Dr Sarah Howling, Consultant Radiologist, Whittington Hospital, London.)

explained to the patient before consent is sought.[3] In addition, although most patients with haemoptysis due to underlying structural lung disease bleed from the bronchial circulation, the pulmonary arterial circulation should be evaluated if the bronchial angiogram is normal. Embolization of bleeding pulmonary arterial vessels has also been shown to be effective at controlling bleeding in such situations.[18]

Other techniques that have been successfully used to halt bleeding in massive haemoptysis include endobronchial balloon tamponade and intrabronchial coagulative treatment with thrombin and fibrinogen instillation.[19–21] A 4 Fr Fogarty balloon catheter is passed through the bronchoscope after localization of the bleeding area, and the balloon is inflated to occlude the region which can additionally be lavaged with cold saline or adrenalin (epinephrine) solution down the lumen of the catheter. Small studies have shown favourable results in individuals with severe haemoptysis, with control and subsequent halting of bleeding in all individuals on whom the technique was used.[22] The infusion of thrombin and fibrinogen-thrombin precursors down the fibreoptic bronchoscope has also been shown to result in favourable outcomes in many individuals with massive haemoptysis. In one study, 28 of 33 patients (85%) with massive haemoptysis had bleeding halted by the infusion of either 5–10 mL of 1000 u/mL thrombin solution or 2% fibrinogen solution.[20] In addition, reports of percutaneous intracavity instillation of antifungals in pulmonary mycetomas have suggested that this is an effective means of treating associated haemoptysis and can also result in complete radiographic resolution of the mycetoma.[23]

For some patients who present with massive haemoptysis active intervention is not suitable because they have recurrent or metastatic neoplasm or end-stage respiratory disease. In these individuals attention should be paid to palliative measures such as appropriate sedation, oxygen therapy, and oropharyngeal suction. In many, however, it may still be appropriate to consider bronchial artery embolization or endobronchial occlusive and coagulative therapy as a means of symptom palliation.

Follow-up

Regular follow of patients who have had a massive haemoptysis is mandatory. As already described, many rebleed and it is important that diagnosis and intervention is prompt in such circumstances. In patients with non-malignant disease and a localized area of lung pathology giving rise to episodic haemoptysis, elective surgery to remove the effected segment or lobe may prove curative and should be considered even in those with moderate impairment of pulmonary function.

Conclusion

Haemoptysis is a common occurrence in many respiratory diseases and is usually self-limiting. Massive haemoptysis, however, is a medical emergency with a significant associated mortality. Rapid intervention in massive haemoptysis by experienced staff is necessary in order to preserve airway function and reduce the considerable associated mortality. Early surgical intervention or embolization is recommended in order to achieve this goal.

References

1 Conlan, A.A., Hurwitz, S.S., Krige, L., Nicolaou, N., and Pool, R. Massive hemoptysis. Review of 123 cases. *J Thorac Cardiovasc Surg* 1983; **85**: 120–4.

2 Hirshberg, D., Biran, I., Glazer, M., and Kramer, M.R. Hemoptysis: etiology, evaluation, and outcome in a tertiary referral hospital. *Chest* 1997; **112**: 440–4.

3 Wedzicha, J.A., and Pearson, M.C. Management of massive haemoptysis. *Respir Med* 1990; **84**: 9–12.

4 Jones, D.K., and Davies, R.J. Massive haemoptysis. *BMJ* 1990; **300**: 889–90.

5 Knott-Craig, C.J., Oostuizen, J.G., Rossouw, G., Joubert, J.R., and Barnard, P.M. Management and prognosis of massive hemoptysis. Recent experience with 120 patients. *J Thorac Cardiovasc Surg* 1993; **105**: 394–7.

6 McGuinness, G., Beacher, J.R., Harkin, T.J., *et al.* Hemoptysis: prospective high resolution CT/bronchoscopic correlation. *Chest* 1994; **105**: 1155–62.

7 Penketh, A.R.L., Wise, A., Mearns, M.B., Hodson, M.E., and Batten, J.C. Cystic fibrosis in adolescents and adults. *Thorax* 1987; **42**: 526–32.

8 Porter, D.K., Van Every, M.J., Anthracite, R.F., and Mack, J.W. Massive hemoptysis in cystic fibrosis. *Arch Intern Med* 1983; **143**: 287–90.

9 Imgrund, S.P., Goldberg, S.K., Walkenstein, M.D., Fischer, R., and Lippman, M.L. Clinical diagnosis of massive haemoptysis using the fibreoptic bronchoscope. *Crit Care Med* 1985; **13**: 438–43.

10 Lederle, F.A., Nichol, K.L., and Parenti, C.M. Bronchoscopy to evaluate hemoptysis in older men with nonsuspicious chest roentgenograms. *Chest* 1989; **95**: 1043–7.

11 Poe, R.H., Israel, R.H., Marin, M.G., et al. Utility of fibreoptic bronchoscopy in patients with hemoptysis and nonlocalizing chest roentgenogram. *Chest* 1988; **93**: 70–5.

12 Addrizzo-Harris, D.J., Harkin, T.J., McGuiness, G., Naidich, D.P., and Rom, W.N. Pulmonary aspergilloma and AIDS. A comparison of HIV-infected and HIV-negative individuals. *Chest* 1997; **111**: 612–8.

13 Naidich, D.P., Funt, S., Ettenger, N.A., and Arranda, C. Hemoptysis: CT-bronchoscopic correlations in 58 cases. *Radiology* 1990; **177**: 357–62

14 Crocco, J.A., Rooney, J.J., Fankushen, D.S., DiBenedetto, R.J., and Lyons, H.A. Massive haemoptysis. *Arch Intern Med* 1968; **121**: 495–8.

15 Fernando, H.C., Stein, M., Benfield, J.R., and Link, D.P. Role of bronchial artery embolization in the management of hemoptysis. *Arch Surg* 1998; **133**: 862–6.

16 Brinson, G.M., Noone, P.G., Mauro, M.A., *et al.* Bronchial artery embolization for the treatment of hemoptysis in patients with cystic fibrosis. *Am J Respir Crit Care Med* 1998; **157**: 1951–8.

17 Ramakantan, R., Bandekar, V.G., Gandhi, M.S., Aulakh, B.G., and Deshmukh, H.L. Massive hemoptysis due to pulmonary tuberculosis: control with bronchial artery embolization. *Radiology* 1996; **200**: 691–4.

18 Santelli, E.D., Katz, D.S., Goldschmidt, A.M., and Thomas, H.A. Embolization of multiple Rasmussen aneurysms as a treatment of hemoptysis. *Radiology* 1994; **193**: 396–8.

19 Bense, L. Intrabronchial selective coagulative treatment of hemoptysis. Report of three cases. *Chest* 1990; **97**: 990–6.

20 Tsukamoto, T., Sasaki, H., and Nakamura, H. Treatment of hemoptysis patients by thrombin and fibrinogen-thrombin infusion therapy using a fibreoptic bronchoscope. *Chest* 1989; **96**: 473–6.

21 Gottlieb, L.S., and Hilliberg, R. Endobronchial tamponade therapy for intractable haemoptysis. *Chest* 1975; **67**: 482–3.

22 Saw, E.C., Gottlieb, L.S., Yokoyama, T., and Lee, B.C. Flexible fiberoptic bronchoscopy and endo-bronchial tamponade in the management of massive haemoptysis. *Chest* 1976; **70**: 589–91.

23 Lee, K.S., Kim, H.T., Kim, Y.H., and Choe, K.O. Treatment of hemoptysis in patients with cavitary aspergilloma of the lung: value of percutaneous instillation of amphoteracin B. *Am J Roentgenol* 1993; **161**: 727–31.

Chapter 24

The therapy of expectoration

Alyn H. Morice

Expectoration, the removal of secretions from the chest, is a symptom that may be triggered by a wide range of respiratory conditions. Because of this diversity, an extensive armamentarium of therapeutic options may be used which are specifically directed at individual causal agents. In general this strategy has a high success rate. Alternatively (and usually less efficaciously), therapy can be given to improve the act of expectoration itself or to suppress the desire to expectorate. Finally, expectoration can be helped by manoeuvres designed to make it easier.

Because treatment of the cause of expectoration is our most successful strategy, efforts should be directed to establishing a diagnosis. Although achieving a precise diagnosis may not be easy, it is helpful to note that there are two major subdivisions of disease leading to expectoration. Firstly, inflammatory conditions such as asthma or bronchiectasis are frequently associated with copious expectoration. Removal of the inflammatory stimulus by either specific therapy aimed at a particular organism or generalized anti-inflammatory therapy (such as the use of inhaled or parenteral corticosteroids for asthma), leads to reduction or abolition of symptoms. Secondly, neoplastic diseases and most notably alveolar cell carcinoma, can produce expectoration through uncontrolled production of mucus. Specific therapy to control expectoration in individual conditions is not be considered further in this chapter other than to list the main therapeutic areas in Table 24.1.

Pathophysiology

Expectoration arises from the collection and progress of secretions from within the bronchial tree to the upper airways. The stimulus for expectoration arises from sensory nerves within the upper airways giving rise to the cough reflex. In the normal lung, airways secretions contain a mixture of submucosal gland products together with secretions of the airways surface cells such as goblet cells. The resultant mixture contains mucous glycoproteins and electrolytes. The airways surface liquid (as it is known) forms two layers, a sol phase which has contact with the cilia and a gel phase which rests on top and traps inhaled particles. The tips of the epithelial cell cilia drive the mucous blanket towards the upper airways and on their return stroke, the cilia dip from the gel phase into the sol phase.[1] As the mucus blanket travels centrally, water and electrolytes are reabsorbed and the volume of secretions is reduced. It has been calculated that approximately 10 mL of secretions are expectorated daily in normal subjects, but in reality it has proved very difficult to measure these.[2]

It has often been debated whether, in disease states, expectoration is due to excessive mucus production, or to poor clearance. In most diseases, however, the excess secretions which are brought up by expectoration are produced by a combination of factors. Thus for example, in cystic fibrosis, excessive sodium absorption may reduce the salt content of the airways surface liquid. This increases mucus viscoelasticity and decreases ciliary motility. In addition,

Table 24.1 Specific disease-related therapy for expectoration

Underlying diagnosis	Specific therapy for expectoration
Bronchiectasis	Antibiotics Intermittent Continuous, (dependent on bacteria sensitivities) or non-specific (e.g. high-dose amoxycillin or amoxycillin with probenecid)
Cystic fibrosis	rhDNAse
Asthma, eosinophilic bronchitis, and chronic obstructive pulmonary disease	Corticosteroids (inhaled or oral) Bronchodilators
Alveolar cell carcinoma	Macrolides, resection, lung transplantation

colonization of the airways by bacteria causes inflammation and abnormal secreted mucins which further impair mucociliary clearance. Release of pro-inflammatory cytokines such as TNFα and the interleukins IL-1β, IL-8, and IL-6 enhance macrophage activity, giving rise to a cycle of lung damage and repair.[3] This causes mechanical obstruction of mucociliary clearance, pooling of mucus, and further inflammation. Thus, a combination of poor clearance and increased mucus production combine to produce excessive mucus needing expectoration. Clearly, therapy can be directed at either the production of mucus or its clearance or both.

Clinical approach to expectorant therapy

Measurement

In many studies of cough and expectoration the endpoints chosen to demonstrate efficacy are difficult to translate into clinical practice. Tracheobronchial clearance as measured by gamma camera studies has been recommended as the gold standard for assessing mucoactive agents,[4] but studies using this method do not accurately assess small airways and are unable to examine the effect of agents on mucus production as opposed to clearance. Measurement of sputum volume is similarly difficult to interpret. A decrease in expectorated volume may indicated clinical improvement, but many patients claim that their inability to expectorate thickened secretions is a major cause of morbidity because of excessive and ineffective coughing. Measures of lung function such as FEV_1 may provide useful information. Exacerbations of airway disease like asthma are characterized by a fall in FEV_1, and it is hypothesized that the improvement in FEV_1 seen in studies of diseases characterized by less reversible airflow obstruction such as COPD and cystic fibrosis are due to reduced mucus secretion. However, simply using spirometry as a measure of the success of expectoration treatment may give false positive results when bronchodilators are used. Although they look at the whole patient and are not focused specifically on expectoration, the two most useful methods of clinical assessment in chronic airflow obstruction are probably quality of life and exacerbation rate. Simple questionnaires can be used to evaluate quality of life in expectoration.[5,6] In the ISOLDE study[7] of inhaled steroids in severe COPD, the St George's Questionnaire demonstrated clinically useful improvements in quality of life which were associated with a reduction in exacerbation rate. Unfortunately very few studies in expectoration provide us with such large numbers of patients, and much of the evidence concerning therapy is of poor quality.

Mucolytic agents

The lysis of pathologically thickened mucus in order to aid expectoration has been attempted by two strategies, each directed at combating the underling pathological processes causing this increased sputum viscosity. Firstly, the abnormal mucins released during airways inflammation can be targeted by preventing cysteine bridging between their glycoprotein molecules, by using sulfydryl moieties. *In vitro*, agents such as acetylcysteine reduce sputum viscosity.[8] However the therapeutic effects of such drugs are debated. There is a marked difference between practice in the UK and North America and that in continental Europe where these agents are widely pre-scribed. Anglophone practice has been influenced by two studies showing no demonstrable effect of oral *N*-acetylcysteine and *S*-carboxymethylcysteine on mucociliary clearance.[9,10] In contrast, European studies using clinical endpoints have pointed to the successful use of sulfydryl mucolytic therapy.[11,12] Oral acetylcysteine reduces the exacerbation rate in chronic bronchitis, reduces days of illness, and has been claimed to improve well-being.[13] Bacterial flora may also be influenced. Can such opposite views of this therapy be reconciled? If oral sulfydryl mucolytic therapy is effective, then perhaps it is not working by an action on mucolysis. These agents are antioxidant and it has been hypothesized that there is a reduction in oxidant stress to the airways. However, it is hard to see how the relatively small quantities of these drugs used in clinical practice (as opposed to *in vitro* studies) could influence the redox status of the lung, particularly when they have undergone first-pass metabolism within the liver. Indeed, oral *N*-acetylcysteine was found to be undetectable in bronchoalveolar lavage fluid, although in this study levels of glutathione, the major determinant of cellular redox state,[14] were altered by therapy. In practice uncertainty remains as to whether this class of mucolytic is clinically effec-tive in expectoration.

The alternate strategy for mucolysis is to disrupt the tangled mesh of DNA derived from dead bacteria and leukocytes. *In vitro*, enzymatic degradation of DNA is a highly effective means of reducing sputum viscosity. Clinical treatment with DNase has a surprisingly long history in airways disease, although the initial use of relatively crude extracts of the bovine enzyme fell out of favour in the late 1960s following a report of hypersensitivity reactions. The advent of human recombinant (hr) DNase produced a renascence of interest in DNase as a mucolytic. Its use has been associated with modest improvements in spirometry and a reduced rate of exacerbations in cystic fibrosis (see Chapter 25).[15] In exacerbations of chronic obstructive pulmonary disease, DNase has not been a success. A multinational study of DNase following admission to hospital with a COPD exacerbation was abandoned because of increased mortality in the active treatment arm. Surprisingly, the results of this study have never been published in full.[16]

In certain circumstances mucolytic therapy might be used in a different way. Patients pre-senting with mucus plugging leading to distal segmented or lobar collapse have been treated with acetylcysteine or hrDNase instilled through the fibreoptic bronchoscope, and the col-lapsed lobe/segment subsequently reexpands. Although it is logical, this therapy has not been subjected to randomized controlled study and it could be difficult to differentiate any mucolytic effects from the effects of the procedure itself, including suction and saline injection.

Secretagogues

The hypothesis that expectoration will be eased by increasing the volume and liquidity of secre-tions is attractive. However, evidence for clinical benefit from the group of substances classed in pharmacopoeias as secretagogues is tenuous. They are mainly compounds that have been used as emetics in previous times. Presumably agents that were capable of inducing emesis were considered capable increasing output from other organs! Guaifenesin, bromhexine, iodide, ipecacuanha, and ammonium chloride have all been used and have remained in the national formularies of many countries, particularly as part of combination over-the-counter cough remedies. Of these agents guaifenesin[17] has been shown to increase mucus secretion in animals, but clinical evidence, mainly in chronic bronchitis, is either of poor quality or negative.[18–20]

Mucokinetic agents

The ideal palliative therapy for intractable expectoration would increase the rate of ciliary mucus transport to enable the patient to clear secretions before bronchial obstruction, infection and inflammation supervenes. Two methods of achieving this therapeutic goal can be envisaged. Either the properties of the mucus itself can be altered to enable more rapid transport or the mucociliary escalator can be stimulated to enhance tracheobronchial clearance. The latter possibility is discussed in the subsequent sections.

Water and saline

Inhalations of water, steam, and saline have been used for centuries to promote expectoration. Most modern interest has centred on the use of hypertonic saline. Even in healthy subjects inhalation of 4–7% saline causes expectoration, and such 'induced' sputum may be used for diagnostic and research purposes. In cystic fibrosis we have used hypertonic saline to induce sputum in patients who are unable or unwilling to provide bacteriological samples (Box 24.1).

Box 24.1 Protocol for sputum induction in patients with airways disease

1 Perform baseline FEV_1/FVC

2 Administer 200 μg salbutamol (by handheld inhaler)

3 Repeat spirometry after 10 min. If $FEV_1 < 60\%$ predicted, check with supervising doctor before proceeding.

4 Give 5 mL 3% saline via a nebulizer with output set at 0.9 mL/min. Instruct the patient to discontinue inhalations if troublesome symptoms develop.*

5 After 5 min, discontinue inhalations, measure FEV_1, ask patient to blow nose and rinse out mouth with water.

6 Patient should then cough sputum into a sterile container.

7 Repeat steps 4–6 with 4% and 5% saline if sputum induction is not successful

8 If after nebulization FEV_1 has fallen by >20%, discontinue sputum induction. If FEV_1 has fallen by <20%, repeat the previous saline inhalation. Do not increase the concentration.

*Note: In step 4, only the FEV_1 is needed if the aim is expectoration rather than the collection of uncontaminated specimens.

The main problem with routine clinical use is the propensity for bronchoconstriction in patients with reactive airways. Pretreatment with bronchodilators will prevent this. Regular treatment with hypertonic saline in cystic fibrosis has been shown to improve FEV_1 when compared with isotonic saline.[21] It is interesting to speculate whether this therapeutic effect has any specific link to the proposed pathophysiological defect in cystic fibrosis, namely an alteration in chloride handling in the airways surface liquid.

The use of isotonic saline and water as expectorants is widespread, either in the form of nebulized solutions or as steam inhalations. In contrast to hypertonic saline the evidence for efficacy of these treatments is poor although a single study has reported benefit when combined with physiotherapy in cystic fibrosis.[22]

β-Agonists and other bronchodilators

The use of nebulized β-agonists to aid expectoration has some rational basis. β-Agonists have been shown to stimulate ciliary beat frequency *in vitro* and some studies *in vivo* have shown effects on mucociliary transport.[23] However, in patients with chest disease as opposed to normal subjects the effects of β-agonists are of doubtful clinical significance.[24] Ipratropium bromide has no effect on mucociliary clearance.[25]

Despite the poor scientific base for the use of bronchodilators as expectorants, they are widely prescribed. Patients with respiratory failure from obstructive pulmonary disease frequently comment that the nebulizers aid expectoration. Whether this is due to any real effect of the β-agonist on mucociliary clearance or, due to the combined bronchodilation and pro-expectorant effect of the co-administered saline is unknown (and very difficult to measure). It is my own practice to offer patients a trial of nebulized saline or bronchodilator and to continue therapy with the preferred substance. If saline is chosen it is cheaper, and does not have side effects such as tremor and the possibility of hypoxemia secondary to alterations in ventilation–perfusion matching after β-agonists.

Triphosphate nucleotides

The use of nucleotides such as uridine-5′-triphosphate has been popularized by studies from Boucher and Knowles. They have demonstrated increased whole-lung clearance in cystic fibrosis and primary ciliary dyskinesia.[26] These agents work both by increasing non-CFTR chloride channel secretion and by stimulation of ciliary beat frequency.[27,28] However, they are not available in the pharmacopoeias of most countries because they are at present unlicensed.

Anticholinergics

The anticholinergic drugs act by blocking muscarinic receptors both on airway smooth muscle and (preganglionically) on airway nerves. Because there is intrinsic cholinergic tone in the airways, particularly in chronic pulmonary disease, these agents are effective bronchodilators, but their effect on expectoration is variable. Tertiary ammonium compounds such as atropine and hyoscine are claimed to reduce bronchial gland secretion, although no change in sputum viscosity is seen.[29] A number of studies have demonstrated a decrease in mucociliary transport with tertiary ammonium compounds given systemically to normal subjects.[30–32] In patients with airflow obstruction, by contrast, a considerable body of evidence suggests either no effect or an increase in mucociliary clearance with quaternary ammonium compounds.[33–35] No effect on sputum rheology is seen in chronic bronchitis.[25]

The contrasting effects on mucociliary clearance seen with the two classes of antimuscarinic agents are difficult to explain. There are minor differences in non-muscarinic receptor binding (the quaternary compounds having a slightly greater affinity for the nicotinic receptor), but these are insufficient to explain the observed disparity. Differing penetration of the compounds in the respiratory tract has been suggested, and indeed the quaternary compounds have been designed to have poor penetration in order to prevent systemic effects. However, both types of compound are effective bronchodilators and so must reach airway smooth muscle receptors. Whatever the explanation, the differential effects can be exploited clinically. If bronchodilation alone is required, then quaternary compounds should be used (e.g. ipratropium bromide, oxitropium bromide). If suppression of mucus secretion is an additional objective, then systemic tertiary ammonium compounds (hyoscine, atropine) are the treatment of choice provided the patient can tolerate the inevitable systemic side effects (e.g. dry mouth).

Glycopyrronium is another quaternary ammonium compound that may offer special advantages for controlling mucus secretion in the advanced stages of disease.[36] It has good antisecretory properties but fewer central nervous system side effects than hyoscine, which make it useful for reducing respiratory mucus or oropharyngeal secretions in terminally ill patients. By subcutaneous infusion it may be helpful for controlling 'death rattle', which can be very distressing for relatives to hear.

Physiotherapy for expectoration

Autogenic drainage

Unlike conventional physiotherapy, autogenic drainage is specifically designed to aid expectoration in a fashion eminently suitable for supportive care. The technique was devised by the Belgian physiotherapist Jean Chevallier and uses inspiration at increasing lung volumes to collect and then expectorate mucus.[37]

It consists of three phases: unstick, collect, and evacuate. Patients begin diaphragmatic breathing at low lung volume. Inspiration is slow and initially terminates with a pause at the end of tidal respiration. Forced expiration is the performed with an open glottis down to expiratory reserve volume. As secretions begin to move the patient is encouraged to breathe at medium and then high lung volumes. When the patient has completed breathing at near total lung capacity and the secretions are felt to have progressed as far as possible, they are asked to expectorate. Coughing is suppressed during the performance of autogenic drainage and the technique is described as physically undemanding and is therefore highly applicable to debilitated patients. Patient cooperation is required, and it may be difficult to teach in children. Ideally a physiotherapist skilled in the technique and trained in its application should be used to initiate treatment.

Studies of autogenic drainage have compared it with conventional physiotherapy such as active cycle of breathing (ACBT). In the largest randomized study in cystic fibrosis, Miller et al.[38] found that autogenic drainage cleared mucus faster than ACBT and that both methods improved ventilation and pulmonary function.

Conclusions

The most effective therapy for expectoration is aimed at the underlying pathophysiological process. If specific therapy is impossible or unhelpful then measures to aid expectoration directly by a combination of pharmacological and physical means can produce clinical benefit. Because the literature supporting the use of individual agents is in general of poor quality and often with conflicting conclusions, individual therapeutic trials should be undertaken to maximize patient benefit. A suggested expectoration care pathway is shown in Figure 24.1.

Suppression of expectoration (as opposed to unproductive cough) is rarely required outside advanced incurable disease. Tertiary ammonium compounds (e.g. hyoscine) are the most useful drugs then.

Methods of affecting mucus production are summarized in Table 24.2.

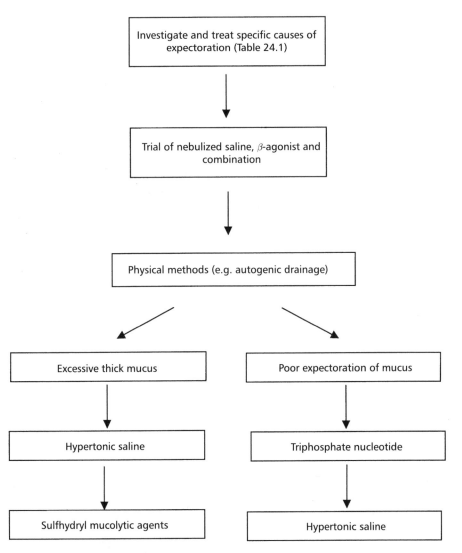

Fig. 24.1 Expectoration care pathway.

Table 24.2 Methods affecting trachobronchial mucus

Increasing mucus production	
Sulfydryl donors (e.g. acetylcysteine)	Debatable
Secretagogues (e.g. guaifenesin)	Weak effect
Increasing mucus clearance	
rhDNase	Effective (CF)
Hypertonic saline	Occasionally useful
Steam/normal saline inhalations	Debatable
Inhaled B agonist	Debatable
Triphosphate nucleotides	Effective? not widely available
Physiotherapy (autogenic drainage)	Effective
Reducing mucus production	
Treat underlying disease	Effective
Tertiary ammonium compounds (e.g. hyoscine)	Effective

Keypoints

♦ Treatment to promote expectoration aims to increase tracheobronchial mucus production, or its clearance, or both

♦ There is no satisfactory method of measuring the effectiveness of expectorants in clinical practice

♦ Proprietary expectorants have not been shown to aid expectoration significantly

♦ Nebulized hypertonic saline (4–7%) is a secretagogue, but normal saline or water is not

♦ Autogenic drainage (huffing) is a physiotherapy technique for aiding in expectoration, and may be particularly suitable for ill patients in the supportive care setting

♦ The most effective strategy for reducing symptoms due to excess sputum production is to treat the underlying disease wherever possible

♦ The anticholinergic tertiary ammonium compounds (e.g. hyoscine) reduce bronchial gland secretion

References

1 Lucas, A.M., and Douglas, M.J. Principles underlying ciliary activity in the respiratory tract. *Arch Otolaryngol* 1934; **20**: 518–41.

2 Rogers, D.F. Airway goblet cells – responsive and adaptable front-line defenders. *Eur Respir J* 1994; **7**: 1690–706.

3 Bonfield, T.L., Panuska, J.R., Konstan, M.W., *et al*. Inflammatory cytokines in cystic-fibrosis lungs. *Am J Respir Crit Care Med* 1995; **152**: 2111–18.

4 Wills, P.J., and Cole, P.J. Mucolytic and mucokinetic therapy. *Pulm Pharmacol Ther* 1996; **9**: 197–204.

5 Curtis, J.R., Deyo, R.A., and Hudson, L.D. Health-related quality-of-life among patients with chronic obstructive pulmonary-disease. *Thorax* 1994; **49**: 162–70.

6 Hansen, N.C.G., Skriver, A., Brorsenriis, L., *et al*. Orally-administered *N*-acetylcysteine may improve general well-being in patients with mild chronic bronchitis. *Respir Med* 1994; **88**: 531–5.

7 Burge, P.S. EUROSCOP, ISOLDE and the Copenhagen City Lung Study. *Thorax* 1999; **54**: 287–8.

8   Scheffner, A.L., Medler, E.M., Jacobs, L.W., and Sarett, H.P. The in vitro reduction in viscosity of human tracheobronchial secretions by acetylcysteine. *Am Rev Respir Dis* 1964; **90**: 721–9.

9   Millar, A.B., Pavia, D., Agnew, J.E., *et al.* Oral *N*-acetylcysteine has no demonstrable effect on mucus clearances in chronic bronchitis. *Thorax* 1984; **39**: 238.

10 Thomson, M.L., Pavia, D., Jones, C.J., and McQuiston, T.A.C. No demonstrable effect of *S*-carboxymethylcysteine on clearance of secretions from the human lung. *Thorax* 1975; **30**: 669–73.

11 Boman, G., Backer, U., Larsson, S., Melander, B., and Wahlander, L. Oral acetylcysteine reduces exacerbation rate in chronic bronchitis – report of a trial organized by the Swedish society for pulmonary diseases. *Eur J Respir Dis* 1983; **64**: 405–15.

12 Rasmussen, J.B., and Glennow, C. Reduction in days of illness after long-term treatment with *N*-acetylcysteine controlled-release tablets in patients with chronic bronchitis. *Eur Respir J* 1988; **1**: 351–5.

13 Grassi, C. Long-term oral acetylcysteine in chronic bronchitis. A double-blind controlled study. *Eur J Respir Dis* 1980; **61**: 93–108.

14 Bridgeman, M.M.E., Marsden, M., Macnee, W., Flenley, D.C., and Ryle, A.P. Cysteine and glutathione concentrations in plasma and bronchoalveolar lavage fluid after treatment with N-acetylcysteine. *Thorax* 1991; **46**: 39–42.

15 Fuchs, H.J., Borowitz, D.S., Christiansen, D.H., *et al.* Effect of aerosolized recombinant human DNase on exacerbations of respiratory symptoms and on pulmonary function in patients with cystic fibrosis. *N Engl J Med* 1994; **331**: 637–42.

16 Anonymous. Pulmonzyme disappoints in COPD. *Script* 1995; **16**: 2043.

17 Perry, W.F., and Boyd, E.M. Method for studying expectorant action in animals by direct measurement of the respiratory tract fluids. *J Pharmac Exp Ther* 1941; **73**: 65–77.

18 Anonymous. Guaiphenesin and iodide. *Drug Ther Bull* 1985; **23**: 62–4.

19 Anonymous. A controlled trial of the effects of bromhexine on the symptoms of out-patients with chronic bronchitis. *Br J Dis Chest* 1973; **67**: 49–60.

20 Guyatt, G.H. A controlled trial of ambroxol in chronic bronchitis. *Chest* 1987; **92**: 618–20.

21 Eng, P.A., Morton, J., Douglass, J.A., *et al.* Short-term efficacy of ultrasonically nebulized hypertonic saline in cystic fibrosis. *Pediatr Pulmonol* 1996; **21**: 77–83.

22 Conway, J.H., Fleming, J.S., Perring, S., and Holgate, S.T. Humidification as an adjunct to chest physiotherapy in aiding tracheobronchial clearance in patients with bronchiectasis. *Respir Med* 1992; **86**: 109–14.

24 Mortensen, J., Hansen, A., Falk, M., Nielsen, I.K., and Groth, S. Reduced effect of inhaled beta 2-adrenergic agonists on lung mucociliary clearance in patients with cystic fibrosis. *Chest* 1993; **103**: 805–11.

23 Wong, L.B., Miller, I.F., and Yeates, D.B. Stimulation of ciliary beat frequency by autonomic agonists – invivo. *J Appl Physiol* 1988; **65**: 971–81.

25 Taylor, R.G., Pavia, D., Agnew, J.E., et al. Effect of 4 weeks high-dose ipratropium bromide treatment on lung mucociliary clearance. *Thorax* 1986; **41**: 295–300.

26 Noone, P.G., Bennett, W.D., Regnis, J.A., *et al.* Effect of aerosolized uridine-5′-triphosphate on airway clearance with cough in patients with primary ciliary dyskinesia. *Am J Respir Crit Care Med* 1999; **160**: 144–9.

27 Olivier, K.N., Bennett, W.D., Hohneker, K.W., *et al.* Acute safety and effects on mucociliary clearance of aerosolized uridine 5′-triphosphate ± amiloride in normal human adults. *Am J Respir Crit Care Med* 1996; **154**: 217–23.

28 Knowles, M.R., Clarke, L.L., and Boucher, R.C. Activation by extracellular nucleotides of chloride secretion in the airway epithelia of patients with cystic fibrosis. *N Engl J Med* 1991; **325**: 533–8.

29 Lopez-Vidriero, M.T., Costello, J., Clark, T.J., *et al.* Effect of atropine on sputum production. *Thorax* 1975; **30**: 543–7.

30 Yeates, D.B., Aspin, N., Levison, H., Jones, M.T., and Bryan, A.C. Mucociliary tracheal transport rates in man. *J Appl Physiol* 1975; **39**: 487–95.

31 Foster, W.M., Bergofsky, E.H., Bohning, D.E., *et al.* Effect of adrenergic agents and their mode of action on mucociliary clearance in man. *J Appl Physiol* 1976; **41**: 146–52.

32 Pavia, D., and Thomson, M.L. Inhibition of mucociliary clearance from the human lung by hyoscine. *Lancet* 1971; **i**: 449–50.

33 Pavia, D., Bateman, J.R., Sheahan, N.F., and Clarke, S.W. Effect of ipratropium bromide on mucociliary clearance and pulmonary function in reversible airways obstruction. *Thorax* 1979; **34**: 501–7.

34 Pavia, D., Bateman, J.R., Sheahan, N.F., and Clarke, S.W. Clearance of lung secretions in patients with chronic bronchitis: effect of terbutaline and ipratropium bromide aerosols. *Eur J Respir Dis* 1980; **61**: 245–53.

35 Bell, J.A., Bluestein, B.M., Danta, I., and Wanner, A. Effect of inhaled ipratropium bromide on tracheal mucociliary transport in bronchial asthma. *Mt Sinai J Med* 1984; **51**: 215–17.

36 Mirakhur, R.K., and Dundee, J.W. Glycopyrrolate: pharmacology and clinical use. *Anaesthesia* 1983; **38**(11): 95–204.

37 Schoni, M.H. Autogenic drainage – a modern approach to physiotherapy in cystic fibrosis. *J R Soc Med* 1989; **82**: 32–7.

38 Miller, S., Hall, D.O., Clayton, C.B., and Nelson, R. Chest physiotherapy in cystic fibrosis – a comparative-study of autogenic drainage and the active cycle of breathing techniques with postural drainage. *Thorax* 1995; **50**: 165–9.

Chapter 25

The management of cystic fibrosis

John W. Wilson and Thomas Kotsimbos

Cystic fibrosis (CF) is a multisystem disorder characterized by chronic airway infection, malnutrition and premature death. It is the most common genetically inherited lethal disorder in white populations, affecting 1 in 2500 births, with a carrier rate of 1 in 25 individuals. The best-characterized genetic abnormality is a phenylalanine substitution at position 508 on chromosome 7 (ΔF508), in the gene which codes for the CF transmembrane regulator protein (CFTR). The CFTR protein facilitates chloride transport at epithelial surfaces and in glands. The resulting abnormalities predominantly affect the respiratory and gastrointestinal tracts, as well as the pancreas.

The major determinant of well-being and longevity is the rate of fall of lung function. It is therefore essential that the aims of therapy in CF are focused on maintenance of good lung function and its determinant factors. In addition, the realization that CF is becoming an adult disease, because of improvements in long-term survival, have identified an essential need to treat long-term factors such as osteoporosis and diabetic microvascular disease in a preventive manner. The treatment plan must therefore incorporate surveillance for complications of CF and its treatment (Table 25.1).

Supportive care in CF

As CF progresses toward respiratory failure and end-organ complications, much can be done to support the patients' needs and improve symptom control. It is as important to be aware of these factors in the management of CF, as it is to optimize lung function, body mass index (BMI) and other quantifiable indices during more stable phases of the disease. The concept of supportive care can be introduced early and will become paramount in the final stages of the illness. This should be borne in mind when reading the following accounts of organ damage and its management.

Respiratory disease

Stable state evaluation and management

Maintenance therapy in CF is aimed at reducing the fall in lung function to below 2% predicted FEV_1 per year, and maintaining BMI (weight in kg/height in m^2) at or above 20 kg/m^2. Ideally, patients should have at least 3-monthly assessment of lung function, BMI, and urinalysis while clinically stable. Each visit involves a medical assessment, and the opportunity to review progress with a physiotherapist, dietitian, and clinic counsellor or social worker. It is likely that survival is enhanced at specialized centres where these facilities are available.[1–3] It is helpful if the CF team meet at least weekly for case management review. If possible, this should include home nurses and a liaison psychiatrist.

Table 25.1 Complications of cystic fibrosis requiring active screening, surveillance or preventive management

Respiratory	Progressive decline in lung function[a]
	Acute exacerbation of airway infection
	Acquisition of resistant airway infections with *Pseudomonas*, *Burkholderia* spp.
	Allergic bronchopulmonary aspergillosis
	Haemoptysis[a]
	Pneumothorax
	Sinus disease and nasal polyposis
	Respiratory failure[a]
	Lung transplantation
Gastroenterological	Reflux oesophagitis
	Peptic ulceration
	Biliary cirrhosis and portal hypertension[a]
	Cholelithiasis
	Pancreatitis
	Meconium ileus equivalent
	Colonic strictures
Nutritional[a]	Voluntary calorie restriction
	Malabsorption
	Maldigestion
	Fat-soluble vitamin malabsortion
Endocrinological	Diabetes mellitus
	Hypogonadism
	Male infertility
	Female infertility
Renal	Renal calculi (oxalate)
	Renal impairment (aminoglycosides, diabetes mellitus)
Rheumatological	Seronegative arthropathy
	Osteoporosis
	Stress fractures
Haematological	Iron deficiency
	Anaemia
	Coagulopathy (vitamin K deficiency, liver disease)
	Hypersplenism (portal hypertension)
	Amyloidosis
Psychosocial[a]	Delayed maturation and adulthood
	Work disability and sick role behaviour
	Identity transition to adulthood
	Response to CF team management
	Depression
	Terminal illness support
Iatrogenic	Venous occlusion (antibiotic therapy)
	Hearing impairment (aminoglycosides)
	Hypercortisonism (oral steroids)
	Genital candidiasis (antibiotics)
	Tendonitis (fluoroquinolonnes)

Table 25.1 (continued)

Terminal care[a]	Dyspnoea and cough
	Airway secretions
	Hypoxaemia and hypercarbia
	Sleep disturbance
	Muscle de-conditioning
	Depression and anxiety
	Family reaction
	Staff reaction

[a] Items that may have a particular requirement for a supportive care approach in advanced disease.

Over 97% of CF patients have lung disease.[4] All patients should be aware of the value of chest physiotherapy in reducing the rate of decline of lung function and its benefits in acute deterioration.[5,6] Several techniques are available, including postural drainage, mechanical percussion, and active breathing techniques. In addition, positive expiratory pressure (PEP) masks may provide the same benefit.[7] Aerobic exercise ability has been correlated with improved survival in cystic fibrosis,[8] but it does not correlate well with lung function assessed by spirometry or other easily measured physiological variables.[9] Although regular exercise maintains muscle tone and exercise, it is important to avoid prolonged desaturation during exercise resulting from airflow obstruction (often responsive to supplemental oxygen) or intrapulmonary shunting (not responsive to supplemental oxygen). A laboratory exercise trial with and without added oxygen will allow the prescription of safe exercise and enable the estimation of correct oxygen flow rates.[10–12] It is important to assess the patient's lifestyle needs in determining goals for physiotherapy and exercise, as many adults will have difficulty achieving unrealistic goals.[13]

Nutritional needs in CF are increased because of an increased resting energy expenditure, maldigestion, and malabsorption. To maintain normal weight, most patients require 20–50% more energy intake than a normal individual, although few are able to maintain this level of intake.[14,15] Where there has been a consistent fall in BMI, a cause should be sought. Specific causes include

- poorly controlled, deteriorating lung function
- inadequate pancreatic enzyme supplementation
- the onset of diabetes mellitus
- inadequate protein–calorie intake
- lifestyle or body image factors
- depression.

Patients with CF should receive an annual influenza vaccination and avoid passive exposure to cigarette smoke.[16] All adults with abnormal lung function in CF will at some time have positive sputum culture with either *Pseudomonas aeruginosa*, *Staphylococcus aureus*, or *Haemophilus influenzae*.[17,18] Most patients in adult life are colonized with *P. aeruginosa* and the objective of therapy is to suppress this organism. Survival in CF has increased because of improved use of antibiotic therapy for *S. aureus* and *P. aeruginosa*.[19–22] There is evidence that long-term suppressive therapy may improve outcome and reduce exacerbation rates with *S. aureus*.[23,24] The situation with *P. aeruginosa* is less clear; where resistance is more common,[25] inducible resistance may occur[26] and response in more severe disease may be reduced.[19] In many patients with *P. aeruginosa* combined treatment with high-dose inhaled tobramycin may be more effective and is recommended to reduce resistance.[27–29] A mean improvement of 12% after 4 weeks treatment with 600 mg three times daily was not sustained when given intermittently over 6 months, and was associated with an initial fall and later rise in numbers of *Pseudomonas* organisms in sputum.[29]

The increased cellular content of airway secretions in CF and the formation of DNA protein fibrils in sputum contribute to increased viscosity.[30] Recombinant human deoxyribonuclease (rhDNase) has been developed specifically to be delivered by inhalation to cleave free DNA, causing mucolysis[31] (see Chapter 24). A 6-month study of multiple doses found that an initial improvement in FEV_1 of 10%, falling to 5% by the end of the study.[32] This study suggested, too, that continuous use might lead to a reduction in the risk of pulmonary exacerbations of CF. A further study, using once-daily treatment in more advanced disease over 12 weeks, found no significant decline in efficacy.[33] There seems to be a spectrum of responsiveness to rhDNase therapy, which can be detected by a 1-month trial. Should this not lead to an improvement of 10% over baseline FEV_1 after 1 month, treatment should be discontinued. Hypertonic saline may be useful as an alternative to other mucolytic therapy.[34]

Many patients with CF show bronchodilator reversibility.[35,36] Nebulized bronchodilators are most helpful prior to chest physiotherapy during acute exacerbations and in those with a proven asthmatic component. The response to β-agonists is variable, and should be determined before therapy to ensure a satisfactory response.[37,38] Some patients may indeed maintain a continued improvement over a long period.[39] There seems to be no clear correlation between responsiveness to either β-agonists or anticholinergic agents, and their combined action may be better than that of each agent alone.[40]

Acute exacerbations

Although a flare of airway infection may be caused by a viral upper respiratory tract infection or infection with atypical organisms, the local bacterial population in the airways is quick to take advantage of any reduction in host defence associated with such events. Knowledge of the dominant organism and previous responsiveness to therapy is therefore important for treatment. For most patients with *P. aeruginosa* infection, a switch to oral ciprofloxacin and the addition of or increase in the dose of inhaled tobramycin may avoid hospital admission. Oral ciprofloxacin may be as effective as intravenous treatment.[41] Precipitating factors including viral infection, gastrooesophageal reflux, and psychological stress should be identified and managed appropriately. It is most helpful to develop a prospective plan and provide patients with supplies of antibiotics and contact details for home nurses in the event of an exacerbation. Although home intravenous antibiotic therapy may be effective, its use is best restricted to selected patients who have had an initial period of management in hospital during an exacerbation.[42]

Acute exacerbations requiring admission to hospital

Pulmonary exacerbations associated with increased sputum production and viscosity, dyspnoea, reduced lung function, temperature, and weight loss may be best managed with high-dose intravenous antibiotics in hospital. The improvement in clinical status and lung function is associated with a fall in sputum content of *P. aeruginosa*.[43] Optimal treatment of a respiratory exacerbation with *P. aeruginosa* infection should include a combination of an antipseudomonal β-lactam antibiotic, together with an aminoglcyoside. Although no clear evidence exists to indicate which of these combinations is most effective, individual patient response to previous therapy is a most useful predictor. Indeed, there is little evidence demonstrating superiority of any specific combination.[18] Two antibiotics are required to reduce the likelihood of resistance.[44] A common combination involves ceftazadime (6 g per day) in two or three divided doses, with tobramycin (10 mg/kg) in one or two doses, depending on levels.[45,46]

The aims of treatment are therefore to

◆ reduce cough and sputum production and systemic symptoms

◆ improve lung function as close as possible to pre-admission levels

◆ restore nutritional indices to pre-admission levels.

Antibiotics should be given by a long-line or implanted venous device,[47] and should continue for 10–14 days.[18] The decision to insert an implantable venous access device must be made only after other options become unsuitable, because the device may become infected and need to be removed.[48] An admission to hospital is an ideal opportunity for the CF team to conduct a detailed case review to consider supportive care, and an agreed action plan should be developed to facilitate management of future exacerbations.

It is essential to provide isolation facilities for patients with methicillin-resistant *S. aureus* (MRSA), *Burkholderia cepacia*, and highly resistant *Pseudomonas* infections. Patients with these infections should be advised appropriately regarding the risk of transmission to others both within the ward environment and in the social setting. In particular, isolation practices should be observed for these patients in any common group setting, such as physiotherapy sessions.

Progressive deterioration

Where the rate of decline of FEV_1 falls away from a projected path, specific causes should be sought. These include:

◆ poor adherence to agreed treatment plans

◆ acquisition of a new or resistant organism (bacterial, fungal, or mycobacterial)

◆ onset or reactivation of allergic bronchopulmonary aspergillosis (ABPA)

◆ onset or exacerbation of aspiration pneumonitis associated with gastrooesophageal reflux

◆ associated airway conditions including asthma or airway plugging, collapse and abscess formation

◆ onset of associated cardiovascular conditions including cor pulmonale, pulmonary hypertension, left ventricular failure.

In many cases, particularly in women, there may be a preterminal drop in lung function without apparent cause. The acquisition of a new organism with a different spectrum of sensitivity, including *B. cepacia* or MRSA, should always be considered.

Burkholderia cepacia

Opinions regarding the specific management of *B. cepacia* are dependent on experience in local settings.[17,18] Significant advances in the understanding of the taxonomy of the organisms known as *B. cepacia* complex indicates a range of transmissibility and virulence.[49,50] Although infection rates are generally higher in adult than paediatric centres and resistance to standard antipseudomonal antibiotics is generally greater, evidence of increased mortality and morbidity occurs in specific subtypes (genomovars I, III, IV)[50,51] in those that have acquired this infection. It is reasonable, however, to institute a single-room isolation policy for hospital management of acute exacerbations and to educate patients regarding the risks of cross-infection in a social environment. Rapid decline in lung function, seen in patients with *B. cepacia* infection, has also been described in those with *P. aeruginosa*.

Allergic bronchopulmonary aspergillosis (ABPA)

Unlike ABPA associated with other conditions such as asthma, CF patients may have bronchiectesis and sputum colonization with *Aspergillus fumigatus* and have bronchiectesis without a classic hypersensitivity response. Up to 50% of CF patients may have *A. fumigatus* in their sputum.[52] Many also have positive skin tests and specific IgE. In addition, some may have non-atopic local airway reactions. Probable ABPA occurs in approximately 10% of CF patients and is associated with a higher concentration of *A. fumigatus* in the sputum.[53,54] It is likely that ABPA is present when there is increased radiological opacity associated with blood eosinophilia, sputum cultures that contain *Aspergillus* and either a positive skin test or specific RAST to *A. fumigatus* is present (see Figures 25.1 and 25.2). Oral prednisolone should be given

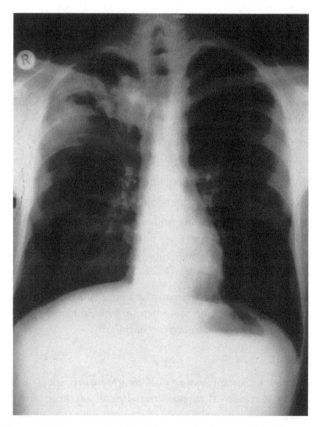

Fig. 25.1 Cystic fibrosis patient with ABPA involving the right upper lobe. The patient had a FEV$_1$ of 82% at the time of the study.

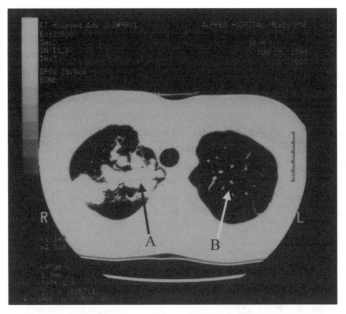

Fig. 25.2 CT scan of the same patient as in Figure 25.1, showing consolidation of the right upper lobe (arrow A) and marked bronchiectasis on the uninvolved, contralateral side (arrow B).

until the IgE falls and radiological opacity clears[55]. In addition, itraconazole 200 mg twice daily may be given. However, eradication of *Aspergillus* is unlikely and long-term effects of this treatment are not yet known[56].

Haemoptysis

Airway bleeding occurs in up to 10% of CF patients and is usually minor, with intermittent episodes of bright bleeding of small volume. Occasionally, massive haemoptysis may occur (>200 mL/24 h). Bleeding is often associated with an exacerbation of infection, microabscess formation, erosion of enlarged bronchial vessels, vitamin K deficiency, biliary cirrhosis, hypersplenism, and antibiotic-associated platelet dysfunction.[57] The importance of airway bleeding can be easily underestimated. Recommendations for radiological intervention have been formulated and include:

* single haemoptysis of over 300 mL within 24 h, associated with ongoing bleeding
* three or more haemoptyses of 100 mL within a week, associated with ongoing bleeding
* chronic, persisting haemoptysis interfering with lifestyle
* haemoptysis preventing other effective therapies, including physiotherapy.[58]

When intervention in required, angiography with embolization of the affected vessel is the treatment of choice.[59] Other options for therapy include pitressin, tranexamic acid, ε-aminocaproic acid, and lobectomy (see Chapter 23). Because of the increased vascularity of the bronchial tree in CF, there are frequently bronchopulmonary anastomoses and aberrant vessels arising from the aorta, intercostal, internal mammary, and subclavian vessels. A diligent search by an experienced radiologist may be required to lateralize and locate the site of the bleeding. Physiotherapy should be continued to remove airway clots and plugs, although vigorous coughing should be discouraged.

Pneumothorax

Pneumothorax is common in CF, and is usually due to rupture of subpleural blebs. It may also occur in association with trauma or insertion of central lines (see Figure 25.3). It occurs in up to 20% of patients and is associated with a poorer outcome.[60,61] Because of the poor compliance of the underlying lung tissue, complications of pneumothorax should be anticipated. Patients should be managed in hospital, with oxygen therapy and intercostal tube drainage where necessary. For a larger pneumothorax, not responding to conservative treatment by tube drainage, or compromising lung function, surgery may be required. Consultation with a surgeon experienced in lung transplantation is recommended, because prior lung surgery may

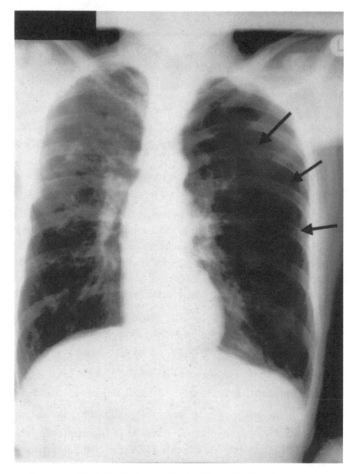

Fig. 25.3 Pneumothorax on the left side in a patient with cystic fibrosis.

cause difficulties with possible future transplantation. Surgical abrasive pleurodesis is recommended where tube drainage with suction has failed.[59]

Respiratory failure

Although FEV_1 is considered the best single predictor of survival in CF, an FEV_1 less than 30% predicted associated with hypoxaemia or hypercarbia (hypercapnia) limits survival to 50% at 2 years.[62] Long-term oxygen therapy (LTOT) has been shown to improve survival in COPD,[63] and this treatment has now been extended to CF. Patients are likely to become hypoxaemic with acute exacerbations during exercise[11] or sleep.[9,64] If chronic hypercarbia occurs, non-invasive positive pressure ventilation may transiently normalize blood gases, but long-term benefits are not proven in CF.[65,66] It is reasonable to recommend domiciliary oxygen where the PaO_2 cannot be maintained above 60 mmHg (8 kPa) after reversible factors have been treated. In addition, where SaO_2 falls more than 4% or below 88% on exercise and there is an improvement of at least 50% in walking distance on supplemental oxygen, it is reasonable to supply oxygen for exercise.

Lung transplantation

Lung transplantation has been an option for the treatment of endstage bronchiectasis and CF for the past decade.[67] Factors to be considered when assessing patients for lung transplantation include

- FEV_1 below 30% predicted after treatment of reversible factors
- quality of life, with four or more admissions to hospital per year for treatment of pulmonary exacerbations
- life-threatening complications including haemoptysis
- other life-threatening co-morbidities including cardiac, renal and hepatic dysfunction.

The assessment of lung function takes into account the rate of decline in lung function and arterial blood gas analysis. The outcome from lung transplantation has gradually improved with an expected survival of 70% at 2 years.[68] Major complications include infection in the early post-transplant period and obliterative bronchiolitis (chronic rejection) in up to 50% of recipients 3 years postoperatively.[69,70] Waiting time for transplantation after listing may be as long as 2 years, depending on size, gender, and blood group. Factors likely to hinder the successful outcome of transplantation include poor pretransplant status, multiply resistant organisms, prior steroid therapy, prior thoracic surgery, and adverse psychosocial factors.

Sinus disease and nasal polyposis

There is evidence of pansinusitis, involving chronic inflammation of paranasal sinuses, on CT scans in almost all CF patients over 1 year of age.[71–73] Often, the ostia draining sinuses become blocked and the frontal sinuses may be hypoplastic or absent. The aetiology of nasal polyposis is unclear. Polyps are more prevalent in younger patients and are rarer in adults.[74] A stepwise approach, involving medical intervention with antibiotics, irrigation, topical decongestants, and corticosteroids is recommended in the first instance.[75] If symptoms persist, surgical intervention is recommended with simple polypectomy for nasal polyps and fibreoptic endoscopic sinus surgery (FESS) for chronic sinusitis. Preoperatively, patients should undergo optimization of lung function with intravenous antibiotics and correction of any coagulopathy.[76] Reoperation rates for polypectomy approach 50% and for sinusitis, may be 100%.[77] Sinuses may act as reservoirs for infection and material removed at the time of drainage should be sent for culture.

Gastrointestinal disease

Gastrooesophageal reflux

Gastro-oesophageal reflux (GER) has been recognized as being common in CF for some time.[78-80] It may occur in 30–50% of patients, and unless associated with distinct features of retrosternal burning, may be easily missed. More recently, it has been recognized that reflux may be a cause of persistent cough.[81] Many factors may contribute to worsening reflux, including smooth muscle relaxants such as β-agonists, 'head down' physiotherapy drainage techniques, and persistent coughing. GER may present in CF patients as persistent cough, retrosternal pain, nutritional decline, or as an exacerbation of respiratory disease. Investigation of suspected reflux should include endoscopy, to exclude the presence of Barrett's oesophagus.[82] A more sensitive test for reflux is 24-h pH monitoring. A range of methods may be effective in treating reflux. Avoidance of provocative factors including prolonged postural drainage and specific foods may be helpful. H2 antagonists may relieve pain. Proton-pump inhibitors may be better in severe oesophagitis.[82] In some patients, reflux may be associated with overt vomiting or progressive lung disease and may require surgical correction. Nissen laparoscopic fundoplication is the treatment of choice, but the long-term outcome may be compromised by persistent coughing.

Biliary cirrhosis and portal hypertension

The findings of postmortem studies[83,84] suggest that it is likely that up to 50% of CF patients have biliary cirrhosis. There may be a degree of selection for survival in those without severe liver disease, given the reduced incidence in older patients. At least 20% of patients have abnormal liver function tests without clinical features; a further 5% will have hepatic cirrhosis and portal hypertension. Oesophageal varices occur in these patients and can be successfully treated by endoscopic sclerotherapy.[85] Abnormal liver function tests will improve with ursodeoxycholic acid (20 mm/kg per day), but evidence of improved liver function is limited.[86-88] Although severe liver disease in CF may require liver transplantation,[89] our experience is that lung transplantation is relatively well tolerated despite poor liver function. The presence of liver disease, suggested by the presence of hepatomegaly, may be as important a prognostic factor for the outcome in CF as lung function and nutritional status.[90]

Cholelithiasis

Gallstones occur in approximately 25% of CF patients,[91] and at least 25% have non-functioning gallbladders.[92] Most stones are of cholesterol origin,[93] although this is not always the case. The presence of gallstones can relatively easily be detected by ultrasonography. When symptomatic, laparoscopic cholecystectomy should be considered, given the serious situation that may arise with impacted stones in the setting of poor lung function.[94]

Pancreatic insufficiency

Both endocrine and exocrine functions of the pancreas are affected in nearly all patients with CF.[17] Reduced pancreatic function may be demonstrated by reduced response after secretin stimulation,[95] steatorrhoea over a 72-h period,[96] or reduced excretion of p-aminobenzoic acid

(PABA) after oral benzyltyrosyl PABA.[97] In adults, pancreatic insufficiency is manifest as weight loss, abdominal discomfort after meals, and offensive low-density bowel motions that are difficult to flush. Fat malabsorption is commonly treated satisfactorily with replacement enzyme preparations. Encapsulated acid-resistant microsphere preparations release enzymes after dosing at the beginning of and during meals. The need for pancreatic enzyme replacement therapy is highly variable. Enzymes may work more effectively at higher pH, which is not easy to ensure in CF because of failure of pancreatic bicarbonate secretion. H2 antagonists may be helpful and in addition, misoprostol, a prostaglandin analogue, may increase bicarbonate secretion.[98] Medium-chain triglycerides have been used to supply dietary fat and may utilize alternate absorption pathways to pancreatic lipase.[99] Although not commonly suspected, pancreatitis may well occur in CF and should be considered as a differential diagnosis in any presentation of abdominal pain.[100]

Colonic strictures

The use of high-lipase-containing pancreatic enzyme replacement therapies has been associated with the presence of colonic strictures in children.[101–103] To date, these lesions have been linked to specific products in localized geographic regions and have not been reported in adults.

Meconium ileus equivalent (MIE)

This condition, also known as **distal intestinal obstruction syndrome** (DIOS) is associated with intestinal obstruction due to inspissated intestinal contents.[104,105] MIE is more common in adults, particularly those on pancreatic enzyme replacement therapy and in those who are dehydrated.[106,107] Often, re-evaluation of dietary intake including fibre content, enzyme therapy,[108] improved hydration, and the use of a laxative may be sufficient to control symptoms. For more severely affected patients, intravenous hydration and the use of oral bowel preparation solutions may be most affective.[109] Although surgical intervention is rarely required, it should be noted that as many as 25% of patients with MIE may have another cause of abdominal pain, including Crohn's disease, volvulus, or appendicitis.

Nutritional factors

Malnutrition is a common feature of CF, at any age. It may arise from reduced food intake, maldigestion of food associated with pancreatic lipase and bicarbonate deficiency, abnormal glucose handling associated with diabetes mellitus, fat-soluble deficiency (vitamins A, D, E, K), and increased energy expenditure. Nutrition may be measured by measuring BMI, which is normally in the range of 20–25. A reduced BMI in CF is associated with reduced survival and poorer lung function. No causative link with ventilatory capacity has yet been described, but improved nutrition may improve respiratory muscle strength, resistance to infection, and exercise tolerance (see Chapter 14). Oral supplements or enteral tube feeding may enable normal weight gain to occur, although the relative advantage of added fat versus lean body weight gain is yet to be determined (see Figure 25.4).

Although poor nutrition in CF is most commonly associated with pancreatic exocrine deficiency, there is often a non-pancreatic component attributable to the reduction of circulating inflammatory factors including TNFα.[110,111]

Because of the difficulty in estimating tissue deficiency from serum levels, fat-soluble vitamins are often prescribed before clinical or biochemical evidence of deficiency becomes apparent. If vitamin deficiencies do occur and cause disease, these can often be corrected by

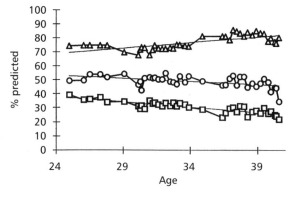

Fig. 25.4 Serial lung function measurements indicate the rate of fall of FEV$_1$ over time. Note percent predicted weight increasing rather than falling with appropriate nutritional supplementation. Triangles, weight (slope 0.79); circles, VC (slope –0.46); squares, FEV$_1$ (slope –0.76).

supplements.[112–114] Vitamin K deficiency is common. Oral supplementation is generally not required unless there is chronic liver disease or a prolonged prothrombin time, or surgical procedures are contemplated.[115]

Endocrine disorders

Diabetes mellitus

Pancreatic destruction in CF generally increases with age. This is reflected in the increasing incidence of diabetes mellitus, with 30% of patients being diabetic by the age of 25.[116,117] The increasing age of the CF population underscores the need for early diagnosis of glucose intolerance and control of microvascular complications including retinopathy and nephropathy[116] as well as increased mortality.[118] There should be no restriction on total energy intake and dietary fat; blood glucose control is best achieved by meal planning, active exercise, and insulin therapy as required. In some instances, patients may be controlled for short periods on oral hypoglycaemic agents.[119]

Osteoporosis

A number of factors have been identified that may contribute to osteoporosis in CF.[120] With the increasing age of patients, long-term complications such as osteoporosis are becoming more evident.[121] The advent of lung transplantation has been associated with accelerated bone loss.[122] Studies in adults with CF have found a mean bone mineral density (BMD) lower by 35% in men and 25% in women compared to controls [123]. In addition, thoracic kyphosis correlates with loss of BMD.[124]

Vitamin D is absorbed with fat, and deficiency may occur with fat malabsorption. Vitamin D levels are reduced in CF[120] and may be improved with the addition of oral vitamin D. Hypercalciuria and osteoporosis may occur if too much vitamin D is given, so replacement should be supervised by an experienced clinician.[125] Calcium absorption in CF is impaired in patients with steatorrhoea and can be improved by the addition of pancreatic enzymes.[126]

Hypogonadism is known to occur in CF[124] and is associated with low BMD. The use of bisphosphonates, well established in the treatment of osteoporosis in postmenopausal women,[127] is not yet well established in CF.[120]

Male infertility

Men with CF are generally considered to be infertile because the vas deferens does not develop normally. The condition of congenital bilateral absence of the vas deferens (CBAVD) is associated with an increased incidence of known CF mutations.[128] Despite distal obstruction, sperm may be produced by the testes and retrieved through an aspiration technique. Successful *in vitro* fertilization (IVF) may occur, resulting in successful pregnancy.[129] Discussion of family planning issues with CF patients must involve partners, an evaluation of their genotype, and a discussion of the risk of CF in the offspring.

Female infertility and pregnancy

Female fertility may be reduced because of thicker cervical mucus[130] or primary and secondary amenorrhoea due to poor lung function and malnutrition.[131]

The longer life expectancy of patients with CF highlights the need to consider family planning at an early stage. There is no increase in fetal loss, although prematurity and perinatal death are more common.[132] With increased survival, the number of women with CF wishing to become pregnant is increasing.[132,133] Pregnancy in CF may have an adverse effect on nutritional status and is likely to result in reduced vital capacity during the last trimester. Often this reduction can be regained *postpartum*, but a decision must be made during family planning discussions as to whether a pregnancy can be safely carried to full term.

Risks during pregnancy include a progressive fall in lung function because of diaphragmatic splinting, nutritional decline because of fetal requirements, increased GER, and poorer blood glucose control. The addition of folic acid supplementation is recommended from the time contraception is ceased. Treatment of any acute exacerbations during pregnancy must take into account the effect on the fetus of medications such as corticosteroids and tobramycin. Although children can be successfully breast-fed by mothers with CF, there is a resultant impact on nutritional status that must be accounted for by increased intake.[134,135] Frequent monitoring and consultation with an obstetrician experienced in CF care can result in high success rates.

Late phase support

Patients with severe respiratory involvement face both physical and psychological stresses that are lifestyle-limiting. Simple activities of daily life may be considerably prolonged and require oxygen. The maintenance of muscle condition requires support from carers and regular assessment by qualified physiotherapists and occupational therapists. Consideration should be given to the quantity and quality of sleep which will maintain a reasonable quality of life. The ability to continue work or education has a significant bearing on self-esteem. Where possible, patients should be supported to continue as long as possible in work and family roles. Frequently, there are difficulties in accepting lifestyle limitations and intervention by a team psychologist or counsellor is often welcomed. It is difficult to judge when the emphasis of care should move from treatment directed at improving prognosis towards supportive care alone. This is made even more difficult for patients on waiting lists for lung transplantation, who may eventually not be transplanted. Anxiety should be managed compassionately with supportive counselling and the judicious use of benzodiazepines. Respiratory distress associated with hypercarbia may benefit from the use of non-invasive ventilation, titrated oxygen, and an experienced physiotherapist.

The wishes of the patient and the attitudes of the family and ward staff are important factors to consider in managing the terminal stages of respiratory failure. It is most important to discuss terminal care with the patient and family, preferably together with the CF team coun-sellor, before the final admission. Concerns that can be dealt with sympathetically in this set-ting include whether a patient wishes to die at home, what sedation will be available, and the likely trajectory of the terminal phase. It is important to recognize that the patient, family members, and staff may all need support during this phase, particularly because of the long time a CF patient may be known to a CF team.

Resources for the CF team

The rapid advances in CF care over the past decade have led to expectations of improved outcome and have outstripped previously acceptable resources. The best outcomes are achieved in specialist centres.[3,4,136] Funding formulae must be accurately constituted to avoid the com-mon pitfall of underestimating the true cost of care[137] and account for patient adherence to treatment plans.[13] The specific attributes of the CF team, the severity of illness in the patient population, and the agreed treatment plans will ultimately determine the cost of care.[138–140]

Key points

- ◆ CF is a multisystem disease and high-quality care needs a team approach
- ◆ Better childhood treatment has led to a large adult population who may have multiple com-plications
- ◆ Management of late disease may be complex and particularly demanding for relatives, carers, and healthcare staff, to whom a patient may have been well known over many years
- ◆ Complications which commonly need a supportive care approach from a relatively early stage include respiratory failure, nutritional depletion, and psychological distress
- ◆ End-of-life planning is important and should not be omitted even if a patient is on a trans-plant list

References

1 Phelan, P., and Hey, E. Cystic fibrosis mortality in England and Wales and in Victoria, Australia 1976–80. *Arch Dis Child* 1984; **59**: 71–3.

2 Walters, S., Britton, J., and Hodson, M. Hospital care for adults with cystic fibrosis: an overview and comparison between special cystic fibrosis clinics and general clinics using a patient questionnaire. *Thorax* 1994; **49**: 300–6.

3 Royal College of Physicians. *Cystic fibrosis in adults: recommendations for care of patients in the United Kingdom.* London: RCP, 1990.

4 Cystic Fibrosis Foundation Patient Registry. *Annual Data Report for 1996.* Bethesda, MD: American Cystic Fibrosis Association, 1997.

5 Reisman, J.J., Rivington-Law, B., Corey, M., *et al.* Role of conventional physiotherapy in cystic fibrosis [see comments]. *J Pediatrics* 1988; **113**: 632–6.

6 Thomas, J., Cook, D.J., Brooks, and D. Chest physical therapy management of patients with cystic fibrosis. A meta-analysis. *Am J Respir Crit Care Med* 1995; **151**: 846–50.

7 McIlwaine, P.M., Wong, L.T., Peacock, D., and Davidson, A.G. Long-term comparative trial of conventional postural drainage and percussion versus positive expiratory pressure physiotherapy in the treatment of cystic fibrosis [see comments]. *J Pediatrics* 1997; **131**: 570–4.

8 Nixon, P.A., Orenstein, D.M., Kelsey, S.F., and Doershuk, C.F. The prognostic value of exercise testing in patients with cystic fibrosis. *N Engl J Med* 1992; **327**: 1785–8.

9 Bradley, S., Wilson, J.W., Solin, P., *et al.* Determinants of respiratory failure during exercise and sleep in cystic fibrosis. *Chest* 1999; **116**: 647–54.

10 Henke, K.G., and Orenstein, D.M. Oxygen saturation during exercise in cystic fibrosis. *Am Rev Respir Dis* 1984; **129**: 708–11.

11 Nixon, P.A., Orenstein, D.M., Curtis, S.E., and Ross, E.A. Oxygen supplementation during exercise in cystic fibrosis. *Am Rev Respir Dis* 1990; **142**: 807–11.

12 Marcus, C.L., Bader, D., Stabile, M.W., *et al.* Supplemental oxygen and exercise performance in patients with cystic fibrosis with severe pulmonary disease [see comments]. *Chest* 1992; **101**: 52–7.

13 Abbott, J., Dodd, M., Bilton, D., and Webb, A.K. Treatment compliance in adults with cystic fibrosis. *Thorax* 1994; **49**: 115–20.

14 Buchdahl, R.M., Fulleylove, C., Marchant, J.L., Warner, J.O., and Brueton, M.J. Energy and nutrient intakes in cystic fibrosis. *Arch Dis Child* 1989; **64**: 373–8.

15 Morrison, J.M., O'Rawe, A., McCracken, K.J., Redmond, A.O.B., and Dodge, J.A. Energy intakes and losses in cystic fibrosis. *J Hum Nutr Diet* 1994; **7**: 39–46.

16 Gilljam, H., Stenlund, D., Ericsson-Hollsing, A., and Strandvik, B. Passive smoking in cystic fibrosis. *Respir Med* 1990; **84**: 298–91.

17 Davis, P.B., Drumm, M., and Konstan, M.W. Cystic fibrosis: State of the art. *Am J Respir Crit Care Med* 1996; **154**: 1229–56.

18 Hodson, G. In: M.E. Hodson, D.M. Geddes (eds) *Cystic fibrosis.* London: Chapman & Hall Medical, 1995.

19 Jensen, T., Pedersen, S.S., Hoiby, N., Koch, C., and Flensborg, E.W. Use of antibiotics in cystic fibrosis. The Danish approach. *Antibiot Chemother* 1989; **42**: 237–246.

20 Stern, R.C., Boat, T.F., Doershuk, C.F., *et al.* Course of cystic fibrosis in 95 patients. *J Pediatr* 1976; **89**: 406–11.

21 Szaff, M., Hoiby, N., and Flensborg, E.W. Frequent antibiotic therapy improves survival of cystic fibrosis patients with chronic *Pseudomonas aeruginosa* infection. *Acta Paediatr Scand* 1983; **72**: 651–7.

22 Ramsey, B.W. Management of pulmonary disease in patients with cystic fibrosis. *N Engl J Med* 1996; **335**: 179–88.

23 Southern, K.W., Littlewood, A.E., and Littlewood, J.M. The prevalence and significance of chronic *Staphylococcus aureus* infection in patients with cystic fibrosis on long term flucloxacillin. In: H. Escobar, C.F. Baquero, and L. Svarez (eds) *Clinical ecology of cystic fibrosis.* Amsterdam: Elsevier Science, 1993; 129–30.

24 Littlewood, J.M., Littlewood, A.E., McLaughlin, S., Shapiro, L., and Connolly, S. 20 years continuous neonatal screening in one hospital; progress of the 37 patients and their families. *Pediatr Pulmonol* 1995; Suppl **12**: 374.

25 Saiman, L., Mehar, F., Niu, W.W., *et al.* Antibiotic susceptibility of multiply resistant *Pseudomonas aeruginosa* isolated from patients with cystic fibrosis, including candidates for transplantation. *Clinl Infect Dis* 1996; **23**: 532–7.

26 Campbell, I.A., Jenkins, J., and Prescott, R.J. Intermittent ciprofloxacin in adults with cystic fibrosis and chronic *Pseudomonas* pulmonary infection. *Med Sci Res* 1989; **17**: 797–8.

27 Steinkamp, G., Tummler, B., Gappa, M., *et al.* Long-term tobramycin aerosol therapy in cystic fibrosis. *Pediatr Pulmonol* 1989; **6**: 91–8.

28 Ramsey, B.W., Dorkin, H.L., Eisenberg, J.D., *et al.* Efficacy of aerosolized tobramycin in patients with cystic fibrosis. *N Engl J Med* 1993; **328**: 1740–6.

29 Ramsey, B.W., Pepe, M.S., Quan, J.M., *et al.* Inntermittent administration of inhaled tobramycin in patients with cystic fibrosis. *N Engl J Med* 1999; **340**: 23–30.

30 Eisenberg, J.D., Aitken, M.L., Dorkin, H.L., *et al.* Safety of repeated intermittent courses of aerosolized recombinant human deoxyribonuclease in patients with cystic fibrosis. *J Pediatrics* 1997; **131**: 118–24.

31 Shak, S., Capon, D.J., Hellmiss, R., Marsters, S.A., and Baker, C.L. Recombinant human DNase I reduces the viscosity of cystic fibrosis sputum. *Proc Nat Acad Sci USA* 1990; **87**: 9188–92.

32 Fuchs, H.J., Borowitz, D.S., Christiansen, D.H., *et al*. Effect of aerosolized recombinant human DNase on exacerbations of respiratory symptoms and on pulmonary function in patients with cystic fibrosis. The Pulmozyme Study Group [see comments]. *N Engl J Med* 1994; **331**: 637–42.

33 McCoy, K., Hamilton, S., and Johnson, C. Effects of 12-week administration of dornase alfa in patients with advanced cystic fibrosis lung disease. Pulmozyme Study Group. *Chest* 1996; **110**: 889–95.

34 Eng, P.A., Morton, J., Douglass, J.A., *et al*. Short-term efficacy of ultrasonically nebulized hypertonic saline in cystic fibrosis. *Pediatr Pulmonol* 1996; **21**: 77–83.

35 Ormerol, L.P., Thomson, R.A., Anderson, C.M., and Stabelforth, D.E. Reversible airway obstruction in cystic fibrosis. *Thorax* 1980; **35**: 768–72.

36 Hordvik, N.L., Konig, P., Morris, D., Kreutz, C., and Barbero, G.J. A longitudinal study of bronchodilator responsiveness in cystic fibrosis. *Am Rev Respir Dis* 1985; **131**: 889–93.

37 Landau, L.I., and Phelan, P.D. The variable effect of a bronchodilating agent on pulmonary function in cystic fibrosis. *J Pediatr* 1973; **82**: 863–8.

38 Zach, M.S., Oberwaldner, B., Forche, G., and Polgar, G. Bronchodilators increase airway instability in cystic fibrosis. *Am Rev Respir Dis* 1985; **131**: 537–43.

39 Konig, P., Gayer, D., Barbero, G.J., and Shaffer, J. Short-term and long-term effects of albuterol aerosol therapy in cystic fibrosis: a preliminary report. *Pediatr Pulmonol* 1995; **20**: 205–14.

40 Sanchez, I., Holbrow, J., and Chernick, V. Acute bronchodilator response to a combination of beta-adrenergic and anticholinergic agents in patients with cystic fibrosis. *J Pediatrics* 1992; **120**: 486–8.

41 Hodson, M.E., Roberts, C.M., Butland, R.J., *et al*. Oral ciprofloxacin compared with conventional intravenous treatment for *Pseudomonas aeruginosa* infection in adults with cystic fibrosis. *Lancet* 1987; **i**: 235–7.

42 Wolter, J.M., Bowler, S.D., Nolan, P.J., and McCormack, J.G. Home intravenous therapy in cystic fibrosis: a prospective randomized trial examining clinical, quality of life and cost aspects. *Eur Respir J* 1997; **10**: 896–900.

43 Smith, A.L. Antibiotic therapy in cystic fibrosis: evaluation of clinical trials. *J Pediatr* 1986; **108**: 866–70.

44 Denton, M., Littlewood, J.M., Brownlee, K.G., Conway, S.P., and Todd, N.J. Spread of β-lactam resistant *Pseudomonas aeruginosa* in a cystic fibrosis unit. *Lancet* 1996; **348**: 1596–7.

45 Conway, S.P. Ceftazidime 3G postop is as effective as ceftazidime 2G t.d.s. in the treatment of respiratory exacerbations in cystic fibrosis. *Israel J Med Sci* 1996; **32**: S256.

46 Whitehead, A., Conway, S.P., and Dave, J. Once daily administration of tobramycin is an effective and safe treatment of acute respiratory exacerbations in adults with cystic fibrosis. *Israel J Med Sci* 1996; **323**: S257.

47 Stead, R.J., Davidson, T.I., Duncan, F.R., *et al*. Use of a totally implantable system for venous access in cystic fibrosis. *Thorax* 1987; **42**: 149–50.

48 Deerojanawong, J., Sawyer, S.M., Fink, A.M., Stokes, K.B., and Robertson, C.F. Totally implantable venous access devices in children with cystic fibrosis: incidence and type of complications. *Thorax* 1998; **53**: 285–9.

49 LiPuma, J.J. *Burkholderia cepacia* epidemiology and pathogenesis: implications for infection control. *Curr Opin Pulm Med* 1998; **4**: 337–41.

50 LiPuma, J.J. *Burkholderia cepacia*. In: S.B. Fiel (ed.) *Clinics in chest medicine*, Vol. 19. Philadelphia: W.B. Saunders, 1998: 473–86.

51 Lewin, L.O., Byard, P.J., and Davis, P.B. Effect of *Pseudomonas cepacia* colonization on survival and pulmonary function of cystic fibrosis patients. *J Clin Epidemiol* 1990; **43**: 125–129.

52 Nelson, L.A., Callerame, M.L., and Schwartz, R.H. Aspergillosis and atopy in cystic fibrosis. *Am Rev Respir Dis* 1979; **120**: 863–73.

53 Hiller, E.J. Pathogenesis and management of aspergillosis in cystic fibrosis. *Arch Dis Child* 1990; **65**: 397–8.

54 Brueton, M.J., Ormerod, L.P., Shah, K.I., and Anderson, C.M. Allergic bronchopulmonary aspergillosis complicating cystic fibrosis in childhood. *Arch Dis Child* 1980; **55**: 348–53.

55 Patterson, R., Greenberger, P.A., and Roberts, M. Allergic bronchopulmonary aspergillosis. *Pediatr Pulmonol* 1992; **8**: 120–2.

56 Denning, D.W., Van Wye, J.E., Lewiston, N.J., and Stevens, D.A. Adjunctive therapy of allergic bronchopulmonary aspergillosis with itraconazole. *Chest* 1991; **100**: 813–19.

57 Wood, R.E. Haemoptysis in cystic fibrosis. *Pediatr Pulmonol* 1992; **8**: 82–4.

58 Cohen, A.M. Haemoptysis – role of angiography and embolisation. *Pediatr Pulmonol* 1992; **8**: 85–6.

59 Schidlow, D.V., Taussig, L.M., and Knowles, M.R. Cystic Fibrosis Foundation consensus conference report on pulmonary complications of cystic fibrosis. *Pediatr Pulmonol* 1993; **15**: 187–98.

60 Penketh, A.R., Knight, R.K., Hodson, M.E., and Batten, J.C. Management of pneumothorax in adults. *Thorax* 1982; **37**: 850–3.

61 Spector, M.L., and Stern, R.C. Pneumothorax in cystic fibrosis: a 26 year experience. *Ann Thorac Surg* 1989; **47**: 204–7.

62 Kerem, E., Reisman, J., Corey, M., Canny, G.J., and Levison, H. Prediction of mortality in patients with cystic fibrosis [see comments]. *N Engl J Med* 1992; **326**: 1187–91.

63 Anon. Continuous or nocturnal oxygen therapy in hypoxemic chronic obstructive lung disease: a clinical trial. Nocturnal Oxygen Therapy Trial Group. *Ann Intern Med* 1980; **93**: 391–8.

64 Tepper, R.S., Skatrud, J.B., and Dempsey, J.A. Ventilation and oxygenation changes during sleep in cystic fibrosis. *Chest* 1983; **84**: 388–93.

65 Gozal, D. Nocturnal ventilatory support in patients with cystic fibrosis: comparison with supplemental oxygen. *Eur Respir J* 1997; **10**: 1999–2003.

66 Cooper, D.M., Piper, A.J., Willson, G., and Sullivan, C.E. Invasive and noninvasive ventilatory assistance in cystic fibrosis. *Pediatr Pulmonol Suppl* 1995; **11**: 72–3.

67 Ramirez, J.C., *et al.* Bilateral lung transplantation for cystic fibrosis. *J Thorac Cardiovasc Surg* 1992; **103**: 287–94.

68 Egan, T., Detterbeck, F., and Mill, M. Improved results of lung transplantation for patients with cystic fibrosis. *J Thorac Cardiovasc Surg* 1995; **109**: 224–235.

69 Madden, B., Hodson, M.E., Tsan, V., *et al.* Intermediate term result of heart-lung transplantation for cystic fibrosis. *Lancet* 1992; **339**: 1583–7.

70 Trulock, E.P. Lung transplantation. *Am J Respir Crit Care Med* 1997; **155**: 790–815.

71 Neely, J.G., Harrison, G.M., Jerger, J.F., Greenberg, S.D., and Presberg, H. The otolaryngologic aspects of cystic fibrosis. *Trans Am Acad Ophthalmol Otolaryngol* 1972; **76**: 313–24.

72 Gharib, R., Joos, H.A., and Hilty, L.B. Sweat chloride concentration; a comparative study in children with bronchial asthma and cystic fibrosis. *Am J Dis Child* 1964; **109**: 66–8.

73 Shwachman, H., Kulczycki, L.L., Mueller, H.L., and Flake, C.G. Nasal polyposis in patients with cystic fibrosis. *Pediatrics* 1962; **30**: 389–401.

74 Stern, R.C., Boat, T.F., Wood, R.E., Matthews, L.W., and Doershuk, C.F. Treatment and prognosis of nasal polyps in cystic fibrosis. *Am J Dis Child* 1982; **136**: 1067–70.

75 Rosenfeld, R.M. Pilot study of outcomes in pediatric rhinosinusitis. *Arch Otolaryngol Head Neck Surg* 1995; **121**: 729–36.

76 Davidson, T.M., Murphy, C., Mitchell, M., Smith, C., and Light, M. Management of chronic sinusitis in cystic fibrosis. *Laryngoscope* 1995; **105**: 354–8.

77 Moss, R.B., and King, V.V. Management of sinusitis in cystic fibrosis by endoscopic surgery and serial antimicrobial lavage. Reduction in recurrence requiring surgery. *Arch Otolaryngol Head Neck Surg* 1995; **121**: 566–72.

78 Feigelsen, J., and Sauvegrain, J. Reflux gastroesophagien dans la mucovisidose. *N Press Med* 1975; **4**: 2729–30.

79 Scott, R.B., O'Loughlin, E.V., and Gall, D.G. Gastroesophageal reflux in patients with cystic fibrosis. *J Pediatr* 1985; **106**: 223–7.

80 Davidson, A.G.F., Wong, L.T.K., and Schoni, M. Gastroesophageal reflux and pulmonary disease in cystic fibrosis patients. *Pediatr Pulmonol Suppl* 1988; **2**: 136.

81 Ing, A.J., Ngu, M.C., and Breslin, A.B. Pathogenesis of chronic cough associated with gastro-esophageal reflux. *Am J Respir Crit Care Med* 1994; **149**: 160–7.

82 Hassall, E., Israel, D.M., Davidson, A.G.F., and Wong, L.T.K. Barrett's esophagus in children with cystic fibrosis: not a coincidental association. *Am J Gastroenterol* 1993; **88**: 1974–8.

83 Oppenheimer, E.H., and Esterley, J.R. Pathology of cystic fibrosis: review of literature and comparison of 146 autopsy cases. *Perspect Pediatr Pathol* 1975; **2**: 241–78.

84 Di Sant Agnese, P.A., and Blanc, W.A. A distinctive type of biliary cirrhosis associated with cystic fibrosis: possible relation to focal biliary cirrhosis. *Paediatrics* 1956; **18**: 387–409.

85 Stringer, M.D., Price, J.F., Mowat, A.P., and Howard, E.R. Liver cirrhosis in cystic fibrosis. *Arch Dis Child* 1993; **69**: 407.

86 Colombo, C., Setchell, K.D.R., Podda, M., *et al.* Effects of ursodeoxycholic acid therapy for liver disease associated with cystic fibrosis. *J Pediatrics* 1990; **117**: 482–9.

87 Colombo, C., Battezatti, P.M., Podda, M., Bettinardi, N., and Giurta, A. UDCA for liver disease associated with cystic fibrosis: a double blind multicentre trial. *Hepatology* 1996; **23**: 1484–90.

88 O'Connor, P.J., Southern, K.W., Bowler, I.M., *et al.* The role of hepatobiliary scintigraphy in cystic fibrosis. *Hepatology* 1996; **23**: 281–7.

89 Noble Jamieson, G., Barnes, N., Jamieson, N., Friend, P., and Caine., R. Liver transplantation for hepatic cirrhosis in cystic fibrosis. *J R Soc Med* 1996; **89**: 31–7.

90 Williams, S., Hayller, K., Hodson, M., and Westaby, D. Prognosis in cystic fibrosis. *N Engl J Med* 1982; **327**: 1244.

91 Roy, C.C., Weber, A.M., McRin, C.C., *et al.* Abnormal biliary lipid composition in cystic fibrosis: effect of pancreatic enzymes. *N Engl J Med* 1977; **297**: 1301–5.

92 Roy, C.C., Weber, A.M., Morin, C.C., *et al.* Hepatobiliary disease in cystic fibrosis: a survey of current issues and concepts. *J Pediatr Gastroenterol Nutr* 1982; **1**: 469–78.

93 Angelico, M., Gandin, C., Canuzzi, P., *et al.* Gallstones in cystic fibrosis: a critical reappraisal. *Hepatology* 1991; **14**: 768–75.

94 Stern, R.C., Rothstein, F.C., and Doershuk, C.F. Treatment and prognosis of symptomatic gallbladder disease in patients with cystic fibrosis. *J Pediatr Gastroenterol Nutr* 1986; **5**: 35–40.

95 Arvanitakis, C., and Cooke, A.R. Diagnostic tests of exocrine pancreatic function and disease. *Gastroenterology* 1978; **74**: 932–48.

96 Goodchild, M.C., and Dodge, J.A. *Cystic fibrosis. Manual of diagnosis and management*, 2nd edn. London: Baillière Tindall, 1989.

97 Puntis, J.W.L., Berg, J.D., and Buckley, B.M. Simplified oral pancreatic function test. *Arch Dis Child* 1988; **63**: 780–4.

98 Robinson, P., and Sly, P.D. Placebo-controlled trial of misoprostol in cystic fibrosis. *J Pediatr Gastroenterol Nutr* 1990; **11**: 37–40.

99 Gracey, M., Bourke, V., and Anderson, C.M. Assessment of medium-chain triglyceridefeeding in infants with cystic fibrosis. *Arch Dis Child* 1969; **44**: 401–403.

100 Shwachman, H., Lebenthal, E., and Khaw, P-T. Recurrent acute pancreatitis in patients with cystic fibrosis with normal pancreatic enzymes. *Pediatrics* 1975; **55**: 86–94.

101 Smyth, R.L., van Velzen, D., Smyth, A.R., Lloyd, D.A., and Heaf, D.P. Strictures of ascending colon in cystic fibrosis and high-strength pancreatic enzymes. *Lancet* 1994; **343**: 85–6.

102 Green, M.R., Southern, K.W., Wolfe, S.P., *et al.* Colonic strictures in children with cystic fibrosis. *Arch Dis Child* 1995; **71**: 191.

103 Sharp, D. High-lipase pancreatin. *Lancet* 1994; **343**: 108.

104 Park, R.W., and Grand, R.J. Gastrointestinal manifestations in cystic fibrosis: a review. *Gastroenterology* 1981; **81**: 1143–61.

105 Jensen, K. Meconium ileus equivalent in a fifteen year old patient with mucoviscidosis. *Acta Paediatr Scand* 1962; **51**: 344–8.

106 Hodson, M.E., Mearns, M.B., and Batten, J.C. Meconium ileus equivalent in adults with cystic fibrosis of the pancreas: a report of six cases. *Br Med J* 1976; **2**: 790–1.

107 Rosenstein, B.J., and Langbaum, T.S. Incidence of distal intestinal obstruction syndrome in cystic fibrosis. *J Paediatr Gastroenterol Nutr* 1983; **2**: 299–301.

108 Rubinstein, S., Moss, R., and Lewiston, N. Constipation and meconium ileus equivalent in patients with cystic fibrosis. *Pediatrics* 1986; **78**: 473–9.

109 Cleghorn, G.J., Stringer, D.A., Forstner, G.G., and Durie, P.R. Treatment of distal intestinal obstruction syndrome in cystic fibrosis with a balanced intestinal lavage solution. *Lancet* 1986; **1**: 8–11.

110 Elborn, J.S., Cordon, S.M., Parker, D., Delamere, F.M., and Shale, D.J. The host inflammatory response prior to death in patients with cystic fibrosis and chronic *Pseudomonas aeruginosa* infection. *Respir Med* 1993; **87**: 603–7.

111 Elborn, J.S., Norman, D., Delamere, F.M., and Shale, D.J. In vitro tumor necrosis factor-alpha secretion by monocytes from patients with cystic fibrosis. *Am J Respir Cell Mol Biol* 1992; **6**: 207–11.

112 Rayner, R.J., Tyrell, J.C., and Hiller, E.J. Night blindness and conjunctival xerosis due to vitamin A deficiency in cystic fibrosis. *Arch Dis Child* 1989; **64**: 1151–6.

113 Stamp, T.C.B., and Gebbes, D.M. Osteoporosis and cystic fibrosis (editorial). *Thorax* 1993; **48**: 585–6.

114 Sitrin, M.D., Leiberman, F., Jensen, W.E., *et al.* Vitamin E deficiency and neurological disease in adults with cystic fibrosis. *Ann Int Med* 1987; **107**: 51–4.

115 Rashid, M., Durie, P., Kalnins, D., *et al.* Prevalence of vitamin K deficiency in children with cystic fibrosis. *Pediatr Pulmonol* 1996; Suppl 13: 313.

116 Laang, S., Thorsteinsson, B., Lund-Andersen, C., *et al.* Diabetes mellitus in Danish cystic fibrosis patients: prevalence and late complications. *Acta Paediatr* 1994; **83**: 72–7.

117 Laang, S., Hansen, A., Thorsteinsson, B., Nerup, J., and Koch, C. Glucose tolerance in patients with cystic fibrosis: five year prospective study. *BMJ* 1995; **311**: 655–9.

118 Finkelstein, S.M., Wielinski, C.L., Elliott, G.R., *et al.* Diabetes mellitus associated with cystic fibrosis. *J Pediatrics* 1988; **112**: 373–7.

119 Culler, F.L., McKean, L.P., Buchanan, C.N., Caplan, D.B., and Meacham, L.R. Glipizide treatment of patients with cystic fibrosis and impaired glucose tolerance. *J Pediatr Gastroenterol Nutr* 1994; **18**: 375–8.

120 Ott, S.M., and Aitken, M.L. Osteoporosis in patients with cystic fibrosis. *Clin Chest Med* 1998; **19**: 555–67.

121 FitzSimmons, S.C. The changing epidemiology of cystic fibrosis. *J Pediatr* 1993; **122**: 1–9.

122 Ferrari, S.L., Nicod, L.P., and Hamacher, J. Osteoporosis in patients undergoing lung transplantation. *Eur Respir J* 1996; **9**: 2378–82.

123 Bachrach, L.K., Loutit, C.W., and Moss, R.B. Osteopenia in adults with cystic fibrosis. *Am J Med* 1994; **96**: 27–34.

124 Aris, R.M., Renner, J.B., Winders, A.D., *et al.* Increased rate of fractures and severe kyphosis: Sequelae of living into adulthood with cystic fibrosis. *Ann Intern Med* 1998; **128**: 186–93.

125 Adams, J.S., and Lee, G. Gains in bone mineral density with resolution of vitamin D intoxication. *Ann Intern Med* 1997; **127**: 203–6.

126 Dingman, S., Lester, G., Aris, R., *et al.* Impaired absorption of dietary calcium by young adults with cystic fibrosis. ASBMR Annual Meeting, 1997.

127 Eastell, R. Treatment of post menopausal osteoporosis. *N Engl J Med* 1998; **338**: 736–46.

128 Chillon, M., Casals, T., Mercer, B., *et al.* Mutations in the cystic fibrosis gene in patients with congenital absence of the vas deferens. *N Engl J Med* 1995; **332**: 1475–80.

129 Schlegel, P.N. Assisted reproductive technologies and sperm aspiration. *Pediatr Pulmonol* 1996; Suppl. 13: 119–120.

130 Kopito, L.E., Kosasky, H.J., and Schwachman, H. Water and elctrolytes in cervical mucus from patients with CF. *Fertil Steril* 1973; **24**: 512–16.

131 Stead, R.J., Hodson, M.E., Batten, J.C., *et al.* Amenorrhoea in cystic fibrosis. *Clin Endocrinol* 1987; **26**: 187–95.

132 Cohen, L.F., Di Sant'Agnese, P.A., and Friedlander, T. Cystic fibrosis and pregnancy: a national survey. *Lancet* 1980; **ii**: 842–4.

133 Geddes, D.M. Cystic fibrosis and pregnancy. *J Roy Soc Med* 1992; **85**: 36–7.

134 Kent, N.E. Cystic fibrosis in pregnancy. *Can Med Assoc J* 1993; 149.

135 Michel, S.H., and Mueller, D.H. Impact of lactation on women with cystic fibrosis and their infants: a review of five cases. *J Am Dietet Assoc* 1994; **94**: 159–65.

136 Walters, S., Britton, J., and Hodson, M.E. Hospital care for adults with c. ystic fibrosis: an overview and comparison between special cystic fibrosis clinics and general clinics using a patient questionnaire [see comments]. *Thorax* 1994; **49**: 300–6.

137 Horn, S.D., Horn, R.A., Sharkey, P.D., *et al.* Misclassification problems in diagnosis-related groups. Cystic fibrosis as an example. *N Engl J Med* 1986; **314**: 484–7.

138 Mahadeva, R., Webb, K., Westerbeek, R.C., *et al.* Clinical outcome in relation to care in centres specialising in cystic fibrosis: cross sectional study. *BMJ* 1998; **316**: 1771–5.

139 Robson, M., Abbott, J., Webb, K., Dodd, M., and Walsworth-Bell, J. A cost description of a cystic fibrosis unit and cost analyses of different categories of patients. *Thorax* 1992; **47**: 684–9.

140 Shale, D.J. The cost of care in cystic fibrosis. *Thorax* 1992; **47**: 673.

Part VI

Pain

Chapter 26

Mechanisms of pain associated with respiratory disease

Carla Ripamonti and Fabio Fulfaro

Chest pain is one of the most frequent reasons for patients to seek medical advice. It can be the symptom of a pathological process that is affecting an intra- or extrathoracic organ, or the thoracic cage and the anatomic structures that form it.[1-3] This chapter covers the pathophysiological mechanisms of pain with particular reference to chest wall, diaphragm, and mediastinal pain, and to brachial plexopathy.

Pain mechanisms

From a pathophysiological point of view, pain can be classified as nociceptive, neuropathic, and mixed or idiopathic.[4] **Nociceptive pain** includes somatic and visceral pain and arises from the stimulation of nociceptors, which are primary afferent neurons that transmit information about noxious stimuli. Nociceptive pain originating from somatic structures (**somatic pain**) is usually well-localized and described as sharp, aching, throbbing, or pressure-like. Typical examples are pains from bones and joints (ribs, shoulder blade, sternum, clavicle), soft tissues (cutaneous and muscular nociceptors) and the parietal pleura. Nociceptive pain that arises from visceral structures (**visceral pain**), by contrast, is poorly localized and is often described as gnawing, cramping, or colicky when due to occlusion of a hollow viscus, and aching, sharp, or throbbing when due to a lesion of a capsule or mesentery.[5] Typical examples of visceral pain are oesophageal mediastinal pain or pulmonary pain due to stimulation of sympathetic and parasympathetic nerves.[6]

Neuropathic pain originates from injury or disease of peripheral or central neural structures or is the result of sustained aberrant somatosensory processing at these sites.[7] The diagnosis is based on the findings of motor, sensory, or autonomic dysfunction due to a neurological lesion and of sensory abnormalities. Neuropathic pain has three cardinal features:

- **dysaesthesia,** a constant, spontaneous, burning pain often associated with aching or cramps in the deep tissues
- **paroxysmal pain,** spontaneous or evoked by movement or tactile stimulation, usually fleeting and intense, electric shock-like or lancinating
- **allodynia,** an aberrant perception of pain in response to a non-noxious stimulus such as light touch.[8]

Autonomic dysregulation sometimes accompanies nerve injury to:

- soft tissues (reflex sympathetic dystrophy or complex regional pain syndrome type I)
- peripheral nerves (causalgia or complex regional pain syndrome type II)

* viscera, or

* the central nervous system.

It can lead to oedema, vasomotor changes, sweating abnormalities, and trophic changes.

Typical examples of neuropathic pain are brachial plexopathy, radiculopathies, and peripheral nerve syndromes due to mediastinal or spinal pressure and postherpetic neuralgia.

Mixed pains which include nociceptive and neuropathic elements often arise from involvement of large nerve branches and surrounding soft tissues, and are felt as cramps or twinges in association with dysaesthesia, allodynia, or an area of hypoaesthesia.

Idiopathic pain can be considered as a pain that is not obviously nociceptive or neuropathic, and cannot be explained by demonstrable organic pathology. It can be due to a psychogenic cause but it is often difficult to tell if psychological distress is the cause of pain or is a consequence of it. So-called 'psychogenic pains' may constitute up to a third of the cases who present to an emergency service for acute chest pains.[9]

In the clinical assessment of pain it is important to consider the following factors:

* mechanisms (nociceptive-somatic or visceral, neuropathic, mixed)

* site and radiation, onset (e.g. acute following injury)

* intensity, duration (recent or long-standing recurrent pain)

* temporal patterns (constant, intermittent, incidental)

* aggravating/relieving factors (stress, weather conditions, posture)

* associated signs (hiccups, nausea, vomiting)

* concomitant disease.

Table 26.1 shows the classification of the pathophysiological mechanisms of pain at the chest wall, pleura, diaphragm, and mediastinum.

Table 26.1 Classification of the pathophysiological mechanisms of pain in the thorax

Site	Mechanism	Clinical syndrome
Bone	M	Infection
	M	Inflammation
	M	Neoplasm
	N-S	Osteoporosis
	M	Trauma
Diaphragm	N-V	Diaphragmatic hernia
	N-V	Irritation due to abdominal pathology
Heart/aorta	N-V	Angina
	N-V	Aortic lesion
	N-V	Pericarditis
Joint	N-S	Infection
	N-S	Neoplasm
	M	Postsurgical lesions
	N-S	Slipping rib syndrome
	N-S	Trauma

Table 26.1 (continued)

Site	Mechanism	Clinical syndrome
Lymph nodes	N-V	Sarcoidosis
Mediastinum	N-V	Infection
	N-V	Inflammation
	N-V	Neoplasm
Muscle	M	Fibromyalgia
	N-S	Myofascial syndrome
	N-S	Trauma
	M	Vascular lesions
Oesophagus	N-V	Hiatus hernia
	N-V	Inflammation
	N-V	Neoplasm
Pleura	N-S	Infection
	M	Inflammation
	M	Neoplasm
	M	Trauma
Skin	M	Breast disease
	N-S	Dercum's disease
	NP	Diabetic neuropathy
	N-S	Herpes zoster infection
	N-S	Mondor's disease
	NP	Scars
	N-S	Trauma
Trachea/bronchi	N-V	Infection
	N-V	Inflammation
	N-V	Neoplasm

M, mixed; N-S, nociceptive – somatic; N-V, nociceptive – visceral; NP, neuropathic.

Pain arising from the skin of the chest wall

The skin of the chest wall is supplied by the intercostal nerves from T1 to T6. A limited area of the lateral chest wall in the axilla is innervated by the intercostobrachial nerve, which includes fibres from the lower roots of the brachial plexus.

Herpes zoster infection is one of the most frequent causes of chest-wall pain.[10] It is characterized by grouped unilateral vesicular eruptions with a dermatomal distribution, and is due to a reactivation within nerve fibres of earlier infection of the varicella virus. The symptomatology is typical, as the pain is limited to the skin covered by usually a single dermatome. It is often preceded by paresthesia and a rash, in the same dermatome, with the appearance of little blisters with clear liquid and grouped on an erythematous background. The pain due to herpes zoster can be acute or chronic. The acute pain precedes the development of the rash by several days. It may occasionally occur without the development of a rash[11] and may be mistaken for musculoskeletal pain or pleurisy. Postherpetic neuralgia is pain that follows resolution of acute zoster, usually more than 1 month after lesion healing.[12] Chronic postherpetic neuralgia is when the pain persists after 3 months. This is a classical neuropathic pain and is characterized by three distinct components:

- continuous spontaneous pain often described as burning
- short attacks of pain described as electric shocks
- an aberrant painful response to a non-noxious stimulus (i.e. allodynia).

Allodynia is due to an exaggerated response of the primary afferent nerve fibres being stimulated by low threshold mechanoreceptors.[13] Acute herpes zoster is associated with a haemorrhagic inflammation affecting the dorsal ganglion and spreading distally down the nerve to the skin and subcutaneous tissues. Atrophy of the corresponding dorsal horn cell is often found and in some cases of refractory pains, persistent and widespread inflammatory changes have been observed.[14]

Cancer patients have about five times the incidence of herpes zoster infection as the general population. The site of the malignancy shows a significant correlation with the dermatomal location of the pain, for example, involvement of thoracic dermatomes is frequently due to breast or lung cancer.[15]

Other causes of cutaneous pain are:

- thoracic scarring with the formation of a neuroma inside the scar (pain is often dull, persistent and sometimes associated with a burning sensation, with exacerbations due to contact, touch and/or movement)
- thoraco-abdominal diabetic neuropathy involving intercostal nerves and with dermatomal distribution (the pain is similar to a simple sunburn or more intensely as after zoster, and is associated with hypoaesthesia, hyperaesthesia, and allodynia)
- breast pathology (benign idiopathic mastalgia, mastitis, tumours)
- thrombosis in a chest-wall vein (Mondor's disease)[16]
- painful cellulitis in which spontaneous pain is generated within subcutaneous fat tissue and is worsened by pressure (neurolipomatosis dolorosa or Dercum's disease).

Muscular pains

Besides the classic causes of muscular pain (bruising, sprains, abscesses, torn tendons) muscular pains may arise from myofascial pain syndromes with trigger points, or from fibromyalgia.[17] Painful muscular syndromes with trigger points are characterized by the following:

- localized muscular pains in a fairly precise muscular area, very often in the muscle body
- a trigger point sometimes separate from the painful area, the stimulation of which produces pain
- an area of more or less limited diffuse pain, muscular spasm, tenderness, stiffness, or limitation of motion.[3]

The rapid onset of these pains, especially over the anterior chest wall, may prompt a doctor to suspect a cardiovascular pathology. Specific myofascial pain syndromes causing chest pain are described in Table 26.2.

Other painful muscular disorders are due to:

- trauma to chest muscles
- the benign precordial catch syndrome (also called chest-wall twinge syndrome)[18,19]
- precordial migraine.

Table 26.2 Myofascial syndromes causing chest pain

Location of pain	Muscle involved
Anterior chest	Sternalis; pectoralis major; pectoralis minor; scalene muscles; sternocleidomastoid (sternal head); subclavius; iliocostalis cervicis
Dorsal chest	
Upper thoracic	Levator scapulae; trapezius
Midthoracic	Latissimus dorsi; rhomboid; serratus posterior superior; trapezius serratus anterior
Low thoracic	Serratus posterior inferior; iliocostalis thoracis multifidi

From Bonica and Sola.[3]1990

The cause of precordial catch syndrome is unknown and it is characterized by episodes of pain that are sudden, brief, sharp, stabbing, and well localized. The pain is unpredictable and not related to exertion, but can be exacerbated by inspiration.[20,21]

In precordial migraine syndrome, the normal migraine crises in some patients are accompanied by precordial chest pain due to vascular changes in the chest-wall muscles.[3,22]

Pleural pain

The visceral and parietal pleura are separated by the pleural space. The parietal pleura lines the thoracic cavity, the chest wall, the diaphragm, and mediastinum and is supplied with somatic pain fibres, whereas the visceral pleura does not contain these and therefore does not sense pain. There are many causes of pleural pain.[23] The most common are inflammation (pleurisy), mechanical distortion, and trauma. Any of these conditions affecting the parietal pleura (which has a somatic innervation) leads to localized pain accompanied by cutaneous hyperalgesia. The pain is unilateral, often more intense in the lower part of the chest, and with a rapid onset; it is accentuated by breathing movements, coughing, sneezing, and laughing. There may be a concomitant tenderness in the overlying muscles, e.g. the pectoralis major. This pain may be referred to the shoulder blade or breast. When the diaphragmatic pleura is involved, the pain can be referred to the neck and shoulder. Clinical examination often reveals cutaneous hyperalgesia, hyperesthesia, and paresthesia in the area of the pain.

Joint pain

Joint pains include rib pain, costochondral pain, sternum injury, and spinal (vertebral) pain. Rib pains are mainly due to traumatic conditions or neoplasm. Costochondral pains include costochondral dislocation, the slipping rib syndrome (due to a fracture or dislocation of the cartilage of floating ribs, probably resulting from trauma),[24] seronegative spondyloarthropathy,[25] and costochondritis.

Costochondritis (also called anterior chest-wall syndrome, costosternal syndrome, or costosternal chondrodynia) is a relatively frequent cause of anterior chest pain, both as a primary condition and in combination with coronary heart disease. Its pathogenesis is unknown; a traumatic cause has been suggested.[26] Costochondritis often affects women over 40 and is characterized by a localized pain at different costochondral joint levels, particularly between the second and the fifth and often on the left side. The pain may simulate cardiac pain, or even abdominal pain when the lower costal cartilages are involved. In 90% of patients, multiple sites are affected and associated conditions may be present such as cervical strain syndrome, coronary heart disease, or myofascial syndrome.[18] Epstein *et al*.[26] describe the diagnosis of this condition.

Teitze's syndrome is the association of a swelling with localized pain, at the level of the second and occasionally the third costochondral joint, in the absence of infection or inflammation.[27–29] It is a rare syndrome, usually presenting under the age of 40 (in 80% of patients). Only one site is involved. Respiratory tract infections often accompany it.[18]

Causes of **sternal pain** include trauma and arthritis of the sternoclavicular joint, manubriosternal arthritis, xiphoidalgia, and sternoclavicular hyperostosis.[30] **Xiphoidalgia** (also called xiphoiditis, painful xiphoid syndrome, hypersensitive xiphoid, and xiphoid cartilage syndrome) is characterized by spontaneous pain in the anterior chest wall and discomfort and tenderness of the xiphoid process of the sternum.[3] The pain may be diffuse because the xiphoid process is innervated by the phrenic nerves and the T4–7 intercostal nerves.

Sternoclavicular hyperostosis is a syndrome only recently recognized, characterized clinically by a painful and chronic swelling of the clavicles, sternum, and first ribs and radiologically by hyperostosis and increased bone density of the clavicles, sternum, ossification of the first costal cartilage, and sternoclavicular synostosis.[30]

It should be remembered that retrosternal pain can derive from the heart, pericardium, aorta, or oesophagus.[31] Oesophageal carcinoma can cause epigastric or retrosternal pain which can radiate towards the dorsal or interscapular areas. The pain worsens when swallowing.

Other causes of pain in the chest wall are **postmastectomy** and postthoracotomy syndromes. After mastectomy a painful burning sensation can arise on the dorsal aspect of the arm and on the anterior chest wall and axilla, accentuated by extension movements which may be limited. It causes frequent paroxysms produced by pressure, rubbing, or lifting the arms together with abnormal sensation in the thoracic–axillary area (distribution T1–2). It arises from surgical damage to the intercostobrachial nerve, and may follow the development of a neuroma.[32,33] The pain can start immediately after surgery or after a few months, rarely after years. In some cases there is an association with lymphoedema of the arm. Phantom breast syndrome can occur after mastectomy, sometimes accompanied by dysesthesic scar pain.[34,35]

In the **postthoracotomy syndrome,** the pain is due to a surgical lesion of the intercostal nerves. It usually decreases over 2–6 months, although one series showed that it persisted after 6 months in 44% of patients.[36] A later exacerbation can point to a relapse of cancer in the lung.[37,38] and is only rarely due to the development of a scar neuroma.

Patients with postthoracotomy or postmastectomy pain may develop a 'frozen shoulder'.[39] Early shoulder mobilization and adequate analgesia may prevent this complication.

Spinal pains are essentially due to lesions of the vertebral body such as traumatic, pathological (metastatic), infective, or osteoporotic fractures. A particular degenerative condition known as **Scheuermann's disease** may be the cause of chronic thoracic pain in adolescents.[1,40] This is osteochondritis of the epiphysis of the vertebral bodies leading to kyphosis, with chronic aching pain, localized over the involved area (usually dorsal and upper lumbar). It is aggravated by exertion, fatigue, and percussion. According to the cause, the pain may be uni- or bilateral, accentuated by spinal movement, by laughing or coughing, and sometimes by breathing movements.

Diaphragmatic pain

The anatomy of the diaphragm is described in Chapter 2. Motor innervation is from the phrenic nerve. Sensory innervation comes from the phrenic nerve (C4–5) for the central part and the intercostal nerves (D9–10) for the peripheral part.

The sensory nerves involved in the diaphragmatic innervation are embryologically derived from the nerves in the brachial plexus. Stimulation of afferents from the diaphragm therefore result in pain being referred to the C4–5 area, e.g. the shoulder tip.

The diaphragm can cause pain in several ways. Diaphragmatic hernia (hernia of abdominal organs through the diaphragm), myositis or sustained spasm of the diaphragm,[41] and acute primary inflammation of the diaphragm (**Hedron's syndrome**) can all give rise to pain in the lower chest, upper abdomen, and shoulder. Diaphragm irritation due to abdominal pathologies, notably subphrenic abscess, can be responsible for pain referred to the shoulder blade and/or the upper thorax. The pain of subphrenic abscess can be exacerbated by breathing movements, and the presence of hiccups may further help to identify phrenic involvement.

Mediastinal pain

For descriptive purposes, the mediastinum is divided into three sections: anterior, middle, and posterior. Acute pain deriving from the mediastinum itself is rare, and is usually due to pathology in an adjacent organ. Examples of acute pathologies arising in or spreading to the mediastinum include pneumomediastinum.[42]

Mediastinal tumours may cause pain by irritation or compression of the surrounding organs according to the anatomical division described above.[43] For example, a mass causing superior vena cava syndrome may cause pain accompanied by other signs and symptoms including oedema and plethora of the face, neck and upper part of the chest; dyspnoea and blurred vision; headache; and failure of the arm veins to empty when lifted.[44]

The speed of any enlargement in the mediastinum is important in determining the symptoms. A mass which expands slowly can be asymptomatic for a long time, whereas a rapidly developing tumour or an inflammatory process can cause pain more quickly, especially if it impinges on the peritracheal and peribronchial nervous plexuses, phrenic nerves, vagus nerves, or paravertebral sympathetic chains.[45] With pathologies in the posterior mediastinum, such as tumour or tuberculosis, there is a tendency to invade the vertebral canal, leading to radicular pain. Pains due to spinal cord compression are often identified too late, even though the treatment should be urgent as the dorsal segments of the spinal cord are at risk due to the occlusion of the peridural space and the fragility of vascular supply. The pain is radicular, often dull, at the dorsal level and is reduced by rest and lying down. If the compression involved the C7–8 roots, the pain involves the pectoral part of the chest and may be accompanied by a cervicobrachial neuralgia.

Early neurological signs should be investigated promptly because of the risk of paraplegia. It is necessary to look for sensory and/or motor signs sometimes occurring far from the presumed site of the lesion. Neurological examination should check for alteration in muscle strength and sphincter functions, unilateral or bilateral Babinski sign, an alteration of the reflexes (e.g. hyperreflexia) and the presence of clonus.[46,47]

Brachial plexopathy

Table 26.3 shows the causes of arm pain (brachialgia) in cancer patients. Of these, brachial plexopathy occurs frequently.[48] This neurological complication occurs most often in patients with lymphoma, breast and lung carcinomas.[46] Pain is aggravated by pressure and movement and can precede neurological signs by as much as 9 months.[49] The plexus can be compressed or infiltrated by tumour in adjacent structures, such as axillary or supraclavicular nodes, or by tumours in the apex of the lung. A classical example is the Pancoast syndrome (Figure 26.1) which is usually caused by a tumour in the apex (or superior pulmonary sulcus) of the lung.[50,51] The pain may increase rapidly with widespread infiltration of the brachial plexus or the Horner's syndrome. Occasionally the tumour may extend into the epidural space via the intervertebral foramina with the likelihood of spinal cord compression.[52]

Other less important causes are: chronic inflammation such as tuberculosis, surgical trauma, postradiation fibrosis, and lung metastases.[53–56] The chest wall and subpleural lymphatic vessels are the first to be invaded. Posteriorly, under the pleura, the tumour can spread due to the paravertebral symphatetic trunk and to the stellate ganglion (cervicothoracic ganglion) producing the characteristic symptomatology of Horner's syndrome: miosis, partial palpebral ptosis, enophthalmos, and anhidrosis in the affected area.

The growing tumour may involve the upper ribs producing local pain mainly in the ipsilateral shoulder. Similarly, the thoracic vertebrae, and rarely the subclavian vein and artery can also be affected. Finally, destruction of the lower trunk of the brachial plexus (C8–T1) may follow with pain in the distribution area of the ulnar nerve (the shoulder joint with radiation to the arm, elbow, medial aspect of the hand with dysaesthesia of the fourth and fifth finger). The upper trunk of the brachial plexus (C5–6) is less often involved, producing pain in the shoulder joint, arm, thumb, and index finger.

Table 26.4 summarizes the main symptoms and signs of brachial plexopathy. It is important to differentiate between metastatic tumour and fibrosis following radiation to this area, e.g. for apical lung cancer or breast cancer. The brachial plexus involves the C5–T1 nerve roots, and the

Table 26.3 Causes of brachialgias

Bony lesions affecting arm, clavicle, and shoulder joint	
Brachial plexopathy	Tumour infiltration
	Postradiation therapy
	Postsurgical
Intercostobrachial nerve neuropathy	
Lymphedema	
Acute brachial neuritis	Non-cancer-related brachial plexopathy
	Thoracic outlet syndrome
	Costoclavicular syndrome
	Hyperabduction syndrome
	Chronic trauma (backpack palsy)
	Acute trauma
Cervical radiculopathy	Metastatic
	Benign
Carpal tunnel syndrome	
Shoulder–hand syndrome	
Non-neurologic brachialgias	Frozen shoulder (e.g. postmastectomy)
	Humeroscapular periarthropathy
	Brachial phlebitis

Reproduced with permission and modified from Caraceni.[6]

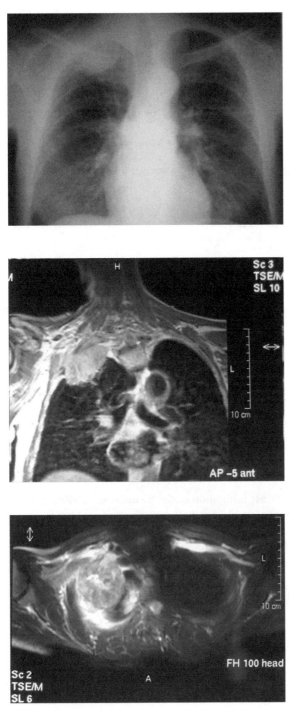

Fig. 26.1 Pancoast syndrome.

Table 26.4 Symptoms and signs of brachial plexopathy[a]

Root	Symptoms	Signs
C5	Cervical pain radiating to the shoulder girdle and lateral aspect of the arm to the elbow	Weakness of arm abduction and external rotation; possible reduced biceps reflex
C6	Cervical pain radiating to the lateral aspect of the arm and forearm to the dorsal aspect of the thumb and index finger	Weakness of forearm flexion; possible reduced brachioradialis reflex
C7	Cervical pain radiating to the dorsal aspect of the arm and forearm to the dorsal aspect of the hand and second, third and fourth fingers	Weakness of extension of the elbow, wrist and fingers; possible reduced triceps reflex
C8–T1	Cervical pain radiating to the medial aspect of the arm and forearm to the fourth and fifth fingers	Weakness of the small muscles of the hand

[a] Innervation of brachial plexus: upper trunk, C5–6; middle trunk, C7; lower trunk, C8–T1.

upper trunk is relatively free of lymph nodes. Consequently, symptoms confined to the upper trunk (C5–6) are rarely due to metastatic disease but are common with radiation fibrosis. Conversely, symptoms confined to the lower trunk (C8–T1) are frequent in metastatic disease involving lymph nodes, but are less likely to be due to radiation fibrosis. According to Cherny and Foley,[49] postradiation fibrosis is more frequent when the dose is greater than 1.9 Gy/day and is characterized by:

- less frequent and less severe pain emerging from 6 months to 5 years after radiotherapy
- absence of Horner's syndrome
- onset of a progressive paresis (C5–6 distribution) with stabilization of pain
- weakness of shoulder abduction and arm flexion
- progressive lymphoedema.

On radiological examination, a diffuse infiltration of the tissues is seen. Moreover, there are rare cases of acute ischemic postradiation plexopathy[57] arising some years after treatment with no pain and a non-progressive acute paralysis and sensory deficit.[49] The best neuroradiological imaging tests are CT and MRI.[58] Electrodiagnostic studies may help in differentiating radiation-induced plexopathy from tumour involvement.[59]

Keypoints

- Thoracic pain can be nociceptive (somatic or visceral), neuropathic, or mixed
- Pain may arise from the thoracic viscera, muscles, bony cage, skin or nerve structures, and may be referred outside the chest
- Thoracic pains are mainly caused by tumour, trauma (including surgery), infection, inflammation
- Difficult pain syndromes arise with postherpetic neuralgia, pleural involvement, mediastinal disease, and brachial plexus infiltration

References

1 Bonica, J.J. General considerations of pain in the chest. In: J.J. Bonica (ed.) *The management of pain*, Vol. 2, 2nd edn. Philadelphia: Lea & Febiger, 1990; 959–83.

2 Richter, J.E. Practical approach to the diagnosis of unexplained chest pain. *Med Clin North Am* 1991; **75**: 1203–8.

3 Bonica, J.J., and Sola, A.F. Chest pain caused by other disorders. In: J.J. Bonica (ed.) *The management of pain*, Vol. 2, 2nd edn. Philadelphia: Lea & Febiger, 1990; 1114–45.

4 Meskey, H. Classification of chronic pain, description of chronic pain syndromes and definition of pain terms. *Pain* 1986; **3** (Suppl): S1

5 Ness, T.J., and Gebhart, G.F. Visceral pain: a review of experimental studies. *Pain* 1989; **41**: 167–234.

6 Caraceni, A. Clinicopathologic correlates of common cancer pain syndromes. *Hematol Oncol Clin North Am* 1996; **10**(1): 57–78.

7 Cherny, N.I. Cancer pain: principles of assessment and syndromes. In: A.M. Berger, R.K. Portenoy, and D.E. Weissman (ed.) *Supportive oncology*. Philadelphia, Pa.: Lippincott-Raven, 1997; 3–42.

8 Moulin, D.E. Neuropathic cancer pain: syndromes and clinical controversies. In: E. Bruera and R.K. Portenoy (eds) *Topics in palliative care*, Vol. 2. New York: Oxford University Press, 1998; 7–29.

9 Wulsin, L.R., and Yingling, K. Psychiatric aspects of chest pain in the emergency department. *Med Clin North Am* 1991; **75**: 1175–88.

10 Gilder, D.H., Dueland, A.N., and Cohrs, R. Preherpetic neuralgia. *Neurology* 1991; **41**: 1215–18.

11 Portenoy, R.K., Duma, C., and Foley, K.M. Acute herpetic and postherpetic neuralgia: clinical review and current management. *Ann Neurol* 1986; **20**: 651–64.

12 Watson, C.P.N. Postherpetic neuralgia. *Neurol Clin* 1989; **7**: 231–48.

13 Bowsher, D. Sensory change in post-herpetic neuralgia. In: C.P.N. Watson (ed.) *Herpes zoster and post-herpetic neuralgia. Pain research and clinical management*, Vol. 8. Amsterdam: Elsevier Science, 1993; 97–107.

14 Bhala, B.B., Ramamoorthy, C., and Bowsher, D. Shingles and post herpetic neuralgia. *Clin J Pain* 1988; **4**: 169–74.

15 Rusthoven, J.J., Ahlgren, P., Elhakim, T., *et al.* Risk factors for varicella zoster disseminated infection among adult cancer patients with localized zoster. *Cancer* 1988; **62**: 1641–6.

16 Mondor, H. Phlebite en cordon de la paroi thoracique. *Mem Acad Chirurg* 1944: 70–96.

17 Mills, K.R., Newham, D.J., and Edwards, R.H.T. Muscle pain. In: P.D. Wall and R. Melzack (eds) *Textbook of pain*, 2nd edn. Edinburgh: Churchill Livingstone, 1989; 420–32.

18 Fam, A.G., and Smythe, H.A. Musculoskeletal chest wall pain. *Can Med Assoc J* 1985; **133**: 379.

19 Sparrow, M.J., and Bird, E.L. 'Precordial catch': a benign syndrome of chest pain in young persons. *N Z Med J* 1978; **88**: 325–6.

20 Reynolds, J.L. Precordial catch syndrome in children. *South Med J* 1989; **82**(10): 1228–30.

21 Pickering, D. Precordial catch syndrome. *Arch Dis Child* 1981; **56**(5): 401–3.

22 Fitz-Hugh, T. Precordial migraine: an important form of 'angina innocens'. *Int Clin* 1940; **3**: 141–4.

23 Jeanfaivre, T., Regnard, O., L'Hoste, P., and Enon, B. Chronic pain of vascular origin caused by a parietopulmonary fistula of the thoracic wall. *Ann Thorac Surg* 1997; **63**: 839–41.

24 Holmes, J.F. A study of the slipping rib cartilage syndrome. *N Engl J Med* 1941; **224**: 928.

25 Olivieri, I., Barozzi, L., Padula, A., De Matteis, M., and Pavlica, P. Clinical manifestations of sero-negative spondylarthropathies. *Eur J Radiol* 1998; **27** (Suppl 1): S3–6

26 Epstein, S.E., Gerber, L.H., and Borer, J.S. Chest wall syndrome: a common cause of unexplained cardiac pain. *JAMA* 1979; **241**: 2793–5.

27 Calabro, J.J., Jeghers, H., Miller, K.A., and Gordon, R.D. Classification of anterior chest wall syndromes. *JAMA* 1980; **243**: 1420–1.

28 Campbell, S.M. Regional myofascial pain syndromes. *Rheum Dis Clin North Am* 1989; **15**: 31–44.

29 Wise, C.M. Chest wall syndromes. *Curr Opin Rheumatol* 1994; **6**: 197–202.

30 Resnick, D., Vint, V., and Poteshman, N.L. Sternocostoclavicular hyperosteosis. *J Bone Joint Surg* 1981; **63**: 1329–32.

31 Rothstein, R.D., and Ouyang, A. Chest pain of esophageal origin. *Gastroenterol Clin North Am* 1989; **18**: 257–73.

32 Vecht, C.J. Arm pain in the patient with breast cancer. *J Pain Symptom Manage* 1990; **5**: 109–17.

33 Watson, C.P.N., Evans, R.J., and Watt, V.R. The post-mastectomy pain syndrome and the effect of topical capsaicin. *Pain* 1989; **38**: 117–86.

34 Kroner, K., Krebs, B., Skov, J., and Jorgensen, H.S. Immediate and long-term phantom breast syndrome after mastectomy: incidence, clinical characteristic relationship to pre-mastectomy breast. *Pain* 1989; **36**: 327–35.

35 Kroner, K., Knudsen, U.B., Lundby, L., and Hvid, H. Long-term phantom breast syndrome after mastectomy. *Clin J Pain* 1992; **8**: 346–50.

36 Kalso, E., Perttunen, K., and Kaasinen, S. Pain after thoracic surgery. *Acta Anaesthesiol Scand* 1992; **36**(1): 96–100.

37 d'Amours, R.H., Riegler, F.X., and Little, A.G. Pathogenesis and management of persistent post-thoracomy pain. *Chest Surg Clin North Am* 1998; **8**: 703–22.

38 Kanner, R., Martini, N., and Foley, K.M. Nature and incidence of postthoracotomy pain. *Proc Am Soc Clin Oncol* 1982; **1**: Abstract 590.

39 Maunsell, E., Brisson, J., and Deschenes, L. Arm problems and psychological distress after surgery for breast cancer. *Can J Surg* 1993; **36**: 315–20.

40 Winter, R.B., and Schellhas, K.P. Painful adult thoracic Scheuermann's disease. Diagnosis by discography and treatment by combined arthrodesis. *Am J Orthop* 1996; **25**: 783–6.

41 Tarver, R.D., Conces, D.J. Jr., Cory, D.A., and Vix, V.A. Imaging the diaphragm and its disorders. *J Thorac Imaging* 1989; **4**: 1–8.

42 Tytherleigh, M.G., Connolly, A.A., and Handa, J.L. Spontaneous pneumomediastinum. *J Accident Emergency Med* 1997; **14**: 333–4.

43 Bonica, J.J., Ventafridda, V., and Twycross, R.G. Cancer pain. In: J.J. Bonica (ed.) *The management of pain,* Vol. 1, 2nd edn. Philadelphia: Lea & Febiger, 1990; 400–60.

44 Zuber, M., Schwamborn, J., and Kramann, B. Thoracic pain and bulky mass in the thoracic wall. *Med Klin* 1998; **93**: 321.

45 Capoferri, M., Furrer, M., and Ris, H.B. Surgical diagnosis and therapy in patients with mediastinal space-occupying lesions. A retrospective analysis of 223 intervention with special reference to long term course. *Swiss Surg* 1998; **4**: 121–8.

46 Elliott, K., and Foley, K.M. Neurologic pain syndromes in patients with cancer. In: R.K. Portenoy (eds) *Neurological clinics: pain, mechanisms and syndromes.* Philadelphia: W. B. Saunders, 1989; 333–60.

47 Faber, L.P. Issues in management of chest malignancies. *Clin Chest Med* 1992; **13**: 113–35.

48 Tsairis, P., Dyck, P.J., and Mulder, D.W. Natural history of brachial plexus neuropathy. *Arch Neurol* 1972; **27**: 109–17.

49 Cherny, N.I., and Foley K.M. Brachial plexopathy in patients with breast cancer. In: J.R. Harris, M.E. Lippman, M. Morrow, *et al.* (eds) *Disease of the breast.* Philadelphia: Lippincott-Raven, 1996; 796–808.

50 Kori, S.H., Foley, K.M., and Posner, J.B. Brachial plexus lesions in patients with cancer – 100 cases. *Neurology* 1981; **31**: 45–50.

51 Tanelian, D.L., and Coisins, M.J. Combined neurogenic and nociceptive pain in a patient with Pancoast tumor managed by epidural hydromorphone and oral carbamazepine. *Pain* 1989; **36:** 85–8.

52 Cascino, T.L., Kori, S., and Foley, K.M. CT scan of brachial plexus in patients with cancer. *Neurology* 1983; **33:** 1553–7.

53 Ben-David, B., and Stahl, S. Prognosis of intraoperative brachial plexus injury: a review of 22 cases. *Br J Anaesthesiol* 1997; **79:** 440–5.

54 Loeser, J.D. Cervicobrachial neuralgia. In: J.J. Bonica (ed.) *The management of pain,* Vol. 1, 2nd edn. Philadelphia: Lea & Febiger, 1990; 868–81.

55 Masson, P., Rigot, A., and Cecile, W. Brachial plexus neuropathy following pyogenic cervical adenophlegmon. *Arch Pediatry* 1994; **1:** 735–7.

56 Lederman, R.J., and Wilbourn, A.J. Brachial plexopathy: Recurrent cancer or radiation? *Neurology* 1984; **34:** 1331–5.

57 Gerard, J.M., Franck, N., Moussa, Z., and Hildebrand, J. Acute ischemic brachial plexus neuropathy following radiation therapy. *Neurology* 1989; **39:** 450–1.

58 Krol, G. Evaluation of neoplastic involvement of brachial and lumbar plexus: imaging aspects. *J Back Musculoskeletal Rehabil* 1993; **3:** 35–43.

59 Harper, C.M., Thomas, J.E., Cascino, T.L., et al. Distinction between neoplastic and radiation-induced brachial plexopathy, with emphasis on EMG. *Neurology* 1989; **39:** 502–6.

Chapter 27

Pain in association with respiratory conditions: assessment in research and clinical practice

Nathan I. Cherny and Sam H. Ahmedzai

The structures in the respiratory system which give rise to painful sensations include the chest wall, diaphragm, parietal pleura, tracheobronchial tree, and vascular structures (Table 27.1). Pain arising from the respiratory system can be caused by somatic or visceral nociceptive mechanisms. Nociceptive stimuli to the chest wall, parietal pleura, and somatic portions of the diaphragm can generate well-localized and sharp somatic pains. Visceral pain is generated by stimuli to the trachea and bronchial tree, pulmonary vascular structures, and lung interstitium. Of the visceral structures, the lung interstitium is relatively insensitive. (For a fuller description of mechanisms of thoracic pain, see Chapter 26.)

Chest pain is an important symptom that requires evaluation. This clinical symptom is important largely because chest pain may be associated with potentially life-threatening conditions such as myocardial ischemia, aortic dissection, pericardial tamponade, and pulmonary embolus. Indeed, the ability to distinguish between these critical events and other causes of respiratory chest pain is an important clinical skill. Recognition of pulmonary pain syndromes can help in the clinical evaluation of such patients, leading to appropriate investigations and rational management.

The evaluation of pain in respiratory disease

In the context of respiratory disease, pain has a dual significance – either as an undifferentiated presenting symptom of an as yet undiagnosed condition, or as a continuing symptom of a known condition.

In most instances, pain is not an isolated clinical symptom; rather, it exists in a clinical context of other symptoms and findings on clinical examination. Diagnostic evaluation begins with review of all reported symptoms and a physical examination. This generally enables the clinician to formulate a clinical hypothesis or differential diagnosis which can subsequently be further refined with appropriate diagnostic investigations.

Pain as a presenting symptom

In many conditions pain may be the first manifestation of respiratory disease. In the absence of a known diagnosis, the character and qualities of the pain may be of critical diagnostic value. Several characteristics of pain need to be evaluated. These are summarized in Box 27.1. Examples are given of how these simple questions can help to make a differential diagnosis of the cause of thoracic pain. The question of severity of the pain does not usually influence this process, but rather helps the clinician to judge the speed of assessment and choose appropriate management.

Table 27.1 Pain arising from respiratory disease with associated pain mechanisms and pathways

Source	Mechanism	Pathway
Chest wall	N-S, NP	Intercostal nerves
Parietal pleura	N-S, NP	Intercostal nerves
Diaphragm muscle	N-V	Intercostal nerve (peripheral) Phrenic nerve (central)
Diaphragmatic pleura	N-V	Phrenic nerve
Trachea	N-V	Midcervical sympathetic ganglion pulmonary plexus of vagus
Bronchial tree	N-V	Pulmonary plexus of vagus
Pulmonary vasculature	N-V	Pulmonary plexus of vagus
Lung interstitium	N-V	Pulmonary plexus of vagus
Visceral pleura	Insensitive to pain	

NS, nociceptive – somatic; N-V, nociceptive – visceral; NP neuropathic (see Chapter 26 for details of classification of pain mechanisms).

Pain as a continuing symptom of a known condition

The adequate relief of pain is an essential element in the overall management of respiratory conditions. At the bedside a simple unidimensional approach to monitoring pain is usually adequate. The two most common approaches in this setting are a **verbal descriptor scale** (mild, moderate or severe);[1] or a **numeric rating scale** in which patients are asked to grade the pain on a 0–10 scale (0 = no pain, 10 = worst pain imaginable).[2] Although **visual analogue scales** (VAS) are useful in more formal and research assessments, they may be more difficult to use in everyday clinical practice.

Box 27.1 Clinical assessment of a new pain

1 **Onset**: sudden, gradual

2 **Severity**: mild, moderate, severe

3 **Site and localization**: Where is the pain? Is it well localized? Is it diffuse? Does it radiate? Is it a referred pain?

4 **Character**: How is it best described? Sharp, dull, tearing, pressure, burning, or discomfort? Is there accompanying abnormal sensation (which could indicate neuropathic component)?

5 **Time course**: Does the pain fluctuate with time? Is it constant?

6 **Exacerbating factors**: Does pain change with respiration or cough? Does it change with posture? Is it worse on lying or standing? Is it worsened by lying on one side or another? Is pain worsened by exertion? Is the area tender?

7 **Relieving factors**: Is the pain relieved by breath holding or by shallow breathing? Is it relieved by changing posture?

When a more comprehensive pain evaluation is needed, a multidimensional pain assessment that evaluates a range of pain parameters as well as pain-related interference with function can be achieved, e.g. the Brief Pain Inventory (BPI).[3] The BPI is a simple and easily administered tool that provides information about pain history, intensity, location and quality. Numeric scales (range 1–10) indicate the intensity of pain in general, at its worst, at its least, and right now. A percentage scale quantifies relief from current therapies. A figure representing the body is provided for the patient to shade the area corresponding to their pain. Seven questions determine the degree to which pain interferes with function, mood and enjoyment of life. Example questions from the BPI are given in Figure 27.1. The BPI is self-administered and easily understood, and has been translated into several languages.[4–6] It is suitable for periodic evaluation of pain in research studies, i.e. weekly or 2-weekly. The short form of the BPI can be used in clinical practice and monitoring of individual patients.[7]

Pain evaluation as part of a comprehensive symptom evaluation

For patients with cancer, several symptom assessment scales have been developed for the clinic and for research. These tools evaluate a range of symptoms that are commonly found among patients with cancer. The most commonly used symptom scales are the Edmonton Symptom

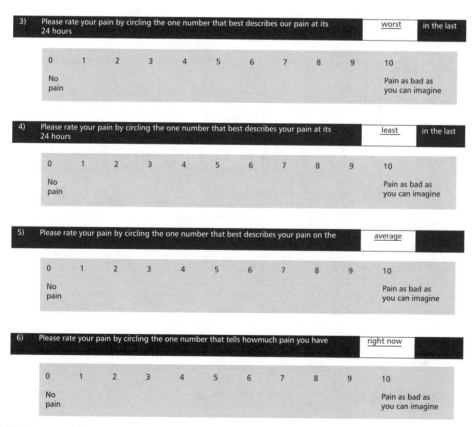

Fig. 27.1 Sample questions from the Brief Pain Inventory (BPI) (short form).

Assessment Scale (ESAS)[8] or the Memorial Symptom Assessment Scale (MSAS).[9] See Chapter 8 for more details of ESAS; example questions from MSAS are shown in Figure 27.2. Both of these symptom scales are validated and easily administered. They contain a single item on pain, but they provide data on prevalence and severity of other symptoms. Of the two scales, the ESAS is more widely used globally and, being shorter, is better adapted for longitudinal follow up in the clinical, as distinct from research, setting.

It is worth recognizing that quality of life (QoL) measures, which are primarily used in research, may also be of value in routine clinical monitoring and evaluation. A QoL scale which has been extensively used in studies of cancer patients is the EORTC QLQ-C30.[10] This 30-item instrument includes two questions on pain (Box 27.2), which ask about the amount and also the degree to which pain interferes with the patient's daily activities. These questions are scored on a 4-point verbal scale, which many patients find easier than VAS scoring. In practice, the patient circles a number in each row of the questionnaire, but these numbers are related to verbal statements. The EORTC QoL measurement approach is modular, and there is a specific module for lung cancer, the LC-13.[11] This has three extra questions on pain, which help to

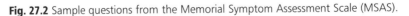

NAME:			DATE:										

SECTION 1
INSTRUCTIONS: We have listed 2 symptoms below. Read each one carefully,
If you have had the symptom during this past week, let us know how <u>often</u> you had it, how <u>severe</u> it was ususlly and how much it <u>distressed or bothered</u> you by circling the appropriate number.
If you did have the symptom, make an "X" in the box marked "DID NOT HAVE"

DURING THE PAST WEEK — Did you have any of the following symptoms?	DID NOT HAVE	IF YES — How OFTEN did you have it?				IF YES — How SEVERE was it usually?				IF YES — How much did it DISTRESS or BOTHER you?				
		Rarely	Occasionally	Frequently	Almost constantly	Slight	Moderate	Severe	Very severe	Not at all	A little bit	Somewhat	Quite a bit	Very much
Difficulty concentrating		1	2	3	4	1	2	3	4	0	1	2	3	4
Pain		1	2	3	4	1	2	3	4	0	1	2	3	4
Lack of energy		1	2	3	4	1	2	3	4	0	1	2	3	4
Cough		1	2	3	4	1	2	3	4	0	1	2	3	4
Feeling nervous		1	2	3	4	1	2	3	4	0	1	2	3	4
Dry mouth		1	2	3	4	1	2	3	4	0	1	2	3	4
Nausea		1	2	3	4	1	2	3	4	0	1	2	3	4
Feeling drowsy		1	2	3	4	1	2	3	4	0	1	2	3	4
Numbness/tingling in hands/feet		1	2	3	4	1	2	3	4	0	1	2	3	4
Difficulty sleeping		1	2	3	4	1	2	3	4	0	1	2	3	4
Feeling bloated		1	2	3	4	1	2	3	4	0	1	2	3	4
Problems with urination		1	2	3	4	1	2	3	4	0	1	2	3	4

Fig. 27.2 Sample questions from the Memorial Symptom Assessment Scale (MSAS).

Box 27.2 Questions on pain in EORTC quality of life instruments

From QLQ-C30 (core questionnaire)

During the past week	Not at all	A little	Quite a bit	Very much
9 Have you had pain	1	2	3	4
19 Did pain interfere with your daily activities?	1	2	3	4

From QLQ-LC13 (lung module)

During the past week	Not at all	A little	Quite a bit	Very much
10 Have you had pain in your chest	1	2	3	4
11 Have you had pain in your arm or shoulder?	1	2	3	4
12 Have you had pain in other parts of your body? If yes, where?	1	2	3	4

localize it anatomically (Box 27.2). As with the general pain questions in the QLQ-C30, these are rated by the patient on a 4-point verbal scale.

Either the QLQ-C30 or the LC-13 may be useful scales to apply in a full clinical assessment of the respiratory patient with pain, or for research projects. However, used together, they will probably be too long for regular monitoring. Other QoL scales which could be used to assess pain, and also gather other data on accompanying symptoms and concerns, include the Lung Cancer Symptom Scale (LCSS)[12] and the FACT-L.[13] These have been more widely used in the North American literature, and as with the EORTC instrument, were designed primarily for research purposes. For further description of measurement scales see Chapter 8.

Recognition of clinical syndromes associated with thoracic pain

As well as formally measuring pain, as described above, the clinician often finds it helpful to assess the symptom in the context of clinical syndromes which arise in respiratory diseases. These syndromes help to put the pain into context with other symptoms and can assist with making a diagnosis. The clinical manifestations of syndromes which commonly occur in respiratory practice are described briefly below. For a fuller description of the aetiology of pain in these situations, see Chapter 26.

Airway-related pain syndromes

Tracheobronchitis

Tracheobronchitis is most commonly due to inflammation or trauma. Inflammation may be caused by infection (most commonly), trauma, chemical irritation, or thermal injury. A common cause of traumatic pain is postintubation pain. Tracheobronchial pain is generally perceived as a retrosternal discomfort and it may be exacerbated by inspiration. Depending on the underlying cause it may be associated with cough, wheeze, or stridor.

Bronchiectasis

Bronchiectasis is characterized by irreversible focal or diffuse dilatation of bronchi. It may be unilateral or bilateral and it has multiple causes. There is little data on the prevalence of pain among patients with bronchiectasis. Among 23 patients with cystic fibrosis, 65% reported chronic chest pain.[15] In a study of patients with chronic sputum production,[16] among 80 patients with bronchiectasis there were 28 separate pains of which 18 were considered to be of respiratory origin. Overwhelmingly, the anatomical location of the pains corresponded to the involved bronchiectatic lobe(s) (Figure 27.3).

Patients with obstructive airways disease (COPD, asthma) often complain of a vague aching chest tightness. This can be retrosternal or more widespread. It is not necessarily related to the severity of the airflow obstruction, but patients may gauge their activity by the development of this pain.

Pleural pain syndromes

Pneumothorax

The most common symptoms of spontaneous pneumothorax are dyspnoea and pain.[17,18] Pleuritic pain is reported in 30–60% of cases.[17–19] Pain may be referred to the chest or the back, and it is usually unilateral. Retrospective data suggest that pain is more likely to be a presenting

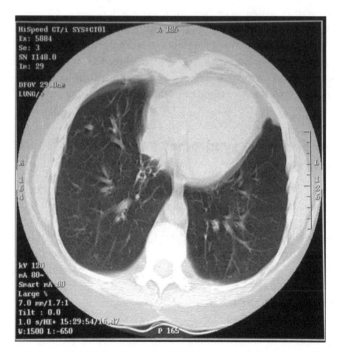

Fig. 27.3 CT scan of bilateral basal bronchiectasis which was causing chronic cough and chest pain. Reproduced by permission of Sheffield Teaching Hospitals NHS Trust.

symptom in younger than older patients.[19] There is no relationship between the severity of the pain and the size of the pneumothorax.

Inflammatory diseases of the pleura

Any inflammatory process involving the parietal pleura may produce pleuritic chest pain. Inflammation of the parietal pleura causes localized pain directly over the affected area, pain referred to the shoulder or neck via the phrenic nerve if the central diaphragmatic surface (C3–5) is involved, or pain referred to the epigastric region if the peripheral diaphragmatic surface is involved. It is characteristically exacerbated by deep inspiration, and coughing or movement of the thorax also exacerbates it. Often the patient demonstrates shallow and rapid respiration to prevent the pain associated with deeper inspiration. On examination, the affected area may be tender and a pleural rub (audible or palpable) may be present. Common causes of pleural inflammation include infection of the underlying lung and chest trauma. Pleurisy may be a manifestation of a polyserositis associated with systemic lupus erythematosus, or familial Mediterranean fever. Bornholm disease, which is caused by group B Coxsackie viruses (occasionally group A, or ECHO virus), can be associated with severe pleuritic-type paroxysmal pain. Asbestos-induced benign pleural fibrosis, which may be associated with linear calcification, may rarely be associated with a chronic dull chest pain.[20,21]

Malignant disease of the pleura

Primary tumours (such as mesothelioma) or metastases may involve the parietal pleura (Figure 27.4). Pleural metastases are commonly associated with cancers of the lung, breast, thymus, and ovary. Pleural tumours commonly present with dyspnea, pleural effusions, or chest pain. Chest pain is caused by involvement of the parietal pleura or adjacent chest-wall structures. It may be exacerbated by breathing or may be constant if there is deeper invasion of adjacent chest-wall tissues.

Empyema

An empyema is a collection of pus in the pleural space. In a recent study of 107 consecutive patients with empyema,[22] the common presenting symptoms were cough, dyspnea and chest pain and pyrexia. Commonly, diagnosis was delayed and the latency between onset of symptoms and diagnosis was almost 2 months. The causes of empyema were pneumonia, malignancy, iatrogenic injury, and trauma. The most frequently isolated organism was *Streptococcus milleri*,[22] and involvement by non-bacterial, non-tuberculous, or fungal infection is uncommon.

Pain associated with chest-wall damage

Post-thoracotomy pain

Pain invariably follows thoracotomy and is mediated by intercostal nerve damage and related chest-wall trauma. It usually follows the line of incision and may be localized in drain sites or related to suture placement. It is usually self-limiting but may last for several months (see Chapter 26 for more details).

(a)

(b)

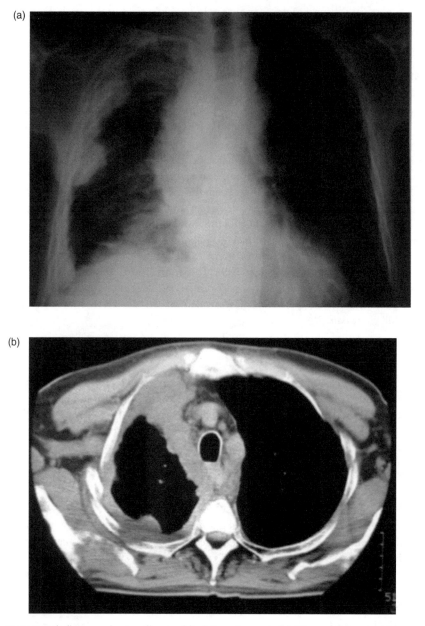

Fig. 27.4 Mesothelioma – chest wall pain: (a) plain radiograph (b) CT scan. Reproduced by permission of Sheffield Teaching Hospitals NHS Trust.

Rib fracture and metastasis

Patients with respiratory disease may have pain arising from the chest wall in association with either a metastasis in the rib or intercostal spaces in the case of cancer, or a 'benign' rib fracture. Rib and intercostal metastasis causes pain arising from the bone, periosteum, and myofascial tissues. Frequently there is subpleural involvement in the thorax and underlying lung. Rib fractures occur occasionally in patients with COPD and osteoporosis (sometimes steroid-induced) after a heavy bout of coughing. Both benign and malignant chest-wall pains can have a 'pleuritic' component, i.e. they are aggravated by deep respiration and coughing. Unlike true pleurisy, they are usually associated with localized tenderness.

Pain syndromes in parenchymal lung disease

Pneumonia

Pain is a feature of pneumonias associated with pleural inflammation. Consequently, it is most commonly associated with lobar pneumonias involving the peripheral lung tissues and it is an uncommon feature of the so-called 'atypical pneumonias'.[23,24] In lobar pneumonia, chest pain usually coexists with fever, tachycardia, tachypnoea, and cough. It may also be associated with cutaneous and deep hyperalgesia.[25] Since pleuritic chest-wall pain may inhibit adequate ventilation or cough, relief of pain is an essential part of treatment of pneumonia.

Lung abscess

Pain is not a major clinical feature of lung abscesses unless the collection is subpleural or is complicated by the development of a bronchopleural fistula.

Lung tumours

Distant metastases to bone and other pain-sensitive structures are the most common causes of pain in patients with lung cancer. Peripheral lung tumours may involve sensitive tissues including the pleura, chest wall, and brachial plexus. Chest-wall invasion is associated with local pain caused by invasion and compression of somatic and neural structures. Involvement of intercostal nerves produces neuropathic pain and may be associated with radicular hypoasthesias, dysesthesias or burning or lancinating pain.[26]

Tumours involving the lung apex (Pancoast tumours) may invade the adjacent neural structures as they pass through the superior sulcus. Most commonly there is involvement of the lower part of the brachial plexus (C7, C8, T1 distribution) with pain distribution involving the elbow, medial forearm, and fourth and fifth fingers.[27–29] Other patterns of distribution are not uncommon, including pain localized to the posterior arm or elbow,[30] in the root of the neck or shoulder,[29–32] or in the scapular region.[30,32] Severe aching is usually reported, but patients may also experience constant or lancinating dysaesthesias along the ulnar aspect of the forearm or hand.

Even in the absence of involvement of the chest wall or parietal pleura, lung tumours can produce a visceral pain syndrome. In a large case series of lung cancer patients pain was unilateral in 80% of the cases and bilateral in 20%. Among patients with hilar tumours the pain was referred to the sternum or the scapula. Upper and lower lobe tumours were referred to the shoulder and to the lower chest respectively.[26,33] Unusually, lung cancers can also generate ipsilateral facial pain.[34–37] It is postulated that this pain syndrome is generated via vagal afferent neurones.

Pain syndromes associated with vascular lung disease

Pulmonary thromboembolism

The clinical manifestation of pulmonary thromboembolism includes the pulmonary infarction syndrome (dyspnoea, tachycardia, and pleuritic pain), isolated dyspnoea or vascular collapse.[38] The pulmonary infarction syndrome is most often caused by small peripheral emboli.[39]

Consequently, diagnostic screening shows a lower likelihood of hypoxemia or abnormalities in the ECG or ventilation–perfusion scan.[38] The predominant symptom of large pulmonary embolism is dyspnoea. Patients may also report a deep visceral sensation of chest pain or pressure reminiscent of that associated with myocardial ischaemia.

Pulmonary hypertension

Primary pulmonary hypertension is an uncommon and poorly understood entity characterized by extensive remodelling of the pulmonary vasculature, with consequent deleterious hypertrophic changes in the right ventricle. It is generally complicated by the development of right heart failure. Symptomatic presentation includes exertional dyspnoea, retrosternal chest pain, and syncope associated with physical signs of right heart failure.[40] Similar symptoms may also be observed in patients with secondary pulmonary hypertension caused by underlying cardiac disease.[41]

Keypoints

- Chest pain is a common feature of many primary thoracic diseases and also systemic diseases involving the lungs or chest wall
- Chest pain can arise from airways, pleural, chest-wall, or visceral structures
- A structural approach to taking a pain history is useful to assess causes and impact on the patient
- Pain can be easily assessed in routine clinical practice using verbal descriptor or numerical scales
- For research studies, several multidimensional symptom scales or QoL measures can be used
- The Brief Pain Inventory (BPI) is currently the best specific instrument for monitoring pain alone
- Recognition of thoracic pain syndromes can be helpful in their clinical assessment

References

1 Jensen, M.P., Karoly, P., and Braver, S. The measurement of clinical pain intensity: a comparison of six methods. *Pain* 1986; **27**(1): 117–26.

2 Paice, J.A., and Cohen, F.L. Validity of a verbally administered numeric rating scale to measure cancer pain intensity. *Cancer Nurs* 1997; **20**(2): 88–93.

3 Daut, R.L., Cleeland, C.S., and Flanery, R.C. Development of the Wisconsin Brief Pain Questionnaire to assess pain in cancer and other diseases. *Pain* 1983; **17**(2): 197–210.

4 Caraceni, A., Mendoza, T.R., Mencaglia, E., *et al.* A validation study of an Italian version of the Brief Pain Inventory (Breve Questionario per la Valutazione del Dolore). *Pain* 1996; **65**(1): 87–92.

5 Cleeland, C.S., and Ryan, K.M. Pain assessment: global use of the Brief Pain Inventory. *Ann Acad Med Singapore* 1994; **23**(2): 129–38.

6 Wang, X.S., Mendoza, T.R., Gao, S.Z., and Cleeland, C.S. The Chinese version of the Brief Pain Inventory (BPI-C): its development and use in a study of cancer pain. *Pain* 1996; **67**(2–3): 407–16.

7 http://www.mdanderson.org/pdf/bpisf.pdf (accessed 19 December 2003).

8 Bruera, E., Kuehn, N., Miller, M.J., Selmser, P., and Macmillan, K. The Edmonton Symptom Assessment System (ESAS): a simple method for the assessment of palliative care patients. *J Palliative Care* 1991; **7**(2): 6–9.

9 Portenoy, R.K., Thaler, H.T., Kornblith, A.B., *et al.* The Memorial Symptom Assessment Scale: an instrument for the evaluation of symptom prevalence, characteristics and distress. *Eur J Cancer* 1994; **30A**(9): 1326–36.

10 Aaronson, N.K., Ahmedzai, S., Bergman, B., Bullinger, M., *et al.* The European Organization for Research and Treatment of Cancer QLQ-C30: A quality of life instrument for use in international clinical trials in oncology. *J Nat Cancer Inst* 1993; **85**(5): 365–76.

11 Bergman, B., Aaronson, N.K., Ahmedzai, S., Kaasa, S., *et al.* The EORTC Study Group on Quality of Life The EORTC QLQ-LC13: a modular supplement to the EORTC core quality of life questionnaire (QLQ-C30) for use in lung cancer clinical trials. *Eur J Cancer* 1994; **30A**(5): 635–42.

12 Hollen, P.J., Gralla, R.J., Kris, M.G., Eberly, S.W., and Cox, C. Normative data and trends in quality of life from the Lung Cancer Symptom Scale (LCSS). *Support Care Cancer* 1999; **7**(3): 140–8.

13 Cella, D.F., Bonomi, A.E., Lloyd, S.R., *et al.* Reliability and validity of the Functional Assessment of Cancer Therapy-Lung (FACT-L) quality of life instrument. *Lung Cancer* 1995; **12**(3): 199–220.

14 Smith, E.L., Hann, D.M., Ahles, T.A., *et al.* Dyspnea, Anxiety, body consciousness, and quality of life in patients with lung cancer. *J Pain Symptom Manage* 2001; **21**(4).

15 Ravilly, S., Robinson, W., Suresh, S., Wohl, M.E., and Berde, C.B. Chronic pain in cystic fibrosis. *Pediatrics* 1996; **98**(4 Pt 1): 741–7.

16 Munro, N.C., Currie, D.C., Garbett, N.D., and Cole, P.J. Chest pain in chronic sputum production: a neglected symptom. *Respir Med* 1989; **83**(4): 339–41.

17 Mayo, P. Spontaneous pneumothorax. A 28-year review. *J Ky Med Assoc* 1984; **82**(8): 369–73.

18 Paape, K., and Fry, W.A. Spontaneous pneumothorax. *Chest Surg Clin N Am* 1994; **4**(3): 517–38.

19 Liston, R., McLoughlin, R., and Clinch, D. Acute pneumothorax: a comparison of elderly with younger patients. *Age Ageing* 1994; **23**(5): 393–5.

20 Fielding, D.I., McKeon, J.L., Oliver, W.A., Matar, K., and Brown, I.G. Pleurectomy for persistent pain in benign asbestos-related pleural disease. *Thorax* 1995; **50**(2): 181–3.

21 Miller, A. Chronic pleuritic pain in four patients with asbestos induced pleural fibrosis. *Br J Ind Med* 1990; **47**(3): 147–53.

22 Galea, J.L., De Souza, A., Beggs, D., and Spyt, T. The surgical management of empyema thoracis. *J Roy Coll Surg Edinb* 1997; **42**(1): 15–18.

23 Cassiere, H.A., and Niederman, M.S. Community-acquired pneumonia. *Dis Mon* 1998; **44**(11): 613–75.

24 Brown, P.D., and Lerner, S.A. Community-acquired pneumonia. *Lancet* 1998; **352**(9136): 1295–302.

25 Bonica, J.J. Painful disorders of the respiratory system. In: J.J. Bonica, (ed.) *The management of pain*, 2nd edn. Philadephia: Lea & Febiger, 1990; 1043–61.

26 Marangoni, C., Lacerenza, M., Formaglio, F., Smirne, S., and Marchettini, P. Sensory disorder of the chest as presenting symptom of lung cancer. *J Neurol Neurosurg Psychiatry* 1993; **56**(9): 1033–4.

27 Kori, S.H., Foley, K.M., and Posner, J.B. Brachial plexus lesions in patients with cancer: 100 cases. *Neurology* 1981; **31**(1): 45–50.

28 Bonica, J.J., Ventafridda, V., and Pagni, C.A. Advances in pain research and therapy. volume 4. management of superior pulmonary sulcus syndrome (Pancoast syndrome). *Adv Pain Res Ther* 1982; **4**.

29 Vargo, M.M., and Flood, K.M. Pancoast tumor presenting as cervical radiculopathy. *Arch Phys Med Rehabil* 1990; **71**(8): 606–9.

30 Wilson, D.S. Pain in the neck and arm. *Rheumatol Rehabil* 1979; **18**(3): 177–80.

31 Kovach, S.G., and Huslig, E.L. Shoulder pain and Pancoast tumor: a diagnostic dilemma. *J Manipulative Physiol Ther* 1984; **7**(1): 25–31.

32 Downs, S.E. Bronchogenic carcinoma presenting as neuromusculoskeletal pain [see comments]. *J Manipulative Physiol Ther* 1990; **13**(4): 221–4.

33 Marino, C., Zoppi, M., Morelli, F., Buoncristiano, U., and Pagni, E. Pain in early cancer of the lungs. *Pain* 1986; **27**(1): 57–62.

34 Shakespeare, T.P., and Stevens, M.J. Unilateral facial pain and lung cancer. *Australas Radiol* 1996; **40**(1): 45–6.

35 Capobianco, D.J. Facial pain as a symptom of nonmetastatic lung cancer. *Headache* 1995; **35**(10): 581–5.

36 Schoenen, J., Broux, R., and Moonen, G. Unilateral facial pain as the first symptom of lung cancer: are there diagnostic clues? *Cephalalgia* 1992; **12**(3): 178–9.

37 Des Prez, R.D., and Freemon, F.R. Facial pain associated with lung cancer: a case report. *Headache* 1983; **23**(1): 43–4.

38 Stein, P.D., and Henry, J.W. Clinical characteristics of patients with acute pulmonary embolism stratified according to their presenting syndromes. *Chest* 1997; **112**(4): 974–9.

39 Dalen, J.E., Haffajee, C.I., Alpert, J.S., *et al.* Pulmonary embolism, pulmonary hemorrhage and pulmonary infarction. *N Engl J Med* 1977; **296**(25): 1431–5.

40 Rubin, L.J. Pathology and pathophysiology of primary pulmonary hypertension. *Am J Cardiol* 1995; **75**(3): 51A–4A.

41 Remetz, M.S., Cleman, M.W., and Cabin, H.S. Pulmonary and pleural complications of cardiac disease. *Clin Chest Med* 1989; **10**(4): 545–92

Chapter 28

Treating severe pain in advanced lung disease

Piotr Sobanski and Zbigniew Zylicz

Pain is one of the most common and distressing symptoms in advanced cancer, with 70–90% of cancer patients experiencing pain at some time during their disease.[1] Moreover, pain is a common problem not only in lung cancer and mesothelioma, but also in other lung diseases such as benign pleural thickening disease, pleurisy, and after thoracotomy for any reason. It is important to note that patients with advanced disease will have their own personal agendas and pain may be relatively low down on their list of priorities, so being pain-free may be not their most important goal. Aggressive treatment, even if it results in freedom from pain, but at the cost of sedation and other adverse effects, may not be appreciated by most patients. Physicians should be aware that being active and independent might, for some patients, be more important than freedom from pain.

Pain treatment should be always individualized, recognizing that any patient may have more than one pain[2] and each of these pains should be addressed separately. No single approach will be helpful for all kinds of pain, and so merely increasing the doses of one agent, e.g. an opioid, until the pain 'disappears' will certainly run the risk of diminishing the quality of life remaining.

Pain treatment is important not only for the patient who is suffering it, but also for family and other carers who will need to cope with their future loss. A peaceful death, free of pain, may help the family to adjust to their bereavement. Conversely, an agonizing death may leave long-term memories that can influence carers' subsequent mental approach to their own serious disease in later life.

In fact, pain is one of the symptoms of cancer that may be controlled successfully. In experienced centres pain control is successful in 95% of patients.[3] This is more likely to happen when pain is seen in the context of the whole person and their needs and priorities. Accurate diagnosis of all symptoms, not only of pain, is essential for good outcomes. Treatment should be individualized, using both pharmacological and non-pharmacological methods of treatment.

Types of pain in relation to respiratory function

In general there are two main categories of pain. The first is **nociceptive** pain, which originates in the vicinity of the nerve endings, which are sensitive to mechanical, chemical, and thermal stimuli. Inflammation sensitizes the nerve endings, both at the periphery and in the dorsal horn of the spinal cord, by a variety of substances released from diverse cells participating in inflammation process. Endogenous opioids released by the same cells can control or limit inflammation.[4,5] Thus it is not surprising that opioids have a specific action in controlling nociceptive or inflammation-related pain.

The other main type of pain originates from damage to nerves and other structures of the central nervous system. This **neuropathic** pain may be to some extent resistant to classical analgesics such as opioids. In this situation additional agents should be given together with classical analgesics to increase the effectiveness of the treatment. (For a review of the assessment and treatment of neuropathic pain, see ref. 6. For a fuller discussion of the classification of nociceptive and neuropathic pain in the respiratory system, see Chapter 26.)

Altered emotional status modifies perception of pain and other symptoms. Pain may be destructive to a patient's morale. It makes the patient feel anxious, depressed, and preoccupied with physical symptoms, and therefore may heighten the awareness of other symptoms such as dyspnoea. The greater the anxiety, the greater the sensitivity to the pain, causing a vicious circle.[7] The anxiety may sometimes increase to fear of suffocation and respiratory panic.[8] Severe chest and abdominal pain after surgical operations may also cause impaired or voluntary shallow respiration. Thus pain management can have a crucial impact on dyspnoea perception and respiratory function control, especially in patients with respiratory problems.[9]

Pain may indirectly cause elevation of inspiratory and expiratory pleural pressures; it may reduce end-tidal volume and vital capacity, and cause a drop in alveolar ventilation accompanied by a rapid respiratory rate. Functional residual capacity may decrease to the level at which small airways collapse, causing atelectasis. Elderly patients, smokers, and those with chronic respiratory diseases are more susceptible to these changes. Pain may make the patient unable to cough and clear airways of secretions, and this in turn may contribute to lobular or lobar collapse and possibly pneumonia. As a result of this, hypoxaemia and hypercapnia may occur. For these reasons, pain relief may help to restore normal pulmonary function.

Opioids such as morphine may reduce respiratory drive, which is a particular concern in the presence of preexisting pulmonary diseases. Altered renal and liver function may modify the drug's actions. Renal failure enhances accumulation of morphine-6- and morphine-3-glucuronides.[10] The first of these may have an additional depressive effect on the respiratory centre; the latter may stimulate it in a rather unpredictable way. To avoid these complications, morphine doses should be modified accordingly to the level of renal function. Sometimes if complete freedom from pain is not possible to achieve, the alleviation of suffering becomes the ultimate goal of treatment. The risks and benefits should ideally be assessed before commencing analgesic therapy, and regularly afterwards.

Main principles of pain treatment

Experience gathered in the field of cancer and chronic pain treatment in the last decades can be summarized in a few important principles:

- ◆ Treatment should be chosen according to the pain mechanism and intensity.
- ◆ Drugs should be preferably administered by mouth and, if that is not possible, subcutaneously, transdermally, or rectally.
- ◆ Drugs should be prescribed regularly in order to prevent pain recurrence; this means that each new drug dose should be given before the effect of the last one wears off.

The WHO three-step analgesic ladder (Figure 28.1) is a recognized method for management of primarily nociceptive pain.[11,12] This decision-making tool was elaborated for cancer pain treatment, but it may also be used in the treatment of chronic non-malignant pain. Step 1 of the WHO analgesic ladder is based on the recognition that mild pain should be treated with

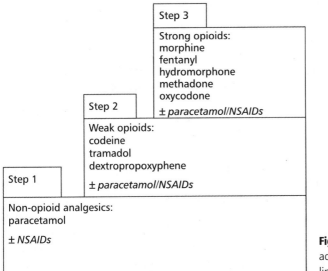

Fig. 28.1 Three-step ladder, adapted from WHO guidelines.

non-opioid analgesics such as **paracetamol (acetoaminophen)** or **NSAIDs**. Paracetamol is a centrally acting weak analgesic. Its benefit increases when combined with opioids. NSAIDs act principally in the periphery where they suppress inflammation, but they may also have central analgesic effects. NSAIDs are very important in cancer pain control,[13] and their usefulness has been formally evaluated.[14,15] NSAIDs work by inhibiting the synthesis of prostaglandins, which sensitize the receptors at the nerve endings.[16] The most useful clinically are ibuprofen, diclofenac, and naproxen.[13] To avoid gastric toxicity, three strategies may be employed:

- protection of gastric mucosa with misoprostol
- inhibition of gastric acid production[17]
- use of NSAIDs which are more specifically COX-2 inhibitors, and are thus less toxic to the gastric mucosa.[18]

Unfortunately, even using these strategies NSAIDs may still be more toxic for old, frail, and terminally ill patients than in ambulant and relatively healthy people.[19] Toxicity of NSAIDs, including COX-2 inhibitors, appears to increase in parallel to the deterioration of patients' condition in advanced disease. In particular, the risk of gastrointestinal and renal toxicity may be increased in dying patients, and these drugs sometimes have to be discontinued.

When the pain becomes moderate and the treatment with NSAIDs and/or paracetamol is insufficient, weak opioids like **codeine, dihydrocodeine**, or **tramadol** are recommended (step 2). When the pain is even more severe, strong opioids should be used (step 3). It is often forgotten that the WHO guidelines recommend that non-opiod analgesics may be combined with opioids, and don't have to be discontinued when changing from step 1 to step 2 or from step 2 to step 3. Paracetamol and codeine is a recognized and validated analgesic combination.[20] There are, however, several problems with using codeine in clinical practice. It is effective only in doses that produce troublesome constipation, so vigorous laxative intervention is usually necessary and this may not always be successful. Codeine also has powerful antitussive properties, which may of course be useful. However, there may be a fear that reducing expectoration could predispose to pneumonia in terminally ill patients, although this is not proven.

An early move to step 3 is recommended, rather than waiting until the patient is dying and then initializing strong opioid therapy, which may be very unsatisfactory for the patient. Some opioid side effects, such as sedation or nausea and vomiting, usually dissipate within a week of commencing therapy, but this may be a significant time for a dying patient.

Use of strong opioids

Opioids have long been known as centrally acting analgesics influencing pain impulse transmission at the spinal and supraspinal level. More recently there has been evidence that inflammation sensitizes not only the spinal neurones but also peripheral nociceptors.[4] These peripheral pain receptors are very sensitive to opioids administered topically. Thus administration of an opioid in a gel directly to the painful area, e.g. skin ulceration, may potentially diminish systemic toxicity.[21] The relevance of these new observations has yet to be explored, but the authors propose that topical opioids, e.g. 0.1–0.3% morphine gel, may be helpful, for example, with cutaneous metastases or wound pain.

Opioids may have different effects and side effects, even if they act principally on the same opioid receptors. Because of to their physicochemical properties, mainly lipophilicity,[22] their availability in the vicinity of the receptor and receptor binding may be different, so changing between different opioids may alter the spectrum of activity and toxicity. Some drugs, such as **fentanyl**, are not metabolized to glucuronides and a switch from **morphine** to fentanyl may therefore reduce those adverse events that are dependent on accumulation of these metabolites in renal insufficiency.[23,24] However, some patients treated with transdermal fentanyl find morphine helpful as an additive analgesic. Thus, the combination of the very lipophilic fentanyl with hydrophilic codeine or morphine may not be irrational, but actually have a logical basis. For example, fentanyl may preferentially accumulate in cerebral fatty white matter and in fat tissue. The spinal grey matter (dorsal horn) may be better penetrated by water-soluble morphine than by fentanyl.[25] So theoretically fentanyl and morphine will not compete for receptors at the same anatomical sites, as fentanyl would preferentially work supraspinally and morphine spinally and peripherally.

Methadone is another strong opioid sometimes used to treat pain in advanced cancer. In practice it is sometimes difficult to use clinically, because of its potentially increasing half-life. Besides its strong opioid activity, methadone is a potent N-methyl-D-aspartate (NMDA) antagonist. Thus it may have a different range of activity to other opioids, especially in morphine-resistant types of pain. However, the clinical relevance of this finding is still uncertain.[26]

Hydromorphone is 5–7 times more potent than morphine. It possesses a similar spectrum of activity and side effects. Because of its good water solubility it is very useful for subcutaneous administration, especially when high doses are necessary. In the UK the drug of choice for this situation is **diamorphine** (diacetyl morphine or heroin), again because of its vastly increased water solubility. The UK is the only country where diamorphine is legally used, and there is no evidence for any other advantage of using this agent, either subcutaneously or orally. Because of its short half-life time hydromorphone has less tendency to accumulate and is especially suitable for use in old and weak patients.[27]

The NMDA channel receptor is known to be crucially important in the generation of chronic pain impulse transmission in neuropathic pain syndromes.[28] Activation of the NMDA receptor by the naturally occurring neurotransmitter glutamate has been shown to cause increased spinal activity, which is seen clinically as the 'wind-up' phenomenon. This means that subsequent afferent pain impulses have increased transmission centrally. NMDA receptor activation is also linked to the development of clinical tolerance to opioids.

By blocking the access of glutamate to the NMDA receptor, it is possible to reduce the severity of neuropathically determined pain, and furthermore, to restore sensitivity to opioids.[29] The most useful NMDA receptor blockers include **ketamine**[30] and **dextromethorphan**.[1,31]

Besides the use of different drugs to enhance analgesic activity of opioids, several other drugs can be given to ease their adverse effects. The most important are laxatives and antiemetics. Use of osmotic laxatives such as **lactulose** is usually not enough to prevent opioid-induced constipation, and in high doses these laxatives may induce gas accumulation and belching. Many patients using osmotic laxatives alone become constipated with soft faeces as the constipating mechanism of opioids relies on inhibition of intestinal motility for expelling faeces, and on changing their consistency.[32] Addition of **sennosides** or **bisacodyl** to lactulose usually solves this problem. Sennosides alone may cause abdominal cramps, nausea, and vomiting. Drugs such as fentanyl are inherently less constipating than morphine, so the change from one opioid to the other may also be considered helpful for this reason.[33,34]

Approximately one third of patients treated with opioids experience nausea and vomiting in the first few days, although fentanyl may induce less nausea and vomiting than morphine.[33] These early symptoms of opioid toxicity at the vomiting centre may be easily treated with dopamine antagonists, such as a low dose of oral **haloperidol** (1–2 mg at night), or metoclopramide orally or by suppositories, 10–20 mg every 8 h. **Metoclopramide** may be particularly useful when nausea and vomiting are due not only to central effects, but also to delay in gastric emptying, as is the case with morphine.

Use of opioids in non-malignant pain

The long-term use of opioids for the treatment of severe non-malignant pain is more controversial. Experience in the field of long-term use of opioids is limited. The risk of subtle cognitive and psychomotor function impairment however exists but seems to be insignificant in patients treated with stable doses of opioids. Nevertheless dose increase may temporarily induce cognitive dysfunction.[35] There is a theoretical risk that long-term use of opioids may impair immune function; however, there is no direct evidence of this in practice. Furthermore, concern has been expressed that using opioids for chronically ill patients may not be advantageous for their psychological and functional status.[36]

Opioids have a bad reputation in some medical fields because of their ability to cause respiratory depression. Patients with severe chronic lung disease may be especially susceptible to this, and if opioids are used carelessly and the respiratory depression is not recognized or remains untreated, it may lead to death. Of course, opioids are not unique among centrally acting agents in having this potential hazard. Moreover, this problem seems to be clinically far less important than was previously thought, as long as the opioids are carefully titrated against the patient's level of pain (see below). Another objection commonly raised to the use of opioids in chronic non-malignant disease is the development of addiction. Considerable experience with cancer patients shows that actual addiction is largely irrelevant, once again if opioids are prescribed responsibly for genuine pain, and it should probably never be the reason to withhold this class of drugs for the purpose of pain relief.[37]

Getting started with morphine

In most situations, morphine is the strong opioid of choice. In chronic pain treatment the oral route of administration is preferred. If the patient has previously been taking weak opioids without adequate pain control, the starting dose of oral morphine should be 10 mg every 4 h (by elixir or normal/immediate release tablets) or 30 mg every 12 h (by slow/controlled-release tablets). In elderly patients it is wise to use half of these doses. The dose may be adjusted upwards every 24 h. If no effect is observed (either on pain or the adverse effects) the next day's doses should be increased by 50%. Most patients achieve satisfactory pain control with doses up to 180 mg/day, but higher doses are occasionally needed. If morphine is effective for pain but nausea, vomiting, or dysphagia are preventing continuing oral administration, it may be given as rectal suppositories or subcutaneously. The rectal route may however be insufficient, as morphine absorption maybe unpredictable in terminal disease.

In developed countries, most morphine is administered orally using controlled-release tablets which release morphine over 8–12 h. Approximately 30% of patients treated with such tablets experience pain recurrence before taking the next scheduled 12-hourly dose, so dividing the total daily requirement of morphine into three rather than two doses may produce more reliable analgesia. Newer products with even more sustained release overcome this problem and they may even be used once daily.[38]

If the patient is unable to take oral medication, the subcutaneous route is often favoured. For short-term use or when titrating upwards to suitable pain control levels, it is reasonable to use this every 4 h. However, for longer-term use when pain is stable, it is usually more convenient to use a continuous subcutaneous infusion. This can be administered by an external battery-powered syringe driver.[39] Carers should check the injection site daily for the presence of swelling (insufficient absorption) or redness and pain (inflammation). Fortunately, both these complications are rare.

Where syringe drivers for subcutaneous infusions are not available, or if the patient does not like needles, the rectal route may be considered. It should be noted that drug absorption from the rectum may be unpredictable, especially in very ill and dehydrated patients. In the past, controlled-release morphine tablets have been used rectally.[40] More recently, controlled-release morphine suppositories have been produced and these are more reliable.[41,42] However, in the authors' experience the rectal route should be limited to situations where subcutaneous infusions are impossible.

Transdermal opioids

The transdermal route is another convenient method for administration of strong opioids. It is useful in patients who need parenteral opioids or have difficulties with regular drug administration. Until recently fentanyl was the only opioid available as a transdermal system, delivering 25, 50, 75 or 100 μg/h over 72 h. A minority of patients require a patch change every 2 days instead of every 3 days. During the first hours after patch application, the drug penetrates the superficial skin layer where a depot reservoir is created. Thus the full analgesic effect cannot be expected until 12–24 h after patch administration. When the patch is removed it may take up to 72 h until fentanyl is cleared from the body. This may be a problem if fentanyl causes toxicity in elderly patients.

The transdermal route of administration offers less gastrointestinal toxicity such as nausea, vomiting, and/or constipation.[33,43] Fine dose titration may be difficult because of the relatively

Table 28.1 Dose conversion from oral morphine to TTS-fentanyl based on manufacturer's recommendations

Oral morphine (mg/24 h)	Initial TTS-fentanyl dose (μg/h)
45–134	25
135–224	50
225–314	75
315–404	100

large dose steps of at least 25 μg/h, equal to 60–80 mg of oral morphine per day. The fentanyl dose may be titrated in two different ways. In the first method, fentanyl is administered through continuous subcutaneous infusion in increasing doses. When the appropriate effect is achieved, the infusion is converted to the equivalent patch dose where 0.6 mg of fentanyl per day by infusion equals 25 μg/h by patch. The subcutaneous administration should then be decreased steadily over 12 h. The second method is cumbersome but safest, and can be easily carried out at home. Initially, the patient is titrated up to analgesia using oral morphine. When the pain relief is stable the morphine is converted to fentanyl patch, using a standard conversion table (Table 28.1).[44]

In the current state of knowledge, fentanyl (patches) should not be used for the treatment of dyspnoea. Although this discussion has focused on the use of transdermal fentanyl for pain control, it should be noted that dyspnoea and apnoea appeared in 3–5% of patients treated with fentanyl patches for cancer pain.[45]

Treatment of neuropathic pain

For the purposes of treatment, neuropathic pain may be divided into two categories: nerve pain associated with oedema and inflammation around the nerve; and nerve destruction without significant inflammation. In the first type of pain, opioids as well as anti-inflammatory drugs (NSAIDs or dexamethasone) may be helpful. If the pain results from nerve damage, these analgesics alone may be insufficient.[46] In this case adjuvants, e.g. anticonvulsants or antidepressants, may be of great help.

Neuropathic pain may be caused by nerve compression or injury. Frequently non-malignant pain is successfully treated with adjuvant analgesics and/or non-drug measures. Cancer neuropathic pain has more complicated mechanisms. Therefore in cancer patients treatment is started with NSAIDs with opioids. About 50% of patients respond satisfactory to combined use of strong opioids and NSAIDs. The rest of them need concurrent adjuvant analgesics.

A symptom-based approach for the treatment of neuropathic cancer pain is the best tool we have at the moment. However, symptoms alone are not a good guide for decision-making, as they are not equivalent to the underlying mechanisms. Therefore, a four-step approach is suggested (Figure 28.2). The first step in the treatment of severe neuropathic cancer pain should be administration of opioids in combination with NSAIDs and/or paracetamol (step 1), even if their usefulness may be limited.[46] If this combination is unsuccessful, specific adjuvant drugs may be tried (step 2). These include anticonvulsants and tricyclic antidepressants.

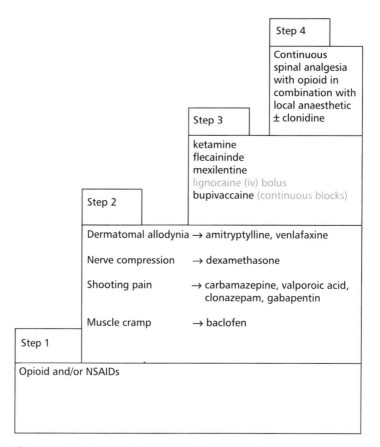

Fig. 28.2 Four-step ladder for neuropathic cancer pain.

Carbamazepine is a prototype drug for this kind of pain, but its interaction with many other drugs makes rational use difficult.[47] A starting dose for carbamazepine is 100 mg every 8–12 h.

Recently **lamotrigine** has been suggested as a better drug; but its use may be compromised by skin reactions that may develop into serious dermatological problems.[48] The usual dose of lamotrigine is 25–50 mg every 24 h for the first 2 weeks. Later the dose can be gradually increased.

Gabapentin is another new drug which is claimed to be effective in several neuropathic pain conditions.[49,50] This can be started at 100 mg every 8 h but if the low dose is well tolerated it can be rapidly increased to as much as 1200 mg every 8 h. Sometimes gabapentin needs to be administered every 4 h instead every 8 h. In the opinion of the authors, gabapentin is one of the most important drugs for the treatment of neuropathic pain. However, the drug is relatively new and probably not all its adverse effects are yet known. In old and frail terminally ill patients this drug should be used with caution, even if it is initially well tolerated.[51] Another problem can arise at the end of life, because gabapentin cannot be given parenterally. Thus, patients who have had their neuropathic pain treated satisfactorily for several months may be at risk of pain recurring if they miss doses, or stop swallowing oral medication altogether. In this situation, patients may need acute intervention with an appropriate parenteral adjuvant analgesics sedative, e.g. clonazepam starting with 1–2 mg/24h continuous subcutaneous infusion (CSCI).

Clonazepam may be a good alternative to use first; however, it should be carefully titrated to avoid sedation. Usually it takes several weeks to find a good dose and diminish sedation. Drops are ideal for titration. **Amitriptyline** is the prototype tricyclic antidepressant used in this context, but it is moderately toxic, especially in old and cachectic patients. For younger patients, the start dose is 25 mg at night. With older, frail patients, these doses should be halved. To avoid unpleasant anticholinergic effects, **desipramine** may be used instead. Drugs with considerable anticholinergic activity, such as tricyclic antidepressants, which are widely used to treat neuropathic pain, may cause thickening of respiratory mucus, which may be more difficult to expectorate. Clinical trials will show in the future if the recently introduced **venlafaxine**, which has no anticholinergic side effects, will be equally potent in the treatment of neuropathic pain. If the pain is accompanied by muscle cramps, **baclofen** or **diazepam** may be a good choice.

In step 3, class 1 antiarrythmic drugs may be used. These are orally active congeners of lignocaine (lidocaine). Their use is, however, limited by their arrhythmogenic and cardiodepressive potential. **Mexiletine** is a prototype of these drugs, but in practice they are rarely used, as their use requires some extra tests and not infrequently clinical admission. In our own experience mexiletine is strongly emetogenic.

Another drug in step 3 is low-dose **ketamine**, or its L-isomer which is now on the market. It may be added to the opioid medication (see above).[52] The dose of ketamine used subcutaneously or intravenously is 150–600 mg/day. Rectal or oral preparations are currently under investigation and may be available in the future.[53] Low, non-sedating doses of benzodiazepines are routinely used to limit hallucinations which are the main ketamine-related adverse effect.

Step 4 of the analgesic ladder is invasive treatment. Spinal opioids and bupivacaine are the standard treatment at this level. However, occasionally other neuroablative techniques are useful (see Chapter 29).

Adverse effects of pain management in patients with respiratory disease

The commonest adverse effects of NSAIDs include gastrointestinal problems and renal salt and water retention. Platelet dysfunction and coagulation disturbances can be especially severe with aspirin, because of irreversible platelet cyclooxygenase acetylation. NSAIDs may also induce bronchospasm in susceptible patients. Patients with asthma, nasal polyposis, or atopic predisposition have a higher risk of this complication. In this regard safer alternatives are choline salicylate or choline magnesium trisalicylate. Paracetamol can be taken by most patients hypersensitive to aspirin. It has also less adverse effect on the gastrointestinal system.

Opioid adverse reactions on respiratory system consist of pulmonary and central effects. It was suggested that morphine used systemically may cause bronchospasm in asthmatic subjects as a result of histamine release, but this reaction is very rare.

The most potentially serious adverse reaction elicited by strong opioids is depression of the respiratory centre. The degree of depression, which may be fatal, is dose related. At equianalgesic doses, all μ-opioid receptor agonists produce an equivalent degree of respiratory depression. Patients receiving long-term opioid therapy usually develop tolerance to the respiratory depressant effect. In practical terms, opioid-induced respiratory depression leads to a reduction in sensitivity to hypercapnia, which is seen in normal volunteers as a shift to the right of the slope of ventilatory response to carbon dioxide.[54]

Patients with impaired respiratory function or advanced chronic obstructive pulmonary disease (COPD) are most susceptible to developing clinically significant respiratory depression with opioids. However, if the opioid dose is carefully titrated up to the point of pain control, significant respiratory depression rarely occurs, because pain itself exerts a stimulatory effect on the respiratory centre and antagonizes respiratory depression.[55] Therefore, respiratory depression due to opioids is more frequent in pain-free patients than in pain-suffering patients. However, it should be noted that postoperative continuous arterial saturation monitoring shows that morphine infusion produces a higher number of hypoxaemic episodes as compared to the equivalent pain control achieved by local or epidural analgesia.[56]

Because pain exerts a stimulatory effect on the respiratory centre in chronic treatment with opioids, patients on high doses of opioids are at risk of severe acute respiratory depression if pain is relieved by other methods such as nerve block or radiotherapy.[55] Far more common is subacute overdosage, in which sedation gradually builds up and is followed by a slowing of the respiratory rate and progressive ventilatory failure. This is a potential risk in patients treated with slow-release opioid formulations such as fentanyl patches, especially if these are started or the dose is increased and then not closely monitored over the following days. There is a practical danger in starting fentanyl patch treatment on Friday or Saturday!

If the respiratory centre is stimulated by any pathological mechanism and the patient is consequently breathing rapidly, low doses at morphine titrated to the respiratory rate, may help to decrease dyspnoea. In other cases, an opioid may induce sufficient respiratory depression and irregular breathing such that the patient may panic, with fear of imminent suffocation. Apart from the known central effects of opioids, their peripheral effects are poorly understood. It has been suggested that they may lead to decrease of inflammation in the bronchi and decrease of mucus production, improved cardiopulmonary performance and decreased oxygen consumption in the peripheral tissues.[5]

Respiratory depression due to opioids may be treated with naloxone. Repeated small doses of this drug (0.02 mg every 2 min or 0.2 mg every 15–30 min) or continuous subcutaneous infusion may reverse respiratory depression without reversing analgesia.

Psychostimulant drugs such as **methylphenidate** or **dextroamphetamine**[57–60] counteract the central depressive effects of opioids, causing decrease in somnolence and improvement of cognitive performance, and with awakening, improved respiration. Methylphenidate appears to enhance the analgesic effects of opioids.[61] The attenuation of sedation permits theoretically administration of larger opioid doses, and thus improves analgesia without loss of alertness. Thus psychostimulants combined with opioids may offer enhanced quality of life among patients with difficult pain syndromes. The oral daily doses used are approximately 15 mg for methylphenidate (10 mg in the morning, 5 mg at noon) and 7.5 mg for dextroamphetamine.[61] Adverse effects of chronic methylphenidate and opioid administration (hallucinations and paranoid aggressive reactions) occur in about 4% of patients. They usually occur early in the treatment and resolve after drug discontinuation. Despite encouraging results, amphetamines are rarely used in clinical practice, probably because of myths surrounding psychostimulants and poor reputation resulting from the abuse of these drugs. They have been successfully used for many years in the management of attention deficit–hyperactivity disorder in children, narcolepsy, and depression refractory to traditional antidepressants. Very few patients treated carefully for these disorders develop psychological dependence or become addicted.[61]

The most common error made by physicians in managing severe pain with opioids is prescribing them in inadequate doses and without careful titration. Since many patients are reluctant to complain, this leads to needless suffering. Many physicians, nurses, and patients refuse to use opioids, perhaps because of an exaggerated fear of addiction. Considerable clinical experience has shown that when titrated to symptom needs, opioids very rarely cause addiction.

Management of pleural pain

Pleural disease with or without effusion may cause severe pain on breathing. **Codeine** as well as **NSAIDs** may be useful in relieving this pain. Intrapleural infusion of **bupivacaine** through a small thoracic catheter may also bring relief.[62] A small drain is inserted intrapleurally and bupivacaine is infused with a pump. This technique helps pleural pain and some other kinds. Good results have been reported with chronic pancreatitis and upper abdominal pains, postherpetic neuralgia, reflex sympathetic dystrophies of the arm or face, frozen shoulder, and invasion of brachial plexus. Skilful intercostal nerve blockade with **lignocaine (lidocaine)** or bupivacaine may be very useful. Intercostal nerve blockade should involve several levels above and beneath the painful spot.

Rib fractures can be of clinical importance in metastatic disease or in osteoporotic patients with chronic cough. Costal pain aggravated by breathing and cough may limit thoracic excursion and thus compromise ventilation and expectoration. Apart from appropriate analgesics intercostal nerve blockade seems to be very useful. In bone metastases palliative radiotherapy should be considered.

Post-thoracotomy chest wall pain can be approached initially using the same methods as for rib fractures. However, it may become chronic and should then be seen and treated as a form of neuropathic pain (see Chapter 26). After some forms of nerve damage, local neuromas may form and these can be difficult to treat. A neuroma is seen as a sprouting on the damaged nerve fibre leading to sensory deficit and allodynia (light touch exacerbates pain) or hyperalgesia (extreme sensitivity to pin pricks) in areas previously innervated by the damaged nerve. They may be treated by local infiltrations with 6% or 10% phenol.

Insertion of an epidural catheter and infusion of morphine and bupivacaine may ease chest pain.

Keypoints

- Knowledge of mechanisms of action, possible adverse reactions and their treatment, permit effective and relatively safe pain management in patients with respiratory illness
- Rational use of opioid analgesics and co-analgesics makes good pain control possible without respiratory failure in most patients
- Not all pain responds to opioids. Especially for neuropathic pain, a sophisticated stepwise approach is necessary
- Respiratory failure with opioids is uncommon when dose is carefully titrated against pain, but treatment should be carefully monitored especially in patients with advanced chronic lung diseases.

References

1 Foley, K.M. The treatment of cancer pain. *N Engl J Med* 1985; **313**: 84–95.

2 Twycross, R., Harcourt, J., and Bergi, S. A survey of pain in patients with advanced cancer. *J Pain Symptom Manage* 1996; **12**: 273–82.

3 Ventafridda, V., Conno F De., Panerai, A.E., *et al*. Non-steroidal anti-inflammatory drugs as the first step in cancer pain therapy: double-blind, within-patient study comparing nine drugs. *J Int Med Res* 1990; **18**: 21–9.

4 Stein, C. The control of pain in peripheral tissue by opioids. *N Engl J Med* 1995; **332**: 1685–90.

5 Krajnik, M., Finlay, L.G., and Zylicz, Z. Opioids affect inflammation and the immune system. *Pain Rev* 1998; **5**: 147–54.

6 Woolf, C.J. and Mannion, R.J. Neuropathic pain: aetiology, symptoms, mechanisms, and management. *Lancet* 1999; **353**: 1959–64.

7 Craig, K.D. Emotional aspects of pain. In: P.D. Wall and R. Melzack (eds) *Textbook of pain*, 2nd edn. Edinburgh: Churchill Livingstone, 1989; 220–9.

8 Sternbach, R.A. Acute versus chronic pain. In: P. Wall and R. Melzack (eds) *Textbook of Pain*, 2nd edn. Edinburgh: Churchill Livingstone, 1989; 242–6.

9 Hotchkiss, R.S. Perioperative management of patient with chronic obstructive pulmonary disease. *Int Anesthesiol Clin* 1988; **26**: 134–42.

10 Mercadante, S. The role of morphine glucuronides in cancer pain. *Palliative Med* 1999; **13**: 95–104.

11 *Cancer pain relief*, 2nd edn. Geneva: World Health Organization, 1996.

12 Hanks, G.W.C. and Cherny, N. Opioid analgesic therapy. In: D. Doyie, G. Hanks, and N. MacDonald (eds) *Oxford textbook of palliative medicine*, 2nd edn. Oxford: Oxford University Press, 1998; 331–52.

13 Ventafridda, V., Tamburini, M., Caraceni, A., De Conno, F., and Naldi, F. A validation study of the WHO method for cancer pain relief. *Cancer* 1987; **59**: 850–6.

14 Moore, R.A., Tramer, M.R., Carroll, D., Wiffen, P.J., and McQuay, H.J. Quantitative systematic review of topically applied non-steroidal anti- inflammatory drugs. *BMJ* 1998; **316**: 333–8.

15 Tramer, M.R., Williams, J.E., Carroll, D., et al. Comparing analgesic efficacy of non-steroidal anti-inflammatory drugs given by different routes in acute and chronic pain: a qualitative systematic review. *Acta Anaesthesiol Scand* 1998; **42**: 71–9.

16 O'Brien, T.P., Roszkowski, M.T., Wolff, L.F., Hinrichs, J.E., and Hargreaves, K.M. Effect of a non-steroidal anti-inflammatory drug on tissue levels of immunoreactive prostaglandin E2, immunoreactive leukotriene, and pain after periodontal surgery. *J Periodontol* 1996; **67**: 1307–16.

17 Roth, S.H. In what circumstances is it justifiable to prescribe concomitant misoprostol and/or H2-receptor blockers with non-steroidal anti-inflammatory drugs? *Br J Rheumatol* 1989; **28**(21): 1.

18 Lane, N.E. Pain management in osteoarthritis: the role of COX-2 inhibitors. *J Rheumatol* 1997; **24**(Suppl 49): 20–4.

19 Hopper, A.H. Non-steroidal anti-inflammatory drugs in elderly people. Treat mild chronic pain with paracetamol initially. *BMJ* 1995; **311**: 391–2.

20 Moore, A., Collins, S., Carroll, D., and McQuay, H. Paracetamol with and without codeine in acute pain: a quantitative systematic review. *Pain* 1997; **70**: 193–201.

21 Krajnik, M., Zylicz, Z., Finlay, I., Luczak, J., and van Sorge, A.A. Potential uses of topical opioids in palliative care – report of 6 cases. *Pain* 1999; **80**: 121–5.

22 Lehmann, K.A. and Zech, D. Transdermal fentanyl: clinical pharmacology. *J Pain Symptom Manage* 1992; **7**: S8–16.

23 Dellemijn, P.L. and Vanneste, J.A. Randomised double-blind active placebo-controlled crossover trial of intraveneus fentanyl in neuropathic pain. *Lancet* 1997; **349**: 753–8.

24 Dellemijn, P.L., van Duijn, H., and Vanneste, J.A. Prolonged treatment with transdermal fentanyl in neuropathic pain. *J Pain Symptom Manage* 1998; **16**: 220–9.

25 Bernards, C.M. Clinical implications of physicochemical properties of opioids. In: C. Stein (ed.) *Opioids in pain control. Basic and clinical aspects.* Cambridge: Cambridge University Press, 1999; 166–87.

26 Ebert, B., Thorkildsen, C., Andersen, S., Christrup, L.L., and Hjeds, H. Opioid analgesics as noncompetitive N-methyl-D-aspartate (NMDA) antagonists. *Biochem Pharm* 1998; **56**: 553–9.

27 Miller, M.G., McCarthy, N., O'Boyle, C.A., and Kearney, M. Continuous subcutaneous infusion of morphine vs. hydromorphone: a controlled trial. *J Pain Symptom Manage* 1999; **18**: 9–16.

28 Payne, R. and Gonzales, G.R. Management of pain: Pathophysiology of pain in cancer and other terminal diseases. Chapter 9.2 in: D. Doyle, G.W.C. Hanks, and N. MacDonald, (eds) *Oxford textbook of palliative medicine*, 2nd edn. Oxford: Oxford University Press, 1999; 299–310.

29 Dickenson, A.H. NMDA receptor antagonists: interactions with opioids. *Acta Anaesthesiol Scand* 1997; **41**(1): 112–15.

30 Cherry, D.A., Plummer, J.L., Gourlay, G.K., Coates, K.R., and Odgers, C.L. Ketamine as an adjunct to morphine in the treatment of pain. *Pain* 1995; **62**: 119–21.

31 Foley, K.M. Pain assessment and cancer pain syndromes. In: D. Doyie, G. Hanks, and N. MacDonald, (eds) *Oxford textbook of palliative medicine*, 2nd edn. Oxford: Oxford University Press, 1998; 310–31.

32 Canty, S.L. Constipation as a side effect of opioids. *Oncol Nurs Forum* 1994; **21**: 739–45.

33 Ahmedzai, S., and Brooks, D. Transdermal fentanyl versus sustained-release oral morphine in cancer pain: preference, efficacy, and quality of life. The TTS-Fentanyl Comparative Trial Group. *J Pain Symptom Manage* 1997; **13**: 254–61.

34 Megens, A., Artois, K., Vermeire, J., *et al.* Comparison of the analgesic and intestinal effects of fentanyl and morphine in rats. *J Pain Symptom Manage* 1998; **15**: 253–7.

35 Pereira, J., Hanson, J., and Bruera, E. The frequency and clinical course of cognitive impairment in patients with terminal cancer. *Cancer* 1997; **79**(4): 835–42.

36 Stein, C. Opioid treatment of chronic nonmalignant pain. *Anesth Analg* 1997; **84**: 912–14.

37 Savage, S.R. Opioid therapy of chronic pain: assessment of consequences. *Acta Anaesthesiol Scand* 1999; **43**(9): 909–17.

38 Gourlay, G.K., Cherry, D.A., Onley, M.M., *et al.* Pharmacokinetics and pharmacodynamics of twenty-four-hourly Kapanol compared to twelve-hourly MS Contin in the treatment of severe cancer pain. *Pain* 1997; **69**: 295–302.

39 O'Doherty, C.A., Hall, E.J., Schofield, L., and Zeppetella, G. Drugs and syringe drivers: a survey of adult specialist palliative care practice in the United Kingdom and Eire. *Palliative Med* 2001; **15**: 149–54.

40 Campbell, W.I. Rectal controlled-release morphine: plasma levels of morphine and its metabolites following the rectal administration of MST Continus 100 mg. *J Clin Pharm Ther* 1996; **21**: 65–71.

41 Bruera, E., Belzile, M., Neumann, C.M., *et al.* Twice-daily versus once-daily morphine sulphate controlled-release suppositories for the treatment of cancer pain. A randomized controlled trial. *Support Care Cancer* 1999; **7**(4): 280–3.

42 Davis, C. A new 24-hour morphine hydrogel suppository. *Eur J Palliative Care* 2000; **7**: 5.

43 Donner, B., Zenz, M., Strumpf, M., and Raber, M. Long-term treatment of cancer pain with transdermal fentanyl. *J Pain Symptom Manage* 1998; **15**(3): 168–75.

44 Ahmedzai, S., Allan, E., Fallon, M., Finlay, I.G., *et al.* Transdermal fentanyl in cancer pain. *J Drug Dev* 1994; **6**(3): 93–7.

45 Jeal, W. and Benfield, P. Transdermal fentanyl. A review of its pharmacological properties and therapeutic efficacy in pain control. *Drugs* 1997; **53**: 109–38.

46 Jadad, A.R., Carroll, D., Glynn, C.J., Moore, R.A., and McQuay, H.J. Morphine responsiveness of chronic pain: double-blind randomised crossover study with patient-controlled analgesia. *Lancet* 1992; **339**: 1367–71.

47 McQuay, H., Carroll, D., Jadad, A.R., Wiffen, P., and Moore, A. Anticonvulsant drugs for management of pain: a systematic review. *BMJ* 1995; **311**: 1047–52.

48 Chaffin, J.J. and Davis, S.M. Suspected lamotrigine-induced toxic epidermal necrolysis. *Ann Pharmacother* 1997; **31**: 720–3.

49 Rowbotham, M., Harden, N., Stacey, B., Bernstein, P., and Magnus-Miller, L. Gabapentin for the treatment of postherpetic neuralgia: a randomised co: trial. *JAMA* 1998; **280**(21): 1837–42.

50 Caraceni, A., Zecca, E., Martini, C., and De Conno, F. Gabapentin as an adjuvant to opioid analgesia for neuropathic cancer pain. *J Pain Symptom Manage* 1999; **17**: 441–5.

51 Zylicz, Z. Painful gynecomastia: an unusual toxicity of gabapentin? *J Pain Sympt Manage* 2000; **20**(1): 2–3.

52 Felsby, S., Nielsen, J., Arendt-Nielsen, L., and Jensen, T.S. NMDA receptor blockade in chronic neuropathic pain: a comparison of ketamine and magnesium chloride. *Pain* 1996; **64**: 283–91.

53 Fisher, K. and Hagen, N.A. Analgesic effect of oral ketamine in chronic neuropathic pain of spinal origin: a case report. *J Pain Symptom Manage* 1999; **18**: 61–6.

54 Daykin, A.P., Bowen, D.J., Saunders, D.A., and Norman, J. Respiratory depression after morphine in the elderly. A comparison with younger subjects. *Anaesthesia* 1986; **41**: 910–14.

55 Borgbjerg, F.M., Nielsen, K., and Franks, J. Experimental pain stimulatesrespiration and attenuates morphine-induced respiratory depression: a controlled study in human volunteers. *Pain* 1996; **64**: 123–8.

56 Choi, H.J., Little, M.S., Garber, S.Z., and Tremper, K.K. Pulse oximetry for monitoring during ward analgesia: epidural morphine versus parenteral narcotics. *J Clin Monit* 1989; **5**: 87–9.

57 Bruera, E., Brenneis, C., Paterson, A.H., and MacDonald, R.N. Narcotics plus methylphenidate (Ritalin) for advanced cancer pain. *Am J Nurs* 1988; **88**: 1555–6.

58 Bruera, E., Fainsinger, R., MacEachern, T., and Hanson, J. The use of methylphenidate in patients with incident cancer pain receiving regular opiates. A preliminary report. *Pain* 1992; **50**: 75–7.

59 Bruera, E., Miller, M.J., Macmillan, K., and Kuehn, N. Neuropsychological effects of methylphenidate in patients receiving a continuous infusion of narcotics for cancer pain. *Pain* 1992; **48**: 163–6.

60 McManus, M.J. and Panzarella, C. The use of dextroamphetamine to counteract sedation for patients on a morphine drip. *J Assoc Pediatr Oncol Nurses* 1986; **3**: 28–9.

61 Dalal, S. and Melzack, R. Potentiation of opioid analgesia by psychostimulant drugs: a review. *J Pain Symptom Manage* 1998; **16**: 245–53.

62 Myers, D.P., O'Leary, K.A., and Lema, M.J. lntrapleural catheters: indication and techniques. In: S. Waldman and A.P. Winnie (eds) *Interventional Pain Management*. Philadelphia: W.B. Saunders, 1996; 319–23.

Chapter 29

Pain in association with respiratory disease management: neurolytic procedures

W.W.A. Zuurmond and J.J. de Lange

In general, therapeutic neural blockades should be performed only after diagnostic and prognostic test procedures.

- **Diagnostic procedures** are applied to localize the pain and help determine its aetiology, by using local anaesthetics and observing the immediate reaction of the patient.
- **Prognostic blockades** allow both patient and doctor to anticipate the likely effects of a destructive block or denervation. A destructive block has to be preceded by a 'prognostic injection' with a local anaesthetic to predict the efficacy of the blockade and its acceptance by the patient. By evaluating the beneficial and harmful effects of the prognostic block, a decision whether to perform an irreversible blockade can then be made.
- **Therapeutic blockades** have to be applied to achieve a definitive decrease of pain. They may be divided into reversible and irreversible blockades:
  - **reversible** blocks may be performed with local anaesthetics with or without corticosteroids, sympathetic blocking drugs, or opioids
  - **irreversible** neurolytic procedures may be performed by administration of neurolytic drugs using alcohol, phenol, or chlorocresol, or by application of cold (cryocoagulation), or heat (thermocoagulation or radiofrequency lesions).

Neural blockades in association with respiratory disease

Pain in association with respiratory disease may be treated with

- intercostal nerve blocks
- selective percutaneous rhizotomy
- intrathecal or epidural administration of neurolytic agents
- cordotomy.

Intercostal nerve or interpleural blocks and intrathecal or epidural administration of neurolytic agents may be performed safely without image-intensifying techniques. However, selective percutaneous rhizotomy and cordotomy must be performed with a C-arm image intensifier which gives continuous fluoroscopic guidance, to provide an excellent insight into the three-dimensional anatomy.

Intercostal nerve blocks

Pain due to growth of tumour into and between ribs, with involvement of the intercostal nerve, is the main indication for this procedure. The technique has been extensively described by Moore.[1] After the patient has been positioned in the prone or lateral position, the needle has to 'walk off the rib' in a caudal direction and then be slowly advanced for 3 mm (Figure 29.1).

The blocks may be performed either at the angle of the rib posteriorly or at the anterior or posterior axillary line. Drugs which can be used for a temporary intercostal nerve block include lignocaine (lidocaine) 1–2% or bupivacaine 0.5%. It is usually necessary to inject local anaesthetics into two or three intercostal spaces, and some malignant lesions may require even more widespread blocks. The total amount of lignocaine 1% which can be injected at one session is 20 mL; lignocaine 2%, 10 mL; and bupivacaine 0.5%, 20 mL. These temporary local anaesthetic blocks be very helpful for diagnostic and prognostic purposes, and in some individuals they may provide longer-term pain relief, especially if backed up by analgesics and TENS (see Chapter 28).

Some practitioners advocate the injection of corticosteroid as well as local anaesthetic around intercostal nerves.[2] There is, however, no clinical trial evidence to show either increased efficacy or prolonged duration of action by adding corticosteroids to the local anaesthetic for intercostal nerve blockade.

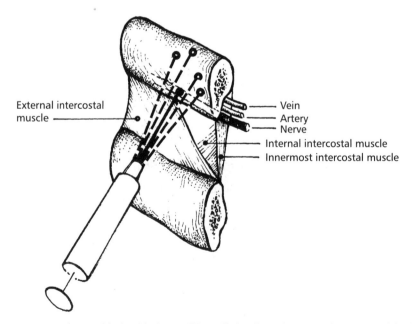

External intercostal muscle

Vein
Artery
Nerve
Internal intercostal muscle
Innermost intercostal muscle

Fig. 29.1 Intercostal nerve block with the 'walking off the rib' technique. After the caudal edge is reached, the needle is advanced 3 mm.

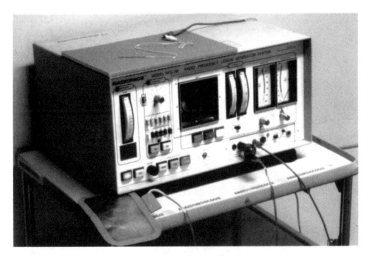

Fig. 29.2 Radiofrequency wave equipment.

In patients suffering from mesothelioma the risk of performing intercostal blocks is increased by the difficulty of performing the puncture because of the loss of anatomical reference points and the risk of tumour growth through the needle tracks in the skin. To prevent these complications, intercostal nerve blocks should be performed proximally from the suspected tumour growth.

Permanent destruction of nerves can also be carried out, using chemicals such as alcohol or phenol, or by physical methods. Chemical destruction of peripheral nerves may often result in a neuritis and deafferentiation pain.[3] Intercostal blockades may be more selectively performed by applying radiofrequency lesions or cryocoagulation. Radiofrequency lesions are produced by inserting a needle adjacent to the nerve to be destroyed. The needle is connected to a device which generates high-energy radiofrequency waves. The area around the tip is then heated to a set temperature by these radiofrequency waves, so that tissues may be destroyed selectively, dependent on temperature and tip length. Cryocoagulation achieves a similar result, but by freezing the inserted needle tip. Both of these techniques require specialized equipment (Figure 29.2) which is readily available, and they do not depend on direct imaging by fluoroscopy. The blocks may be repeated after weeks or months if necessary.[4] Pneumothorax may occur as a complication, but in experienced hands the incidence is low.

Selective percutaneous rhizotomy

In patients suffering from thoracic segmental pain as a result of tumour growth which is difficult to reach by the intercostal approach, a percutaneous selective rhizotomy may be performed according to the technique of Uematsu[5] (Figure 29.3). A very localized rhizotomy using the radiofrequency technique or a small lesion is more like to be successful.[6,7] This gives better results than applying neurolytic agents in these areas, because producing a lesion by the radiofrequency technique is more selective than performing the same blockade using neurolytic agents. According to the study of Van Kleef et al.,[7] if more than two

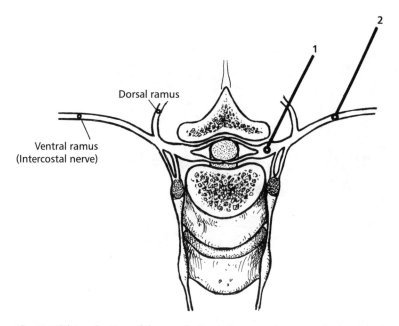

Fig. 29.3 (1) Localization of the needle tip during percutaneous selective rhizotomy. (2) Localization of the needle tip during intercostal block.

segments are involved this technique is less effective in pain treatment. The complications include pneumothorax and – rarely – damage to the spinal cord by penetration of the dura.

Intrathecal or epidural administration of neurolytic agents

Intrathecal or epidural instillation of a neurolytic solution (phenol or alcohol) may be performed for intractable cancer pain which has not responded to analgesics and the procedures described above. The relevant nerve roots are first localized by injecting local anaesthetic. This is followed by intermittent injections of 0.1–0.2 mL alcohol or phenol into the subarachnoid space, up to a maximum of 0.5–1.0 mL. The patient is then placed in the 45° neurosurgical sitting position, to allow the agents to have prolonged contact with the nerve roots to be destroyed.[4]

An alternative technique is to insert an epidural catheter and administer 0.1–0.2 mL of neurolytic agents via the catheter after a successful blockade with local anaesthetics.

Distorted anatomy resulting from growth of tumour into the epidural space is a relative contra-indication for this block. Complications may vary in severity and include hypotension, motor paresis or paralysis, and postdural puncture headache. Because of these, and the possibility of incomplete analgesia in 15–28%,[8] the spinal administration of neurolytic agents has been more or less replaced by the continuous spinal administration of opioids, often in combination with local anaesthetics. The reversibility and greater ease of control with the latter procedure is safer for patients.

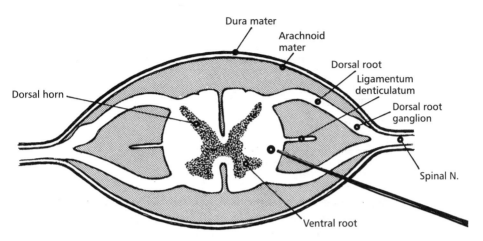

Fig. 29.4 Localization of the needle tip between C1 and C2 in performing cordotomy.

Cordotomy

Cordotomy is the unilateral destruction of the lateral spinothalamic tract in the anterolateral column of the cervical cord for the purpose of pain relief (Figure 29.4). This procedure may be indicated in patients suffering from unilateral pain not responding to previous treatments, including intrathecal administration of opioids in combination with local anaesthetics. In patients suffering from incident pain (e.g. movement-related), from lung carcinoma, neuropathic and somatic pain due to mesothelioma, or brachial plexus pain due to a Pancoast tumour, cordotomy may result in better pain control. The unilateral pain should not extend above the C5 dermatome, because the nerve fibres ascend three or four segments before crossing the spinal cord to the opposite anterolateral quadrant. When the lesion is made at the C1–C2 level, analgesia on the opposite side will normally only occur up to and including C5.[9] A less destructive alternative to cordotomy for brachial plexus pain is the continuous administration of a local anaesthetic through a catheter, which is placed percutaneously so that the tip is adjacent to the relevant nerve trunk.

For decades the axillary block of the brachial plexus has traditionally been performed by insertion through the skin overlying the axillary artery in the abducted arm. However, a 'posterior approach' may be used. In this technique, the patient is placed in the lateral or sitting position, with the arm adducted. From the dorsal side of the top of the axilla, the entry point is marked 2 cm cranially and 2 cm laterally. With the aid of a neurotracer and an insulated regional block needle, the brachial plexus is located and the local anaesthetic can be administered. For long-term continuous administration of local anaesthetic, a needle-over-needle method has to be employed: after location of the brachial plexus, the needle has to be removed to allow the axillary catheter to be inserted. The catheter may then be tunnelled to the ventral side and may be left for many days or weeks.[10,11]

Jackson *et al.*[12] recommend unilateral percutaneous cervical cordotomy in patients suffering from mesothelioma when pain due to chest wall involvement, the **costo-pleural syndrome**, is first suspected. Sanders and Zuurmond[13] have shown in a study of 62 terminally ill patients suffering from cancer that percutaneous cervical cordotomy, using a

Table 29.1 Possibilities for neurolytic blockade during respiratory disease and desirability of the procedure

Type of block	Neurolytic agents	Cryocoagulation	Radiofrequency lesion
Intercostal	±	+	+ +
Percutaneous selective rhizotomy	−	−	+
Intrathecal/epidural neurolysis	±	−	−
Unilateral cordotomy	−	−	+ +

Key: −, not recommended; ±, indifferent, 'pros and cons'; +, recommended; + +, highly recommended.

two-needle technique, resulted in 54 patients having satisfactory pain relief, 6 patients partial relief, and 2 patients no relief. They also found that major permanent complications can occur, such as urinary retention (6.5%), hemiparesis (8.1%), and mirror image pain (6.5%).

In this study *bilateral* percutaneous cervical cordotomy was evaluated in 18 patients. After this procedure 9 patients had satisfactory pain relief, 6 patients partial relief, and 3 patients no relief. The major permanent complications were the same as after unilateral percutaneous cervical cordotomy, being respectively 11.1%, 11.1%, and 5.6%.

Sleep-induced apnoea, due to the loss of the carbon dioxide drive for respiration (Ondine's curse), was not observed in any patient. When these results and complications are compared with previously reported studies, there is a noticeable variation in benefits and adverse effects (see Table 29.2).

The relative high incidence of severe motor deficit after percutaneous cervical cordotomy, especially after a bilateral procedure, has also been encountered by other authors.[14–16] This complication, together with urinary retention and mirror-image pain, may decrease the patient's quality of life. Nevertheless, in the treatment of intractable malignant pain which is localized unilaterally, and which has failed to respond to other symptomatic management, unilateral percutaneous cordotomy can be recommended, particularly for incident pain due to movement. However, considering the high incidence of complications combined with the high failure rate (50%), bilateral percutaneous cervical cordotomy cannot be recommended. Table 29.2 summarizes the possibilities for neurolytic blockade during respiratory disease.

Keypoints

♦ Thoracic pain in association with respiratory disease may be treated with the following neurolytic blocks:
  – intercostal nerve blocks
  – selective percutaneous rhizotomy
  – intrathecal or epidural administration of neurolytic agents
  – unilateral cervical percutaneous cordotomy

♦ Nerves may be destroyed by drugs (alcohol, phenol), by radiofrequency or cryocoagulation

♦ More destructive procedures such as cervical cordotomy are associated with more adverse effects

Table 29.2 Comparison of published long-term results from percutaneous cervical cordotomy and bilateral percutaneous cervical cordotomy (BPCC)

Reference	n	Success rate[a]	Respiratory depression (%)	Urinary retention (%)	Mirror-image pain (%)	Motor deficit (severe) (%)
Percutaneous cervical cordotomy						
16	62	61.3	3.9	n/a	16.5	8
15	103	32	3.9	8.7	54.5	3.9
14	76	80	n/a	10	14.5	9
17	n/a	89	1.5?	6	n/a	0.4
13	62	87.1	0	6.5	6.5	8.1
Bilateral percutaneous cervical cordotomy						
15	36	47	0	38.9	n/a	6.9[b]
18	100	80	4	2	n/a	3
16	41	48.8	n/a	n/a	1[2]	26.8
17	n/a	66	1.5?	21	n/a	0.4
13	18	50	0	11.1	5.6	11.1

[a] The success rate was defined as 'no pain after the procedure, resulting in total withdrawal of opioids'. From Sanders and Zuurmond.[13]

[b] Not all patients could be evaluated.

n/a, not available (Tasker[16] studied 264 patients, but did not differentiate between PCC and BPCC).

References

1 Moore, D.C. *Regional block*, 4th edn. Springfield, IL.: Charles, C. Thomas, 1973; 123–37.

2 Waldman, S.D., Feldstein, G.S., Donohoe, C.D., and Waldman, K.A. The relief of body wall pain secondary to malignant hepatic metastases by intercostal nerve block with bupivacaine and methylprenisolone. *J Pain Symptom Manage* 1988; **3**: 39–43.

3 Ramamurthy, S., Walsh, N.E., Schoenfield, L.S., and Hoffman, J. Evaluation of neurolytic blocks using phenol and cryogenic block in the management of pain. *J Pain Symptom Manage* 1989; **4**: 72–5.

4 Coles, P.G., and Thompsom, G.E. The role of neurolytic blocks in the treatment of cancer pain. *Int Anesthesiol Clin* 1991; **29**: 93–104.

5 Uematsu, S., Udvarhelyi, G.B., Benson, D.W., and Siebens, A.A. Percutaneous radiofrequency rhizotomy. *Surg Neurol* 1974; **2**: 319–25.

6 Sluijter, M.E., and Mehta, M. Percutaneous thermal lesions in the treatment of back and neck pain. In: S. Lipton and J. Miles (eds) *Persistent pain. Modern methods of treatment*, vol. 3. London: Academic Press, 1981.

7 van Kleef, M., Barendse, G.A.M., Dingemans, W.A.A.M., *et al.* The effects of producing a radio-frequency lesion adjacent to the dorsal root ganglion (RF-DRG) in patients with thoracic segmental pain. *Clin J Pain* 1995; **11**: 325–32.

8 Bonica, J.J., Buckley, F.P., Moricca, G., *et al.* Neurolytic blockade and hypophysectomy. In: J.J. Bonica (ed.) *The management of pain*, 2nd edn. Philadelphia: Lea & Febiger, 1990; 1980.

9 Lipton, S. *The control of chronic pain*. London: Edward Arnold, 1979; 97–103.

10 Zuurmond, W.W.A., Wagemans, M.F.M., and de Lange, J.J. A posterior approach of the brachial plexus for axillary block. *Br J Anaesth* 1999; **82**(Suppl 1): 112.

11 Vranken, J.H., Zuurmond, W.W.A., and de Lange, J.J. Continuous brachial plexus block as treatment for the Pancoast syndrome. *Clin J Pain* 2000; **16**: 327–33.

12 Jackson, M.B., Pounder, D., Price, C., Matthews, A.W., and Neville, E. Percutaneous cervical cordotomy for the control of pain in patients with pleural mesothelioma. *Thorax* 1999; **54**: 238–41.

13 Sanders, M., and Zuurmond, W.W.A. Safety of unilateral and bilateral percutaneous cervical cordotomy in 80 terminally ill cancer pain patients. *J Clin Oncol* 1995; **13**: 1509–12.

14 Broggi, G., Franzini, A., Giorgi, C., and Servello, D. The role of cervical percutaneous antero-lateral cordotomy in malignant low-back pain. *Acta Neurochirurgica, Suppl* 1984; **33**: 427–40.

15 Ischia, S., Luzzani, A., Ischia, A., and Maffezzoli, G. Bilateral percutaneous cervical cordotomy: immediate and long-term results in 36 patients with neoplastic disease. *J Neurol Neurosurg Psychiatry* 1984; **47**: 141–7.

16 Nathan, P.W. Results of antero-lateral cordotomy for pain in cancer. *J Neurol Neurosurg Psychiatry* 1963; **26**: 353–62.

17 Tasker, R.R. Percutaneous cervical cordotomy. *Appl Neurophysiol* 1976; **39**: 114–21.

18 Rosomoff, H.L., Carroll, F., Brown, J., and Sheptak, P. Percutaneous radiofrequency cervical cordotomy: technique. *J Neurosurg* 1965; **23**: 639–44.

Part VII

Specific diseases

Chapter 30

Assessment and management of respiratory symptoms of malignant disease

Peter Hoskin and Sam H. Ahmedzai

Supportive care is a major component in the management of malignant diseases that affect the respiratory system. It should be included in the overall management plan for the patient from the very outset. Even in cancers that are potentially curable, the burden of respiratory symptoms and their psychosocial consequences can be significant for the patient and family carers, and supportive care should be instituted alongside the anticancer intervention. It is no longer justified to wait for anticancer treatments with curative intent to be tried and seen to fail before the patient is considered for expert symptom palliation and the family as a whole is offered supportive care. (See Chapter 1 for a detailed discussion on the timing of supportive care with respect to anticancer therapy.)

Many patients who present with new respiratory or systemic symptoms of lung cancer will need urgent palliation of these problems, even before a definitive histological diagnosis can be made. Indeed, some patients who present late with advanced disease may be too ill for invasive diagnostic investigations, and palliative interventions will be planned on the basis of a working diagnosis of lung cancer, guided on radiological findings and clinical history. However, as will be seen below, it is helpful to pursue the histology if primary lung cancer is suspected, even in quite elderly and frail patients, because the differentiation into small-cell lung cancer (SCLC) or non-small-cell lung cancer (NSCLC) can be a very helpful guide to palliative therapeutic decisions. NSCLC is the commoner of these two main types of lung cancer.

Prevalence of symptoms in cancer

Although this chapter concentrates on supportive care needs of patients with primary thoracic cancers, much of the assessment and therapeutic content applies equally well to patients with extrathoracic primary cancers. Several studies have shown that respiratory symptoms and systemic consequences of malignancy are common to many solid tumours. Portenoy et al.[1] investigated patients with a variety of primary cancer types attending a cancer hospital in New York. Using their own Memorial Symptom Assessment Scale, they found that dyspnoea, fatigue, and pain were prevalent in most cancer patients, although there are of course variations relating to specific sites (Table 30.1). Thus, dyspnoea affected 28% of patients with colon cancer, 26% of those with breast cancer, and 12% of patients with ovarian cancers.

Hopwood and Stephens[2] reported on symptom prevalence in large numbers of patients with lung cancer who entered the UK Medical Research Council (MRC) clinical trials (Table 30.2). The data on symptoms were derived from the Rotterdam Symptom Checklist (RSCL),[3] a quality-of-life instrument that was widely used in Europe in the mid-1990s. It is worth noting that as these

Table 30.1 Prevalence of symptoms in patients attending a cancer hospital

Symptom	Prevalence (%) by primary site				
	Colon	Prostate	Breast	Ovary	Overall
Shortness of breath	28.3	25.4	25.7	12.0	23.5
Cough	22.2	25.8	37.1	28.0	28.6
Lack of energy	78.3	66.7	80.0	68.0	73.7
Pain	61.7	68.3	60.0	67.3	64.0

Source: Modified with permission from Portenoy et al.[1]

Table 30.2 Prevalence (%) of symptoms in patients with early lung cancer. See text for discussion of gender differences in symptom prevalence

Symptom	SCLC	NSCLC
Shortness of breath	87	86
Cough	81	87
Haemoptysis	26	36
Lack of energy	88	87
Chest pain	52	50

Source: Modified with permission from Hopwood and Stephens.[2]

patients were being entered in clinical trials of anticancer treatments, those who were considered too ill for such interventions will have been excluded, so the true picture of symptom and psychosocial burden at presentation may be even worse. In general there was little difference between SCLC and NSCLC, but it is interesting to note that gender differences were detectable using the RSCL.[2] Thus, women with early NSCLC reported an average of 16.8 symptoms, whereas men reported an average of 13.8 symptoms. The prevalence of general symptoms was similar but women tended to declare more psychological problems (difference of 20%). In contrast, men reported slightly more physical symptoms, e.g. 12% more haemoptysis, 7% more cough, 3% more dyspnoea, and 2% more chest pain. In early SCLC, these differences were not noted.

There are several published reports on symptom prevalence in patients with advanced lung cancer.[4,5] Once again, it is important to be aware of potential selection bias in these studies, as the criteria for including patients will vary. Many of the patients were recruited from palliative care services, and the data will therefore undoubtedly reflect differences between countries (and within countries) regarding how they select patients with advanced disease. Table 30.3 shows prevalence of symptoms in a large international study, conducted on behalf of WHO, of patients with advanced cancer who were receiving specialist palliative care.[4]

Few studies have tried to map the progression of respiratory symptoms from diagnosis to advanced disease and death. Higginson and McCarthy[6] followed a cohort of patients with a variety of primary cancer sites over several months, using a staff-rated assessment tool. These patients were not recruited at diagnosis, however, but from the point of referral to palliative care services in

Table 30.3 Prevalence (%) of symptoms in patients with advanced cancer

Symptom	Primary site						
	Lung	Breast	Oesophagus	Prostate	Gynaecological	Colorectal	Overall[a]
Dyspnoea	46	24	19	16	11	10	19
Weakness	60	57	64	53	56	68	51
Pain	52	60	44	66	75	64	57

Source: Modified from Vainio and Auvinen.[4]

[a] Represents mean percentage of all patients in survey (including four other sites)

the UK. Their important finding was that during the months that the patients had contact with specialist palliative care teams, pain was reported as coming under control over the same time course that breathlessness became more troublesome. Thus it seemed that, even in specialist hands, the respiratory aspects of palliation were not as successful as pain control.

Causes and assessment of symptoms in cancer

The main symptoms that will be considered in this chapter are dyspnoea, cough, haemoptysis, and pain. The causes of these symptoms are often complex, and the symptoms themselves may come in patterns, which together with clinical findings and evidence from imaging such as chest radiographs and ultrasound, can help to make a working diagnosis. Table 30.4 list the common patterns of symptoms which are seen in patients who have or are suspected of having problems related to cancer or its treatments.[7]

Patients with malignant disease often have other reasons for having respiratory and other systemic problems, and it is important to be able to separate the symptoms of co-morbidity

Table 30.4 Patterns of respiratory symptoms in patients with cancer: symptoms and their anatomical–pathological bases

Anatomical 'site'	Pathological change	Symptom
Pulmonary	Tracheal tumour	Dyspnoea, stridor, cough
	Lung collapse	Dyspnoea, cough
	Airway collapse	Dyspnoea, cough
	Tracheo-oesophageal fistula	Cough, haemoptysis
	Consolidation	Dyspnoea, cough, pleurisy
	Infection	Dyspnoea, cough, pain, haemoptysis
	Lymphangitis carcinomatosa	Dyspnoea, cough
	Thromboembolism	Dyspnoea, cough, pain
	Radiation damage	Dyspnoea, cough
Pleural	Effusion	Dyspnoea
	Thromboembolism	Dyspnoea, pain
	Tumour	Pain, pleurisy
Thoracic cage	Chest wall tumour	Pain, 'fungating' cancer
	Carcinoma en cuirasse	Dyspnoea, pain, 'fungating' cancer
	Diaphragmatic tumour	Dyspnoea, pain, hiccups

Source: Modified from Ahmedzai.[7]

from those of the cancer. This is particularly relevant with elderly and frail patients, as embarking on a course of management aimed at palliating malignant symptoms can expose them to potentially major side effects, when in fact less harmful treatments may be needed for coexisting chronic or acute conditions. Table 30.5 lists the common co-morbid conditions that arise in patients with cancer who complain of respiratory symptoms.

The symptoms caused by these co-morbid conditions can easily mimic those that arise directly from malignant disease. Compared with disorders producing chronic airflow limitation, i.e. asthma and chronic obstructive pulmonary disease (COPD), the onset and pattern of breathlessness related to exertion may for some patients be identical to the picture seen in malignant obstruction. Others with asthma or COPD, however, may be able to differentiate the sensations, especially if the new dyspnoea associated with cancer is not provoked by the usual factors that aggravate their chronic airflow problem. Table 30.6 shows the time course of breathlessness with different causes in such patients.

Other clues which can help to separate dyspnoea caused by cancer from the same sensation arising with non-malignant conditions come from accompanying symptoms that the patient may report. These include the presence of wheezing, cough, purulent sputum, haemoptysis, chest pain, and oedema (of lower or upper limbs). As can be seen from Table 30.7, even these clues may not be foolproof in making a secure diagnosis and in many cases further investigations will be needed, unless the patient is very ill. The detailed approaches to investigation and assessment of dyspnoea, cough, and pain are discussed elsewhere in this volume (Chapters 8 and 27).

Table 30.5 Common problems coexisting in patients with cancer (co-morbidity)

Problem	Cause
Pain	Arthritis; ischaemia; osteoporosis
Dyspnoea	COPD; heart failure; panic attacks
Cough	COPD; ACE-inhibitor; neurogenic
Fatigue	Anaemia; nutritional deficit; chronic fatigue syndrome

Table 30.6 Causes of dyspnoea in patients with cancer: relationship to time course of symptom

	Onset Acute (h)	Subacute (days or weeks)	Chronic (months)	Recurrent episodes	Nocturnal attacks
Pulmonary					
Asthma	+	+		++	++
COPD	+	++	++		
Infection	+	++			
Pleural effusion		+		+	
Bronchial obstruction	++	+			
Pulmonary embolism	+	++		+	

Source: Modified from Ahmedzai.[7]

Key: ++, common; +, occasional.

Table 30.7 Causes of dyspnoea in patients with cancer: associated clinical features

	Wheeze	Purulent sputum	Cough	Haemop- tysis	Chest pain	Oedema	
Pulmonary							
Asthma	++	(+)	++				
COPD	++	++	++	(+)		+	(Cor pulmonale: legs)
Infection	+	++	++	(+)	(+)		
Pleural effusion		+		+			
Bronchial obstruction	+	+	++	+	+	(+)	(Superior vena cava obstruction: arms/face)
Pulmonary embolism	(+)		+	+	++	+	(Deep vein thrombosis: leg)

Source: Modified from Ahmedzai.[7]

Key: ++, common; +, occasional; (+), unusual

Table 30.8 list the minimal useful investigations for dyspnoea, which may help in making a diagnosis before embarking on new therapy. The table also indicates which tests may be helpful in monitoring progress and in estimating prognosis. For example, serial lung volumes can be helpful in assessing response to bronchodilator or steroid therapy. Pericardial effusion, detected by cardiac ultrasound, and pulmonary embolism, which is confirmed by ventilation–perfusion scanning, are both poor prognostic findings.

Table 30.8 Investigation of dyspnoea in patients with cancer

Recommended test	Useful for Making diagnosis	Monitoring progress	Determining prognosis
Imaging			
Chest radiograph	++	+	(+)
CT scan of thorax	++	+	(+)
Ultrasound (to localize pleural or pericardial effusion)	+	(+)	(+)
Ventilation-perfusion lung scan (for pulmonary embolism)	+	(+)	+
Blood			
Full blood count	++	(+)	
Skin oxygen saturation (SaO_2)	++	+	
Pulmonary function			
Dynamic lung volumes (FEV_1, FVC) preferably with bronchodilator	++	+	

Source: Modified from Ahmedzai.[7]

Key: ++, essential for comprehensive assessment; +, desirable; (+) optional or limited value.

Approaches to symptom management

Once the causes of symptoms have been established, it is possible to make a rational plan for their management. Table 1.2 (page 6) presents a generic model for differentiating symptom palliation interventions on the basis of the intention to treat, for both cancer and non-malignant conditions. These categories of treatment intention (prevention/prophylaxis, targeting of primary disease process, manipulation of pathophysiological consequences, and alteration of perception) are exemplified further in the case of cancer-related symptoms in Table 30.9. Thus, where respiratory symptoms are directly related to progressive malignancy, selective use of anticancer treatment (type 2 palliation) is an important component of the management of such patients, even in the setting of advanced incurable disease. Indeed, in the context of lung cancer less than 10% of patients presenting with NSCLC will be suitable for radical (i.e. potentially curative) treatment.

Mesothelioma is another malignancy that is increasing in some parts of the world. It arises in the thorax (and also less commonly in the abdomen) and causes significant symptom load. Palliation and supportive care of these cancers and also metastatic disease from primary sites elsewhere are reviewed here, but the infrequent instances of mediastinal disease due to progressive lymphoma, germ-cell tumour, or tumours of the thymus are not considered in detail.

Which anticancer treatments are available?

The two principal modalities of treatment available in the management of cancer-related respiratory symptoms are chemotherapy and radiotherapy. In general, radiotherapy has a larger role with NSCLC and most non-thoracic primary cancers, whereas chemotherapy is the treatment of choice for SCLC, as well as breast and colorectal cancer. This partly reflects the relative sensitivities of these tumours to chemotherapy and also the differences in their natural history.

Table 30.9 Classification of palliative intervention in patients with thoracic cancers

Type of palliation	Intention	Example of intervention
Type 1	Prevention/prophylaxis	Prophylactic cranial irradiation (PCI) to prevent brain metastases in SCLC
Type 2	Direct targeting of the primary disease process	Resection of tumour Radiotherapy (RT) for bone destruction Chemotherapy for primary SCLC RT for primary NSCLC
Type 3	Manipulation of the pathophysio-logical consequences of the primary disease process	Bisphosphonate for symptoms of hypercalcaemia Haemostatic treatments for haemoptysis Pleural aspiration
Type 4	Alteration of the perception or secondary effects of the symptom	Analgesia for pain Oxygen for breathlessness Opioid for cough

Radiotherapy

Non-small-cell lung cancer

Palliative radiotherapy for NSCLC has been the subject of a series of phase III randomized controlled trials (RCTs) performed by the UK MRC and other collaborative groups in Europe and USA (such as the European Organization for Research and Treatment of Cancer [EORTC] and the South Western Oncology Group [SWOG]) over the last decade or more. These studies have extensively investigated the efficacy of radiotherapy in the management of symptoms from advanced inoperable disease and explored optimal radiation dose schedules. From these results it appears clear that for less fit patients, symptom control can be achieved either with single doses of 10 Gy, or with two treatments given 1 week apart delivering 17 Gy in two fractions.[8,9] One trial suggests that in patients with good performance status a more protracted treatment delivering 39 Gy in 13 fractions can achieve similar symptom control with a small but statistically significant improvement in survival.[10] Estimates of rates of symptom control from these trials are shown in Table 30.10. The issue of deferring treatment in the absence of symptoms has also been explored in a recent MRC trial in which 230 patients with inoperable NSCLC were randomized to immediate palliative radiotherapy or supportive care and later radiotherapy only if symptoms arose. This study showed that there was no disadvantage in avoiding treatment in the asymptomatic patient.[11]

Radical radiotherapy may be indicated in some patients presenting with locally advanced inoperable NSCLC, typically those with stage IIIA or IIIB disease and good performance status and pulmonary function. Extensive trials have been undertaken in recent years evaluating the role of dose escalation and acceleration in NSCLC.[12] Studies by the Radiation Therapy Oncology Group (RTOG) in the USA have explored dose escalation demonstrating a plateau for response and survival at 69.6 Gy using treatment delivered twice daily in 58 fractions of 1.2 Gy over 5.5 weeks. In the UK continuous hyperfractionated accelerated radiotherapy (CHART) has been evaluated in a large randomized trial of 563 patients. This schedule treats patients three times daily using fractions of 1.5 Gy to a total dose of 54 Gy. Radiotherapy is given continuously, including over weekends, so that the entire course is completed in 12 days. The results of the RCT comparing this to standard conventional radiotherapy delivering 60 Gy in 6 weeks has

Table 30.10 Symptom response and survival in lung cancer following radiotherapy

| | Trial 1[a] | | Trial 2[b] | | Trial 3[c] | |
	17 Gy	10 Gy	39 Gy	17 Gy	30 Gy	EBRT
Dyspnoea	41%	43%	51%	46%	49%	38%
Cough	48%	56%	36%	48%	45%	65%
Haemoptysis	75%	72%	89%	95%	90%	71%
Fatigue	NS	NS	40%	48%	65%	30%
Chest pain	59%	72%	58%	65%	77%	43%
Median survival (days)	100	122	270	216	287	250

[a] MRC (1992):[9] 17 Gy in 2 fractions, 10 Gy in 1 fraction.

[b] MRC (1996):[10] 39 Gy in 13 fractions; 17 Gy in 2 fractions.

[c] Stout et al. (2000):[14] 30 Gy in 8 fractions: 15 Gy endobronchial radiotherapy.

NS, not stated.

shown a consistent improvement in survival, with 30% alive at 2 years compared to 21% and a 5-year survival of 12% compared to 7%.[13] In the UK CHART has been recommended by the Department of Health as the radiotherapy schedule of choice in the treatment of early inoperable NSCLC. Current efforts are being focused on evaluating chemo-radiation in the radical treatment of NSCLC; similar gains to those seen using CHART are being reported using cisplatin-based schedules concomitantly with high-dose thoracic irradiation.

Small-cell lung cancer

Radiotherapy is also effective in SCLC; indeed, SCLC is a highly radioresponsive tumour in which rapid regression is often seen. However, systematic trials have not been performed on the role of radiotherapy for palliation of symptoms from SCLC. In general, therefore, an analogy between NSCLC and SCLC is assumed, with similar doses being used for both.

Mesothelioma

Treatment of mesothelioma with radiotherapy is usually undertaken for chest pain. Other symptoms such as pleural effusion, cough, and dyspnoea reflecting diffuse chest-wall disease are not helped by radiotherapy because of the difficulties in localization and the toxicity from delivery of radiation to large volumes of the thorax. Palliation has been reported in 60–70% of patients, although this may be maintained for only a few months.[15,16] Retreatment may be effective and no dose–response relationship for palliation has been shown, standard doses being 20–30 Gy in 5–10 daily fractions over 1–2 weeks.

Endobronchial therapy

The trials discussed above concerned external beam radiotherapy, but radiation can also be delivered internally to endobronchial tumours using **brachytherapy**. This is a technique whereby a radiation source is directly introduced into the bronchus. High dose rate (HDR) afterloading brachytherapy may now be delivered using a high-activity source (iridium). Because of its high specific activity, iridium requires only a small amount of isotope to provide sufficient radiation for clinical use. A typical source is 1.6 mm in diameter, which allows fine-bore catheters to be used to direct its delivery. The standard HDR afterloading catheters for endobronchial use are 2 mm in outside diameter, which means they can pass easily through the suction channel of a fibreoptic bronchoscope and be placed readily within the bronchial tree without causing physical disruption (Figure 30.1).

A common problem in the larger bronchi is to ensure that the source is centred in the lumen and not alongside one wall or the other. This is sometimes managed by using self-centring catheters which have side wings to stabilize their position. Catheters are placed under direct vision at fibreoptic bronchoscopy and their position is verified, following removal of the bronchoscope, by radiography or CT scan (Figure 30.2). The length of catheter to be treated is then defined on the film and the afterloading machine is programmed to pass its source into the catheter and deliver an effective radiation dose along that segment. This is achieved by moving the source in 5 mm steps along the defined length, keeping it for a few seconds in each position to deliver its radiation dose at that site.

The usual dose for a single endobronchial treatment is 15 Gy defined at 1 cm from the catheter; points inside that 1-cm envelope will receive much higher doses. This technique is usually performed as a daycase procedure, but requires fibreoptic bronchoscopy under sedation or light general anaesthetic to place the catheter which carries the radiation source. Single-centre studies

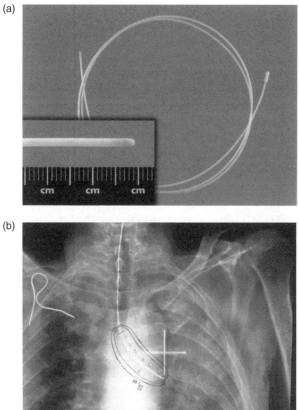

Fig. 30.1 HDR brachytherapy catheter. (a) Coiled catheter; (b) catheter placed in bronchus.

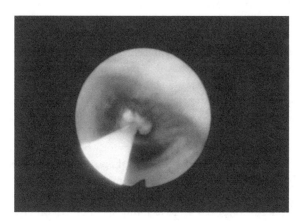

Fig. 30.2 HDR catheter *in situ* following removal of broncho-scope.

have shown this to be effective in palliation of endobronchial symptoms. A recent RCT compared endobronchial brachytherapy with external beam radiotherapy and concluded that fractionated external beam therapy is to be preferred in patients with good performance status.[14] External beam radiotherapy gave better and more sustained overall palliation, but it caused greater acute toxicity, in particular dysphagia. As would be expected, there was no survival difference between the two techniques. The relative efficacies for symptom palliation are shown in Table 30.10.

Initial experience suggested that brachytherapy was associated with a high incidence of later death from massive intrapulmonary haemorrhage, but this has not been confirmed in more recent studies and was not a feature of the randomized trial by Stout et al.[14] The main acute toxicity is in the form of increased cough from the irritant effect of the catheter and later endobronchial radiation reaction. This is typically short-lived and self-limiting over a few days. The place of endobronchial brachytherapy in the overall management of advanced lung cancer remains unclear. The Stout et al. trial suggests that for most patients external beam therapy should be considered initially, and the main role of brachytherapy is in those patients relapsing with chest symptoms after previous palliative or radical external beam treatment. (See Chapter 16 for more on brachytherapy.)

Chemotherapy

Non-small-cell lung cancer

A role for chemotherapy in NSCLC has emerged in recent years, with randomized trials showing both efficacy and possible survival advantages from the use of combination chemotherapy. A number of drugs are effective, the most commonly used schedules in the palliative setting being **cisplatin, vinblastine, and mitomycin-C (MVP)**, **cisplatin with gemcitabine**, **cisplatin with paclitaxel**, and **cisplatin with vinorelbine**. A recently completed RCT comparing cisplatin and paclitaxel with cisplatin and gemcitabine, cisplatin and docetaxel, and carboplatin and paclitaxel in 1207 patients with stage IIIB or IV NSCLC has shown no overall difference in efficacy or toxicity between these four schedules for palliation in advanced NSCLC.[17] There are fewer data on the role of further second-line chemotherapy after relapse, but one randomized study of **docetaxel** against 'best supportive care' in this setting suggested that there was an improvement in quality of life in the chemotherapy arm and an increase in median survival from 4.6 months with best supportive care, to 7.5 months with chemotherapy.[18]

One important observation is the dissociation between objective tumour response rates and symptom response, especially in NSCLC. This is illustrated in the results of MVP which gives a 32% objective response yet a substantial improvement in symptoms in 69% of a series of 110 patients.[19] Further studies from this group have shown that in a randomized trial three cycles of MVP produced the same degree of palliation as six cycles: the objective symptom response was 31% after three cycles and 32% after six cycles with median response duration 7 months and 8 months respectively.[20] In patients unable to tolerate cisplatin or where renal function is poor, similar results are achieved with the substitution of carboplatin. RCTs comparing chemotherapy with so-called 'best supportive care' demonstrate modest gains in survival of 2–4 months (see Table 30.11).[19,21–23] Together with improved quality of life in the chemotherapy arms of these trials, this survival advantage has led to recommendations in North America and the UK that 'best supportive care' only should no longer be considered the 'standard of care' for patients with advanced NSCLC. However, it should be stressed that the term 'best supportive care' in the studies quoted above was usually employed as a euphemism or shorthand for 'standard oncology follow-up care', and not as the package of comprehensive multidisciplinary supportive care described in Chapter 1. In the UK the National Institute for Clinical

Table 30.11 Symptom response rates (%) with chemotherapy in NSCLC

Treatment	PV + M or I[a]	MIP[b]	MVP[c] All	Gemcitabine[d]	Mod./severe
Dyspnoea	78	46	59	26	51
Cough	45	70	66	44	73
Haemoptysis	91	92	–	63	100
Anorexia	50	58	–	29	38
Pain	47	77	60	32	37
Malaise	–	–	53	–	–

Source: Modified from Thatcher et al. (1993)[23] and Ellis et al.(#1995).[19]

PV, cisplatin, vindesine with either mitomycin (M) or ifosfamide (I); MIP, mitomycin, ifosfamide, cisplatin. MVP (also called CMV), cisplatin, mitomycin C and vinblastine.

'All' refers to the percentage of patients with symptoms (mild, moderate and severe) who had relief; 'Mod./severe' refers to the percentage of patients with only moderate and severe symptoms who improved.

Excellence (NICE) has recently given approval for the use of docetaxel, vinorelbine, and gemcitabine in combination with cisplatin for first-line palliative chemotherapy in NSCLC and docetaxel alone for second-line chemotherapy.

Small-cell lung cancer (SCLC)

SCLC is highly chemosensitive, although responses may be only short-lived. The role of chemotherapy in palliation has been the subject of many randomized phase III trials. A comparison of four cycles of single-agent oral **etoposide**, with one of two combination chemotherapy schedules, either **etoposide and vincristine (EV)** or **cyclophosphamide, doxorubicin, and vincristine (CAV)** reported equivalent palliation, seen in 41% of patients receiving etoposide and 46% with EV or CAV.[24] There was, however, a small statistically significant survival advantage with the two combination chemotherapy regimes, median survival being 130 days with etoposide compared to 183 days with EV or CAV. A randomized trial of three versus six courses of chemotherapy using **ECMV (etoposide, cyclophosphamide, methotrexate, and vincristine)** reported palliation of major symptoms (cough, haemoptysis, chest pain, anorexia, and dysphagia) in 63% with no difference between the regimes and no statistically significant difference in survival.[25] In patients presenting with extensive disease or limited disease but poor performance status a comparison of three cycles of ECMV with EV found no difference in response or survival rates with median survivals of 141 days (ECMV) and 137 days (EV) and similar rates of palliation, with less treatment-related toxicity associated with EV.[24]

Mesothelioma

Chemotherapy for mesothelioma is, by contrast, extremely disappointing. Single agents appear as effective as combination chemotherapy and overall response rates are of the order of 20%. The most effective agents are probably the antimetabolites, with response rates of over 30% reported with high-dose methotrexate. Adriamycin, epirubicin, mitozantrone, mitomycin C, cisplatin, and alkylating agents are all broadly equivalent as single agents.[26,27] The combination of MVP as used in NSCLC has been reported to have a 20% objective response rate and 62% symptomatic response rate in a small series of 39 patients.[28] Intracavitary chemotherapy using instillation of cisplatin, mitomycin, or cytosine arabinoside into the pleural space has been reported, but currently remains an investigational approach. Temporary control of recurrent pleural effusions has been seen but this may simply reflect a local irritative pleurodesis rather than a true cell-killing effect, and further trials of this approach are required. (See below for more on management of pleural effusions.)

Radiotherapy or chemotherapy for palliation?

Symptoms of breathless, haemoptysis, cough, and pain due to either NSCLC or SCLC can be effectively palliated in the previously untreated patient with either radiotherapy or chemotherapy. The choice between the two is often difficult and, as shown in Tables 30.10 and 30.11, response rates are similar. Chemotherapy may be seen as a more debilitating treatment with more associated systemic toxicity, but radiotherapy may also cause acute effects, typically transient dysphagia due to radiation oesophagitis. Chemotherapy may be more effective where symptoms are multiple and due to widespread disease, where there is metastatic disease outside the lung, and where other symptoms such as cachexia and anorexia are prominent. Comparison of RCTs suggests that better quality of life will be achieved with chemotherapy than so-called 'best supportive care' alone, not to mention the observed survival advantage.

Radiation therapy is predominantly a locoregional treatment, and where symptoms are due to locoregional tumour progression, for example isolated haemoptysis from the bronchus or obstruction secondary to endobronchial tumour growth, then local radiotherapy is effective and simple with toxicity usually limited to a short period of dysphagia. Phase III evidence supports its use in short pragmatic schedules delivering one or two large doses where performance status is poor. These doses are close to normal tissue tolerance, however, in particular that of the spinal cord, and in general these treatments cannot be repeated. Brachytherapy localizes the radiation dose within the bronchus and offers an alternative means of retreatment for patients with cough, dyspnoea, or haemoptysis due to recurrent endobronchial tumour.

No direct phase III comparison of chemotherapy versus radiotherapy has been undertaken in the management of symptoms from advanced NSCLC or SCLC. Phase III trials in NSCLC suggest that chemotherapy has advantages over supportive care alone, although difficulties in the definition and delivery of so-called 'best supportive care' leave these conclusions open to debate. (See Chapter 1 for further discussion of definitions and the proposed composition of a truly comprehensive supportive care programme.)

Both radiotherapy and chemotherapy have been shown to have a small survival advantage, of the order of 3 months. However, this must be viewed in the light of the time taken to undergo a course of treatment and recover from its treatment-related side effects. A cost-benefit analysis from Canada addressing the role of chemotherapy in NSCLC found a benefit from both cisplatin and vinorelbine and gemcitabine when survival and quality of life were considered against so-called 'best supportive care' alone.[29]

A 'scripted interview' study in the US exploring the views of patients who had had previous cisplatin-based chemotherapy for NSCLC found that although there was considerable individual variation, chemotherapy would be accepted by these patients if there was median survival threshold of 4.5 months for mildly toxic chemotherapy and 9 months for chemotherapy with severe toxicity.[30] When considering the effect of chemotherapy on symptoms, 68% would choose chemotherapy if it would substantially reduce symptoms.

Perhaps the most important single factor to take into consideration for planning therapy is performance status. Patients with good performance status (i.e. WHO grade 0 or 1) may gain a survival advantage from protracted radiotherapy (i.e. >5 fractions) or chemotherapy

(>3 courses) whereas patients with poor performance status are generally best served by single-fraction palliative radiotherapy, or in SCLC, short (three-course) combination chemotherapy.

Treatment choices will also be influenced by previous exposure to treatment. Previous radiation may exclude further exposure if tolerance doses to critical normal tissues are exceeded. This will usually relate to the spinal cord rather than intrathoracic structures. Spinal cord tolerance is generally perceived to be around an equivalent dose of 40–50 Gy given in 2 Gy fractions over 4–5 weeks. The palliative schedule of 17 Gy in two fractions has been demonstrated to result in fewer episodes of myelitis, with an estimated risk of about 2% across the 1042 patients treated in MRC trials with this schedule.[31] Most patients are therefore very close to or at the limits of spinal cord tolerance after palliative radiotherapy, and retreatment after such schedules carries significant hazards.

A different principle applies to re-exposure to chemotherapy relating to drug-resistance. In general re-exposure to a previously administered chemotherapy agent is avoided, on the basis that residual cells progressing after that exposure will be resistant to the original chemotherapy drug. Since in most circumstances there are two recognized effective treatment chemotherapy schedules, this limits the need for repeating treatments. The palliative efficacy of second-line chemotherapy has been formally evaluated in a randomized trial in SCLC confirming an advantage for second-line chemotherapy over 'supportive care' in patients responding to an initial four cycles of treatment.[32]

Comprehensive palliation of symptoms

Apart from treatments directed at the cancer itself (type 2 palliation) which have been extensively discussed above, management of symptoms can also be considered using the other types of palliative interventions described in Chapter 1. Examples of these approaches include:

♦ endobronchial tumour causing obstruction or cough (types 3, 4 palliation)

♦ lung parenchymal disease which will typically cause breathlessness and may also be associated with cough (types 3, 4 palliation)

♦ chest wall invasion, predominantly pain (type 4 palliation)

♦ systemic illness, e.g. fatigue, distant metastases (types 3, 4 palliation)

These are shown in Figure 30.3, along with examples of types 1 and 2 palliation (preventive and direct anticancer intervention).

Breathlessness

Breathlessness due to endobronchial obstruction may be associated with stridor or lung collapse. Initially this may be treated with an endobronchial clearing procedure such as laser therapy,[33–35] photodynamic therapy,[36] or cryotherapy.[37,38] These are all strictly speaking type 2 palliative interventions, as they work by destruction of the tumour. Airway stenting may also be useful where tumour outside the bronchi is causing external compression.

Airway stenting can give very rapid and dramatic relief of dyspnoea, especially if it is caused by extrinsic compression of bronchi or trachea. Figure 30.4 shows two such examples of extrinsic airways compression arising in mesothelioma and primary lung cancer. Figure 30.5 shows a patient with recurrent NSCLC who was previously treated with external beam radiotherapy, and was successfully palliated with a bronchial stent after complete lung collapse. (For a fuller discussion of these techniques and the role of endobronchial stenting, see Chapter 16.)

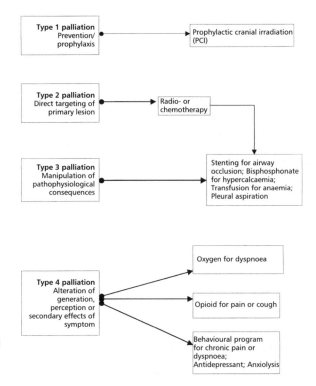

Fig. 30.3 Model of palliative intervention for cancer-related symptoms. See Chapter 1 for explanation.

For both NSCLC and SCLC, external beam radiotherapy or endobronchial brachytherapy is effective and should be considered. Where breathlessness is due to diffuse parenchymal infiltration or multiple lung metastases or lymphangitis then chemotherapy is indicated and radiotherapy has no role. Lymphangitis due to primary lung cancer is usually resistant to both types of intervention; however, chemotherapy may be helpful when lymphangitis arises in breast cancer.[39]

Where pleural effusion secondary to malignancy is the cause of breathlessness then initial treatment will include drainage and possibly pleurodesis – the methods for these are discussed below. Radiotherapy does not have a significant role in this situation, but chemotherapy may be helpful where recurrent effusions are a problem. One study of 37 patients receiving chemotherapy for malignant pleural effusion using mitomycin C and cisplatin with either 5FU (MCF) or vinblastine (MVP) reported a symptomatic response rate of 78% and objective improvement of the effusion radiologically in 86%.[40]

Where breathlessness is due to diffuse pleural infiltration with multiple deposits of mesothelioma, radiotherapy may be tried if the disease is relatively localized. For more generalized disease, chemotherapy can be considered, but as stated before, the response rate for mesothelioma is very disappointing.

Haemoptysis

Haemoptysis is most commonly due to endobronchial tumour and is more common in NSCLC.[41] It is more likely to occur with centrally placed tumours, and with primary lung cancer than with lung metastases (see Figure 23.1).

(a)

(b)

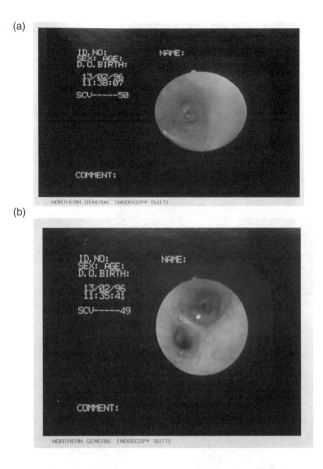

Fig. 30.4 Bronchoscopic appearance of extrinsic compression: (a) Bronchoscopic appearance in a 51-year-old man with extensive left sided pleural mesothelioma. This picture shows narrowing of the left main bronchus due to external compression, arising from mesothelioma infiltration around bronchial roots. (b) Bronchoscopic appearance of left upper lobe bronchus showing marked external compression. Endobronchial biopsies were normal.

Patients who have had many years of COPD may well cope with breathlessness if it becomes worse on development of lung cancer; however, the same patients may be very fearful if haemoptysis develops. They can usually distinguish the fresh blood expectorated from a cancer from the dark staining of sputum associated with an exacerbation of COPD. The bleeding from a cancer may indeed be aggravated by intercurrent infections with increased coughing, and it is helpful to offer the patient antibiotics early on if there are signs of a new respiratory infection developing.

Haemoptysis that is intermittent and mild (often described by the patient as 'specks', 'streaks', or 'small blobs' of blood) may be managed by simple pharmacological means. Two drugs are helpful in this situation. **Tranexamic acid** works by inhibiting the breakdown of fibrin clots, primarily by blocking the binding of plasminogen and plasmin; it is given orally at a dose of 1 g four times daily. Alternatively, **ethamsylate** works not by interfering with coagulation directly, but rather through increasing capillary vascular wall resistance and platelet adhesiveness. This agent is also given orally, at a dose of 500 mg four times daily. It is possible to use both ethamsylate and tranexamic together for resistant haemoptysis; the drugs should be continued for a week after the bleeding subsides. There are no published trials of the use of these agents for haemoptysis.

If haemoptysis is not controlled by these means, or if the patient is unduly at risk of major bleeding, it may be readily controlled with local radiotherapy either given by external beam

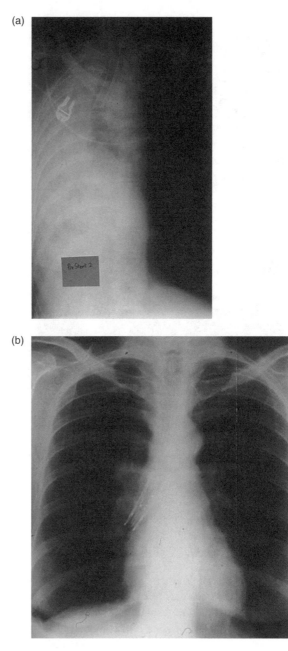

Fig. 30.5 Female patient with recurrent NSCLC treated with endobronchial stent: (a) Complete collapse of right lung. (b) Re-expansion of right lung 1 week after stent placement in right main bronchus.

treatment or endobronchial treatment given in standard palliative doses. Chemotherapy may also be effective, particularly in SCLC.[42]

Occasionally haemoptysis may be due to parenchymal lung metastasis. Localized treatment such as radiotherapy is then of less value unless a definite segment of the lung can be identified at bronchoscopy from which haemorrhage is occurring. For a discussion on the role of arterial embolization for major haemoptysis, see Chapter 23.

Cough

Cough due to malignancy is often a difficult symptom to palliate. Many patients with long-standing lung disease who later develop a primary lung cancer will be familiar with chronic cough which is exacerbated by infective episodes. It is important to allow cancer patients access to antibiotics if infection is definitely the cause of increased cough. The pharmacological management of cough is described fully elsewhere in this volume (Chapter 24). The drug of choice for reducing the cough reflex is an opioid. Often patients with cancer are already on analgesic doses of opioids: in this situation it does not necessarily help to add another opioid for cough, but it may help to give long-acting forms, especially by night.

When cough is due to endobronchial tumour then palliative external beam radiotherapy, endobronchial brachytherapy, and chemotherapy may all be effective. Overall efficacy rates are similar, as shown in Tables 30.10 and 30.11. It should be recognized that in the short term cough may be made worse both by external beam radiotherapy and by endobronchial irradiation, which produce localized radiation tracheitis or bronchitis. Patients should therefore be warned of the possibility and they should be offered a short course of opioid linctus, e.g. codeine.

Where cough is due to diffuse parenchymal infiltration, lymphangitis, or multiple pulmonary metastases then chemotherapy may help. Cough may also be due to pleural effusion, and the appropriate therapy for that should be offered (see below).

Pain

Pain is a very common symptom arising in thoracic malignancy. Chapter 26 describes the causes in terms of anatomical lesions and Chapter 27 covers typical pain syndromes. Patients who have had thoracotomy for attempted or curative resection of tumour will have added surgical scar pain, which is predominantly neuropathic. The pharmacological management of pain is covered in Chapter 28 and in other palliative medicine texts.[43,44] It is always useful to try a combination of NSAID and opioid (codeine, dihydrocodeine, or more potent agents such as morphine, fentanyl, or hydromorphone) before considering anticancer measures. Even after the latter have been successful, it is likely that the patient will continue to use analgesics, at reduced dose or for usage as required. It is important that patients who have had pain associated with cancer always have access to suitable analgesics at home, should the pain recur or progress. Patients should also be instructed to report worsening pain, which does not respond to their usual regular or as-required medication, sooner rather than later.

Chest pain due to primary lung cancer can be effectively treated, as with other symptoms, by either local radiotherapy using external beam or by chemotherapy; response rates are shown in Tables 30.10 and 30.11. Pleuritic pain due to peripheral lesions may be more difficult to localize and treat, and it may be more appropriate to refer to a pain clinic for local anaesthetic or neurolytic intercostal or paravertebral blockade, rather than for anticancer therapy. Chapter 29 describes these techniques and other invasive approaches for the management of refractory pain.

Patients with lung cancer often develop peripheral metastases which cause local pain. Bone metastases respond well to single fractions of external beam radiotherapy. In some situations, e.g. metastasis to head and neck of femur, very good palliation and restoration of function may be achieved by surgical intervention, e.g. pinning or total hip replacement (see Figure 30.6).

(a)

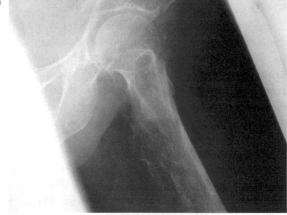

(b)

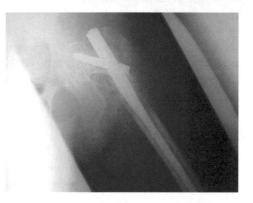

Fig. 30.6 Radiological appearance of left femur affected by metastatic cancer: (a) Multiple lytic lesions in proximal end of femur causing severe pain on weight-bearing and presenting risk of pathological fracture. (b) Prophylactic pinning of the proximal end of femur. The patient had reduced pain on mobility and risk of fracture was eliminated.

Management of effusions

Pleural effusion frequently arises from primary lung cancer, in the early stages of mesothelioma, and occasionally with metastases affecting the pleura. If it is a presenting feature of a new illness, then it is quite likely that the effusion may be drained for diagnostic purposes. Usually this is done fairly simply using a simple percutaneous needle and syringe with a three-way valve apparatus. If the effusion is large and produces significant dyspnoea at the outset, or if it recurs soon after diagnostic drainage, then a pleural catheter should be considered. It is common now to use a so-called 'pigtail' catheter in the interpleural space, as this adopts a pronounced curvature on removal of the metal guide from the chest wall, which prevents the catheter from falling out (see Figure 30.7). Alternatively, a conventional intercostal drain may be inserted and sutured in well.

A substantial effusion may require 24–48 h to drain fully. When it is dry, or there is minimal fluid, it may be helpful to instil a sclerosing agent to prevent recurrence. This is not usually necessary until the effusion has recurred two or more times, or if it recurs quickly with a large volume. The purpose of instilling a sclerosing agent is to induce pleural inflammation, which allows the parietal and visceral pleura to adhere, thus preventing further fluid leakage. Various agents have been used, notably talc, but tetracycline (with local anaesthetic to cover for the pain

(a)

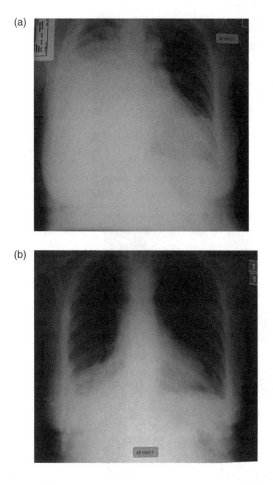

(b)

Fig. 30.7 (a) Large malignant pleural effusion before aspiration. (b) After aspiration – residual effusion.

of inflammation) is cheap and reliable.[45,46] Anticancer drugs such as bleomycin do not offer significant advantages for most recurrent malignant pleural effusions.

Pericardial effusions may occur, often developing rapidly, causing patients to be extremely breathless. For rapid relief, they can be drained directly or a catheter may be left *in situ*; see Figure 30.8 for an example of this in a patient with mesothelioma. Pericardial effusion can occur with breast cancer, and may then respond to appropriate chemotherapy. For recurrent pericardial effusion, a permanent 'window' may be placed surgically between the pericardial sac and the interpleural space.

Rarely, a pleural effusion recurs in spite of attempts at chemical pleuradhesis. In this case, it can be helpful to seek the help of a thoracic surgeon to perform a pleurectomy. This can be done under direct vision using a thoracoscope, and allows the surgeon to peel off the affected area of pleura. This technique may be particularly helpful in mesothelioma, but should be reserved for patients with relatively good expected survival.[45] In a prospective cohort study of 51 patients with malignant mesothelioma, video-assisted thoracic surgery (VATS) was used to achieve pleurectomy in 17 (34%), but decortication was required for the remainder (using

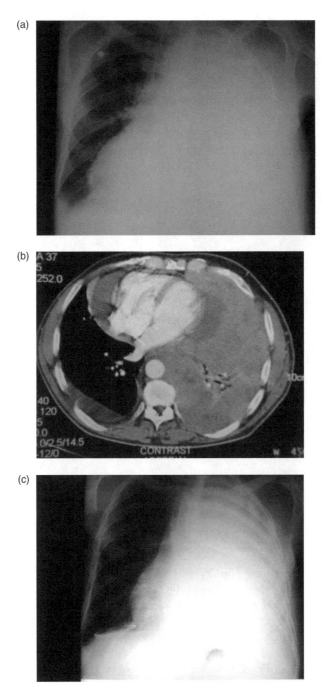

Fig. 30.8 Mesothelioma causing pericardial effusion: (a) A huge left-sided solid mass consisting of mesothelioma, causing mediastinal shift to the right side. Also pericardial effusion which is more clearly demonstrated in (b). The right costophrenic angle is obliterated, indicating a small pleural effusion. (b) CT scan showing complete filling of left hemithorax with mesothelioma. There is a pericardial effusion and also small right pleural effusion. (c) Radiographic appearance after a catheter was placed in the pericardial sac (seen lying at base of right lung). The space between right chest wall and cardiac border was increased indicating loss of pericardial volume. Note that the small pleural effusion has also been drained.

VATS in 3 and thoracotomy in 31).[47] is suggested that debulking surgery should be reserved for patients who have the epithelial cell type of mesothelioma, and who have not yet suffered significant weight loss.

Keypoints

- Dyspnoea, cough, haemoptysis and chest pain are common symptoms in patients with thoracic malignancy
- For mild symptoms, pharmacological methods are usually helpful
- Small-cell lung cancer, non-small-cell lung cancer and metastatic cancers may be palliated by means of radiotherapy; for endobronchial disease, brachytherapy or laser therapy may be helpful
- Chemotherapy is effective in patients with small-cell lung cancer, breast and colorectal cancer and for selected patients with non-small-cell lung cancer
- Invasive mechanical procedures including pleural drainage, pleurectomy, and endobronchial stenting can give useful palliation of dyspnoea

References

1 Portenoy, R.K., Thaler, H.T., Kornblith, A.B., *et al.* Symptom prevalence, characteristics and distress in a cancer population. *Qual Life Res* 1994; **3**: 183–9.

2 Hopwood, P., and Stephens, R.J. Symptoms at presentation for treatment in patients with cancer; implications for the evaluation of palliative treatment. The Medical Research Council (MRC) Lung Cancer Working Party. *Br J Cancer* 1995; **71**(3): 633–6.

3 de Haes, J.C.J.M., van Knippenberg, F.C.E., and Neijt, J.P. Measuring psychological and physical distress in cancer patients: structure and application of the Rotterdam Symptom checklist. *Br J Cancer* 1990; **62**: 1034–8.

4 Vainio, A., and Auvinen, A. Prevalence of symptoms among patients with advanced cancer: An international collaborative study. *J Pain Symptom Manage* 1996; **12**(1): 3–10.

5 Donnelly, S., and Walsh, D. The symptoms of advanced cancer: Identification of clinical and research priorities by assessment of prevalence and severity. *J Palliative Care* 1995; **11**(1): 27–32.

6 Higginson, I., and McCarthy, M. Measuring symptoms in terminal cancer: are pain and dyspnoea controlled? *J Roy Soc Med* 1989; **82**: 264–7.

7 Ahmedzai, S. Palliation of respiratory symptoms. Chapter 9.5 in: D. Doyle, G.W.C. Hanks, and N. MacDonald (eds) *Oxford textbook of palliative medicine*, 2nd edn. Oxford: Oxford University Press, 1998; 583–616.

8 Medical Research Council Lung Cancer Working Party. Prepared on behalf of the working party and all its collaborators by: N.M. Bleehen, D.J. Girling, D. Machin, and R.J. Stephens. Inoperable non-small-cell lung cancer (NSCLC): a Medical Research Council randomised trial of palliative radiotherapy with two fractions or ten fractions. *Br Jr Cancer* 1991; **63**: 265–70.

9 Medical Research Council Lung Cancer Working Party. Prepared on behalf of the working party and all its collaborators by: N.M. Bleehen, D.J. Girling, D. Machin, and R.J. Stephens. A Medical Research Council (MRC) randomised trial of palliative radiotherapy with two fractions or a single fraction in patients with inoperable non-small-cell lung cancer (NSCLC) and poor performance status. *Br J Cancer* 1992; **65**: 934–41.

10 Medical Research Council Lung Cancer Working Party. Randomized trial of palliative two-fraction versus more intensive 13-fraction radiotherapy for patients with inoperable non-small cell lung cancer and good performance status. *Clin Oncol* 1996; **8**: 167–75.

11 Falk, S.J., Girling, D.J., White, R.J., *et al.* on behalf of the Medical Research Council Lung Cancer Working Party. Immediate versus delayed palliative thoracic radiotherapy in patients with unresectable locally advanced non-small cell lung cancer and minimal thoracic symptoms: randomised controlled trial *BMJ* 2002; 325 (7362): 465.

12 Saunders, M.I. Programming of radiotherapy in the treatment of non small cell lung cancer – a way to advance care. *Lancet Oncol* 2001; **2**: 401–8.

13 Saunders, M.I., Dische, S., Barrett, A., *et al.* Continuous hyperfractionated accelerated radiotherapy (CHART) versus conventional radiotherapy in non small cell lung cancer: mature data from the randomised multicentre trial. *Radiother Oncol* 1999; **37**: 137–48.

14 Stout, R., Barber, P., Burt, P., *et al.* Clinical and quality of life outcomes in the first United Kingdom randomized trial of endobronchial brachytherapy vs external beam radiotherapy in the palliative treatment for inoperable non-small cell lung cancer. *Radiother Oncol* 2000; **56**: 323–7.

15 Bissett, D., Macbeth, F.R., and Cram, I. The role of palliative radiotherapy in malignant mesothelioma. *Clin Oncol* 1991; **3**: 315–17.

16 Davis, S.R., Tan, L., and Ball, D.L. Radiotherapy in the treatment of malignant mesothelioma of the pleura, with special reference to its use in palliation. *Australas Radiol* 1994; **38**: 212–14.

17 Shepherd, F.A., *et al.* Prospective randomised trial of docetaxel versus best supportive care in patients with non small cell lung cancer previously treated with platinum based chemotherapy. *J Clin Oncol* 2000; **18**: 2095–103.

18 Schiller, J.H., *et al.* for the ECOG. Comparison of four chemotherapy regimens for advanced non-small-cell lung cancer. *N Engl J Med* 2002; **346**: 92–8.

19 Ellis, P.A., *et al.* Symptom relief with MVP (mitomycin C, vinblastine and cisplatin) chemotherapy in advanced non-small cell lung cancer. *Br J Cancer* 1995; **71**: 366–70.

20 Smith, I.E., O'Brien, M.E.R., Talbot, D.C., *et al.* Duration of chemotherapy in advanced non small cell lung cancer: a randomized trial of three versus six courses of mitomycin C, vinblastine and cisplatin. *J Clin Oncol* 2001; **19**: 1336–43.

21 Fernandez, C., Rosell, R., Abad-Esteve, A., *et al.* Quality of life during chemotherapy in non-small cell lung cancer patients. *Acta Oncol* 1989; **28**: 29–33.

22 Cullen, M.H. The MIC regimen in non-small cell lung cancer. *Lung Cancer* 1993; Suppl 2: 81–9.

23 Thatcher, N., Anderson, H., Betticher, D.C., and Ranson, M. Symptomatic benefit from gemcitabine and other chemotherapy in advanced non-small cell lung cancer: changes in performance status and tumour-related symptoms. *Anti Cancer Drugs* 1995; **6**(Suppl 6): 39–48.

24 Medical Research Council Working Party. Randomised trial of four-drug vs less intensive two-drug chemotherapy in the palliative treatment of patients with small cell lung cancer (SCLC) and poor prognosis. *Br J Cancer* 1996; **73**: 406–13.

25 Bleehan, N.M., Girling, D.J., Machin, D., and Stephens, R.J. A randomised trial of three or six courses of etoposide cyclophosphamide methotrexate and vincristine or six courses of etoposide and ifosfamide in small cell lung cancer (SCLC). *Br J Cancer* 1993; **68**: 1157–66.

26 Ong, S.T., and Vogelzang, N.J. Chemotherapy in malignant pleural mesothelioma: a review. *J Clin Oncol* 1996; **14**: 1007–17.

27 Ryan, C.W., Herndon, J., and Vogelzang, N.J. A review of chemotherapy trials for malignant mesothelioma. *Chest* 1998; **113**: 66–73S.

28 Middleton, G.W., Smith, I.E., O'Brien, M.E.R., *et al.* Good symptom relief with palliative VP (mitomycin C, vinblastine and cisplatin) chemotherapy in malignant mesothelioma. *Ann Oncol* 1998; **9**: 269–73.

29 Berthelot, J.M., Will, B.P., Evans, W.K., *et al.* Decision framework for chemotherapeutic interventions for metastatic non-small-cell lung cancer. *J Natl Cancer Inst* 2000; **92**: 1321–9.

30 Silvestri, G., Pritchard, R., Welch, G., *et al.* Preferences for chemotherapy in patients with advanced non small cell lung cancer: descriptive study based on scripted interviews. *BMJ* 1998; **317**: 771–5.

31 Macbeth, F.R., Wheldon, T.E., Girling, D.J., *et al.* Radiation myelopathy: estimates of risk in 1048 patients in three randomized trials of palliative radiotherapy for non small cell lung cancer. *Clin Oncol* 1996; **8**: 176–81.

32 Spiro, S.G., Souhami, R.L., Geddes, D.M., *et al.* Duration of chemotherapy in small cell lung cancer: a Cancer Research Campaign trial. *Br J Cancer* 1989; **59**: 578–83.

33 George, P.J., *et al.* Laser treatment for tracheobronchial tumours: local or general anaesthesia? *Thorax* 1987; **42**: 656–60.

34 Tobias, J.S., and Brown, S.G. Palliation of malignant obstruction – use of lasers and radiotherapy in combination. *Eur J Cancer* 1991; **27**: 1352–5.

35 George, P.J.M., Clarke, G., Tolfree, S., Garrett, C.P.O., and Hetzel, M.R. Changes in regional ventilation and perfusion of the lung after endoscopic laser treatment. *Thorax* 1990; **45**: 248.

36 Lam, S. Photodynamic therapy of lung cancer. *Thorax* 1993; **48**: 469.

37 Walsh, D.A., *et al.* Bronchoscopic cryotherapy for advanced bronchial carcinoma. *Thorax* 1990; **45**: 509–13.

38 Walsh, D.A., Nath, A.R., and Maiwand, M. Authors' reply. *Thorax* 1990; **45**: 150.

39 Isaacs, C. Lymphatic spread of breast cancer. In: J.R. Harris, M.E. Lippman, M. Morrow, and S. Hellman, (ed.) *Diseases of the breast.* Philadelphia, Pa.: Lippincott-Raven, 1996; 827–33.

40 Bonnefoi, H., and Smith, I.E. How should cancer presenting as a malignant pleural effusion be managed? *Br J Cancer* 1996; **74**: 832–5.

41 Salajka, F. Occurrence of haemoptysis in patients with newly diagnosed lung malignancy. *Schweiz Med Wochenschr* 1999; **129**(41): 1487–91.

42 James, L.E., Gower, N.H., Rudd, R.M., *et al.* A randomised trial of low dose high frequency chemotherapy as palliative treatment of poor prognosis small cell lung cancer: a Cancer Research Campaign trial. *Br J Cancer* 1996; **73**: 1563–8.

43 Twycross, R.G., and Wilcock, A. *Symptom management in advanced cancer,* 3rd edn. Abingdon: Radcliffe Medical Press, 2001.

44 Twycross, R., Wilcock, A., and Thorp, S. *PCF1 palliative care formulary.* Abingdon: Radcliffe Medical Press, 1998.

45 Sahn, S.A. Management of malignant pleural effusions. *Monaldi Arch Chest Dis* 2001; **56**(5): 394–9.

46 Paz-Ares, L., and Garcia-Carbonero, R. Medical emergencies. In: F. Cavalli, HH. Hansen, SB. Kaye (eds), *Textbook of medical oncology,* 2nd edn. London: Martin Dunitz, 2000; 619–50

47 Martin-Ucar, A.E., Edwards, J.G., Rengajaran, A., Muller, S., and Waller, D.A. Palliative surgical debulking in malignant mesothelioma. Predictors of survival and symptom control. *Eur J Cardiothorac Surg* 2001; **20**(6): 1117–21.

Chapter 31

Comprehensive supportive care in HIV pulmonary disease

Elizabeth Bjorndal and Sam H. Ahmedzai

AIDS has become a chronic disease, treatable but ultimately fatal.[1] Since the 1980s, more than 40 million people have become infected with HIV and almost 12 million have died. Although 90% of those infected live in the developing countries, over 90% of the money for prevention and treatment is spent in developed countries. Deaths from AIDS have been declining in these countries since 1996, and the outlook of those infected with HIV has been transformed.

This is due to the advent of two major treatment advances, highly active antiretroviral therapy (HAART) and also the HIV RNA viral load assay, an important tool in clinical decision-making. Before this, HIV infection was almost invariably a progressive and rapidly fatal disease mainly affecting young adults. It occurred in an age when it was believed that antimicrobial therapy could control the majority of life-threatening infections.[2] Faced with this situation, the care of those infected required viewing the disease in its broadest context and palliative medicine therefore had a vital role to play.

Treatment regimes containing protease inhibitors, in addition to previously available antiretroviral agents, entered clinical trials in 1995, and by 1996 impressive results were emerging. These results were replicated in the general patient population by 1997–1998, so much so that phrases such as the 'Lazarus syndrome' and 'a second life' were being coined.[3] The results were indeed most impressive. Most AIDS-defining illnesses (Table 31.1), particularly the opportunistic infections, occur when the CD4 lymphocyte count falls below 200 cells/mL. Increases in the CD4 count, which were transient before the advent of HAART, now persist over long periods of time with a consequent reduction in morbidity and mortality. These reductions occur regardless of sex, race, age, and risk factors for the transmission of HIV. Although the incidence of lymphoma, cervical cancer, and the HIV wasting syndrome have not declined,[4] a reduction of more than 70% in all other AIDS-defining illnesses was observed between 1992 and 1996.[5]

Admissions to hospital have also declined.[6] A downward trend was noted before the introduction of HAART, thought to be due to routine prophylaxis against *Pneumocystis carinii* pneumonia (PCP) and increased experience in treating HIV infection itself within specialist units, but this decline became strikingly obvious during 1996 and 1997.

The impact of improved treatment has also been seen in falling mortality rates. In the USA, the number of AIDS-related deaths fell by 46% in 1997 compared to the previous year.[7] In Europe as a whole, death rates have been falling since 1995 and at the start of 1998 were less than one fifth of their previous level.[8] The impact of HIV on adult mortality in central London has been studied and the results indicate that HIV is the leading cause of death in men aged between 15 and 54 and the second leading cause of death in women of the same age.[9]

Table 31.1 Conditions included in the 1993 AIDS surveillance case definition

Candidiasis of bronchi, trachea, or lungs
Candidiasis, esophageal
Cervical cancer, invasive[a]
Coccidioidomycosis, disseminated or extrapulmonary
Cryptococcosis, extrapulmonary
Cryptosporidiosis, chronic intestinal (>1 month's duration)
Cytomegalovirus disease (other than liver, spleen, or nodes)
Cytomegalovirus retinitis (with loss of vision)
Encephalopathy, HIV-related
Herpes simplex: chronic ulcer(s) (>1 month's duration); or bronchitis, pneumonitis, or oesophagitis
Histoplasmosis, disseminated or extrapulmonary
Isosporiasis, chronic intestinal (>1 month's duration)
Kaposi's sarcoma
Lymphoma, Burkitt's (or equivalent term)
Lymphoma, immunoblastic (or equivalent term)
Lymphoma, primary, of brain
Mycobacterium avium complex or *M. kansasii*, disseminated or extrapulmonary
Mycobacterium tuberculosis, any site (pulmonary[a] or extrapulmonary)
Mycobacterium, other species or unidentified species, disseminated or extrapulmonary
Pneumocystis carinii pneumonia
Pneumonia, recurrent[a]
Progressive multifocal leukoencephalopathy
Salmonella septicaemia, recurrent
Toxoplasmosis of brain
Wasting syndrome due to HIV

Source: MMWR **41** RR 17: 1–19.

[a] Added in the 1993 expansion of the AIDS surveillance case definition.

The effect of the infection in sub-Saharan Africa has been catastrophic. AIDS is now the leading cause of death in the continent.[10] Life expectancy has decreased from 64 to 47 years.[11] The effect of HIV infection in Asia, where data collection and projection are less accurate, is less clear.

In order to understand the modern approach to comprehensive supportive care for HIV-related disease, it is important to appreciate the current strategies used to control CD4 levels and thus the mortality of the disease. Not only has the reduction in mortality and extension of survival led to a larger number of people living for longer with the physical and psychosocial sequelae of HIV disease, but also the toxicities and demands of the powerful new treatments themselves can substantially add to the burden of illness.

HAART

HAART has become acknowledged as the best HIV care and is widely available in North America and western Europe. The aim of therapy is to stop viral replication (Figure 31.1) so as to enable some immune reconstitution to occur and hence allow clinical improvement or at least stabilization.[12] Where this can be achieved for prolonged periods of time with therapy, partial

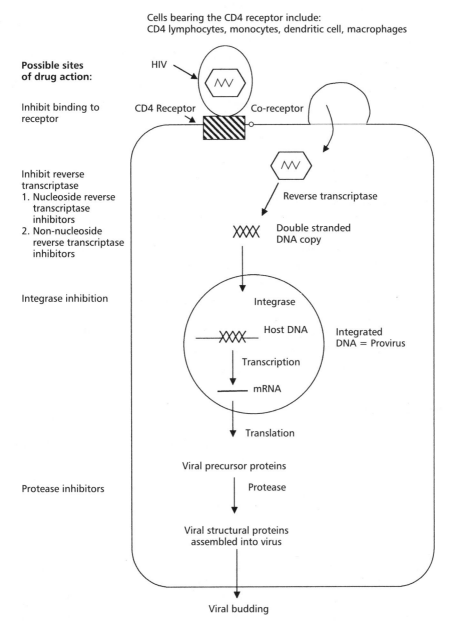

Fig. 31.1 HIV replication.

immune restoration has been shown to occur.[13] Even during clinically asymptomatic periods, which may last for many years, the virus is not latent. The situation has been likened to that of trench warfare where neither side gains ground but nevertheless continues to suffer casualties. Continuously high levels of viral replication persist with the destruction, replenishment, and reinfection of lymphocytes. It is only when viral replication exceeds the host capacity for regeneration that a critical point is reached and AIDS-defining illnesses occur. Effective antiretroviral therapy must therefore be started early with a potent combination of drugs. When such therapy is begun, there is a profound initial fall in viral load (usually 100-fold) within the first 1–2 weeks. This is followed by a slower rate of decline over subsequent weeks and viral load should be undetectable by 24 weeks (<50 copies/mL). Although there is considerable debate as to the best way of achieving this, experts are agreed that initial therapy must be hard hitting enough to achieve a viral load below the detection level of current assays. The emergence of resistance, the main cause of treatment failure, is less likely in this case. The British HIV Association published revised treatment guidelines in 1998 and 1999 and these are summarized in Table 31.2.

Reverse transcriptase inhibitors

These agents block viral replication by inhibiting the enzyme reverse transcriptase and so prevent the incorporation of viral genetic material into host DNA. Two classes exist:

+ The **nucleoside analogues** are phosphorylated within cells to their active form and disrupt construction of the proviral DNA strand which is then left incomplete. This group includes the first anti-HIV agent, zidovudine, introduced in 1987. The **nucleotide analogues** are a recently introduced group of agents, the drug adefovir being an example. These agents are monophosphated nucleosides designed to avoid the first phosphorylation step required for activation of the nucleoside analogues.

+ The **non-nucleoside reverse transcriptase inhibitors** bind directly and specifically to the enzyme in a non-competitive way. They have a low toxicity profile and a long half-life and hence low pill burden, which facilitates compliance. They are probably most useful in patients who have not previously been exposed to many different agents and are not failing on current regimes.

Table 31.2 Revised BIHVA guidelines: initiation of antiretroviral therapy in HIV infected adults

When?	Patient agrees to treatment
	Possible risks of therapy outweighed by likely benefit
	CD4 count > 350 cells/mL
	Viral load value associated with risk of disease progression
What?	<50 000 RNA copies/mL: two nucleoside analogues plus non-nucleoside reverse transcriptase inhibitor or protease inhibitor
	>50 000 RNA copies/mL: two nucleoside analogues plus one or two protease inhibitors
Aim of therapy in treatment-naive patients	Plasma viral load to be less than 50 copies/mL by 24 weeks of therapy
	Improve and extend length and quality of life

Source: Pozniak A, Gazzard B, Anderson J et al. British HIV Association (BHIVA) guidelines for the treatment of HIV-infected adults with retroviral therapy. *HIV Med* 2003; **4**(suppl.1): 1–41.

Hydroxyurea is used as an adjunct to the nucleoside analogues, and the combination has been found to be effective. Hydroxyurea inhibits the cellular enzyme ribonucleotide reductase rather than any viral protein. This enzyme represents the rate-limiting step in the production of deoxynucleoside triphosphates. These triphosphates normally compete with the nucleoside analogues, which are themselves phosphorylated to their active form within cells, for incorporation into HIV DNA. The addition of hydroxyurea therefore reduces the intracellular levels of the deoxynucleoside triphosphates and hence more phosphorylated nucleoside analogue is available to be used to inhibit HIV DNA synthesis.

Protease inhibitors

Competitive inhibition of the HIV protease enzyme prevents the maturation of infective virus within the host cell. Each of the drugs currently licensed can cause significant side effects and result in clinically relevant interactions with other common medications.

Immunotherapy

Approximately 50% of those who initially respond to HAART fail treatment within the first year, with falling CD4 counts and rebound of viral load to baseline levels. Various mechanisms for this have been suggested and have led to the search for immune-based therapies to preserve and restore immune competence. Interleukin (IL)-2 is the most studied agent, though other cytokines such as GM-CSF, TNF-1α and interferon-α have also received attention. Recent studies of IL-2 given as an adjunct to HAART have shown a significant increase in CD4 cell counts. Ultimately, however, preventive vaccination will be the best way of stopping the spread of HIV. The requirements of a therapeutic vaccine to prevent further disease progression are different from those of a prophylactic vaccine to prevent the initial infection. HIV is the most variable virus ever studied, and the obstacles to effective vaccine production are formidable.

Much effort has been placed into the development of vaccines based on the envelope glycoprotein, gp120. Indeed this vaccine, known as AIDSVAX,[14] has entered clinical trials in the USA though evidence from animal studies has indicated that it is unlikely to control the epidemic. Inactivated and live attenuated virus vaccines are more promising, though concerns remain about safety.[15]

Viral load

The development of an assay for HIV RNA viral load has been a major development in the management of HIV infection. The variable course of the disease itself as well as the increasing numbers of drugs available makes it important to identify failing regimes before signs of disease progression become apparent. The CD4 lymphocyte count was the first useful such marker but it is a weak predictor of disease progression over a prolonged period. The level of HIV RNA is directly related to the production of virus in the body, mainly within the lymphatic system, and has been found to be the single best predictor of clinical outcome. Even single measurements of viral load are of use in assessing disease progression, but sequential changes over time are much better predictors of drug failure. Lowering the viral load results in a decrease in morbidity and mortality.

When information from viral load assay is combined with CD4 cell counts, a more accurate prognosis is possible. This situation has been likened to a runaway train heading down the track to an abyss. The CD4 count represents the length of track remaining and the viral load indicates the speed of travel.[16]

Drawbacks of HAART

Compliance

The semantic debate over 'compliance' or 'adherence' continues, but there is no doubt that the tablet burden associated with HAART can be enormous and must not be underestimated, although, with pharmacokinetically better agents, it is now improving. Patients often have to take many other medications in addition to their antiretrovirals. Even the most efficient, organized, and motivated patient may have difficulty remembering which drug to take before meals and which to take after, and the meticulous timing required may result in scheduling of the whole day around taking the medication correctly. Various strategies have been developed to improve compliance, and examples are given in Table 31.3.

Compliance has become a crucial issue in the emergence of resistant virus. Failure to take medication correctly may result in periods when plasma drug concentrations fall below the critical level needed to suppress viral replication and so allow the emergence of resistance. It is therefore vital that patients are educated and take their medication correctly from the start. Compliance must be encouraged at every clinic visit and is most important during the initial stages of therapy when the patient is unfamiliar with the drugs and when start-up adverse reactions are most likely. It has been estimated that non-compliance accounts for approximately 50% of treatment failures, and some departments have started compliance clinics to address this.

Resistance

HAART is very unforgiving of non-compliance, particularly with regard to the development of resistance. Mutant virus, which can replicate even in the presence of drug, is selected, and it has

Table 31.3 Strategies to improve compliance

Strategy	Example
Combining medication	Combivir (zidovudine and lamivudine in one tablet)
Pharmaceutical manipulation to improve convenience of dosing and drug bioavailability	Didanosine combined with antacids and available as a once daily preparation Saquinavir soft gel formulation
Once daily dosing due to a long half-life	Nevirapine Efavirenz
Exploitation of drug interactions	Ritonavir increases the plasma concentrations of drugs metabolised by the cytochrome P450 system by inhibiting the enzyme function. These drugs are often prescribed together, e.g. ritonavir and saquinavir
Use drugs with similar dietary requirements together	Nelfinavir and saquinavir with food

been argued that such virus is actually a new and distinct organism as far as treatment is concerned. The nucleoside and non-nucleoside reverse transcriptase inhibitors each have distinct binding sites on the enzyme and if they are used as monotherapy, resistance will develop to any of these agents within days to months, particularly in patients with more advanced disease.[17] The viral protease system consists of 99 amino acids, and substitutions at 18 or more positions have been associated with lack of response to protease inhibitor therapy. The sequence of mutations may be drug and patient specific but this confers cross-resistance to all of the currently available protease inhibitors. The pattern of cross-resistance between the nucleoside and non-nucleoside reverse transcriptase inhibitors is different. The non-nucleosides select identical or near identical mutations in the enzyme. This process effectively restricts the number of non-nucleosides to one per patient. As far as the nucleoside analogues are concerned, although some mutations are shared many are not and it is therefore possible to switch from one agent to another within this group.

Mega-HAART is a term used to describe a drug regime used in patients who are treatment-experienced and by implication have resistant virus populations. It involves taking six or sometimes as many as nine different drugs, alternatively known as 'kitchen sink therapy'. This approach is relatively new, and early results show some benefit. It will only be suitable for well-motivated patients and, not surprisingly, is associated with frequently reported side effects.[18] When HAART first arrived on the scene, trends in viral load and CD4 lymphocyte count prompted calculations as to how long it would take to completely eradicate HIV from any particular patient. Estimates were between 2.3 and 3.1 years,[19] providing there were no sanctuary sites for the virus. One such site has been found: the reservoir of latently infected CD4 lymphocytes in the blood. Another component of the reservoir is infection of the eye, the central nervous system, and testes, these sites being relatively protected from the normal immune response and difficult for antiviral drugs to access.[20] Undetectable viral load may lead many patients to believe that the virus has been cleared and they may then falsely believe that there is no longer such a pressing need to maintain compliance with therapy. Furthermore, safe sex practices may be abandoned and there are reports of the sexual transmission of multidrug resistant virus, which is possibly an important clinical and public health issue.[21]

Side-effects and interactions

As more HIV-infected patients are now starting potent combination therapy early in the course of their disease, the side effects and interaction of the drugs, particularly in the long term, are becoming apparent and more of an issue. These effects range from those that manifest at the start and then subside, to those that are potentially life threatening.

Nucleoside analogues

Over the years that these drugs have been available, it has emerged that most of the serious side effects associated with them are due to organ-specific manifestations of mitochondrial toxicity (Table 31.4).[22] Mitochondrial failure is the mechanism which links such diverse effects as bone marrow toxicity, peripheral neuropathy, myopathy, pancreatitis, lactic acidosis, and hepatic steatosis (fatty change). Each of the drugs appears to have a different toxicity profile, with zidovudine causing mainly marrow toxicity and myopathy whereas didanosine and zalcitabine cause primarily pancreatitis and peripheral neuropathy. Deficiency of L-acetylcarnitine may contribute to the development of neuropathy, and

Table 31.4 Nucleoside reverse transcriptase inhibitors

Drug name	Most reported side-effects	Significant drug interactions	Caution
Nucleoside reverse transcriptase inhibitors			
Zidovudine (AZT)	Nausea and vomiting, headache, fatigue, myopathy, cardiomyopathy, myelosupression, macrocytosis, lactic acidosis, hepatic steatosis	Levels increased by opioids (~50%)	Other myelosuppressive drugs
Stavudine (d4T)	Peripheral neuropathy, headache, fever, diarrhoea, constipation, macrocytosis, lactic acidosis, hepatic steatosis		Other drugs causing peripheral neuropathy or pancreatitis
Didanosine (ddI)	Peripheral neuropathy, diarrhoea, pancreatitis, mental changes, lactic acidosis, hepatic steatosis		Other drugs causing peripheral neuropathy or pancreatitis, tetracyclines, H2 blockers, proton pump inhibitors
Zalcitabine (ddc)	Peripheral neuropathy, stomatitis and mouth ulcers, pancreatitis, lactic acidosis, hepatic steatosis		Other drugs causing peripheral neuropathy or pancreatitis
Lamivudine (3TC)	Headache, fatigue, peripheral neuropathy, alopecia	Levels increased by co-trimoxazole	Other drugs causing peripheral neuropathy
Abacavir	Hypersensitivity reactions including rash, fever, malaise and GI upset, headache, nausea and vomiting		
Non-nucleoside reverse transcriptase inhibitors			
Efavirenz	Skin reactions, headache, dizziness and syncope, diarrhoea, insomnia,vivid dreams and nightmares, agitation, hallucinations, delusions, euphoria or depression	Avoid terfenadine, astemizole, triazolam, midazolam because of potentially fatal arrhythmias	Clarithromycin
Nevirapine	Rash, Stevens–Johnson syndrome, hepatotoxicity		Increased risk of side-effects if taken with:amoxycillin, clarithromycin, orerythromycin Reduces levels of beta-blockers: doxycycline, methadone, metronidazole, nifedipine, steroids, theophylline, warfarin

Table 31.4 (continued)

Drug name	Most reported side-effects	Significant drug interactions	Caution
Delavirdine	Rash, leg cramps, fever, headache	Increases blood levels of: clarithromycin, warfarin, Ca^{2+} channel blockers Delavirdine level increased by: clarithromycin, itraconazole, ketoconazole, fluoxetine	
Nucleotide analogues Adefovir	Proximal renal tubular acidosis, GI intolerance, elevated liver enzymes		
Ribonucleotide reductase inhibitors Hydroxyurea	Nausea, mouth ulcers, hair loss		Other drugs causing peripheral neuropathy Pregnancy
Protease inhibitors Saquinavir	Abdominal discomfort, diarrhoea, nausea and vomiting, headache, lipodystrophy, hyperglycaemia, hyperlipidaemia	Avoid: terfenadine, astemizole, carbamazepine, phenytoin, dexamethasone, ergot derivatives	
Ritonavir	Nausea and vomiting, diarrhoea, anorexia and taste disturbance, tingling round the mouth, lipodystrophy, hyperglycaemia, hyperlipidaemia	Inhibits cytochrome P450 and therefore has a large number of potentially life-threatening interactions. Seek expert advice	
Indinavir	Kidney stones, nausea and vomiting, elevated liver enzymes, paronychia, lipodystrophy, hyperglycaemia, hyperlipidaemia		Maintain high fluid intake
Nelfinavir	Diarrhoea, rash, pruritis, lipodystrophy, hyperglycaemia	Avoid: terfenadine, astemizole, midazolam, pimozide, amiodarone, quinidine, ergot derivatives	Reduced level of oral contraceptive pill
Amprenavir	Headache, nausea, rash, fatigue Not yet clear if associated with metabolic disturbance	Avoid: terfenadine, astemizole	

supplements may be useful in treating some patients suffering from this problem. Toxicity arising from mitochondrial dysfunction is reversible if the drug is discontinued. Lamivudine is the only agent of this class that does not have the above toxicity profile, but it may cause alopecia, the mechanism of which is unclear.

Non-nucleoside reverse transcriptase inhibitors

This relatively new group of drugs has rapidly gained a place in the treatment of HIV. Three agents are currently licensed for use. Nevirapine was the first, its major side effect being dermatological. A dose-escalating regime over the first 2 weeks of therapy is recommended to reduce the frequency of this. Rashes have been found to occur in up to 17% of patients but are usually mild and self-limiting. Severe rashes may occur in 6–7%[23] and the Stevens–Johnson syndrome is seen in 0.3% of treated patients.[24] Abnormal liver function tests and hepatitis have also been reported. Delavirdine was the second agent from this group to be licensed, and again rash is the most frequently reported side effect. Dose escalation does not reduce its frequency. Efavirenz is a particularly useful drug as it is potent and well tolerated and, because of its long half-life, can be given once daily. All these agents are metabolized by the hepatic CYP 3A enzyme system and there is potential for interaction with other medications that are metabolized by this route.

Protease inhibitors

This group of drugs has important side effects. Long-term use has revealed a range of metabolic disturbances including lipodystrophy, dyslipidaemias, insulin resistance, and diabetes mellitus.

Body fat changes in patients taking the protease inhibitors fall into three distinct patterns: fat loss only, fat gain only, and a combination of the two. Lipodystrophy may occur in up to 60% of those taking protease inhibitors and the change in appearance that it causes – preservation of central fat stores relative to peripheral stores – may be severe enough to render the patient superficially cachexic and so lead to body-image problems. The mechanism is unknown, and recent reports have suggested that the syndrome may not in fact be specific to the protease inhibitors. The non-nucleoside reverse transcriptase inhibitor nevirapine was found to cause lipodystrophy in 16% of patients taking it as part of their regime (nevirapine plus two nucleoside analogue HAART regime).[25] Stavudine may also contribute to these changes.[26]

Hyperlipidaemia may occur in up to one third of those treated with protease inhibitors. This effect may be transient, but may confer an increased risk of vascular events in already predisposed individuals.[27] Treatment is by dietary modification, exercise, and attention to other cardiovascular risk factors. The use of lipid-lowering agents such as gemfibrozil has been shown to be effective but should be reserved for those with significant risk.[28]

Hyperglycaemia has been reported as a consequence of treatment with protease inhibitors.[29] This may occur in patients without a previous history of glucose intolerance, between 1 and 7 months of starting therapy. The hyperglycaemia may be controlled by dietary modification or the use of oral hypoglycaemic agents and does not usually require discontinuation of the drug. It has been suggested that the cause is insulin resistance and this is more commonly found in patients with lipodystrophy. In them, levels of insulin and c-peptide are raised.[30] Overt diabetes mellitus is rare. All the protease inhibitors are metabolized by the cytochrome P450 enzyme system, mainly the 3A3/4 isoform, within the liver. This is a common pathway for the metabolism of many other compounds, and advice should be sought before commencing other medication.

Immune restoration syndrome

As well as restoring immune function, HAART may paradoxically cause disease in some patients. The syndrome occurs in a proportion of patients, mainly those who are severely immunocompromised at the start of therapy and usually during the first few months after its commencement. The syndrome was first described with reference to cytomegalovirus (CMV) retinitis which was exacerbated after HAART was commenced despite an absolute CD4 count of more than 195 cells/mL.[31] AIDS-related CMV retinitis usually occurs in patients with CD4 counts of 50 cells/mL or less. Since then, the syndrome has been recognized in case reports of *Mycobacterium tuberculosis* with the paradoxical expansion of intracranial tuberculomas,[32] and with *Mycobacterium avium* complex where the addition of indinavir therapy in patients with CD4 counts of less than 50 cells/mL and subclinical infection resulted in fever, leukocytosis, and lymphadenitis, hepatitis B and C, cryptococcal disease, and herpes simplex disease.[33]

The precise mechanism of this syndrome is unknown but is probably related to enhanced immunological reaction at the site of a previous infection due to an improvement in T cell function.

Pulmonary disease

Along with HAART, the treatment of the infections and malignancies associated with AIDS forms the basis of comprehensive care. The lungs are one of the principal target organs of HIV-associated pathology, and lung disease is a major source of morbidity and mortality in patients with AIDS (Table 31.5). Over two thirds of patients will experience at least one respiratory episode during the course of their disease.[34] Experience has shown that only a few diseases account for most respiratory pathology, but vigilance must be maintained as less common problems still arise and there is always the possibility of new manifestations as the disease process evolves. The incidence of pneumonia from *P. carinii*, which is now known to be a fungus,[35] has decreased markedly but it still remains the most common AIDS-defining illness in developed countries whereas tuberculosis (TB) is by far the most common in developing countries.[36]

HIV probably enters the lung during the early stages of infection. It can be detected in lung tissue during the asymptomatic phase and this lung burden increases as the disease progresses. Lung function tests have been shown to be useful in identifying patients in whom further investigation is indicated.[37] The interpretation of these tests may, however, be complicated by the impact of intravenous drug abuse, infections, malignancy, and the impact of HIV itself. The most consistent finding demonstrated on serial testing has been a continuous decline in

Table 31.5 Pulmonary disorders associated with HIV infections

	Common	Less common
Bacteria	S. pneumoniae, H. influenzae, S. aureus, P. aerugirosa	Gram –ve organisms, Moraxella catarrhalis, Rhodococcus equi, Nocardia steroides,
Mycobacteria	M. tuberculosis	Mycobacterium avium complex, M. kansasii, M. gordonae, M. xenopi
Parasites		Strongyloides stercoralis, Toxoplasma gondii
Fungi	P. carinii	Cryptococcus neoformans, Histoplasma capsulatum, Coccidioides immitis, Aspergillus spp.
Inflammatory process	Lymphoid interstitial pneumonitis Non-specific interstitial pneumonia	
Neoplasms	Kaposi's sarcoma	B cell lymphoma, carcinoma

Source: Walker PA, White DA. Management of HIV-infected pulmonary disease. *Med Clin N Am* 1996; **80**(6): 1337–62.

the transfer factor for carbon monoxide (TL_{CO}) or the transfer coefficient (K_{CO}).[38] This is related to the severity of the HIV-associated complication but also occurs where there is little clinical evidence of pulmonary pathology, suggesting that there is specific pulmonary involvement by HIV and consequent damage to the alveolar-capillary membrane as part of the infectious process. Smoking is associated with a decrease in lung function beyond that expected from HIV infection alone. In patients recovering from PCP, smoking may slow or even prevent recovery.

As HIV infection is associated with a decline in immune function with time, lung disease becomes more common and severe as the immune system fails (Figure 31.2).

Sinusitis, bronchitis, and bacterial pneumonia

The clinical features of these infections are the same as those of the general population but they occur more frequently in HIV-infected people even at relatively high CD4 counts. Sinusitis is commonly caused by *Streptococcus pneumoniae* and *Haemophilus influenzae*, but *Pseudomonas aeruginosa* may cause problems in the later stages of HIV infection as may *Aspergillus* and *Cryptococcus neoformans*. Symptoms are often non-specific and may be chronic or recurrent especially as the CD4 lymphocyte count falls.

Acute bronchitis is the most common disorder of the lower respiratory tract. Bacterial pneumonia often occurs early in the course of HIV infection, though the rate of infection increases with falling CD4 counts.[39] Recurrent bacterial pneumonia, i.e. more than two episodes per year, is now recognized as an AIDS-defining illness. HIV infection primarily results in reduced cell-mediated immunity but is also associated with significant dysfunction of humoral immunity and predisposes to infection, particularly with encapsulated bacteria. Pneumonia is a particular problem in HIV-infected drug abusers where again *S. pneumoniae* and *H. influenzae* are the most common pathogens but *S. aureus* and *P. aeruginosa* are found increasingly. Treatment is directed towards the causative organism and outcome is good in most cases. Patients receiving co-trimoxazole as prophylaxis against PCP have a 67% decrease in the incidence of bacterial pneumonia. Vaccination with the polyvalent pneumococcal vaccine has been recommended for all HIV-infected persons.[40] In particular cases, the haemophilus vaccine may be useful. Vaccines should be given early in the disease when an antibody response is more likely.

Pneumocystis carinii pneumonia (PCP)

The incidence of this infection has declined as a result of the widespread use of primary and secondary prophylaxis but it still remains a common pathogen in those with AIDS. Primary prophylaxis should be recommended to all patients with:

- CD4 lymphocyte count <200 cells/mL and/or
- persistent oral thrush
- an AIDS diagnosis

Stopping primary prophylaxis appears to be safe in patients receiving HAART who have had a CD4 lymphocyte count of at least 200 cells/mL for at least 12 weeks. Secondary prophylaxis should be given to all patients following an infection with *P. carinii*. Discontinuation of therapy in this group may also be reasonable, though fewer data are available to support this.

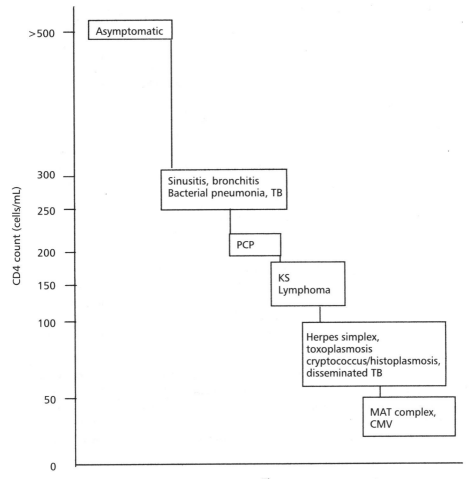

Fig. 31.2 Spectrum of pulmonary disease with declining CD4 count. The decline in CD4+ lympho-cytes among people with HIV infection is associated with the development of opportunistic dis-eases. Although several disorders occur at a wide range of CD4 counts, such as tuberculosis and Kaposi's sarcoma, the approximate CD4 levels depicted here provide a guide for anticipating the appearance of HIV-related conditions and are helpful when planning prophylactic strategies. Reproduced with permission from: Walker. P.A., White. D.A. Management of the HIV infected patient with pulmonary disease. *Med Clin N Am* 1996; **80**(6): 1337–1362.

Co-trimoxazole is the drug of choice for both prophylaxis and treatment and every effort should be made to enable patients to take it regularly. The regime is 960 mg daily or three times weekly. If treatment needs to be discontinued due to side effects, between one third and one half of patients will have no recurrence of effects on re-challenge. Prophylactic doses may be tolerated adequately in those who are unable to take treatment doses. Where there is documented mild to moderate allergy, e.g. rash or itching with the use of co-trimoxazole, a desensitization regime may be tried. This should not be considered in cases of severe reaction, i.e. Stevens–Johnson syn-drome, anaphylaxis, hepatitis, or pancreatitis. Table 31.6 summarizes PCP prophylaxis.

Table 31.6 Drugs for prophylaxis of PCP

	Agent	Main side-effects
1st choice	Co-trimoxazole	Nausea, vomiting, diarrhoea, skin reactions, mild → severe, tremor, anaemia, neutropaenia, thrombocytopaenia, raised liver enzymes, jaundice, hepatitis, pancreatitis
Others	Dapsone	Nausea, vomiting, anorexia, headache, psychosis, hepatitis, haemolysis, aplastic anaemia, methaemoglobinameia, skin reactions (mild → severe), peripheral neuropathy
	Pyrimethamine	Rash, vomiting, abdominal pain, pancytopaemia, megaloblastic anaemia. CNS effects: headache, dizziness, insomnia
	Pentamidine nebulized	Cough, dyspnoea, wheeze, bronchospasm, pneumothorax.
	Pentamidine IV	Hypotension, cardiac arrhythmias, hypo/hyper glycaemia, pancreatitis, acute renal failure, hyperkalaemia, hypocalcaemia, anaemia, leucopenia, thrombocytopaenia, abnormal liver function tests
	Dapsone and trimethoprim	Skin rash, nausea and vomiting; decreased haemopoiesis secondary to folate deficiency
	Azithromycin	Nausea and vomiting, diarrhoea, abdominal discomfort, skin reactions, jaundice, cardiac arrhythmias

PCP is insidious and usually presents with fever, dry cough, and dyspnoea on exertion. Systemic symptoms such as weight loss, night sweats, fatigue and malaise may also occur. The serum lactate dehydrogenase (LDH) is frequently elevated in PCP infection. Studies report the sensitivity of this to be in the range 83–100%. Serum LDH is, however, not specific for PCP and a raised level may be due to other causes. Despite this, many studies have

Table 31.7 Grading of severity of PCP

	Mild	Moderate	Severe
Symptoms and signs	Increasing exertional dyspnoea with or without cough and sweats	Dyspnoea on minimal exertion. Occasional dyspnoea at rest. Fever with or without sweats	Dyspnoea at rest. Tachypnoea at rest. Persistent fever. Cough
Blood gas tensions (room air)	PaO_2 normal SaO_2 falling on exercise	PaO_2 8.1–11.0 kPa	$PaO_2 \leq 8.0$ kPal
Chest radiograph	Normal or minor interstitial shadowing	Diffuse interstitial shadowing	Extensive interstitial shadowing with or without diffuse alveolar shadowing (whiteout) sparing the costophrenic angles and apices

Source: Miller RF, Mitchell DM. *Thorax* 1992; **47**: 305.

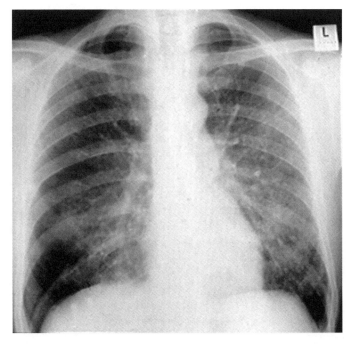

Fig. 31.3 Mild PCP showing interstitial shadowing superimposed on the vascular markings with no lymphadenopathy or pleural effusion. The changes are predominantly perihilar and there is peripheral sparing.

shown a strong relationship between survival and the LDH level. An initial high value or a rising value despite treatment correlates with treatment failure, a poor prognosis and increased mortality. A falling LDH correlates with a good response to treatment.

Treatment for PCP (Table 31.7) can be based on its division into mild (Figure 31.3), moderate, and severe infection (Figure 31.4). Mild to moderate cases may be treated with oral therapy. Moderate to severe cases may benefit from the addition of steroids. The regimen (Table 31.8) used varies from centre to centre but commonly includes intravenous methylprednisolone, 1 g for the first 3 days, 500 mg for the next 2 days, then converting to oral prednisolone given in a reducing dose, starting at 60 mg daily, tailing down to zero over the next 10 days. Steroids should be started at the same time as specific anti-PCP therapy in patients developing respiratory failure. Any delay markedly reduces their effectiveness.

Kaposi's sarcoma (KS)

KS is the most common tumour seen in HIV-positive patients and among the groups at risk for HIV, it occurs most commonly in homosexual men. KS results in a wide spectrum of disease ranging from asymptomatic skin lesions to extensive skin disease with ulceration and oedema (Figure 31.5). Visceral involvement may occur in up to 50% of cases with gastrintestinal haemorrhage, bowel obstruction, cough, haemoptysis, and respiratory failure. Those with symptomatic lung involvement (Figure 31.6) have the poorest prognosis, usually less than 6 months.[41]

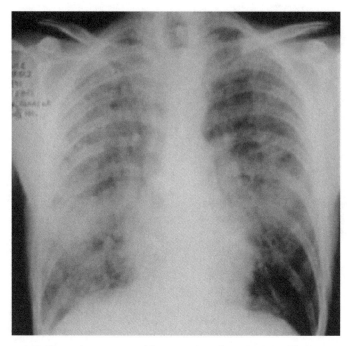

Fig. 31.4 Severe PCP. The patient presented *in extremis* and required ventilatory support. Short-term mortality is high in this group, but long-term survival is similar to those patients with less severe episodes.

A new herpesvirus has recently been identified as the likely cause of KS. It is known as human herpesvirus type-8 (HHV-8) or KS-related herpesvirus (KSHV). Experimental data suggests that in the early stages KS is not a true sarcoma but an angiohyperplastic inflammatory lesion stimulated by cytokines and growth factors produced by HHV-8 infected cells. These early lesions may regress but with time they become monoclonal in nature, and progression to a true sarcoma probably requires immunodeficiency.

Table 31.8 Drugs for treatment of PCP

	Drug
1st choice	Co-trimoxazole
2nd choice	Clindamycin and primaquine
Others	*Mild disease*:
	Dapsone and trimethoprim
	Atovaquone
	Severe disease:
	Pentamidine
	Trimetrexate (with folinic acid rescue)
	Corticosteroids

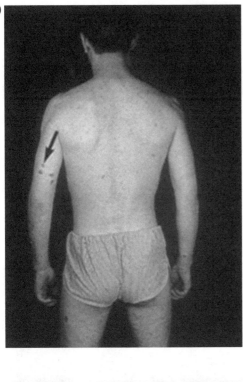

Fig. 31.5 Cutaneous Kaposi's sarcoma. The progression of cutaneous disease is demonstrated. Note the small purple lesions on the patient's left upper arm (a, arrow) which slowly grow over 12 months (b). New skin lesions start to appear symmetrically and line up along the skin creases. The patient showed features of marked weight loss, particularly muscle bulk, and he died from pulmonary KS after a further 4 months.

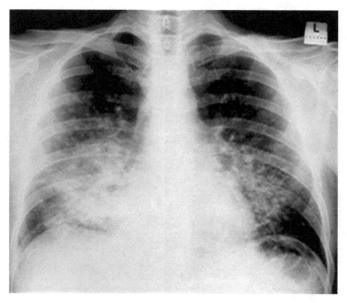

Fig. 31.6 Pulmonary KS. This produces parenchymal reticulonodular opacities in a perivascular or bronchocentric distribution. Hilar or mediastinal adenopathy and pleural effusion are common.

Treatment
HAART

Antiretroviral therapy with protease inhibitors has led to a clinical response of up to 80% in those suffering from HIV-associated KS and its complications.[42] This response occurs regardless of whether the patients had received antineoplastic chemotherapy. Indeed, the response may be so good that chemotherapy can be discontinued.

Antineoplastic chemotherapy

This is indicated for those with progressive or disseminated disease causing problems such as oedema, ulceration, or pain or effects related to the site of the lesions, e.g. biliary obstruction or gastrointestinal bleeding. Pulmonary KS is usually treated as it is invariably progressive and causes symptoms. Patients present with progressive dyspnoea (69%), cough (92%), pleuritic pain (20%), and haemoptysis (13%).[43] It is almost always seen in conjunction with cutaneous or lymphadenopathic KS, palatal disease being a particularly strong predictor for the presence of pulmonary disease. Chest radiograph findings are non-specific, but the commonest findings are bilateral interstitial infiltrates which follow septal lines and are located towards the hilae; nodular infiltrates with focal consolidation and pleural effusions, usually bilateral.

- ◆ **Liposomal anthracyclines:** Liposomal daunorubicin and doxorubicin are used extensively in the treatment of HIV-related KS and are now considered first-line therapy. Response rates are approximately 50%. Cellular toxicity is enhanced as the drugs accumulate in KS tissue. Dose limiting toxicity is marrow suppression with an increased incidence of infection, particularly candidiasis.[44]

- **Paclitaxel:** The cellular target of this compound is similar to that of the vinca alkaloids and it is known to be an inhibitor of endothelial cell proliferation. Recent studies with paclitaxel have shown response rates of up to 71%[45] in patients who had extensive KS and who had received previous chemotherapy. Even those with pulmonary KS had an objective response of their lung disease.[46] Neutropenia is the most frequent dose-limiting effect, but new toxic effects occur in this patient population, e.g. fever, rash, decreased renal function, eosinophilia, and cardiomyopathy.

- **Vinca alkaloids:** Vinblastine was the first such agent used and it induces a response of more than 90%. However, this is usually short-lived and may be complicated by myelosupression. Vincristine is less toxic to the marrow but may cause peripheral neuropathy. The newer agent vinorelbine has also been used with some success. These agents may be injected directly into lesions as well as being given parenterally, but such local injections are often painful, tissue necrosis may occur, and the technique is only practically useful for the treatment of a limited number of small lesions.

- **Bleomycin:** This is another effective agent and again may be given parenterally or intralesionally. Response is usually short lived and the risk of pulmonary fibrosis may be dose limiting.

- **Doxorubicin:** Response rates vary from 10 to 48%. The major side effects are nausea, vomiting, mucositis, and neutropenia. Combinations of doxorubicin, bleomycin, and vincristine (ABV) used to be the best standards of care with response rates of 25% but with significant toxicity,[47] and newer agents have replaced these.

Lymphomas

Lymphomas affecting HIV-positive patients are predominantly of the high-grade B-cell type and they occur late in the course of the disease. Histology should be pursued in all cases and staging will often reveal the involvement of extranodal sites such the central nervous system, skin, and marrow. Intrathoracic involvement is generally uncommon but may present radiologically as pleural effusion, interstitial and alveolar disease, pulmonary nodules, and less commonly as lymphadenopathy. The diagnosis should be considered where the clinical presentation is with pleural effusion or non-infective interstitial or alveolar process.[48] Treatment is with conventional chemotherapy regimes and radiotherapy. Doses may need to be adjusted if the level of immune function is very compromised.

Mycobacterial infection

It has been estimated that globally 1 in 7 cases of TB are associated with HIV infection. Pulmonary TB can develop at all stages of HIV infection. The manifestations depend on the level of immune function. In the early stages, there is typical post-primary disease, but where HIV is more advanced, the diagnosis may be difficult as symptoms and signs may be non-specific and the disease is often disseminated. TB is a notifiable disease and a public health issue as it is communicable. Control has proved difficult and multidrug resistant organisms have emerged. The treatment of TB and HIV together can be difficult, and priority should be given to treating the TB effectively in the shortest time.[49] Drug interactions with the antiretrovirals may be complex, and cases are best managed by experts from each field working together. (For further details on the management of pulmonary TB, see Chapter 32.)

Table 31.9 Treatment of *Mycobacterium avium intra-cellulare*

1st choice	2nd choice
Rifabutin	Rifampicin
Ethambutol	
Clarithromycin	Azithromycin
±Amikacin	Ciprofloxacin

Infection with atypical mycobacteria is an increasing problem, and disseminated *Mycobacterium avium intra-cellulare* (MAI) is now a cause of significant morbidity and mortality in those with advanced disease. Clinical features are non-specific with fevers, sweats, malaise, anorexia, and weight loss. The diagnosis is made by culturing the organism from blood and sputum or from bronchial washings and biopsy material from liver, lymph nodes or marrow. Treatment may involve the use of many agents depending on sensitivities. Conventional antituberculous therapy is not effective in this infection. Steroids may be of benefit where symptoms do not respond well to first-line therapy (Table 31.9).

Evidence is emerging that primary MAI prophylaxis may improve survival where the CD4 lymphocyte count is below 100 cells/mL. First choice for this is azithromycin given weekly or alternatively rifabutin given daily.

Fungi

Infection with *Cryptococcus* is the most frequent systemic fungal disease in HIV-positive patients. Cryptococcal pneumonia may occur as a focal infection but more commonly occurs as disseminated infection with central nervous system disease. Standard therapy for pulmonary disease is the same as for that of cryptococcal meningitis and is with amphotericin B or liposomal amphotericin where renal function is impaired. Flucytosine may be added, depending on the severity of the infection. If infection is mild, fluconazole alone may be sufficient. Secondary prophylaxis is with fluconazole, itraconazole or amphotericin with or without the addition of flucytosine. *Aspergillus* infection is becoming more common. This may present as pulmonary infiltrates or cavitating nodules, though necrotizing tracheobronchitis may also occur.

Certain fungal species are endemic to various areas of the world. Histoplasmosis and coccidioidomycosis both occur as complications of immunosupression, either as a new disease in those living in endemic areas or as reactivation of latent previously acquired infection.

Viruses

Cytomegalovirus (CMV), a member of the herpes group, is the most common cause of viral pneumonia and is often associated with other pathogens and coexisting lung disease. CMV is usually regarded as 'more of a passenger than a pathogen' [36] in the lung. It may cause a disseminated illness with hepatitis, colitis, retinitis, or encephalitis in late-stage HIV infection.

Figure 31.7 shows a chest radiograph of a patient with CMV pneumonitis. There is ill-defined consolidation in the right mid-zone extending down the right heart border (arrow). The patient presented with cough, dyspnoea, and a CD4 count of <200 cells/mL.

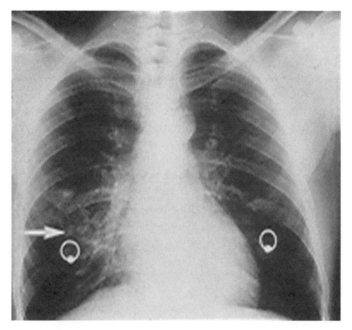

Fig. 31.7 CMV pneumonitis. There is ill-defined consolidation in the right mid-zone extending down the right heart border (arrow).

Although CMV infection is often found in AIDS patients, it is not usually clear if it contributes to respiratory symptoms and therefore whether it always needs to be treated when found in the lungs.

Interstitial pneumonitis

Lymphocytic interstitial pneumonia is very much more common in infants and children and is AIDS-defining in those under the age of 13. Non-specific interstitial pneumonitis is more commonly found in adults and its course is chronic and indolent. Symptoms are generally mild and include cough, dyspnoea, or fever. The condition needs to be distinguished from PCP, which presents with similar symptoms. The diagnosis is made histologically via transbronchial or open lung biopsy, as the condition has no distinguishing features clinically or radiologically. The cause is unknown but may be related to the direct effect of HIV on the lung. Epstein–Barr virus has also been implicated. Treatment if required is with steroids.

Symptom management

The natural history of HIV disease has radically changed in recent years, but as treatment options continue to expand and clinical decision-making becomes more complex, there is a real danger that attention will be focused only on the CD4 count, viral load, and complicated algorithms of antiretroviral agents. This may be further compounded by the centralization of HIV services to specialist units, although an increasing body of literature suggests that patients managed by the experts in these units have a better clinical outcome.[50] The personal needs of the patient must never be overlooked, and a multidisciplinary approach to care from time of diagnosis is crucial. In this respect the comprehensive supportive care of HIV patients and their circle of family or friends is very similar to that of the classical palliative care scenario for advanced cancer patients. The settings in which the multidisciplinary, multimodality care is given, however, is usually very different because of the demographics of the patients and the types of interventions required.

Symptoms may be associated with HIV infection itself, or due to the infections and malignancies associated with it and to the therapies used to treat them. Involvement of the lungs may range from mild to fulminant respiratory failure. The principles of symptom management in HIV are the same as for any other condition. Indeed, good symptom management is required from the initiation of antiretroviral therapy to enable patients to comply with their drug regimes. An important caution required in this patient group is possible drug interaction between commonly used palliative care drugs and antiretroviral therapy. Attention to psychosocial factors is known to influence compliance, as is the relationship between patient and clinician and the quality of the communication between them. Empathy is also considered important in encouraging compliance.[51] In those patients unable to benefit from, or unable to adhere to HAART, for whatever reason, the temptation to criticize and blame the patient must be resisted. It is not the patient who has failed the medication, rather the medication that has failed the patient.

Pain control

Pain is a common symptom in patients with HIV-related diseases, particularly in the more advanced stages. Several pain syndromes have been identified,[52] including soft tissue (myofascial), visceral, neuropathic, and musculoskeletal/joint pains. The common types of nociceptive pain are summarized in Table 31.10. Neuropathic pains may be classified according to the stage of HIV progression, as shown in Table 31.11. From these tables, it can be seen that although most causes of pain are disease-related, iatrogenic causes should also be looked for. Thus in one study, the aetiology of pain was found to be related to pre-existing conditions in 24%, the direct effects of HIV in 30%, secondary effects of therapy in 4%, and unknown causes in 37%.[53]

Several studies have shown a significant undertreatment of symptoms, particularly pain, in HIV-infected patients,[54] with opioids in particular rarely being prescribed.[55] Reasons given for

Table 31.10 Sources of nociceptive pain in HIV/AIDS

Cutaneous superficial causes	Kaposi's sarcoma
	Oral cavity pain
Deep somatic causes	Rheumatologic (e.g. arthralgias)
	Back pain
	Myopathies
Visceral causes	Tumour
	Gastritis
	Pancreatitis
	Infection
	Biliary tract disorders
Headache	HIV-related (e.g. meningitis, encephalitis, neoplasm)
	HIV-unrelated (e.g. tension, migraine)
	Iatrogenic (e.g. azidothymide)

Reproduced with permission from Daniel B. Carr.

Table 31.11 Painful neuropathies according to stage of HIV

Acute or seroconversion phase	Mononeuritides, brachial plexopathy
	Acute demyelinating polyneuropathy (Guillain–Barré syndrome)
Latent (asymptomatic) phase	Acute demyelinating polyneuropathy (Guillain–Barré syndrome)
(CD4 + T lymphocytes >500/mm³)	Chronic inflammatory demyelinating polyneuropathy
Transition phase	Herpes zoster (shingles)
(200 − 500 CD4 + cells/mm³)	Mononeuritis multiplex
Late phase	Predominantly sensory polyneuropathy
(<200 CD4 + cells/mm³)	Autonomic neuropathy
	Cytomegalovirus polyradiculopathy
	Mononeuritis multiplex (severe)
	Mononeuropathies associated with aseptic meningitis
	Mononeuropathies secondary to lymphomatous meningitis
	Nucleoside (dideoxyinosine, dideoxycytidine) toxicity

this from the patient's point of view include the perceived addictive potential of opioids, side effects and fear of injections although these are rarely needed for pain control. On the other hand, doctors may be reluctant to prescribe strong opioids especially for those patients who abuse drugs, and reports indicate that this patient group is more likely to receive inadequate analgesia and so suffer a greater level of psychological distress.[56]

Studies have shown that up to 60% of patients report 'frequent or persistent' pain and related functional impairment. Advanced HIV disease is associated with the presence of pain and its intensity is associated with the demographic factors of female gender and being of non-white ethnicity. The number of HIV-related physical symptoms present are also positively associated with pain intensity.[57] Significant associations have been demonstrated between pain and psychological distress, depression, hopelessness, and quality of life in this patient group.[58] The management of pain in HIV patients is similar to that of pain in other progressive and life-limiting diseases. Thus, the WHO cancer pain three-step ladder approach has been advocated as a suitable model for treating pain in HIV patients.[52] This model is covered in detail in Chapter 28.

As with cancer, there is sometimes reluctance on the part of physicians (and corresponding fears on the side of patients) about the use of strong opioids.[54] Morphine has been the main drug used in advanced disease, but oxycodone and fentanyl have also been advocated.[52]

An open label comparison of transdermal fentanyl with oral morphine in patients with severe AIDS-related chronic pain found good results with fentanyl.[59] Interestingly, in this non-randomized study, AIDS patients with a history of chemical dependence required lower doses of transdermal fentanyl to active similar pain control.

Supportive care in HIV/AIDS

A recent survey of the use of specialist palliative care services in the UK has found that although teams are in place, services are underused for a variety of reasons. These include poor information exchange between the acute units and specialist palliative care providers which, not surprisingly, often leads to misunderstanding about what each has to offer. Furthermore, the printed information available to HIV-infected patients often fails to mention palliative care services at all. However, it has been shown that where good links exist misunderstandings can be avoided.

Issues of access by minority groups are not new. Hospices may be perceived as being 'middle class' and 'religious' and therefore not welcoming to HIV-infected patients. This patient group may also have different needs from the more traditional users of palliative care services. For example, HIV patients need provision of longer-term respite admissions and daycare facilities tailored to younger adults.[60]

As with palliative care in malignant disease, attention must also be focused on psychosocial and existential distress. There is no doubt that treatment with HAART improves clinical measures such as CD4 count, RNA viral load, and body weight, and can maintain functional capacity. However, a recent study has shown that there is little corresponding improvement in psychological measures or in general distress levels, whether physical or psychological cause. Overall quality of life measures were unchanged by therapy.[61]

Dedicated clinical nurse specialists, social workers, and counsellors are available in most treatment centres to address all aspects of care, and in some countries there are numerous charitable organizations dedicated to providing support for those with HIV and AIDS.

As those with HIV disease approach the terminal phase of their illness, the need for supportive care increases. One study observed that there has been a trend towards a more aggressive approach to interventions at the end of life, with a 200% increase in resuscitation attempts between 1987–1990 and 1990–1993. However, no patient had been discharged alive from hospital after resuscitation since 1988. Another study showed that an increase in the use of drugs and diagnostic procedures has tended to reflect persistent efforts towards 'cure' rather than allowing a palliative attitude to prevail.[62] This has occurred despite a wish on the part of patients for end-of-life issues to be openly discussed and their wishes sought and respected. Where these issues were shared, 54% requested a palliative approach, only 29% an aggressive approach, and 9% a combination of the two.[63]

The interface between curative and palliative treatment is much less clear-cut in HIV disease than in cancer, and palliation of symptoms and psychosocial distress should be addressed throughout the course of the illness, using a comprehensive supportive approach such as the Sheffield model (see Chapter 1). Many of the symptoms, including those arising in the respiratory system, may in fact best be palliated by aggressive antiviral or other disease-specific therapies, i.e. by using type 2 (anti-HIV) or type 3 (against local/systemic effects of HIV infection) palliation, according to the classification given in Chapter 1. The palliative management of these symptoms (i.e. type 4 palliation) is described in detail elsewhere in this volume. By using a supportive care model, both life-prolonging and palliative interventions may coexist for the patient's best interests.

Keypoints

♦ Infection with HIV is now considered a chronic condition

♦ Best practice involves the appropriate treatment of associated infections and malignancies as well as the use of antiretroviral agents

♦ Symptoms, particularly pain, are often inadequately treated and their management may well be required from diagnosis

♦ Respiratory symptoms are a common source of distress and should be treated using standard approaches from palliative care

♦ Prolonging life with HIV and relieving symptoms and psychosocial distress should coexist, using a supportive care approach

References

1 Roberts, J. AIDS now more chronic than fatal. *BMJ* 1996; 312, 796–7.

2 Selwyn, P.A., and Arnold, R. From fate to tragedy: the changing meanings of life, death and AIDS. *Ann Intern Med* **129**(11): 899–902.

3 Rabkin, J.G., and Ferrando, S. A second life agenda. *Arch Gen Psychiatry* 1997; **54**: 1049–1053.

4 Moore, R.D., and Chaisson, R.E. Natural history of HIV infection in the era of combination antiretroviral therapy *AIDS* 1999; **13**: 1933–42.

5 Brodt, H.R., Kamps, B.S., Gute, P., *et al.* Changing incidence of AIDS-defining illnesses in the era of antiretroviral combination therapy. *AIDS* 1997; **11**: 1731–8.

6 Morcroft, A., Barry, S., Saloin, C.A., *et al.* The changing pattern of admissions to a London hospital of patients with HIV: 1988–1999. *AIDS* 1999, **13**: 1255–61.

7 Gottlieb, S. AIDS deaths fall by nearly one half. *BMJ* 1998; **317**: 1032.

8 Mocroft, A. Changing patterns of mortality across Europe in patients infected with HIV-I. *Lancet* 1998; **352**: 1725–30.

9 Hickman, M., Bardsley, M., DeAngelis, D., and Ward, H. Impact of HIV on adult (15–54) mortality in London: 1979–96. *Sex Transm Infect* 1999; **75**(6): 385–8.

10 Stephenson, J. Apocalypse now: FHV/AIDS in Africa exceeds the experts' worst predictions. JAMA 2000; **284**(5): 556–7.

11 Logie, D. AIDS cuts life expectancy in sub-Saharan Africa by a quarter. *BMJ* 1999; **319**: 806.

12 O'Brien, W.A., Hartigan, P.M., Daar, E.S., Simberkoff, M.S., and Hamilton, J.D. Changes in plasma HIV RNA levels and CD4+lymphocyte counts predict both response to antiretroviral therapy and therapeutic failure. *Ann Intern Med* 1997, **126**(12): 939–45.

13 Arno, A., Ruiz, L., Juan, M., *et al.* Impact on the immune system of undetectable plasma HIV-1 RNA for more than 2 years. *AIDS* 1998, **12**: 697–704.

14 Josefson, D. Approval given for trials of AIDS vaccine. *BMJ* 1998, **316**: 1769.

15 Stolt, E.J., and Schild, G.C. Strategies for AIDS vaccines. *J Antimicrob Chemother* 1996; 37 (Suppl B): 185–98.

16 Saag, M.S. Use of HIV viral load in clinical practice: back to the future. *Ann Intern Med* 1997; **126**: 983–5.

17 Chen, P., Schmit, J-C., Arendt, V., *et al.* Drug resistance mutations as predictors of phenotypic Zidovudine resistance in HIV-1 infection. *AIDS* 1997, **11**(12): 1528–9.

18 Poppa, A. *AIDS treatment update.* 1999;**79**: 1–4.

19 Grant, R.M., and Abrams, D.I. Not all is dead in HIV-1 graveyard. *Lancet* 1998; **351**: 308–9.

20 Graham, B. Infection with HIV-1. *BMJ* 1998; **317**: 1297–301.

21 Hecht, F.M., Grant, R.M., Petropoulos, C.J., *et al.* Sexual transmission of an HIV-1 variant resistant to multiple reverse transcriptase and protease inhibitors. *N Engl J Med* 1998; **339**: 307–11.

22 John, M., Mallal, S., and French, M. Emerging toxicity with long-term antiretroviral therapy. *J HIV Therapy* 1998, 3(3): 58–61.

23 Havlir, D., and Lange, J.M.A. New antiretrovirals and new combinations. *AIDS* 1998; **12**(suppl A): 5165–74.

24 Pollard, R.B., Robinson, P., and Dransfield, K. Safety profile of nevirapine, and a nucleoside reverse transcriptase inhibitor for the treatment of human immunodeficiency virus infection. *Clin Therapeut* 1998; **20**(6): 1071–92.

25 Aldeen, T., Wells, C., Hay, P., Davidson, F., and Lau, R. Lipodystrophy associated with nevirapine containing antiretroviral therapies. *AIDS* 1999; **13**: 865–6.

26 Alcoin, K. Body fat changes. *AIDS Treatment Update* 1999; **80**: 4–6.

27 Henry, K., Melroe, H., Huebsch, J., *et al.* Severe premature coronary artery disease with protease inhibitors. *Lancet* 1998; **351**: 1328.

28 Hewitt, R.G., Shelton, M.J., and Esch, L.D. Gemfilorozil effectively lowers protease inhibitor associated hypertriglyceridemia in HIV-1 positive patients. *AIDS* 1999, **13**: 868–9.

29 Dube, M.P., Johnson, D.L., Currier, J.S., and Leedom, J.M. Protease inhibitor associated hyperglycaemia. *Lancet* 1997, **350**: 713–14.

30 Carr, A., Samaras, K., Burton, S., *et al.* A syndrome of peripheral lipodystrophy, hyperlipidaemia and insulin resistance in patients receiving HIV protease inhibitors. *AIDS* 1998; **12**: F51–8.

31 Jacobson, M.A., Zegan, S.M., Pavan, P.R., *et al.* Cytomegalovirus retinitis after initiation of highly active antiretroviral therapy. *Lancet* 1997, **349**: 1443–5.

32 Crump, J.A., Tyrer, M.J., Lloyd-Owen, S.J., *et al.* Miliary tuberculosis with paradoxical expansion of intracranial tuberculomas complicating human immunodeficiency virus infection in a patient receiving highly active anti-retroviral therapy. *Clinl Infect Dis* 1998; **26**: 1008–9.

33 Lundgren, J., and Masur, H. New approaches to managing opportunistic infections. *AIDS* 1999, **13**(suppl A): 5227–34.

34 Miller, R. HIV associated respiratory diseases. *Lancet* 1996; **348**: 307–12.

35 Wakefield, A.E., Peteis, S.E., Baneiji, S., *et al.* *Pneumocystis carinii* shows DNA homology with the ustomycetous red yeast fungi. *Mol Microbiol* 1992; **6**(14): 1903–11.

36 Murray, J.F. Pulmonary complications of HIV infection. *Annu Rev Med* 1996; **47**: 117–26.

37 Camus, F., de Picciotto, C., Gerbe, J., *et al.* Pulmonary function on tests in HIV-infected patients. *AIDS* 1993; **7**: 1075–9.

38 Huang, L., and Stansell, J.D. AIDS and the lung. *Med Clin N Am* 1996; **80**(4): 775–801.

39 Hirschtick, R.E., Glassroth, J., Jordan, M.C., *et al.* Bacterial pneumonia in persons infected with the human immunodeficiency virus. *N Engl J Med* 1995; **333**: 845–51.

40 Guerrero, M., Krugers, S., Saitoh, A., *et al.* Pneumonia in HIV-infected patients: a case-control survey of factors involved in risk and prevention. *AIDS* 1999; **13**: 1971–5.

41 Mihalcea, A.M., Smith, D.L., Monini, P., *et al.* Treatment update for AIDS-related Kaposi's sarcoma. *AIDS* 1999; **13**(Suppl A): 5215–25.

42 Lebbe, C., Blum, L., Pellet, C., *et al.* Clinical and biological impact of antiretroviral therapy with protease inhibitors on HIV-related Kaposi's sarcoma. *AIDS* 1998; **12**: F45–9.

43 Hannon, F.B., *et al.* Bronchopulmonary Kaposi's sarcoma in 106 HIV-1 infected patients. *Int J Sex Transm Dis AIDS* 1998; **9**(9): 518–25.

44 Stewart, S., Jablouowski, H., Goebel, F.D., *et al.* Randomised comparative trial of pegylated liposomal doxorubicin versus bleomycin and vincristine in the treatment of AIDS-related Kaposi's sarcoma. *J Clin Oncol* 1998; **16**(2): 683–91.

45 Welles, L., Saville, M.W., Lietzau, J., *et al.* Phase II trial with does titration of paclitaxel for the therapy of human immunodeficiency virus associated Kaposi's sarcoma. *J Clin Oncol* 1998; **16**(3): 1112–21.

46 Saville, M.W., Lietzau, J., Pluda, J.M., *et al.* Treatment of HIV-associated Kaposi's sarcoma with paclitaxel. *Lancet* 1995; **346**(8966): 26–8.

47 Northfelt, D.W., Dezube, B.J., Thommes, J.A., *et al.* Pegylated-liposmal doxorbicin versus doxorubicin bleomycin and vincristine in the treatment of AIDS-related Kaposi's sarcoma: results of a randomised phase III clinical trial. *J Clin Oncol* 1998; **16**(7): 2445–51.

48 Sider, L., Weiss, J.A., and Smith, M.D. Varied appearance of AIDS related lymphoma in the chest. *Radiology* 1989; **171**: 629–32.

49 Pozniac, A.L., Miller, R., and Ormerod, L.P. The treatment of tuberculosis in HIV-infected persons. *AIDS* 1999; **13**: 435–45.

50 Zuger, M., and Sharp, V.L. HIV specialists: The time has come. *JAMA* 1997; **278**: 1131–32.

51 Squier, R.W. A model of empathic understanding and adherence to treatment regimens in practitioner-patient relationships. *Soc Sci Med* 1990; **30**(3): 325–39.

52 Carr, D.B. Pain in HIV/AIDS. Editorial review. *Curr Opin Anaesthesiol* 1995; **8**; 441–4.

53 Hewitt, D.J., McDonald, M., Portenoy, R.K., *et al*. Pain syndromes and aetiologies in ambulatory AIDS patients. *Pain* 1997; **70**(2–3): 117–23.

54 Larue, F., Fontaine, A., and Colleau, S. Underestimation and under treatment of pain in HIV disease: multicentre study. *BMJ* 1997; **314**: 23–8.

55 Breitbart, W., Passik, S., McDonald, M.V., *et al*. Patient-related barriers to pain management in ambulatory AIDS patients. *Pain* 1998; **76**(1–2): 9–16.

56 Breitbart, W., Rosenfeld, B., Passik, S., *et al*. A comparison of pain report and adequacy of analgesic therapy in ambulatory AIDS patients with and without a history of substance abuse. *Pain* 1997; **72**(1–2): 235–43.

57 Breitbart, W., McDonald, M.V., Rosenfeld, B., *et al*. Pain in ambulatory AIDS patients. Pain characteristics and medical correlates. *Pain* 1996; **68**(2–3): 315–21.

58 Rosenfeld, B., Breitbart, W., McDonald, M.V., *et al*. Pain in ambulatory AIDS patients. Impact of pain on psychological functioning and quality of life. *Pain* 1996; **68**(2–3): 323–8.

59 Newshan, G., and Lefkowitz, M. Transdermal fentanyl for chronic pain in AIDS: a pilot study. *J Pain Symptom Manage* 2001; **21**(1): 69–77.

60 Salt, S., Wilson, L., and Edwards, A. The use of specialist palliative care services by patients with human immunodeficiency virus-related illness in the Yorkshire Deanery of the Northern and Yorkshire region. *Palliative Med* 1998; **12**: 152–60.

61 Brechtl, J.R., Breitbart, W., Galietta, M., Krivo, S., and Rosenfeld, B. The use of highly active anti-retroviral therapy (HAART) in patients with advanced HIV Infection: impact on medical, palliative care, and quality of life outcomes. *J Pain Symptom Manage* 2001; **21**(1): 41–51.

62 Manfredi, R., Mastroianni, A., Coronado, O., and Chiodo, F. Therapeutic and diagnostic procedures in hospitalized AIDS patients with a terminal illness. *AIDS Care* 1996; **8**(3): 373–6.

63 Teno, J.M. and Mor, V. Preferences of HIV-infected patients for aggressive versus palliative care. *N Engl J Med* 1991; **324**: 1140.

Chapter 32

Chronic infections: pulmonary tuberculosis

Suresh Kumar, Martin F. Muers, and Sam H. Ahmedzai

About 8 million people worldwide develop tuberculosis (TB) every year and 3 million die of it. It is the fourth leading cause of death, according to the World Health Organization (WHO).[1] TB is a disease that is known to have affected humans since time immemorial. Egyptian mummies and similar ancient human relics show the evidence of tubercular damage to body structures, and we may presume that the infection affected the respiratory system then as much as it does now.

Epidemiology and socio-economic issues

Across the world and through time, TB has been associated with social and economic factors that determine its distribution. It is strikingly associated with poverty, particularly urban poverty.[2,3] A strong association has been found between all TB mortality statistics and overcrowding in households.[4]

The epidemiology of TB has changed drastically over the last few decades. More than 90% of all cases of TB and 95% of all deaths arising from it now occur in developing countries. Incidence rates estimated by WHO vary from 23 per 100 000 population in industrialized countries to 191 per 100 000 in Africa and 237 per 100 000 in south-east Asia.[5] In addition, several factors such as multidrug resistant TB (MDRTB), HIV, and immigration from areas with high rates of TB[6] (and high frequencies of MDRTB) have altered the epidemiology. These factors are operating both in the developing and developed worlds.

The control of TB remains as much a social and political issue as a medical one. The typical patient with TB is usually someone who is already marginalized in society and is in need of support. Public health programmes in this area have to be sensitive to the different needs and concerns of the men and women who are affected.

At the level of the individual, the person or family affected by TB needs a holistic approach to physical symptoms, psychological problems, economic deprivation, and educational needs, as well as the best antimycobacterial chemotherapy. TB can be seen as a chronic and life-threatening disease, and it then fits into the 'Sheffield model' of supportive care, which emphasizes the need to support the individual and family at the same time as tackling the primary pathological process (see Chapter 1).

In many ways, the campaign against TB in developed countries can be seen as a forerunner of the modern approach to comprehensive supportive care for patients with cancer. For example, 'chest clinics' were very common in Britain from the 1930s to the 1980s, and a large part of their workload was the longer-term management of TB and patient and family support.

Table 32.1 Global health situation: leading causes of mortality, morbidity and disability, selected causes for which data are available, all ages (1996 estimates)

Leading selected causes of mortality	Deaths Rank	Number (000)
Ischaemic heart disease	1	7200
Cerebrovascular disease	2	4600
Acute lower respiratory infection	3	3905
Tuberculosis	4	3000
COPD	5	2888
Diarrhoea (including dysentery)	6	2473
Malaria	7	1500–2700
HIV/AIDS	8	1500
Hepatitis B	9	1156
Prematurity	10	1150
Measles	11	1010
Cancer of trachea, bronchus, and lung	12	989

Source: Adapted from Table 3 of the 1997 *World Health Report* (WHO, 1997).[1]

Adopting a public health model, these clinics employed nurses who spent much of their time (and still do) in the community following up families, both for screening and to ensure treatment compliance. Social workers (previously known as hospital almoners) were involved in cases of poverty, and also tried to provide psychological support. As TB became less prevalent in Britain in the 1980s and 1990s many of these chest clinics were closed down and in their place have appeared the lung cancer clinics which now form a major part of the workload for respiratory services.

In developing countries, where hospital-based clinics have never been so well developed, the approach to TB control and management has tended to be more sporadic and largely community-based. Because of the lack of resources, not only medication but also the support services have been rationed in just those countries and deprived strata of society which could benefit most.

The resurgence of TB in developed countries in the past decade is largely due to medical factors, notably the emergence of multidrug resistant strains and the increased number of immunosuppressed individuals, particularly from HIV/AIDS. Immigration has always played an important part in the persistence of cases of TB in developed countries, and this brings the added factor of communication difficulties. The most susceptible members of immigrant groups are the elderly and very young; language and cultural barriers are particularly problematic with older people. Healthcare workers and social workers may need to rely heavily on professional interpreters rather than young family members to communicate about symptoms, other concerns, and the instructions for complying with medication. Poverty and cultural requirements may compromise the dietary intake of elderly immigrants, and this is also relevant for drug abusers with HIV/AIDS in large cities in developed countries.

Standard antituberculous treatment for pulmonary TB with regimens containing rifampicin usually needs to run for 6 months. Longer periods may occasionally be needed, depending on drug sensitivities, the immune status of the patient, and the site of disease. Compliance with an effective medication regimen leads to cure in >97% of cases – yet many patients with TB fail to comply. Non-compliance is thus a major problem undermining TB control today. The causes of non-compliance are diverse: it can be a significant problem in patients who are homeless, who are drug abusers or who for various psychological or cultural reasons cannot or will not complete a course of therapy.[7] Important economic barriers to regular treatment may include transport costs, cost of prescribed nutritional supplements, and lost income. These barriers may be reduced through public health interventions that reduce the number of health encounters, travel distances, and duration of illness before diagnosis.[8]

The struggle against TB is now seen as a worldwide emergency, but the experience of many TB control programmes has shown that the solution for eradication may be beyond the general framework of routine medical practice.[9] Public-health-based programmes therefore have the best chance of achieving good cure rates, especially in developing countries and rural communities.[10] For comprehensive care of patients and families affected by TB, this needs to be combined with the best antitubercular regimen and a supportive care approach to palliating individual symptoms and concerns.[11]

Natural history of pulmonary disease

The natural history of pulmonary disease in an immunocompetent person is for infection to occur as a result of inhalation of infected particles from an index case with pulmonary TB, who is usually sputum smear-positive. The likelihood of infection depends on the duration and intensity of 'contact' between the index case and the patient. For example in some studies more than a quarter of family members were infected by smear-positive cases, and about 3% where the index case was smear-negative. Casual contact by contrast had an infection rate of probably 10% for smear-positive and 1% for smear-negative index cases.[12]

Infection of a person by TB organisms does not always result in clinical disease, and the cumulative risk of disease in infected cases is about 15%. Within 3 months of infection, there is a systemic immunological reaction with a rise in temperature and occasionally flu-like symptoms, and at this time the tuberculin skin test is positive. A minority of people who are infected develop primary disease in which there is a tiny locus of disease in the lung with enlarged hilar lymph nodes. This 'primary' complex usually resolves leaving a small scar (Ghon focus) in the affected lung. The hilar nodes shrink and may become calcified later. Occasionally very large nodes may obstruct adjacent bronchi and lead to persistent non-bacterial infection and perhaps bronchiectasis (e.g. 'middle lobe syndrome' affecting the right lung). It is at this primary stage that miliary TB may occur in some patients as a result of haematogenous spread of the bacilli to distant organs of the body. These organisms may remain dormant, but if they later multiply locally then post-primary non-pulmonary TB develops, e.g. in the kidneys, bones, and gut.

Post-primary TB (classical TB) is said to occur usually within 5 years of the primary infection, although this may be delayed. The patient usually presents with a combination of systemic symptoms such as fever, malaise, anorexia, weight loss, and respiratory symptoms – notably cough with sputum, haemoptysis, and breathlessness. Most cases of adult post-primary TB are due to reactivation of quiescent primary disease, but a minority may occur in immunocompetent individuals as a result of reinfection from another index case.

Untreated post-primary pulmonary TB leads to death usually from a combination of the systemic effects and unchecked destruction of lung tissue leading to respiratory failure. With

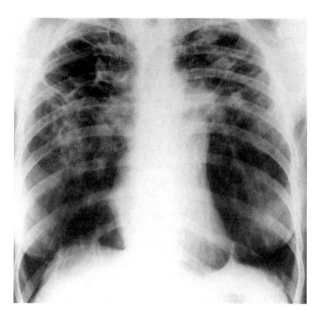

Fig. 32.1 Chronic fibrotic scarring in upper lobes. Courtesy of Rotherham General Hospitals NHS Trust.

effective treatment, healing occurs and there is contraction and fibrosis of the affected part of the lung, which may lead in the long term to persistent cavitation. This process commonly results in shrinkage of the upper lobes, and consequent elevation of the hila, and upwards traction on the bronchovascular bundles of the lower lobes (Fig. 32.1). Pleural effusions may occur as a consequence of primary infection and occasionally post-primary infection. If promptly treated they may resolve completely, but if not, persistent infection (tuberculous empyema) and pleural thickening with calcification may ensue.

As a result of pulmonary damage lobes of the lung may become bronchiectatic with secondary infection, and residual cavities may become colonized by fungi, e.g. *Aspergillus*, inhaled from the environment producing a ball in the affected cavity (a mycetoma) (see Figure 23.2, Chapter 23).

Drug treatment

Combination chemotherapy is essential. Details of the drugs used, modes of administration, side-effect profiles, and combinations can be found in standard texts.[13] The following is a brief summary of current best practice.

A 6-month short course of chemotherapy is standard, usually **rifampicin, isoniazid, pyrazinamide, and ethambutol** for 2 months and then **rifampicin and isoniazid** for a final 4 months for fully sensitive organisms. If pyrazinamide cannot be used or tolerated, ethambutol, rifampicin, and isoniazid are given for 2 months and then rifampicin and isoniazid for a further 7 months. Short-course chemotherapy like this is effective for all pulmonary TB with fully sensitive organisms, and in addition, non-pulmonary TB except for central nervous system and tuberculous meningitis which need a year of treatment.

In cases of likely non-compliance, treatment should be fully supervised (directly observed therapy, DOT). For example, isoniazid, rifampicin, and pyrazinamide with ethambutol or streptomycin are given 3 times weekly for 2 months and then rifampicin and isoniazid 3 times weekly for 4 months.

In countries where the cost of rifampicin is still a problem, adapted regimens can be used where rifampicin is either given for 2 months only or omitted. A standard text should be consulted for details.

The impact of HIV

Pulmonary TB is an AIDS-defining illness in HIV-positive patients, and in the HIV-positive individual the risk of TB in those who are positive on tuberculin testing is increased by about 100-fold. The pattern of TB in HIV-positive individuals is different: they are more likely to present with disseminated or lymph node-positive TB and to be sputum smear-negative. They are treated with standard regimens, but the incidence of drug reactions is increased. There are important interactions between some TB drugs and antiretroviral drugs (see Chapter 31).

Multidrug resistant TB

Essentially, multidrug resistance implies resistance to rifampicin and one of the other standard drugs used for treatment. The usual cause is inadequate drug treatment – for example because of monotherapy, poor compliance, or short intermittent treatment periods.

The consequences of the emergence of resistant strains are that cure rates fall from >97% in fully sensitive organisms to about 50%. Successful outcome relies on good laboratory services to identify drug sensitivities, and then a prolonged period of treatment (usually 2 years after cultures are negative) using second-line drugs to which the organisms are sensitive *in vitro*. It is usual for the therapy of these patients to be directly observed (DOT).

A patient with sputum-positive, fully sensitive pulmonary TB can be rendered non-infectious within 2 weeks of starting standard treatment, but a patient with multidrug-resistant TB may not 'sputum-convert' for many months and during this time they are potentially infectious. This means that patient isolation has to be organized for much longer periods of time, against the background of a much higher probability of treatment failure. It is worrying that MDRTB is becoming increasingly common particularly in disadvantaged sectors of communities, such as prison populations and the very poor.

Supportive care

Isolation

Although an otherwise well sputum-positive individual can be treated at home, and is likely to become non-infectious after 2 weeks, patients with unstable or unsatisfactory domestic circumstances and particularly patients with multidrug resistant disease may need segregation for far longer periods of time. This can inevitably lead to further psychological stresses.

Compliance

Issues underlying poor compliance are multifactorial and are a particular problem in developing countries where drug treatment can be expensive. Some people may erroneously believe that they are cured when they feel better after a short course of treatment. It is particularly for these reasons and, also because multidrug resistance strongly correlates with poor compliance, that DOT has become the recommended standard treatment in the third world and is recommended by the WHO.

Employment

Historically TB has had a stigma attached to it, but in the developed world this is receding. There are no reasons to proscribe or adapt employment, providing that the patient has good pulmonary function and no complications at the end of therapy.

Travel

It is necessary to advise patients not to travel on public transport while they are infectious. This may be particularly difficult, but it is necessary where individuals are identified as having sputum-positive TB away from home.

Contact tracing

The perceived stigma of TB may affect people's feelings when they are requested to provide information about their close contacts or work contacts. Some individuals may need detailed counselling about the importance of contact tracing and the social responsibility of helping to control the spread of disease.

Unvaccinated children are highly susceptible to tuberculous infection, and families need advice from experienced health visitors and other healthcare workers about the risks to children, particularly neonates, and the appropriate tuberculin testing and segregation, and prophylactic regimens – usually isoniazid. Again, details of the action to be taken in particular cases can be obtained from standard texts.[14] In some circumstances, a mother with TB may need to be kept in hospital with her children.

Nutrition

Patients with advanced TB lose weight, but with the onset of effective treatment, systemic symptoms resolve relatively rapidly and weight gain can be expected without the use of partic-ular supplements.

Symptoms and their management in acute disease

Haemoptysis

Haemoptysis may occur during active TB or after chemotherapy for it, and the usual causes are post-tuberculous bronchiectasis, secondary infection, or mycetomas in cavities. The combined use of bronchoscopy and thoracic CT has the best yield in evaluating such cases.

During active TB, bleeding is usually streaky and small in quantity. However, from the patient's point of view any bleeding may be frightening and care should be taken to explain what is happening and to provide reassurance. In most cases a combination of meticulous antituber-culous chemotherapy, rest and sedation (if necessary) will control bleeding.[15] If the bleeding becomes more persistent and severe (e.g. >200 mL/24 h) active investigation and treatment may be necessary (see Chapter 23).[16–18]

Breathlessness

A variety of factors can cause breathlessness during a course of TB treatment. These may include anaemia, a pleural effusion, airflow obstruction, and muscular weakness. The man-agement must therefore be individualized, focusing on the underlying cause and particular situations. Specific management should always be supplemented with general measures like reassurance, pain relief and on occasion breathing exercises. The psychological components of breathlessness may need attention.[19]

Fever

Fever usually responds to antituberculous drugs in a fortnight or so. If it is more prolonged, alternative explanations such as drug hypersensitivity, coexisting infection, poor compliance, or occasionally concomitant neoplasm should be considered. Paracetamol, fans, and tepid sponging may help to overcome major distress if the fever is high.

Pain

Acute pulmonary TB is normally painless. Occasionally pleurisy can occur, and needs treatment with analgesics such as paracetamol or a NSAID. It will resolve as the disease improves. Occasionally pain may occur elsewhere as a result of extrapulmonary involvement, particularly in bones such as the spine, and joints. Correct diagnosis is essential. It is uncommon for severe pain to occur, and an alternative diagnosis should be considered rather than immediate application of stronger analgesics. If these are required the WHO analgesic ladder, which was developed for cancer pain, is an appropriate model.[20]

Anorexia

As indicated above, anorexia and weight loss usually respond rapidly to successful chemotherapy. Nasogastric or enteral feeding is hardly ever required, except in a very sick patient. Pharmacological approaches for increasing appetite and weight gain such as megestrol acetate or dronabinol (a cannabinoid) have not been studied in TB, as opposed to the anorexia associated with cancer or HIV.[21–23]

Symptoms of drug toxicity

Important toxic effects of antituberculous drugs include visual damage from ethambutol, hepatotoxicity from pyrazinamide and isoniazid, rashes, puritis, and hepatitis, thrombocytopenic purpura and gastrointestinal reactions to rifampicin, and vestibular toxicity from streptomycin. Appropriate drug monitoring and clinical and ocular examinations are necessary to minimize these. Patients with these particular symptoms may need palliation with antiemetics, antipruritics such as antihistamines, and analgesics.[24]

Symptoms arising from complications of treated disease

Breathlessness

Severe pulmonary TB, even if successfully treated, may result in considerable lung damage with extensive fibrosis particularly in the upper lobes. This commonly causes fixed airflow obstruction. Current or previous smoking may exacerbate this problem. Physical signs and physiology are similar to those of chronic obstructive pulmonary disease (COPD), but the patient is far less likely to respond well to simple bronchodilator medication. Inhaled or oral corticosteroids are not required, unless there is good evidence of asthma as a separate disease. Although the airflow obstruction is likely to be 'fixed', a trial of bronchodilators should nevertheless be considered, but they should be withdrawn if no improvement ensues. Inhaled corticosteroids are

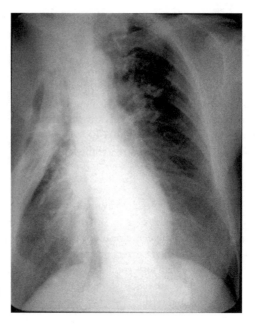

Fig. 32.2 Thoracoplasty of right side.

not contraindicated in the management of airflow obstruction in patients with pulmonary TB, especially if full antituberculous therapy is applied. If chronic airflow obstruction develops, the supportive care of such patients should be along the lines discussed in Chapter 17. There is no contraindication to the use of spirometry for the diagnosis and management of these patients providing they have been fully treated.

It is uncommon for patients to develop purely restrictive lung disease after treatment for TB, but in some cases pleural disease and diffuse pleural thickening may occur. Furthermore, other patients may have required lung resection perhaps for drug resistant or atypical mycobacterial infections, and occasionally thoracoplasties are still required under these circumstances (Figure 32.2).

In patients who are breathless as a result of previous pulmonary TB, pulmonary rehabilitation is entirely appropriate.

Cor pulmonale

Patients with both severe obstructive and restrictive lung disease secondary to TB and its complications may develop cor pulmonale. This needs treatment in the standard fashion with the correction of any existing hypoxaemia and diuretic therapy.

Haemoptysis

The usual causes of this in treated patients are post-tuberculous bronchiectasis, occasionally intercurrent infection, and more commonly the erosion of vessels in a post-tuberculous cavity as a result of colonization by a fungus ball (a mycetoma). Bleeding from post-tuberculous bronchiectasis is usually treated by broad-spectrum antibiotics, and general nursing measures. If bleeding is from a mycetoma, nursing measures usually suffice. More severe bleeding needs active management as detailed in Chapter 23. Repetitive haemoptysis require further investigation, usually nowadays with bronchial artery angiography. Embolization may be needed for definitive treatment.

Lung cancer

Concomitant lung cancer can occasionally be the cause of an apparent relapse after successful treatment, particularly in a patient who has smoked. It is essential to exclude true relapse of TB or the development of its respiratory complications, before assuming that cancer is the cause of the deterioration.

Empyema thoracis

Empyema thoracis most commonly occurs 3–7 months after the primary infection, but may occur any time during the natural course of the disease. It presents with chest pain, dyspnoea, cough with expectoration, fever and toxaemia. It can be managed with intercostal tube drainage, antibiotics, and appropriate antituberculous treatment.[25]

The aim of treatment is to relieve symptoms and to prevent fibrothorax. Aspiration of pleural fluid to dryness or administration of antituberculous drugs should suffice to solve the problem.[11] Aspiration of the pleural fluid seldom needs to be undertaken more than twice. Prednisolone 20 mg/day for 2–3 weeks may be useful in preventing adhesions.

Bronchopleural fistula

Bronchopleural fistula (BPF) is an important complication of TB in the developing world. The patient usually presents with a history of violent cough and expectoration accompanied by quick deterioration in general condition. When the patient turns in bed with the affected lung uppermost, violent bouts of coughing occur. The management of spontaneous BPF is controversial. Opinions differ as to whether to combine chemotherapy with intercostal drainage or surgical intervention (e.g. decortication, pleuropneumonectomy, pleurolobectomy, saucerization or local evacuation, closure of the fistula with a muscle graft, or thoracoplasty). Thoracoscopic and bronchoscopic closure of the fistula may also be attempted. A thoracic surgical opinion is always needed.

Conclusions

In the developed world, the focus of supportive care has moved away from TB towards cancer which has become more prevalent and has a far higher public profile. However, for many patients in the developed world and for the millions in the developing world, the same supportive principles underlying the successful management of patients with cancer can be applied to patients with TB. The importance of a multidisciplinary team approach, involving the physician, nurses, health visitor, and social worker needs to be emphasized. Appropriate management of patients with TB involves attention to the psychosocial circumstances of the patients as well as their physical illness. This means that supportive care needs to be directed also towards the family. Support may be needed not only at the beginning of the illness, but for some time afterwards and for people who are immunocompromised or have fatal multidrug resistant TB, need to continue into the terminal stages.

Keypoints

♦ Pulmonary TB is an important cause of mortality and morbidity worldwide, especially in the developing world

♦ Modern principles of antituberculous therapy including multidrug regimens should achieve a high cure rate

♦ Multidrug resistance and HIV are important factors in failure to control TB

♦ Respiratory and systemic symptoms are common, but can be relieved by effective antibiotic therapy and palliative drugs

♦ A holistic patient and family approach is needed to support them through antituberculous therapy and in advanced disease which has not responded

References

1 WHO. *The state of world health. The world health report. Conquering suffering, enriching humanity.* Geneva: World Health Organization, 1997.

2 Terris, M. Relation of economic status to tuberculosis mortality by age and sex. *Am J Public Health* 1948; **38**: 1061–70.

3 Spence, D.P.S., Hotchkiss, J., and Davies, P.D.O. Tuberculosis and poverty. *BMJ* 1993; **307**: 759–761.

4 Elendes, F., Benthain, G., and Laryford, I. Tuberculosis mortality in England and Wales during 1982–1992: its association with poverty, ethnicity and AIDS. *Soc Sci Med* 1998; **46**(6): 673–81.

5 Billo, N.E. Epidemiologic trends in tuberculosis. *Rev Prat* 1996; **46**(11): 1332–5.

6 Onorato, I.M. and Ridzon, R. In: A.P. Fishman, *et al.* (eds) *Fishman's Pulmonary Diseases and Disorders*, 3rd edn. New York: McGraw-Hill, 1998; 2432.

7 McDermott, L.J., Glassrotes, J., Mehta, J.B., and Dutt, A.K. Tuberculosis Part I. *Dis Mon* 1997; **3**: 113–80.

8 Needham, D.M., Godfrey-Faussett, P., and Foster, S.D. Barriers to tuberculosis control in urban Zambia: the economic impact and burden on patients prior to diagnosis. *Int J Tuberc Lung Dis* 1998; **2**(10): 811–17.

9 Abel, E.K. Taking the cure to the poor: patients' responses to New York City's tuberculosis program, 1894 to 1918. *Am J Public Health*, 1997; **87**(11): 1808–15.

10 Chowdhury, A.M., Chowdhury, S., Islam, M.N., Islam, A., and Vaughan, J.P. Control of tuberculosis by community health workers in Bangladesh. *Lancet*, 1997; **350**(9072): 169–72.

11 *Global tuberculosis control – WHO report.* Geneva: World Health Organization, 1999.

12 Grzybowski, S., Barnett, G.D., and Styblo, K. Contacts of cases of active pulmonary tuberculosis. *Bull Int Union Tuberc* 1975; **50**: 90–106.

13 Joint Tuberculosis Committee of the British Thoracic Society. Chemotherapy and Management of tuberculosis in the United Kingdom 1998. *Thorax* 1998; **53**: 536–48.

14 Joint Tuberculosis Committee of the British Thoracic Society. Control and prevention of tuberculosis in the United Kingdom: Code of Practice 2000. *Thorax* 2000; **55**: 887–901.

15 Corey, R. and Hla, K.M. Major and massive hemoptysis: re assessment of conservative management. *Am J Med Sci* 1987; **294**: 301–9.

16 Garzon, A.A., Cerruti, M.M., and Goldring, M.E. Exsanguinating hemoptysis. *J Thorac Cardiovasc Surg* 1982; **84**: 829–33.

17 Coulan, A.A., Hurwitz, S.S., Krige, L., *et al.* Massive hemoptysis: Review of 123 cases. *J Thorac Cardiovasc Surg* 1983; **85**: 120–4.

18 Mal, H. *et al.* Immediate and long term results of bronchial artery embolisation for life threatening hemoptysis *Chest* 1999; **115**(4): 996–1001.

19 Ahmedzai, S.H. Palliation of respiratory symptoms. In: D. Doyle, W.C.G. Hanks, and N. MacDonald (eds) *Oxford textbook of palliative care*, 2nd edn. Oxford: Oxford Medical Publications, 1998; 589.

20 WHO. *Cancer pain relief and palliative care*, 2nd edn. Geneva: World Health Organization, 1990.

21 Loprinzi, C.L., Ellison, N.M., Schaid, D.J., *et al.* A controlled trial of megestrol acetate treatment of cancer anorexia and cachexia. *Semin Oncol* 1990; **17**(suppl.9): 8–12.

22 Wadleigh, R., *et al.* Dronabinol enhancement of appetite and cancer patients (abstract). *Proc Am Soc Oncol* 1990; **9**: 1280–331.

23 Nelson, K., Walsh, D., Deeter, P., and Sheenan, F. A phase II study of delta-9-tetrahydrocannabinol for appetite stimulation in cancer-associated anorexia. *J Palliative Care* 1994; **10**(1): 14–18.

24 Chan, S.L. Chemotherapy of tuberculosis. In: P.D.O Davies (ed.) *Clinical tuberculosis*. London: Chapman & Hall, 1994; 141–56.

25 Ravikumar, R., and Satya Sri, S. Pleural complication: tuberculous pleural effusion. In Satya Sri, S. (ed.) *Textbook of pulmonary and extra pulmonary tuberculosis*, 2nd edn. NewDelhi: Interprint, 1995; 82–6.

Index

abacavir 494
abdominal muscles 41
ACEI (angiotensin converting enzyme
    inhibitor) 366, 369
acetylcysteine 294, 383
acidosis 110
acinus 43–4
active cycle of breathing (ACBT) 386
activities of daily living
    assessment 124–7, 137–8
    breathing retraining 192
    exercise 202
acupuncture 67
    for advanced cancer-related dyspnoea 73
    for asthma 68–9
    for COPD 73
acute respiratory distress syndrome
    (ARDS) 299
adefovir 490, 495
advance directives 30, 57, 321
age factors 7
AIDS see HIV/AIDS
AIDSVAX 491
air hunger 328, 331, 332
airway lining fluid (ALF) 53–4
airways
    anatomy and physiology 41–5, 49–50
        lung defence mechanisms 55
    cough 344–5
        inflammation 350–2
    parenchymal receptors 98–100
    resistance 49–50
alcohol 156
allergic bronchopulmonary aspergillosis 396–7
allergies 70, 71
allodynia 413, 416
almitrine 150
alprazolam 150
alternative therapies see complementary medicine
alveolar cell carcinoma 381, 382
alveoli 43, 44–5, 50–1
ambulatory oxygen therapy
    definition 165
    diffuse airflow obstruction 294
    equipment 165, 182
    evidence 169
    guidelines 178
    restrictive lung disease 301
    smokers 290, 294
amitriptyline 447
amoxicillin 86
amphetamines 448–9
amprenavir 495
amyloidosis 266

amyotrophic lateral sclerosis see motor neurone
    disease/amyotrophic lateral sclerosis
anaemia 108
analgesia see pain, management
anatomy and physiology 39, 55
    airway resistance 49–50
    airways 41–5
    breathing
        during exercise 52–3
        regulation 51–2
    bronchial circulation 46
    diaphragm 39
    dyspnoea 95–105
    hyperventilation 323
    innervation 46–7
    integration 47–9
    intercostal muscles 39–41
    lungs
        defence mechanisms 53–5
        inflammation 55
    lymph 45–6
    pleura, pleural space, and pleural fluid 41–7
    pulmonary gas exchange 50–1
    pulmonary vessels 46
    ribcage, respiratory muscles, and respiratory
        'pump' 39–41
    ventilation 47–9
angina 6
angiotensin converting enzyme inhibitor
    (ACEI) 366, 369
ankylosing spondylitis 48–9
anticholinergics 385–6
antidepressants 293, 312, 330
antihistamines 156, 295
antimuscarinics 386
anxiety
    diffuse airflow obstruction 293, 295
    hyperventilation 327, 328, 329
    motor neurone disease 317, 318
    occupational therapy 254–5
anxiolytics 293, 295, 318
appendicitis 401
Armstrong–Workman nomogram 197–8
Arnold's nerve 345
aromatherapy 71
art therapy 23, 234, 235, 236
asbestos 54
aspergillomas 372–3
Aspergillus 396–7, 507
asphyxia 265
aspirin
    adverse effects 447
    overdose 328
assisted suicide 32–3

Association for Palliative Medicine of Great
    Britain and Ireland 12
asthma
    alveolar gas exchange 51
    complementary therapies 67–73
    cough
        airways inflammation 350, 351
        bronchial hyperresponsiveness 352
        chronic, with 'normal' chest radiograph
            366, 367–8, 369
        gastrooesophageal reflux 345
        neuropeptides 346, 346
        tracheobronchial tree 344
    cystic fibrosis 394
    dyspnoea 215, 216
        diffuse airflow obstruction 283
        drug therapies 148
        hyperventilation 327, 330
        oxygen therapy 172, 186
        psychosocial therapies 229
        respiratory muscle training 226
    expectoration 381, 382
    forced expiration 50
    pain 432
    quality of life 59–62
Asthma Bother Profile 59, 60, 64
Asthma Quality of Life Questionnaire 59, 60
atelectasis 111, 317
atropine 385
Australia, complementary medicine 68
autogenic drainage 386
autogenic training 72, 255
autohypnosis 72

baclofen 348, 356, 447
Balker–Ware protocol 198
Barrett's oesophagus 400
Barthel Index 251
Baseline Dyspnoea Index 125, 126–7, 137, 288
Belgium
    cost-effectiveness analysis 82
    euthanasia, decriminalization of 32
benzodiazepines
    dyspnoea 150–1, 157, 160, 293, 334
    haemoptysis 375
bereavement counselling 31
β-agonists 385, 394
beta-blockers 333–4
biliary cirrhosis 400
biofeedback, asthma 72
bisacodyl 443
bisphosphonates 402
bleomycin 481, 505
body composition 242
body weight 239, 240
    cystic fibrosis 401
    nutritional intervention 243
    see also nutrition
Borg scale, dyspnoa assessment 129, 130,
    136, 137, 138
    diffuse airflow obstruction 288
    exercise intensity 202

Bornholm disease 433
brachytherapy
    brachial plexopathy 419–22
    cancer 470–2, 474
    upper airflow obstruction 267, 270–1
bradykinin 351
breast cancer
    chemotherapy 476
    chest-wall pain 416
    pericardial effusions 481
    postmastectomy syndrome 418
    prevalence of symptoms 463, 464, 465
breast-feeding by mothers with cystic fibrosis 403
Breathe Easy programme 22, 27–8, 259, 294
breath holding, dyspnoa assessment 138
breathing
    anatomy and physiology 47–9
    Buteyko breathing technique 72–3
    deep 311
    diaphragmatic 311
    emergency 192–4
    during exercise 52–3
    frog 311, 312
    mechanical ventilation 87
    neuromuscular and skeletal diseases 311
    pacing 192, 193, 196, 207
    pursed-lip 191–2, 206–7
        diffuse airflow obstruction 292
    regulation of 51
    retraining 191–4, 196, 206–7
        hyperventilation 333
    support
        motor neurone disease 319–21
        neuromuscular and skeletal diseases 313–15
Breathing Problems Questionnaire 59, 60
Breathing Space Kit 318–19
breathlessness see dyspnoea
Brief Pain Inventory (BPI) 429
British Lung Foundation, Breathe Easy programme
    22, 27–8, 259, 294
bronchi and bronchioles 41–3, 44
bronchial arterial angiography and
    embolization 375–7
bronchial circulation 46
bronchial hyperresponsiveness (BHR) 352
bronchiectasis
    chronic cough with 'normal' chest
        radiograph 368
    cystic fibrosis 396, 397
    diffuse airflow obstruction 283
    expectoration 381, 382
    haemoptysis 375, 376
    pain 432
    surfactant IgA, congenital lack of 54
bronciolitis obliterans 283
bronchitis, chronic see chronic obstructive
    pulmonary disease
bronchitis, eosinophilic
    cough
        airways inflammation 350–1
        with 'normal' chest radiograph 368
    expectoration 382

bronchodilators
  cystic fibrosis 394
  dyspnoea 104, 148
  economic issues 86–7
  expectoration 385
  tuberculosis 521
bronchomalacia 265, 266
bronchopleural fistula (BPF) 523
bronchoscopy
  haemoptysis 375
  upper airflow obstruction 265, 266, 269
Bruce Protocol 197, 198
bupivacaine 447, 449, 454
Burkholderia cepacia 395–6
burn-out, healthcare professionals 32
Buteyko breathing technique (BBT) 72–3
butyrophenones 6, 156

cachexia 239, 245–6
  medication 243
  nutritional intervention 243–4
  nutritional supplementation strategy 244–5
  weight loss and inflammatory mediators
      in COPD 242–3
  weight loss and muscle wasting, pathogenesis
      of 240–2
calcitonin gene related peptide (CGRP) 346, 347
Calicut model 9
Canadian Occupational Performance Measure
    (COPM) 252
cancer 463, 483
  approaches to symptom management 468
  available anticancer treatments 468
  causes and assessment of symptoms 465–7
  chemotherapy 472–5
  cough 479
  dyspnoea 93, 475–6
    complementary medicine 73–4
    drug therapies 149, 150, 151, 153
    oxygen therapy 166, 167, 168, 182
  earlier stages 27–8
  effusions, management of 480–3
  haemoptysis 476–8
  information needs and resources 22, 27–8
  medicine, changing aims of 4
  pain
    brachial plexopathy 419–22
    evaluation 429–30
    herpes zoster infection 416
    management 445–6, 479–80
  palliation 6, 11–12, 15, 19–20, 474–80
  prevalence of symptoms 463–5
  prevention 4
  radiotherapy 469–72, 474–5
  supportive care
    composition of networks 23
    comprehensive 18, 19–20, 21, 22
    concept 16, 17
    opportunities for interventions 24, 25
    and palliative care, relationship between 27
    transfer to 25
  see also specific cancers

CancerBACUP 27
CancerLink 27
cannabis, therapeutically administered 150
capsaicin 355–6
carbamazepine 446
cardiac disease 106–7
cardiopulmonary resuscitation 26–7
cardiovascular endurance exercise *see* exercise,
      cardiovascular endurance
cardiovascular system dyspnoea 106–8
carers, family and friends
  end-of-life care 9, 29, 30, 31
  motor neurone disease 320–1
  occupational therapy 257–9
  Sheffield model of comprehensive supportive care 18
category scaling, dyspnoea assessment 128–9
cefaclor 86
ceftazadime 395
central processing
  cough reflex 348
  dyspnoea 100–5, 110, 116
central sleep apnoea 307
C-fibres 345
charities 3
chemoreceptors 95, 96, 109–10, 116
chemotherapy 468, 472–5
  antineoplastic 505
  cough 479
  haemoptysis 478
  tuberculosis 515, 518–19
chest clinics 515–16
chest-wall pain 415–16
chest-wall twinge syndrome (precordial catch
      syndrome) 416, 417
Cheyne–Stokes respiration 307, 327
Childhood Asthma Questionnaires 60–1, 62
children
  asthma, complementary medicine for 68, 70–1, 72
  Harrison's sulcus 39
  quality of life, measuring 60–1, 62
  tuberculosis infection, susceptibility to 520
Chinese herbal medicine 70
chiropractic 70
chlorpromazine 156
choking 318
cholelithiasis 400
chronic airflow limitation *see* diffuse airflow
      obstruction
chronic fatigue syndrome 331
chronic obstructive pulmonary disease (COPD)
  alveolar damage 44, 51
  anatomy and physiology
    airways 44
    diaphragm 39
    forced expiration 50
    ventilation 48
  'blue bloaters' 110, 239
  'Breathe Easy' programme 22
  complementary medicine 73
  complications, possible 282
  cough
    airways inflammation 350

chronic obstructive pulmonary disease (*continued*)
  with 'normal' chest radiograph 366
  tracheobronchial tree 344
  dyspnoea 215, 216
    'blue bloaters' 110
    breathing retraining 191, 194
    diffuse airflow obstruction 281–98
    drug therapies 148, 149, 150, 151, 152, 155
    exercise 197, 198, 218, 221
    nutrition and cachexia 239, 240, 241, 242–5
    oxygen therapy 165, 166, 167–74, 182, 183
    respiratory muscle function 219
    respiratory muscle training 223–6
    restrictive lung disease 298, 300–2
    ventilatory pump 111
  earlier stages 28
  economies of 85–7
  expectoration 382, 383
  haemoptysis 477
  HIV 498
  pain 432, 448
  palliation 6, 26
  'pink puffers' 239
  quality of life 62
  supportive care
    comprehensive 18, 19
    opportunities for interventions 24, 25
    and palliative care, relationship between 26, 27
    transfer to 25
Chronic Respiratory Disease Questionnaire (CRQ)
    59–62, 125, 127–8, 138
  diffuse airflow obstruction 288
  occupational therapy 251
cigarette smoking *see* smoking
ciliary dyskinesias 54
ciprofloxacin 86, 394
cisplatin 472, 473, 474
citric acid 354, 355, 356
clonazepam 446–7
coal dust 54
codeine 441–2, 449
cognitive impairment 30
cognitive techniques 216, 293
colonic strictures 401
colorectal cancer 463, 464, 465
communication problems 180
  see also speech problems
co-morbidity, Sheffield model 18
complementary medicine 67, 74
  for advanced cancer-related breathlessness 73–4
  for asthma 67–73
  for COPD 73
  composition of supportive care networks 23
  definition 67
  earlier stages of illness 28
  see also specific therapies
computed tomography (CT) scanning,
    haemoptysis 375, 376
congenital bilateral absence of the vas deferens
    (CBAVD) 403
constipation 154, 443
contact tracing, tuberculosis 520

continuous hyperfractionated accelerated
    radiotherapy (CHART) 469–70
cordotomy 453–4, 457–8, 459
cor pulmonale 522
corticosteroids
  cystic fibrosis 403
  dyspnoea 148–50
    muscle wasting 243, 293
    respiratory muscle function 218
    restrictive lung disease 301
  intercostal nerve blocks 454
  tuberculosis 521–2
cost-benefit analysis 80, 81
cost-effectiveness acceptability curve 84
cost-effectiveness analysis 80, 81–5
cost issues *see* financial issues
cost-minimization analysis 80, 81
costochondritis 417–18
costopleural syndrome 457
cost-utility analysis 80
co-trimoxazole 499, 500
cough
  anatomy, physiology and pathophysiology
    341, 359–60
    abdominal muscles 41
    airways inflammation 350–2
    bronchial hyperresponsiveness 352
    central processing of cough reflex 348
    cough receptors 47
    cough reflex 341–51
    disease 350–2
    efferent limb of cough reflex 348–50
    inflammatory mediators 351–2
    larynx 343–4
    neuropeptides 345–8
    quantification and measurement 352–9
    tracheobronchial tree 344–5
  assistance 312
  cancer 479
  challenge 353–5, 358
  chronic, with 'normal' chest radiograph 365–9
  diaries 352, 353, 358
  non-productive 350
  phases 348–50
  productive 350
  psychogenic 348, 368
counselling
  bereavement 31
  dyspnoea 189–91
  psychosexual 28
creative art therapy 23, 234, 235, 236
Crohn's disease 401
cryocoagulation 455, 458
cryotherapy 269
Cryptococcus infection 506–7
cryptogenic fibrosing alveolitis (CFA) 298, 299
cultural issues, end-of-life care 30
cyclophosphamide 473
cystic fibrosis (CF) 391, 404
  allergic bronchopulmonary aspergillosis 396–7
  biliary cirrhosis and portal hypertension 400
  Burkholderia cepacia 395–6

cholelithiasis 400
colonic strictures 401
complications 391, 392–3
diabetes mellitus 402
diffuse airflow obstruction 283
endocrine disorders 402–3
expectoration 381–2, 383, 384–5
female infertility 403
gastrointestinal disease 400–2
gastrooesophageal reflux 400
haemoptysis 372, 397–8
late phase support 403–4
lung transplantation 399
male infertility 403
meconium ileus equivalent 401
nutritional factors 401–2
osteoporosis 402
oxygen therapy 178
pancreatic insufficiency 400–1
pneumothorax 398–9
pregnancy 403
resources for CF team 404
respiratory disease 391–400
respiratory failure 399
sinus disease and nasal polyposis 399–400
supportive care 391
cystic fibrosis transmembrane regulator
    (CFTR) 54, 391
cytokines 54, 55
cytomegalovirus (CMV) 507–8
    retinitis 496–7

Daily Adjustable Progressive Resistance Exercise
    (DAPRE) 195, 196
death rattle 158
    drug therapies 158, 386
deconditioning 108, 218, 253
deep breathing 311
delavirdine 495, 496
depression 149, 190, 293
Dercum's disease 416
desaturation during exercise 205
desipramine 447
dexamethasone 149–50, 445
dextroamphetamine 448
dextromethorphan 443
diabetes mellitus
    cystic fibrosis 402
    ketoacidosis 328
diamorphine (diacetyl morphine) 442
    dyspnoea 152, 154, 157, 158, 160
        motor neurone disease 319
diaphragm
    anatomy and physiology 39
    and hyperventilation 218
    neuromuscular and skeletal diseases 308, 309
    pain 418–19
    paralysis 308
diaphragmatic breathing 311
diathermy 269
diazepam 150, 293, 295, 315, 447
diclofenac 441

didanosine 493, 494
diet see nutrition
dietary intake 240
difficult breathlessness 159–60
diffuse airflow obstruction 281–3, 302
    assessing disease severity 285
    assessing supportive care needs 288–9
    disease-modifying treatment 283–5
    effectiveness of supportive care components 290–5
    organization of supportive care 289
    problem areas 295–6
    prognosis and end-of-life planning 296–8
    supportive care needs, fitting to conventional
        management 285–90
diffuse parenchymal lung disease (DPLD) 298–9
diffuse pleural thickening 298, 299
diffusing capacity for carbon monoxide (DL_{CO}) 51
dihydrocodeine 151, 152, 441
disproportionate breathlessness 323, 331–3
distal intestinal obstruction syndrome (DIOS) 401
DNase 383, 394
docetaxel 472, 473
doctrine of double effect 159–60
dorsal respiratory group (DRG) 348
doxapram 51, 150
doxorubicin 473, 505
Duchenne muscular dystrophy see muscular
    dystrophy
dying patients see end-of-life care
dysaesthesia 413
dysphagia 317
dyspnoea
    airway damage 44
    assessment in clinical practice and audit 135–42
    assessment in research 123–32
    cancer 466–7, 475–6
    clinico-pathological links 105–12
    clinics 24
    complementary medicine 73–4
    comprehensive supportive care network 19
    descriptors of 113–14
    diffuse airflow obstruction 281–98, 302
    disproportionate 323, 331–3
    drug therapies 147–60
    in exercise 52
    hyperventilation 323–35
    language 112–15, 123, 139
    measurement, during activities of daily living 124–7
    mechanisms 93–117
    motor neurone disease 317–21
    nature of 94–5
    neuromuscular and skeletal diseases 307–15
    nutrition and cachexia 239–46
    occupational therapy and environmental
        modifications 249–60
    oxygen therapy 165–86
    physiological correlates of 131
    physiology of 95–105
    psychological response to 231–2
    psychosocial therapies 229–36
    quality of life 127–8
    rehabilitation and exercise 189–211

dyspnoea (*continued*)
respiratory muscle training 215–27
restrictive lung disease 281, 298–302
supportive care and palliative care, relationship
between 27
therapeutic implications 115–16
tuberculosis 520–2
underlying causes 135–6
upper airflow obstruction 265–77
dyspnoeic index 131
dystrophia myotonica 307, 308

ear–cough reflex 345
early disease detection 18, 20
economic issues *see* financial issues
Edmonton Symptom Assessment Scale
(ESAS) 141, 429–30
education, dyspnoea 189–91, 232, 291
efavirenz 494, 496
effusions, in cancer 480–3
emergency breathing 192–4
emphysema *see* chronic obstructive pulmonary disease
empyema 433, 523
endobronchial balloon tamponade 377, 475
endobronchial brachytherapy 470–2, 476, 478, 479
end-of-life care 7–10, 29
cystic fibrosis 403–4
dyspnoea 156–8
diffuse airflow obstruction 296–8
drug therapies 160
motor neurone disease 319–20
oxygen therapy 177
restrictive lung disease 302
family/carers' needs 31
healthcare professionals' needs 31–2
HIV 510
physical symptoms 29–30
psychological aspects 30
social aspects 30
spiritual and cultural aspects 30
energy conservation 253–4, 292
environmental modifications 256–7, 258, 259
EORTC (European Organization for Research and
Treatment of Cancer) 61, 138, 251, 430–1
eosinophilic bronchitis
cough
airways inflammation 350–1
with 'normal' chest radiograph 368
expectoration 382
eosinophils 55
ephedrine 70
epidural administration of neurolytic
agents 453, 456, 458
Epstein–Barr virus 508
equipment provision 256–7, 258, 259, 292
ergoreceptors 96, 100
ergoreflex 100
error signal processing, dyspnoea 101, 102–3, 110, 116
ethambutol 518, 521
ethamsylate 375, 477
ethical issues
dyspnoea, drug therapies 158
'n of 1' trials, oxygen therapy 177

etoposide 473
European Organization for Research and Treatment
of Cancer (EORTC) 61, 138, 251, 430–1
euthanasia 32–3
evening primrose oil 71
exercise 189, 194, 211
breathing during 52–3
cardiovascular endurance 195–6
duration 205
frequency 205
limitations 205–7
mode 205
prescription 201–5
testing 197–201
effects 216–18, 220–2
flexibility 194–5
follow-up 210
interval 207
mild to moderate disease 208–10
moderate to severe disease 208, 209
neuromuscular and skeletal diseases 311–12
occupational therapy 253
restrictive lung disease 300
severe disease 207–8
strengthening 195, 196
testing 131, 138, 177, 197–201
contraindications 200
oxygen therapy 169, 175, 177
see also respiratory muscles, training
expectoration 381, 387–8
clinical approach to therapy 382–6
pathophysiology 381–2
physiotherapy 386
external beam radiotherapy
cancer 472, 476, 477–8, 479
upper airflow obstruction 265–6
extrinsic allergic alveolitis 283

facial cooling 294, 301
fans 168, 169, 175, 186, 317
FACT-L 431
family *see* carers, family and friends
fans 168, 169, 175, 186, 317
fat-free mass (FFM) 240, 243
body composition 242
nutritional intervention 244
pathogenesis of weight loss and muscle wasting 240
feedback processing, dyspnoea 101, 102–3, 116
feedforward processing, dyspnoea 101–3, 110, 116
fentanyl 442, 443, 444–5, 510
adverse effects 448
fibrinogen infusion 377
fibrosing alveolitis 51, 55, 298, 299
financial advice 28, 31
financial issues 79–80, 87–8
chronic obstructive pulmonary disease 85–7
complementary medicine 67
cost-benefit analysis 80, 81
cost-effectiveness analysis 80, 81–5
cost-minimization analysis 80, 81
cost-utility analysis 80
economic evaluation 79, 80–1
oxygen therapy 180–1

fire hazards, oxygen therapy
    178, 179, 180, 185
fish oil 71
flexibility exercise 194–5
forced expiration 49–50
foreign bodies, inhaled 265
Friedreich's ataxia 307
friends *see* carers, family and friends
frog breathing 311, 312
frozen shoulder 418
functional residual capacity (FRC) 48–9

gabapentin 446
gallstones 400
γ-amino butyric acid (GABA) 348
gas exchange 50–1, 109, 111–12
gastrooesophageal reflux 345, 400
    chronic cough with 'normal' chest radiograph
        366, 368, 369
gemcitabine 472, 473, 474
gemfibrozil 496
gender factors, symptom perception 7
genetic screening 18, 20
Germany, cancer rehabilitation model 28
Ghon focus 517
gingko 70
glycopyrrolate 158
glycopyrronium 319, 386
growth hormone therapy 244, 293
guaifenesin 384

HAART *see* highly active antiretroviral
    therapy
Haemophilus influenzae 393
haemoptysis 371, 378
    aetiology 371–3
    assisted suicide and euthanasia 33
    cancer 476–8
    cystic fibrosis 372, 397–8
    diagnosis and treatment 373–7
    follow-up 378
    tuberculosis 372, 374, 520, 522–3
    upper airflow obstruction 265
haloperidol 6, 156, 293, 443
Harrison's sulcus 39
healing (complementary medicine) 70
healthcare professionals, needs 31–2
heart failure 178
Hedron's syndrome 419
helium/oxygen (heliox) mixtures 186, 265
Henderson–Hasselbach equation 323
herbalism 70–1
Hering–Breuer reflex 47, 99, 344
heroin *see* diamorphine
herpes zoster infection 415–16
highly active antiretroviral therapy (HAART)
    487, 489–90, 508
    drawbacks 492–7
    immunotherapy 491
    Kaposi's sarcoma 505
    protease inhibitors 491
    reverse transcriptase inhibitors 490–1
    viral load 491–2

HIV/AIDS 487–8, 510–11
    HAART 489–92, 505
        drawbacks 492–7
    haemoptysis 373
    lung defence mechanisms 55
    pain control 508–10
    palliation 26
    pulmonary disease 497–508
    replication 489, 490
    symptom management 508–10
    tuberculosis 516, 519
HIV RNA viral load assay 487, 491–2
Holter monitor 356
homeopathy 71
Horner's syndrome 420
hospices
    arts therapy 23
    complementary therapies 23
    end-of-life care 7–8, 9
    HIV/AIDS 510
    medicine, changing aims of 3
    supportive care and palliative care, relationship
        between 26–7
Hospital Anxiety and Depression (HAD) Scale 255, 289
humidification, oxygen therapy 181
hydromorphone 152, 442
hydroxyurea 491, 495
hyoscine 158, 318, 319, 385, 387
hypercalcaemia 5, 6
hypercapnia
    dyspnoea 110, 116
        neuromuscular and skeletal diseases 308
        oxygen therapy 180
        physiology 96–7, 104–5
        respiratory muscle function 218
    pain 440
hyperglycaemia 149
hyperinflation 215
    breathing retraining 192, 206–7
    and dyspnoea perception, relationship
        between 217–18
    exercise 206–7
    respiratory muscle function 218
hyperventilation 323, 334–5
    acute 330, 333
    aetiology 326
    chronic 331
    clinical syndromes 329–31
    diagnosis 325–6
    empirical treatment 332
    initiating factors 327–8
    physiology 323
    screen 325–6
    signs 324
    subacute 330
    sustaining factors 328–9
    symptomatic management 333–4
    symptoms 323–4
    syndrome 329–30
hypnotherapy 51, 72
hypocapnia 323–4, 327, 330
hypoglycaemia 328
hypogonadism 402

hypopnoea 307
hypoxaemia 165, 168, 169–75, 440
hypoxia 97–8, 110, 116, 218, 308

ibuprofen 441
ICIDH-2 249–50
immune restoration syndrome 496–7
immunotherapy, HIV 491
immunoglobulins 54
incremental cost-effectiveness ratio (ICER) 83–4
India, end-of-life care 9
indinavir 495
indomethacin 352
infertility 403
information needs and resources 22, 27–8
inhaled steroids 150
inspiratory flow resistive training 222–3
inspiratory muscle training (IMT) 222
    effects 223–7
    inspiratory flow resistive training 222–3
    inspiratory threshold loading 222, 223
    target flow and target pressure 222, 223
    voluntary isocapnic hyperpnoea 222
inspiratory threshold loading 222, 223
insufflator–exsufflator 312
intercostal muscles 39–41
intercostal nerve blocks 453, 454–5, 458
interdisciplinary work 17, 32
interleukin-2 (IL-2) 491
intermittent oxygen therapy 165, 169, 179
International Union against Cancer (UICC) 3
internet 24, 28, 301
interstitial lung disease (ILD) 112, 155, 167, 171
interstitial pneumonitis 508
interstitium 43
interval exercise 207
intrathecal administration of neurolytic agents
    453, 456, 458
ipratropium bromide 86–7, 385, 386
isoniazid 518, 520, 521
itraconazole 397

joint pain 417–18

Kaposi's sarcoma (KS) 501–5
Kartagener's syndrome 54
Karvonen equation 201
ketamine 443, 447
ketoacidosis, diabetic 328
Klebsiella pneumonia 55
kyphoscoliosis 49

lactate dehydrogenase (LDH) 500–1
lactulose 443
lamivudine 494, 495
lamotrigine 446
Langerhans cell histiocytosis (LCH) 283
larynx
    anatomy and physiology 41, 42
    cough reflex 343–4
lasers, tumour resection 267–9
laxatives 154, 443

legal issues 302
leptin 240–1
levomepromazine 156
lignocaine (lidocaine) 449, 454
Lindsell, Annie 318
liposomal anthracyclines 505
liquid oxygen 182
liver disease 400
living wills 30, 57, 321
Living with Asthma Questionnaire 61
lobectomy 375
lobes, anatomy and physiology 43
local anaesthetics, nebulized 150
Logan–Sinclair cough monitor 356, 357, 358–9
London Chest Activity of Daily Living
    (LCADL) 253
long-term oxygen therapy (LTOT)
    adverse effects 180
    cystic fibrosis 399
    definition 165
    evidence 169
    guidelines 178
    humidification 181
    oxygen production and storage devices 182, 183
    role 165
lorazepam 150–1, 293, 295, 375
lung cancer 463
    approaches to symptom management 468
    chemotherapy 468, 472–3, 474–5
    cough 479
    dyspnoea 475–6
        drug therapies 148, 155
        non-pharmacological nursing intervention 229–31
        oxygen therapy 166
    effusions, management of 480
    haemoptysis 372, 476, 478
    pain 479
        chest wall 416
        evaluation 430–1
    palliation 26, 468–70, 474–6, 478, 479
    prevalence of symptoms 464, 465
    radiotherapy 468–70, 474–5
    restrictive lung disease 299
    tuberculosis 523
Lung Cancer Symptom Scale (LCSS) 431
lungs
    abscesses 435
    anatomy and physiology
        airway resistance 49–50
        defence mechanisms 53–5
        definitions 43
        gas exchange 50–1
        inflammation 55
        innervation 46–7
        ventilation 47–9
        see also specific structures
    surgical reduction of volume 87, 215
    transplantation
        cystic fibrosis 398–9, 402, 403
        economic issues 87
        restrictive lung disease 301–2
    tumours 435

lymph 45–6
lymphangioleiomyomatosis (LAM) 283, 301
lymphocytes 55
lymphoedema clinics 24
lymphomas 506
lyzozyme 54

Macmillan Cancer Relief 27
magnesium 70
malnutrition 218, 401–2
Manchester Respiratory Activities of Daily
    Living (MRADL) 253
manubrium 39, 40
massage 71
mastectomy 418
McGill Quality of Life Questionnaire 62, 63
mechanical ventilation 87
mechanoreceptors 96, 98–100, 110, 116
meconium ileus equivalent (MIE) 401
mediastinal pain 419
Medical Outcome Study (MOS) Short Form 36
    (SF-36) 63, 125, 127, 252
Medical Research Council (MRC) dyspnoea scale
    124, 125, 126, 137, 138
medicine, changing aims of 3–6
meditation 71
Mediterranean fever, familial 433
Medtronic Digitrapper 356
mega-HAART 493
Memorial Symptom Assessment Scale (MSAS) 430, 463
mesothelioma 299
    approaches to symptom management 468
    chemotherapy 473–4
    dyspnoea 476
    effusions 481–3
    pain 433, 434
        cordotomy 457
        intercostal nerve blocks 455
    radiotherapy 470
metabolic equivalents (METs) 199–200, 203, 204
metaboreceptors (ergoreceptors) 96, 100
metaboreflex 100
metastases 433, 434–5, 479–80
methacholine inhalation challenge (MIC) 367
methadone 442
methicillin-resistant *Staphylococcus aureus*
    (MRSA) 395
methotrexate 473
methylphenidate 448
metoclopramide 443
mexiletine 447
Microselection afterloading machine 270–1
midazolam
    dyspnoea 151
        diffuse airflow obstruction 295
        motor neurone disease 318, 319
        terminal phase 157, 158, 160
    haemoptysis 375
mind/body techniques 71–2
minimally invasive techniques, upper airflow
    obstruction 265, 266–77
misoprostol 149

Missoula-VITAS quality of life index 62, 63
mitomycin-C 472
Mondor's disease 416
morphine 5–6, 440, 442, 443, 444, 445
    adverse effects 447, 448
    dyspnoea 151, 152–3, 154, 155, 156
        diffuse airflow obstruction 295
        terminal phase 158, 160
    HIV 510
    supportive care and palliative care, relationship
        between 27
motivation problems, dyspnoea 253
motor neurone disease/amyotrophic lateral sclerosis
    (MND/ALS) 111, 317–21
    cough assistance 312
    supportive care
        charitable organizations 28
        opportunities for interventions 24, 25
        and palliative care, relationship between 26
        transfer to 26
    ventilatory support 314
Motor Neurone Disease Association 318–19
Mounier–Kuhn anomaly 266
MRC scale 288
mucokinetics 384
mucolytics 294–5, 383, 394
multidisciplinary work 17, 32
muscle wasting 240–2, 243
muscular dystrophy
    clinical features 307, 308
    cough assistance 312
    dyspnoea 111
    exercise training 312
    frog breathing 311
    ventilatory support 314
muscular pains 416–17
music therapy 233–4
myasthenia gravis 111
mycetomas 372–3, 377, 518, 522
mycobacterial infection 506
Mycobacterium avium intra-cellulare (MAI) 506
myofascial pain syndromes 416, 417

nabilone 150
naloxone 348, 448
nandrolone decanoate 244
naproxen 441
nasal passages, anatomy and physiology 41, 42
nasal polyposis 399–400
nausea and vomiting 5, 6
nelfinavir 495
neoplastic diseases 381
Netherlands, decriminalization of euthanasia 32
neural blockades 453–4, 458
    cordotomy 457–8, 459
    intercostal nerve blocks 454–5
    intrathecal/epidural administration of
        neurolytic agents 456
    selective percutaneous rhizotomy 455–6
neurokinin 1 (NK1) 346, 347
neurokinin A (NKA) 346, 347
neurokinin B (NKB) 347

neurolipomatosis dolorosa 416
neuromuscular and skeletal diseases 111, 307, 315
  clinical features 307–8
  pathophysiology 309–10
  treatment 310–15
neuropeptides 345–8
neutrophils 55
nevirapine 494, 496
Nissen laparoscopic fundoplication 400
N-methyl-D-aspartate (NMDA) receptor 18–19, 442–3
nocturnal non-invasive ventilation (NIPPV) 295–6
'n of 1' trials, oxygen therapy 177–9
non-governmental organizations 3
non-nucleoside reverse transcriptase inhibitors
    490, 493, 494–5, 496
non-obstructive lung disease *see* restrictive lung disease
non-small-cell lung cancer (NSCLC) 463
  approaches to symptom management 468
  chemotherapy 472–3, 474–5
  dyspnoea 475–6
  haemoptysis 476
  prevalence of symptoms 464
  radiotherapy 468–70, 474–5
non-steroidal anti-inflammatory drugs (NSAIDs)
    149, 441, 445, 447, 449
Nottingham Extended Activities of Daily Living
    (NEADL) 252
Nottingham Health Profile 63
nucleoside reverse transcriptase inhibitors 490, 493–5
nucleotide reverse transcriptase inhibitors 490, 495
nursing and nurses 25, 229–32
nutrition 239, 245–6
  asthma, dietary treatments 70–1
  cystic fibrosis 393, 401–2
    pregnancy 403
  dietary intake 240
  diffuse airflow obstruction 293–4
  interventions 243–4
  medication 243
  supplementation strategy 244–5
  tuberculosis 520
  weight loss and inflammatory mediators
      in COPD 242–3
  weight loss and muscle wasting, pathogenesis
      of 240–2

obstructive sleep apnoea 41, 307
occupational therapy 249–50, 259–60
  assessment 251–3
  carer's role 257–9
  earlier stages of illness 28
  intervention 253–7, 258
  sexual dysfunction 257
oesophageal cancer 465
omega-3 fatty acids 71
omega-6 fatty acids 71
Ondine's curse 458
opioids 5–6, 439–40, 441–5, 447–9
  adverse effects 442, 443, 447–9
  cough
    cancer 479
    challenge 355
    reflex 348

dyspnoea 151–6
  diffuse airflow obstruction 295
  motor neurone disease 318, 319
  terminal phase 157, 158, 160
  HIV 509, 510
  nebulized 154–6, 295
  supportive care and palliative care, relationship
      between 27
  transdermal 444–5
  see also specific opioids
opportunity costs 79
orthopnoea 308
osteopathy 70
osteoporosis 402
ovarian cancer 463, 464, 465
Oxford Technique for resistance exercise 195
oxitropium bromide 386
oxycodone 510
oxygen addiction 180
oxygen concentrators 182
oxygen-conserving techniques 183–4
oxygen cylinders 182
Oxygen Cost Diagram (OCD) 124–5, 137, 138
oxygen masks 184–5
oxygen therapy 165, 186
  adverse effects 179–81
  assessment of patient 175–6
  costs 180–1
  cystic fibrosis 399
  definitions 165
  diffuse airflow obstruction 294
  evidence 166–75
  exercise 196, 205–6
  guidelines 176–9
  inhalation devices 184–6
  neuromuscular and skeletal diseases 312–13
  production and storage devices 181–4
  respiratory muscle function 218
  restrictive lung disease 301
  role 165–6
  withdrawal 180
Oxymizer 183

pacing, breathing 192, 193, 196, 207
paclitaxel 472, 505
Paediatric Asthma Caregiver's Quality of Life
    Questionnaire 61
Paediatric Quality of Life Questionnaire 61
pain 413, 422
  adverse effects of pain management 447–9
  arising from chest-wall skin 415–16
  assessment 427–31, 436
  brachial plexopathy 419–22
  cancer 479–80
  clinics 24, 67
  as continuing symptom of known
      condition 428–9
  diaphragmatic 418–19
  HIV 508–10
  hyperventilation induced by 327–8
  idiopathic 414
  joint 417–18
  language of 113, 139

management 5–6, 7
  acupuncture 67
  in advanced lung disease 439–40
  motor neurone disease 318
  preemptive analgesia 19
  supportive care and palliative care, relationship
    between 26
mechanisms 413–15
mediastinal 419
mixed 414
muscular 416–17
neurolytic procedures 453–9
neuropathic 413–14, 440
  HIV 508–9
  treatment 445–7
nociceptive 413, 439, 508–9
opioids 442–5
paroxysmal 413
perception 7
pleural 417, 432–3, 449
as presenting syndrome 427, 428
psychogenic 414
recognizing associated clinical syndromes 431–6
somatic 413
supportive care, comprehensive 18–19
tuberculosis 521
visceral 413
wind-up problem 19
palliation 33
  assisted suicide and euthanasia 32
  cancer 464–5, 468–9, 470, 474–80
  composition of supportive care networks 23
  definitions 5
  dyspnoea
    COPD 289
    drug therapies 147, 149
    motor neurone disease 319
    oxygen therapy 165–6, 169, 175, 176–9, 183
  end-of-life care 7–10, 29–32
  HIV 510–11
  leadership of supportive care teams 25
  medicine, changing aims of 3–6
  models 10–15
  patients who benefit from 21–2
  quality of life 62
  as a specialty 15–16
  success, factors determining 7, 8
  and supportive care, relationship between 26–7
  transfer to 26
Pancoast syndrome 420, 421, 435
pancreatic insufficiency 400–1
panic attacks and panic disorder 150–1, 327
pansinusitis 399
paracetamol 441, 445, 447
parenchymal lung disease, pain associated with 435
parenteral medication 29
partners see carers, family and friends
Pendant 183
peptic ulceration 149
percutaneous selective rhizotomy
  453–4, 455–6, 458
pericardial effusions 481, 482
pertussis infection 365–6

phantom breast syndrome 418
pharynx 41, 42
phenothiazines 156
phosphodiesterase inhibitors 148
photodynamic therapy (PDT) 267, 271
physical aids 256–7, 258, 259, 292
physiology see anatomy and physiology
physiotherapy
  cystic fibrosis 393, 394, 398
  expectoration 386
  hyperventilation 330
  leadership of supportive care teams 25
  motor neurone disease 317
  neuromuscular and skeletal diseases 311
Pink City Lung Exerciser 72
platypnoea 308
pleura, pleural space, and pleural fluid
  anatomy and physiology 41–7
    airways 41–5
    bronchial circulation 46
    innervation 46–7
    lymph 45–6
    pulmonary vessels 46
  inflammatory diseases 433
  malignant disease 433
pleural effusions 480–1
pleural pain 417, 432–3
pleurisy 417, 433, 521
pneumoconiosis 299
pneumonia
  HIV/AIDS 497, 498–501, 502, 506–8
  Klebsiella 55
  pain 435
  Pneumocystis carinii (PCP) 487, 497, 498–501, 502
  streptococcal 55
pneumothorax
  cystic fibrosis 398–9
  pain 432–3, 455, 456
poliomyelitis 311
portal hypertension 400
postmastectomy syndrome 418
postnasal drip syndrome (PNDS) 366, 367, 368
postthoracotomy syndrome 418, 433, 449
posture 292
Poznan declaration 9
precordial catch syndrome 416, 417
precordial migraine 416, 417
prednisolone 149, 396–7, 523
pregnancy 110, 403
pressure-dependent airway collapse 50
preventive palliation 6
primary care teams 21–2, 24
primary lobule 43
progestagens 150
progesterone 293, 328
progressive relaxation 71, 255
promethazine 156
prostaglandins 351–2
prostate cancer 464, 465
protease inhibitors 487, 491, 495, 496
proton pump inhibitors 149
Pseudomonas aeruginosa 393–4, 396
psychiatric illness 149

psychogenic dyspnoea 331–3
psychological issues
  complementary medicine 73
  comprehensive supportive care network 19
  cystic fibrosis 403
  diffuse airflow obstruction 289
  end-of-life care 30
  HIV/AIDS 510
  individualization of treatment 65
  neuromuscular and skeletal diseases 312
  pain 440
  palliation 6
psychophysics 128
psychosexual counselling 28
psychosis 149
psychosocial therapies and needs 229–32, 236
  alternative feedback model 232–3
  art therapy 234, 235, 236
  diffuse airflow obstruction 288
  music therapy 233–4
  non-pharmacological nursing intervention 229–32
  staff support 234–6
pulmonary alveolar macrophages (PAMs)
    43, 44, 54, 55
pulmonary embolus 327
pulmonary fibrosis 155
Pulmonary Functional Status and Dyspnoea
    Questionnaire 251
Pulmonary Functional Status Scale 251
pulmonary gas exchange 50–1
pulmonary hypertension 327, 436
pulmonary infarction syndrome 435–6
pulmonary parenchymal receptors 98–100
pulmonary thromboembolism 435–6
pulmonary vascular diseases 107–8
pulmonary vessels 46, 47
pursed-lip breathing 191–2, 206–7
  diffuse airflow obstruction 292
pyraxinamide 518, 521
pyrexia 328

quality of life (QoL) 57–9, 65
  definitions 57, 58
  dyspnoea 125, 127–8, 138, 390
  implications for treatment selection and patient
      management 64–5
  individual conceptualizations of 7
  measuring 59–63
    disease-specific scales 59–62
    generic scales 62, 63
    idiographic scales 62
  pain 430–1
  palliative care 13
  quantity of life vs. 4, 57
  response options 64
  statistical matters 64

radiofrequency lesions 455, 458
radiograph, chest
  chronic cough with a 'normal' radiograph 365–9
  haemoptysis 375, 376
radiotherapy 468–72, 474–5
  cough 479

haemoptysis 477–8
  upper airflow obstruction 265–6
rapidly adapting receptors (RARs) 99, 345
radio scaling, dyspnoea assessment 128
reflexology 71
refractory breathlessness 159–60
rehabilitation 189, 210–11
  breathing retraining 191–4
  diffuse airflow obstruction 290–1, 292
  education and counselling 189–91
  medicine, changing aims of 4–5
  see also exercise
relaxation techniques
  asthma 71–2
  diffuse airflow obstruction 293
  hyperventilation 330
  music therapy 234
  occupational therapy 255
  progressive relaxation 71, 255
religious issues
  end-of-life care 30
  loss of faith, case study 232
  music therapy 233
repetition maximum (RM), in resistance exercise 195
resection techniques, upper airways
    obstruction 266–9
resistance exercise 195, 196
respiratory bronchioles 43
respiratory controller 109–10
respiratory drive abnormalities 310
respiratory muscles
  anatomy and physiology 39–41
  function 218–20
  motor neurone disease 317
  neuromuscular and skeletal diseases 309, 311–12
  training 227
    diffuse airflow obstruction 293
    effects 223–6
    inspiratory muscle training 222–3
    neuromuscular and skeletal diseases 311–12
    restrictive lung disease 301
    see also exercise
respiratory pump
  anatomy and physiology 39–41
  dyspnoea 109, 110–11
  failure 218
respiratory secretions 318
respiratory sedative drugs 150–6
respiratory stimulant drugs 150
respiratory system dyspnoea 106, 109–12
respite care 259
restrictive lung disease 281, 298–9, 302
  assessment and treatment 300
  medicolegal issues 302
  prognosis and end-of-life planning 302
reverse transcriptase inhibitors 490–1, 493–6
rhinitis 345, 367
ribcage 39–41
rib fracture 434–5, 449
rifampicin 516, 518–19, 521
riluzole 317
ritonavir 495
Rotterdam Symptom Checklist (RSCL) 463–4

St George's Respiratory Questionnaire (SGRQ) 59, 61
  dyspnoea 125, 128, 251, 288
  expectoration 382
salbutamol 86–7
saline 384–5, 394
saquinavir 495
sarcoidosis 266, 283, 372
scalene muscles 41
Schedule for the Evaluation of Individual Quality
  of Life (SEIQoL) 62
Scheuermann's disease 418
scoliosis 309, 310
screening programmes 18, 20
secondary lobule 43, 44–5, 46
secretagogues 383–4
sedation 29–30, 315, 375
segments, lung 43
selective percutaneous rhizotomy 453–4, 455–6, 458
selective serotonin reuptake inhibitors (SSRIs) 330, 333
selenium 70–1
self-esteem problems 253
self-help groups 294, 301
semi-permanent indwelling studs 73–4
sennosides 443
serotonergic neurones 348
sexual counselling 28
sexual dysfunction 257
SF-36 63, 125, 127, 252
Sheffield model of comprehensive supportive
  care 17–18, 19–21
  earlier stages of disease 27
  end-of-life care 29
  palliative care 26
  tuberculosis 515
short-burst oxygen therapy 165, 169, 179
Short Form 36 (SF-36) 63, 125, 127, 252
Shortness of Breath Questionnaire (SOBQ) 137
shuttle walk test 198, 199, 288
Sickness Impact Profile (SIP) 63, 125, 127
sighing 324, 328
Silver Lining Questionnaire 62, 63
sinus disease 399–400
sinus imaging studies 367
sinusitis 498
skeletal diseases *see* neuromuscular and skeletal diseases
sleep problems
  apnoea 41, 307, 458
  cough 352
  motor neurone disease 317
  neuromuscular and skeletal diseases
    307, 308, 310, 313
  respiratory muscle training 226
slowly adapting receptors (SARs) 99, 344–5
small-cell lung cancer (SCLC) 463
  chemotherapy 468, 473, 474–5
  dyspnoea 476
  haemoptysis 478
  prevalence of symptoms 464
  radiotherapy 470, 474–5
smoking
  cessation advice 285, 290, 300
  chronic cough with 'normal' chest radiograph 366
  cystic fibrosis 393

HIV 498
  and lung function 282
  and oxygen therapy 178, 179, 180
  passive exposure to 393
social isolation 190
social issues, end-of-life care 30
social services 28, 292
speech problems 138, 328
  see also communication problems
spinal pains 418
spiritual issues
  end-of-life care 30
  loss of faith, case study 232
  music therapy 233
spouses *see* carers, family and friends
squamous cell cancer of the lung 5
Staphylococcus aureus 393
  methicillin-resistant (MRSA) 395
stavudine 494, 496
stents 267, 272–5, 276
sternal pain 418
sternoclavicular hyperostosis 418
sternum 39, 40
St George's Respiratory Questionnaire (SGRQ) 59, 61
  dyspnoea 125, 128, 251, 288
  expectoration 382
strengthening exercise 195, 196
streptococcal pneumonia 55
streptomycin 521
stress 329
  see also anxiety
strictures 265, 266
stridor 265
studs, semi-permanent indwelling 73–4
substance P (SP) 346–7
suicide, assisted 32–3
sulfydryl mucolytic therapy 383
sulindac 352
support
  for healthcare staff 236
  for patient and family 234–5
supportive care 33
  assisted suicide 32–3
  composition of network 23–6
  comprehensive network, implementation 17–21
  concept, need for 16–17
  at earlier stages of illness 27–8
  end-of-life care 29–32
  euthanasia 32–3
  and palliative care, relationship between 26–7
  patients who benefit from 21–2
swallowing problems 317
Sweden, economics of COPD 85
systemic hypertension 107
systemic lupus erythematosus 433
systemic sclerosis 301

talc 480
target flow inspiratory muscle training 222, 223
target pressure inspiratory muscle training 222, 223
teamwork 17, 32
Teitze's syndrome 418
terminal bronchioles 43

terminal care *see* end-of-life care
tetracycline 480–1
tetraplegia 311
theophylline 148
thoracotomy 418, 433, 449
thrombin infusion 377
timed walk tests 198–9, 202
tobacco *see* smoking
tobramycin 394, 395, 403
trachea 41, 42
tracheobronchial tree 344–5
tracheobronchitis 431–2
tracheobronchomegaly 266
tracheomalacia 265, 266
tracheopathia osteoplastica 266
tracheostomy 314, 320
tramadol 441
tranexamic acid 375, 477
transcendental mediation 71
transfer coefficient for carbon monoxide (TL$_{CO}$) 51
Transition Dyspnoea Index (TDI) 125, 126–7
transtracheal oxygen therapy 183–4
treadmills 202
triphosphate nucleotides 385
tuberculosis 515, 523–4
    anorexia 521
    bronchopleural fistula 523
    compliance 519
    contact tracing 520
    cor pulmonale 522
    diffuse airflow obstruction 283
    drug treatment 518–19
    dyspnoea 520–2
    employment 520
    empyema thoracis 523
    epidemiology and socio-economic issues 515–17
    fever 521
    haemoptysis 372, 374, 520, 522–3
    HIV/AIDS 497, 506, 519
    isolation 519
    lung cancer 523
    lung inflammation 55
    multidrug resistant (MDRTB) 519
    natural history of pulmonary disease 517–18
    nutrition 520
    pain 521
    symptoms of drug toxicity 521
    travel 520
tumours
    pain 435
    upper airflow obstruction 265, 266–71
    see also cancer; *specific cancers*

ubiquitin–proteasome pathway 242
UICC 28
ultrasonically nebulized distilled water (UNDW) 356
United States of America
    assisted suicide 32
    chronic obstructive pulmonary disease 182
    complementary medicine 67
    oxygen therapy 182
    rehabilitation programmes 28

unmyelinated nerve fibres 345
upper airflow obstruction 265, 275–7
    brachytherapy 270–1
    causes 265–6
    photodynamic therapy 271
    resection techniques 266–9
    stents 272–5, 276

vagotomy 99
vascular disease 107–8, 373
vasoactive intestinal polypeptide (VIP) 347
venlafaxine 447
ventilation *see* breathing
ventilatory pump 109, 110–11
ventral respiratory group (VRG) 348
verbal category descriptive scoring systems (VCDs)
    cough 352, 353, 358
    pain 428
video-assisted thoracic surgery (VATS) 481–3
vinblastine 472, 505
vinca alkaloids 505
vincristine 473, 505
vinorelbine 472, 473, 474, 505
virtual team 17
visual analogue scale (VAS)
    cough 352, 353
    dyspnoea 129–30, 136, 138
        oxygen therapy 177
    pain 428
visual imagery 255
vitamins 70, 401–2
volume-dependent airway narrowing 50
voluntary isocapnic hyperpnoea 222
volunteers in health and social care 3
volvulus 401
vomiting and nausea 5, 6

walking distance tests 288
websites 24, 28, 301
weight loss 239, 242–3
    diffuse airflow obstruction 293–4
    medication 243
    nutritional intervention 243–4
    pathogenesis 240–2
    restrictive lung disease 301
    tuberculosis 520, 521
whooping cough 365–6
wills, living 30, 57, 321
World Health Organization (WHO)
    analgesic ladder 440–2, 510, 521
    medicine, changing aims of 3
    palliative care 11–12, 14, 19–20
    quality of life 59
world wide web 24, 28, 301

xiphoidalgia 418

yoga 72–3

zalcitabine 493, 494
zidovudine (AZT) 490, 493, 494